Sex and Gender Differences in Alzheimer's Disease

Women's Brain Project

About the Women's Brain Project: The Women's Brain Project (WBP) is an international non profit organization studying sex and gender determinants to brain and mental health. Founded in 2016, the WBP is composed by a group of scientists hailing from various disciplines including medicine, neuroscience, psychology, pharmacology, and communication who work together with caregivers, patients and their relatives, policymakers, and other stakeholders. The WBP aims to identify how sex and gender factors impact diseases, diagnostics, drug and novel technologies development, and to achieve precision medicine for sustainable and inclusive healthcare. http://www.womensbrainproject.com/

About the Women's Brain Project Book Series: The purpose of the series is to provide comprehensive references on different topics in basic/clinical research being conducted on the influence of sex and gender in brain and mental health and precision medicine research.

Editorial Advisory Board: Maria Teresa Ferretti, Ph.D., Cofounder and Chief Scientific Officer, Women's Brain Project, Switzerland; Annemarie Schumacher Dimech, Ph.D., Cofounder and President, Women's Brain Project, Switzerland; Program Manager CAS Palliative Care, University of Lucerne, Switzerland; Antonella Santuccione Chadha, Ph.D., CEO pro bono and co-founder Women's Brain Project, Guntershausen, Switzerland; Vice-President at Euresearch, Switzerland.

Sex and Gender Differences in Alzheimer's Disease edited by Maria Teresa Ferretti, Annemarie Schumacher Dimech, and Antonella Santuccione Chadha, 9780128193440

Sex and Gender Bias in Technology and Artificial Intelligence: Biomedicine and Healthcare Applications edited by Davide Cirillo, Silvina Catuara Solarz, and Emre Guney, 9780128213926

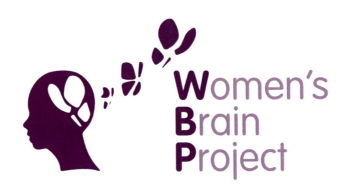

Sex and Gender Differences in Alzheimer's Disease
The Women's Brain Project

Edited by

Maria Teresa Ferretti, Ph.D.
Co-founder and Chief Scientific Officer, Women's Brain Project,
Guntershausen, Switzerland

Annemarie Schumacher Dimech, Ph.D.
Co-founder and President, Women's Brain Project,
Guntershausen, Switzerland
Program Manager, Palliative Care, University of Lucerne,
Lucerne, Switzerland

Antonella Santuccione Chadha, MD
CEO pro bono and Co-founder Women's Brain Project,
Guntershausen, Switzerland
Vice-President at Euresearch, Switzerland

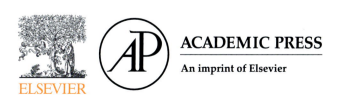

Academic Press is an imprint of Elsevier
125 London Wall, London EC2Y 5AS, United Kingdom
525 B Street, Suite 1650, San Diego, CA 92101, United States
50 Hampshire Street, 5th Floor, Cambridge, MA 02139, United States
The Boulevard, Langford Lane, Kidlington, Oxford OX5 1GB, United Kingdom

Copyright © 2021 Elsevier Inc. All rights reserved.

No part of this publication may be reproduced or transmitted in any form or by any means, electronic or mechanical, including photocopying, recording, or any information storage and retrieval system, without permission in writing from the publisher. Details on how to seek permission, further information about the Publisher's permissions policies and our arrangements with organizations such as the Copyright Clearance Center and the Copyright Licensing Agency, can be found at our website: www.elsevier.com/permissions.

This book and the individual contributions contained in it are protected under copyright by the Publisher (other than as may be noted herein).

Notices
Knowledge and best practice in this field are constantly changing. As new research and experience broaden our understanding, changes in research methods, professional practices, or medical treatment may become necessary.

Practitioners and researchers must always rely on their own experience and knowledge in evaluating and using any information, methods, compounds, or experiments described herein. In using such information or methods they should be mindful of their own safety and the safety of others, including parties for whom they have a professional responsibility.

To the fullest extent of the law, neither the Publisher nor the authors, contributors, or editors, assume any liability for any injury and/or damage to persons or property as a matter of products liability, negligence or otherwise, or from any use or operation of any methods, products, instructions, or ideas contained in the material herein.

Library of Congress Cataloging-in-Publication Data
A catalog record for this book is available from the Library of Congress

British Library Cataloguing-in-Publication Data
A catalogue record for this book is available from the British Library

ISBN : 978-0-12-819344-0

For information on all Academic Press publications
visit our website at https://www.elsevier.com/books-and-journals

Publisher: Nikki Levy
Acquisitions Editor: Joslyn Chaiprasert-Paguio
Editorial Project Manager: Tracy I. Tufaga
Production Project Manager: Kiruthika Govindaraju
Cover Designer: Victoria Pearson

Typeset by SPi Global, India

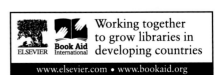

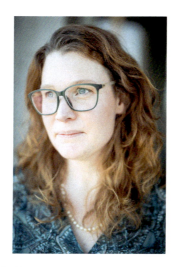

We would like to dedicate this book to Sofia Petersson, a woman living with familial Alzheimer's disease and Cause Ambassador of the Women's Brain Project.

Sofia has inspired this book in multiple ways: as a patient, as a lifelong caregiver against an illness that has run in her family for generations, but also as an inquisitive person who never stops asking questions and expressing hope. Sofia is also actively contributing to science, helping the research community understand Alzheimer's natural history by studying individuals like her who carry Alzheimer's-causing mutations.

Her courage and determination gave us the strength to pursue the topic of sex and gender and precision medicine in Alzheimer's disease; like her, we will never stop hoping and asking questions with the goal of helping millions of patients and caregivers.

Maria Teresa Ferretti
Annemarie Schumacher Dimech
Antonella Santuccione Chadha

Photo credit: Fabienne Wild

Contents

Contributors xxi
Acknowledgments xxvii
Introduction xxix
Editors' biography xxxi
Foreword xxxiii

SECTION 1 Sex differences in fundamental neurobiological processes that are relevant to Alzheimer's disease

Maria Teresa Ferretti, Annemarie Schumacher Dimech, and Antonella Santuccione Chadha

CHAPTER 1 Sex differences in Alzheimer's disease animal models 3
Stefania Ippati, Lars Matthias Ittner, and Yazi Diana Ke

Overview of Alzheimer's disease 3
AD animal models 3
   Mutant APP mouse models 4
   Mouse models with multiple FAD mutations 4
   Mouse models of tau pathology 5
   Other AD mutant models 5
Evidence for sex differences in AD animal models 6
   The triple transgenic AD mouse model: 3xTg-AD 6
   APP and PSEN1 transgenic mouse models: TgCRND8, APPswe/PSEN1dE9, APPPS1, and PS2APP/Trem2KO 8
   ApoE transgenic mouse models: ApoE4/3xTg, 5xFAD/ApoE3, and 5xFAD/ApoE4 10
   Tau mouse models: P301S, rTg4510, JNPL3 11
   Nontransgenic animals 12
Limitations 12
Conclusion 13
Chapter highlights 14
References 18

CHAPTER 2 **Sex and sex hormone differences in hippocampal neurogenesis and their relevance to Alzheimer's disease** 23
Bonnie H. Lee, Tanvi A. Puri, and Liisa A.M. Galea

Introduction 23
Adult neurogenesis in the dentate gyrus..................................24
The function of adult neurogenesis in the hippocampus..........26
Neurogenesis and aging..28
Sex differences in neurogenesis 30
Sex differences in neurogenesis in the context of
 cognitive training..32
Alzheimer's disease..33
Sex differences in Alzheimer's disease 34
Animal models for Alzheimer's disease and
 sex differences..35
Neurogenesis in Alzheimer's disease 37
Neurogenesis in models of Alzheimer's disease 38
Estrogens and aging..39
Estrogens and neurogenesis...41
Estrogens and neurogenesis in the context of aging................43
Estrogens, aging, and cognition 44
Estrogens and neurogenesis in the context of Alzheimer's
 disease 45
Parity and neurogenesis..46
Parity and Alzheimer's disease...48
Testosterone and neurogenesis 49
Testosterone and neurogenesis in the context of
 aging and Alzheimer's disease 51
Conclusion..52
Chapter highlights 52
References 53

CHAPTER 3 **Sex differences in microglia as a risk factor for Alzheimer's disease**...79
Charlotte Delage, Danielle N. Rendina,
Karen E. Malacon, Marie-Ève Tremblay,
and Staci D. Bilbo

Introduction 79
Microglia: Protection and pathology in Alzheimer's
 disease 80

Protective functions of microglia in Alzheimer's disease 80
  TREM2 and Aβ plaques 80
  TREM2 and tau 82
Detrimental roles of microglia in Alzheimer's disease 82
  Complement and synapse elimination 83
Neuroinflammation 84
Sex differences in the immune system 85
Sex differences in microglia 87
Aging microglia 89
Interactions between AD, sex, and inflammation in the
  aged brain 91
Conclusion 94
Chapter highlights 94
References 95

SECTION 2 Sex and gender differences in clinical aspects of Alzheimer's disease

Maria Teresa Ferretti, Annemarie Schumacher Dimech, and Antonella Santuccione Chadha

CHAPTER 4   Sex differences in CSF biomarkers of Alzheimer's disease 107

Michelle M. Mielke

Introduction 107
Sex differences in brain structure and function 109
Sex differences in the core AD-related biomarkers 110
  Amyloid-beta 110
  Phosphorylated tau and total tau 111
  Neurofilament light chain 112
  Neurogranin 112
Sex differences in CSF biomarkers of other mechanisms
  related to the development and progression of AD
  pathology and clinical symptoms 112
  Inflammatory markers 113
Examples of sex-related factors that can influence the
  interpretation of AD-related biofluid biomarker results 113
  Genetic factors 114
  Sex differences in the permeability of the blood-brain
    barrier 115
  Consideration of study design 115

Future potential of blood-based biomarkers...........................116
Conclusion...116
Chapter highlights...117
References..117

CHAPTER 5 **Sex differences in neuroimaging biomarkers in healthy subjects and dementia**.................................125

Federico Massa, Dario Arnaldi, Michele Balma, Matteo Bauckneht, Andrea Chincarini, Pilar M. Ferraro, Matteo Grazzini, Caterina Lapucci, Riccardo Meli, Silvia Morbelli, Matteo Pardini, Enrico Peira, Stefano Raffa, Luca Roccatagliata, and Flavio Nobili

Introduction...126
Structural MRI..127
    Structural MRI sex differences in healthy subjects............128
    Structural MRI sex differences in dementia.......................129
    Conclusion...131
Functional MRI...131
    fMRI sex differences in healthy subjects............................132
    fMRI sex differences in dementia.......................................135
    Conclusion...135
Perfusion SPECT...136
    Perfusion SPECT sex differences in healthy subjects........136
    Perfusion SPECT sex differences in dementia...................137
    Conclusion...140
DAT SPECT..140
    DAT SPECT sex differences in healthy subjects................141
    DAT SPECT sex differences in dementia............................142
FDG-PET..145
    FDG-PET sex differences in healthy subjects....................145
    FDG-PET sex differences in dementia................................146
Amyloid PET...148
    Amyloid PET sex differences in healthy subjects..............148
    Amyloid PET sex differences in dementia.........................148
    Conclusion...149
Emerging PET modalities..150
    Tau PET sex differences in healthy subjects and dementia...150
    Neurotransmission PET sex differences in healthy subjects and dementia...151
    Neuroinflammation PET sex differences in healthy subjects and dementia...152

Conclusion 152
Chapter highlights 153
References 153

CHAPTER 6 Sex and gender differences in neuropsychological symptoms for clinical diagnosis of Alzheimer's disease 163
Emnet Z. Gammada, Rhoda Au, and Nancy S. Foldi

Introduction 163
Memory 165
   Introduction 165
   Sex/gender differences in verbal memory in healthy adults 165
   Sex/gender differences in verbal memory in mild cognitive impairment 166
   Sex/gender differences in verbal memory in AD 167
   Sex/gender differences and rates of verbal memory decline 167
   Summary 168
Language 168
   Introduction 168
   Laterality, handedness, and connectivity of the language system 169
   Semantic dysfunction in neural disorders other than AD 170
   Critical semantic disruption in AD 170
Executive function 171
   Introduction 171
   Sex/gender differences in executive function 172
   Sex/gender differences in cognitive reserve mechanisms 174
Conclusion 175
Chapter highlights 177
Support 177
References 177

CHAPTER 7 Sex differences in psychiatric disorders and their implication for dementia 187
Ewelina Biskup, Valeria Jordan, Beatrice Nasta, and Katrin Rauen

Psychiatric disorders matter as modifiable risk factors for dementia over the entire life span 187

Major depression: A relevant modifiable risk factor for
   dementia with sex- and gender-related implications 190
   Social signal transduction theory of depression: A
      hypothesis to explain the female's increased
      vulnerability during childhood and puberty 193
   Late life versus earlier life depression and risk of
      developing dementia 193
   Depression or dementia? A key diagnostic challenge
      in the elderly 195
Pharmacotherapy in the elderly: A major challenge with
   the risk of detrimental polypharmacy 197
   Antidepressants in dementia 197
   Polypharmacy 198
Behavioral and psychological symptoms of dementia 199
   Treatment of BPSD: A key challenge in dementia care 200
   Benzodiazepines in the elderly 200
Conclusion 201
Chapter highlights 201
References 202

CHAPTER 8   **Sleep disorders and dementia** 207
Beatrice Nasta, MaryJane Hill-Strathy,
Ewelina Biskup, and Katrin Rauen

Why do we spend a third of life sleeping? An introduction
   to sleep and its main characteristics 207
Sleep disorders and physiological sleep changes during
   aging 209
Sex- and gender-related differences in sleep and sleep
   disorders 210
Sleep disorders in Alzheimer's disease 211
   Sleep architecture in Alzheimer's disease 212
   Treating sleep disorders in Alzheimer's disease 213
   Sleep disorders and Alzheimer's disease: The
      caregiver's burden 214
Key points 215
Insomnia: An independent risk factor for cognitive
   impairment 215
   Treating sleep disorders in the elderly 217
Key points 218

    Obstructive sleep apnea syndrome: A risk factor for
       cognitive impairment and Alzheimer's disease 218
    Obstructive sleep apnea syndrome and the different
       clinical pictures in male and female patients 218
    Obstructive sleep apnea syndrome in relation to
       cognitive impairment and Alzheimer's disease 219
    Biomarkers in OSAS and Alzheimer's disease 220
Key points 221
REM sleep behavior disorder: A relevant parasomnia and
  an early clinical biomarker for neurodegenerative
  ldiseases 221
    REM sleep behavior disorder and sex- and
       gender-related differences 223
    REM sleep behavior disorder and the risk of clinical
       manifestation of a neurodegenerative disease 223
    Sundown syndrome in Alzheimer's disease is
       associated with RBD 224
Key points 225
Conclusion 226
Chapter highlights 226
References 226

CHAPTER 9   **Hormones and dementia** 233
Cassandra Szoeke, Sue Downie, Susan Phillips,
and Stephen Campbell

Sex differences are hormone differences 233
Hormones and cognition 234
    Estrogen 235
    Progesterone 235
    Testosterone and DHEA 236
Menopause and cognition 237
    Natural menopause 237
    Surgical menopause 239
Observational studies of hormone therapy use 239
Interventional HT use 240
    Hormone therapy and cognition 241
Hormone therapy in younger women 242
    The timing hypothesis 243
    Side-effect profile 245

Hormones and cognition in men 246
Gaps in knowledge 248
   The impact of hormones on known key risk factors
      for cognitive decline 248
   Midlife to late-life longitudinal prospective studies
      including hormone, cognitive, and neuropathological
      biomarkers 252
Conclusion 254
Chapter highlights 256
References 256

CHAPTER 10 Sex and gender differences in genetic and lifestyle risk and protective factors for dementia 269

Shireen Sindi, Sima Toopchiani, Mariagnese Barbera, Krister Håkansson, Jenni Lehtisalo, Anna Rosenberg, Ruth Stephen, Chinedu Udeh-Momoh, and Miia Kivipelto

Introduction 269
APOE allele 270
Hormones, menopause, and andropause 272
   Hormone replacement therapy 273
   Reproductive history and timing of menopause 274
Andropause 275
Cardiometabolic risk factors 275
Smoking and alcohol consumption 277
Physical activity and exercise 278
Nutrition 279
Sleep disturbances 280
Neural reserve and resilience 282
   Sex and gender dichotomies in cognitive aging research ... 282
The stress axes 283
   Implications of sex and gender differences in relation
      to stress 284
Loneliness and social isolation 285
Depression 286
Response and adherence to multidomain lifestyle
   interventions 288
Discussion 290
Chapter highlights 291
Funding 292
References 292

CHAPTER 11 **Sex and gender considerations in clinical trials for Alzheimer's disease: Current state and recommendations** 309

Maitee Rosende-Roca, Carla Abdelnour,
Ester Esteban, Mercè Boada Rovira,
Julie N. Martinkova, Simona Mellino, and
Antonella Santuccione Chadha

Introduction 309
Sex considerations in preclinical stages of clinical trials 310
Sex and gender considerations in clinical trial stages
    involving human subjects 311
Sex and gender considerations in Alzheimer's disease
    clinical trials 312
    Prevalence and pathophysiology of the disease in men
        and women 312
    Differences in AD biomarkers between men and women 313
    Efficacy of AD drugs in men and women 315
    Safety and pharmacokinetics of AD drugs in men and
        women 316
    Participation of women in AD clinical trials 317
    The role of biomarkers in selection/stratification of
        men/women 319
    Digital biomarkers 320
Conclusion 321
Recommendations for considering sex and gender in
    clinical trials 321
Chapter highlights 322
References 323
Further reading 327

SECTION 3 Gender differences in the socio-economic factors linked to Alzheimer's disease

Maria Teresa Ferretti, Annemarie Schumacher Dimech, and
Antonella Santuccione Chadha

CHAPTER 12 **Gender and socioeconomic differences in modifiable risk factors for Alzheimer's disease and other types of dementia throughout the life course** 333

Stefania Ilinca and Elina Suzuki

Inequality in early educational achievement 335
  Cognitive resilience and dementia risk are associated with
    early childhood outcomes 335
  Gender and socioeconomic inequalities in educational
    attainment 335
  Reducing inequalities in cognitive reserve 337
Inequality in behavioral risk factors: Obesity and physical
  activity 337
Inequality in clinical risk factors: Hypertension and
  diabetes 340
  Gender and socioeconomic inequalities in hypertension
    among current adult cohorts 340
  Gender and socioeconomic inequalities in diabetes
    among current adult cohorts 342
  Inequalities in awareness, access to care, and rate of
    complications 343
Social support, social isolation, and depression 345
  Old-age poverty 346
  Gender and socioeconomic inequalities in clinical
    depression among current adult cohorts 347
  Gender and socioeconomic inequalities in social
    isolation and loneliness 350
Discussion 353
Chapter highlights 354
References 355

**CHAPTER 13 Living with dementia and caregiving:
Psychosocial considerations through the
gender lens 361**
Charles Scerri, Angela Abela, and Anthony Scerri

Introduction 361
Family dynamics in the context of caregiving in
  individuals living with dementia 361
  Spouses as caregivers of individuals living with
    dementia 362
  The adult child caregiver of a parent living with
    dementia and the effect of gender on expectations 364
  Family dynamics and residential long-term care for
    persons living with dementia 367
Psychosocial interventions for individuals living with
  dementia and their caregivers 368
  Psychosocial interventions targeting cognitive function 369

Activity-based psychosocial interventions 370
Other nonpharmacological therapies for dementia 372
The influence of gender on psychosocial interventions for
behavioral and psychological symptoms in dementia
and Alzheimer's disease 374
   Gender differences in behavioral and psychological
     symptoms of individuals living with dementia 375
   Gender differences in psychosocial interventions
     for individuals living with dementia 376
   Gender differences in psychosocial interventions
     for informal caregivers 376
   Gender differences in psychosocial interventions for
     formal caregivers 378
Conclusion 380
Chapter highlights 380
References 381

CHAPTER 14   **Sex and gender differences in caregiving patterns and caregivers' needs** 393
Klara Lorenz-Dant and Mary Mittelman

What are the patterns of care? 393
   Women continue to be expected to care whether they
     want to or not 394
   Men become an increasingly important caregiver group 395
   Sex and gender differences in the care provided 396
What are the implications of providing dementia care? 398
   Positive outcomes 398
   Negative outcomes of caregiving 399
Why do we observe different outcomes for male and
   female caregivers? 401
   Gender differences in coping mechanisms 401
   Complexity of care situations 402
   Societal demands and caregiving 403
   Support structures for unpaid caregivers 404
Identified key support needs 405
   Need for information 405
   Time for themselves—Improved access to caregiver
     allowance and respite care 406
   Recognition by relevant professionals 407
Barriers to support 407
   Designing and delivering effective interventions is
     not that straightforward 408

Is this likely to change in future? 409
Chapter highlights 413
References 413

CHAPTER 15 **Gender barriers to communication in Alzheimer's disease** 421
Sara Rubinelli and Nicola Diviani

Introduction 421
Communication: Grounding concepts 422
Ethical implications of effective communication 423
Gender issues in IHC in general and implications for AD 424
General strategies for communication with dementia and
    Alzheimer's patients 426
Communicating with caregivers of AD patients 428
A research agenda in AD, gender, and communication 430
Ten lessons learned about health communication
    avoiding gender biases in AD 432
Conclusion 434
Chapter highlights 434
References 434

CHAPTER 16 **Women and dementia policy: Redressing imbalance through gender transformative policies** 439
Wendy Weidner, Paola Barbarino, and Chris Lynch

Acknowledging the imbalance: Where we are now 440
    One: More women have dementia 440
    Two: More women are carers 441
    Three: Women with dementia experience added stigma 441
    Four: Early education for girls is key for risk reduction 442
Understanding the imbalance: How did we get here 442
    Data bias—Women are invisible 443
    Research—Patchy progress 444
    Policy and gender—Giving women a voice 445
Addressing the imbalance: How do we change and move
    forward? 446
    International frameworks 447
    Global action plan on the public response to dementia
        2017–2025 450
    Toward a gender-transformative global action plan 452
    Encouraging and empowering female leadership 455

    Advocacy from the bottom-up: The role of civil
        society 458
    Gender-based data 459
Conclusion 460
Chapter highlights 462
References 462

Index 469

Contributors

Carla Abdelnour
Research Center and Memory Clinic, Fundació ACE, Institut Català de Neurociències Aplicades, Universitat Internacional de Catalunya, Barcelona; Networking Research Center on Neurodegenerative Diseases (CIBERNED), Instituto de Salud Carlos III, Madrid, Spain

Angela Abela
Department of Family Studies, Faculty for Social Wellbeing, University of Malta, Msida, Malta

Dario Arnaldi
Department of Neuroscience (DINOGMI), University of Genoa; Department of Neurology, IRCCS Polyclinic Hospital San Martino, Genoa, Italy

Rhoda Au
Departments of Anatomy & Neurobiology, Neurology and Framingham Heart Study, Boston University School of Medicine; Department of Epidemiology, Boston University School of Public Health, Boston, MA, United States

Michele Balma
Department of Health Sciences (DISSAL), University of Genoa, Genoa, Italy

Paola Barbarino
Alzheimer's Disease International, London, United Kingdom

Mariagnese Barbera
Institute of Clinical Medicine, Neurology, University of Eastern Finland, Kuopio, Finland

Matteo Bauckneht
Department of Health Sciences (DISSAL), University of Genoa; Nuclear Medicine Unit, IRCCS Polyclinic Hospital San Martino, Genoa, Italy

Staci D. Bilbo
Department of Neurobiology; Department of Psychology and Neuroscience, Duke University, Durham, NC, United States

Ewelina Biskup
Women's Brain Project, Guntershausen, Switzerland; Department of Advanced Biomedical Sciences, Federico II University of Naples, Naples, Italy; College of Clinical Medicine, Shanghai University of Medicine and Health Sciences, Shanghai, China

Stephen Campbell
Australian Healthy Ageing Organisation, Melbourne, VIC, Australia

Antonella Santuccione Chadha
Women's Brain Project, Guntershausen, Switzerland

Andrea Chincarini
National Institute for Nuclear Physics (INFN), Genoa Section, Genoa, Italy

Charlotte Delage
Division of Medical Sciences, University of Victoria, Victoria, BC, Canada

Annemarie Schumacher Dimech
Women's Brain Project, Guntershausen; Program Manager, Palliative Care, University of Lucerne, Lucerne, Switzerland

Nicola Diviani
Department of Health Sciences and Medicine, University of Lucerne, Lucerne; Person-Centered Health Care and Health Communication Group, Swiss Paraplegic Research Nottwil, Switzerland

Sue Downie
Department of Medicine (RMH), University of Melbourne, Melbourne, VIC, Australia

Ester Esteban
Research Center and Memory Clinic, Fundació ACE, Institut Català de Neurociències Aplicades, Universitat Internacional de Catalunya, Barcelona, Spain

Pilar M. Ferraro
Department of Neuroradiology, IRCCS Polyclinic Hospital San Martino, Genoa, Italy

Maria Teresa Ferretti
Women's Brain Project, Guntershausen, Switzerland

Nancy S. Foldi
Department of Psychology, Queens College and The Graduate Center, City University of New York, New York; Department of Psychiatry, NYU Langone Hospital—Long Island, NYU Langone Health, Mineola, NY, United States

Liisa A.M. Galea
Graduate Program in Neuroscience; Djavad Mowafaghian Centre for Brain Health; Department of Psychology, University of British Columbia, Vancouver, BC, Canada

Emnet Z. Gammada
Department of Psychiatry and Biobehavioral Sciences and Semel Institute for Neuroscience and Human Behavior, David Geffen School of Medicine at UCLA, Los Angeles, CA, United States

Matteo Grazzini
Department of Neuroscience (DINOGMI), University of Genoa, Genoa, Italy

Krister Håkansson
Division of Clinical Geriatrics, Center for Alzheimer Research, Karolinska Institutet, Stockholm, Sweden

MaryJane Hill-Strathy
Department of Geriatric Psychiatry, Psychiatric Hospital Zurich, University of Zurich, Zurich, Switzerland

Stefania Ilinca
San Raffaele Scientific Institute, San Raffaele Hospital, Milan, Italy

Stefania Ippati
Experimental Imaging Center, San Raffaele Hospital, Milano, MI, Italy

Lars Matthias Ittner
Dementia Research Centre, Department of Biomedical Sciences, Faculty of Medicine Health and Human Sciences, Macquarie University, Sydney, NSW, Australia

Valeria Jordan
Women's Brain Project, Guntershausen, Switzerland

Yazi Diana Ke
Dementia Research Centre, Department of Biomedical Sciences, Faculty of Medicine Health and Human Sciences, Macquarie University, Sydney, NSW, Australia

Miia Kivipelto
Division of Clinical Geriatrics, Center for Alzheimer Research, Karolinska Institutet, Stockholm, Sweden; Ageing Epidemiology (AGE) Research Unit, School of Public Health, Imperial College London, London, United Kingdom; Theme Aging, Karolinska University Hospital, Stockholm, Sweden; Institute of Public Health and Clinical Nutrition and Institute of Clinical Medicine, Neurology, University of Eastern Finland, Kuopio, Finland

Caterina Lapucci
Department of Neuroscience (DINOGMI), University of Genoa; Laboratory of Experimental Neurosciences, HNSR, IRCCS Polyclinic Hospital San Martino, Genoa, Italy

Bonnie H. Lee
Graduate Program in Neuroscience; Djavad Mowafaghian Centre for Brain Health, University of British Columbia, Vancouver, BC, Canada

Jenni Lehtisalo
Institute of Clinical Medicine, Neurology, University of Eastern Finland, Kuopio; Population Health Unit, Finnish Institute for Health and Welfare, Helsinki, Finland

Klara Lorenz-Dant
Care Policy and Evaluation Centre, The London School of Economics and Political Science, London, United Kingdom

Chris Lynch
Alzheimer's Disease International, London, United Kingdom

Karen E. Malacon
Department of Psychology and Neuroscience, Duke University, Durham, NC, United States

Julie N. Martinkova
Memory Clinic, Department of Neurology, Second Faculty of Medicine, Charles University and Motol University Hospital, Prague, Czech Republic; Women's Brain Project, Guntershausen, Switzerland

Federico Massa
Department of Neuroscience (DINOGMI), University of Genoa, Genoa, Italy

Riccardo Meli
Department of Neuroscience (DINOGMI), University of Genoa, Genoa, Italy

Simona Mellino
Women's Brain Project, Guntershausen, Switzerland

Michelle M. Mielke
Departments of Health Sciences Research and Neurology, Mayo Clinic, Rochester, MN, United States

Mary Mittelman
Department of Psychiatry, NYU Grossman School of Medicine, New York, NY, United States

Silvia Morbelli
Department of Health Sciences (DISSAL), University of Genoa; Department of Neuroradiology, IRCCS Polyclinic Hospital San Martino, Genoa, Italy

Beatrice Nasta
Women's Brain Project, Guntershausen; Department of Geriatric Psychiatry, Psychiatric Hospital Zurich, University of Zurich, Zurich, Switzerland

Flavio Nobili
Department of Neuroscience (DINOGMI), University of Genoa; Department of Neurology, IRCCS Polyclinic Hospital San Martino, Genoa, Italy

Matteo Pardini
Department of Neuroscience (DINOGMI), University of Genoa; Department of Neurology, IRCCS Polyclinic Hospital San Martino, Genoa, Italy

Enrico Peira
Department of Neuroscience (DINOGMI), University of Genoa; National Institute for Nuclear Physics (INFN), Genoa Section, Genoa, Italy

Susan Phillips
Department of Medicine (RMH), University of Melbourne, Melbourne, VIC, Australia

Tanvi A. Puri
Graduate Program in Neuroscience; Djavad Mowafaghian Centre for Brain Health, University of British Columbia, Vancouver, BC, Canada

Stefano Raffa
Department of Health Sciences (DISSAL), University of Genoa, Genoa, Italy

Katrin Rauen
Women's Brain Project, Guntershausen; Department of Geriatric Psychiatry, Psychiatric Hospital Zurich, University of Zurich, Zurich, Switzerland; Institute for Stroke and Dementia Research, University Hospital, LMU Munich, Munich, Germany

Danielle N. Rendina
Department of Psychology and Neuroscience, Duke University, Durham, NC, United States

Luca Roccatagliata
Department of Health Sciences (DISSAL), University of Genoa; Department of Neuroradiology, IRCCS Polyclinic Hospital San Martino, Genoa, Italy

Anna Rosenberg
Institute of Clinical Medicine, Neurology, University of Eastern Finland, Kuopio, Finland

Maitee Rosende-Roca
Research Center and Memory Clinic, Fundació ACE, Institut Català de Neurociències Aplicades, Universitat Internacional de Catalunya, Barcelona, Spain

Mercè Boada Rovira
Research Center and Memory Clinic, Fundació ACE, Institut Català de Neurociències Aplicades, Universitat Internacional de Catalunya, Barcelona; Networking Research Center on Neurodegenerative Diseases (CIBERNED), Instituto de Salud Carlos III, Madrid, Spain

Sara Rubinelli
Department of Health Sciences and Medicine, University of Lucerne, Lucerne; Person-Centered Health Care and Health Communication Group, Swiss Paraplegic Research Nottwil, Switzerland

Anthony Scerri
Department of Nursing, Faculty of Health Sciences, University of Malta, Msida, Malta

Charles Scerri
Department of Pathology, Faculty of Medicine and Surgery, University of Malta, Msida, Malta; Alzheimer Europe, Luxembourg

Shireen Sindi
Division of Clinical Geriatrics, Center for Alzheimer Research, Karolinska Institutet, Stockholm, Sweden; Ageing Epidemiology (AGE) Research Unit, School of Public Health, Imperial College London, London, United Kingdom

Ruth Stephen
Institute of Clinical Medicine, Neurology, University of Eastern Finland, Kuopio, Finland

Elina Suzuki
Organization for Economic Co-operation and Development, Directorate for Employment, Labour and Social Affairs, Paris, France

Cassandra Szoeke
Centre for Medical Research, Royal Melbourne Hospital, University of Melbourne, Melbourne, VIC, Australia

Sima Toopchiani
Ageing Epidemiology (AGE) Research Unit, School of Public Health, Imperial College London, London, United Kingdom

Marie-Ève Tremblay
Division of Medical Sciences, University of Victoria, Victoria, BC, Canada

Chinedu Udeh-Momoh
Ageing Epidemiology (AGE) Research Unit, School of Public Health, Imperial College London, London, United Kingdom

Wendy Weidner
Alzheimer's Disease International, London, United Kingdom

Acknowledgments

This book would have not been possible without the support, encouragement, and feedback of so many team members, authors, and collaborators of the Women's Brain Project (WBP), who worked amidst a global COVID-19 pandemic and several personal and societal challenges to complete their tasks.

First, we would like to thank the contributing authors for their enthusiasm in joining the project and their dedication to the chapters. Many of them hail from leading organizations that are long-standing collaborators of WBP, including the European Academy of Neurology, Alzheimer Europe, Alzheimer's Disease International, the Organisation for Economic Co-operation and Development (OECD), the Framingham Heart Study, and Fundació ACE, whom we wholeheartedly thank.

Second, we would like to thank the supporters and persons living with Alzheimer's disease and their family caregivers, who have encouraged and motivated us to pursue this project even when it looked impossible.

Special thanks go to all the team members and advisors of WBP who fostered the project, believed in us, and helped in the revision of the chapters. In particular, Mara Hank Moret, our honorary president, has been instrumental in developing WBP, believing in our work since day one and accompanying our growth.

WBP is indebted to a number of collaborators, across various fields, who have shared our journey and joined our vision. A special mention to the Leaders Engaged on Alzheimer's Disease (LEAD) Coalition, the World Dementia Council, the Alzheimer's Drug Discovery Foundation, the World Economic Forum, the Global CEO Initiative on Alzheimer's Disease (CEOi), Prof. Andrea Pfeifer, UsAgainstAlzheimer's (in particular, Meryl Comer and George Vradenburg), Prof. Ed Constable and Prof. Thorsten Schwede from the University of Basel. The support provided by the WBP corporate sponsors in 2020 (Roche, Eli Lilly, and Biogen) has allowed us to grow and to undertake many exciting projects, like this one.

We are particularly grateful to Dr. Lukas Engelberger from the Regierungsrat of the Canton Basel-Stadt (Governing Council of Canton Basel City) for authoring the foreword of this book. His support of our project is a continuous source of motivation for us.

Our gratitude goes to our Senior Acquisitions Editor, Melanie Tucker, who envisioned this book and accompanied us on this journey, together with Tracy Tufaga, who has been assisting us in every step.

Finally, our heartfelt thanks go to our families for supporting our long working hours, the stress, and the worries, but also for partaking in our excitement and pride.

Maria Teresa Ferretti
Annemarie Schumacher Dimech
Antonella Santuccione Chadha

Introduction

Women's Brain Project

The Women's Brain Project, a nonprofit organization studying sex and gender differences in brain and mental diseases, is very proud to present the book "Sex and Gender Differences in Alzheimer's Disease." This book aims, for the first time, to gather available evidence on sex and gender differences in Alzheimer's disease and related dementias and indicate avenues for future research and policy actions that could benefit both men and women. Eminent international experts have been invited to contribute to this work, thus representing the state of the art in this field.

As the recognition and consideration of sex and gender differences is increasing in significance at all levels, from basic neuroscience to patient care, the need has arisen for a reference text that can be used across disciplines to guide research and practice based on a precision medicine paradigm. This book is meant for clinicians and other health care providers, students, policymakers, academic researchers, and other stakeholders to encourage and promote a precision medicine approach in basic research and clinical practice, as well as novel policy actions. While this book focuses on Alzheimer's disease, it will provide, whenever appropriate, references to other dementia types, as many sex and/or gender differences go beyond Alzheimer's disease.

The book is made up of three parts:

Part 1. Sex differences in fundamental neurobiological processes that are relevant to Alzheimer's disease

This part offers the foundation for some biologically driven differences that are observed in animal models, related to inflammation and synaptic plasticity, between males and females. These processes are likely to underlie the clinical differences observed in patients and could represent novel targets for tailored treatment.

Part 2. Sex and gender differences in clinical aspects of Alzheimer's disease

The second part will delve into aspects of relevance for clinicians and clinical researchers, in terms of sex and, when appropriate, gender differences in biomarkers, disease presentation, risk/protective factors, and response to treatment.

Part 3. Gender differences in the socioeconomic factors linked to Alzheimer's disease

This section provides a comprehensive discussion of the various aspects related to socioeconomic factors (from caregiving to health communication and transformational policy) and gender inequity in Alzheimer's disease and puts forward recommendations for shaping future policies and strategies that consider individual needs and characteristics while addressing existing inequities.

This is the first book of an innovative series, led by the Women's Brain Project in collaboration with Elsevier, that will look at sex and gender differences in various aspects of medicine and healthcare. Indeed, the integration of sex and gender related factors has significant implications for clinical practice, research methods, data analysis, and policy writing, which will be covered by this series. The second book of the series is edited by Cirillo, Catuara, and Guney; entitled "Sex and Gender Bias in Technology and Artificial Intelligence: Biomedicine and Healthcare Applications," it details the integration of gender and sex factors in exponential technologies (artificial intelligence, digital medicine, robotics) for healthcare applications.

Editors' biography

Maria Teresa Ferretti, PhD
Co-founder and Chief Scientific Officer, Women's Brain Project, Guntershausen, Switzerland

Dr. Maria Teresa Ferretti is a neuroscientist and neuroimmunologist, expert in Alzheimer's disease and gender medicine. In 2016, together with Dr. Schumacher-Dimech, Dr. Santuccione Chadha and Gautam Maitra, she co-founded the nonprofit organization "Women's Brain Project" (where she currently serves as Chief Scientific Officer), a world leader in the study of sex and gender characteristics in brain and mental health as the gateway to precision medicine.

After graduating in Chemical and Pharmaceutical Technologies at University of Cagliari (Italy), she studied and worked in England, Canada (where she earned a PhD in Pharmacology and Pharmacological Therapy at McGill University in Montreal), Switzerland and Austria. Her studies have been published in numerous peer-reviewed journals, including Nature, and she is regularly invited by leading scientific conferences to lecture on Alzheimer's disease, precision medicine and the differences between men and women in neurology and psychiatry. She has taught in numerous university courses and is currently 'External Teacher' at the Medical University of Vienna; in addition, Dr. Ferretti is responsible for continuous medical education courses in the field of gender and precision medicine.

Passionate about scientific communication and motivated by the desire to break the stigma on mental and brain diseases, she was a TED-x speaker in 2019 and in 2021; in 2021, together with Antonella Santuccione Chadha, she wrote the book for the general public 'Una bambina senza testa' (Edizioni Mondo Nuovo).

Annemarie Schumacher Dimech, PhD
Co-founder and President, Women's Brain Project, Guntershausen, Switzerland
Program Manager, Palliative Care, University of Lucerne, Lucerne, Switzerland

Dr. Annemarie Schumacher Dimech obtained her first psychology degree with honors from the University of Malta, and holds an MSc in Health Psychology from the University of Surrey (UK) as a Chevening Scholar. In 2010, she obtained her PhD at the University of Bern.

Her fascination with the interaction between body and mind motivates her to study physical and environmental factors affecting brain and mental health. The sex and gender differences in various socioeconomic and psychological factors affecting brain and mental health was Dr. Schumacher Dimech's motivation to join forces with Antonella Santuccione Chadha, Maria Teresa Ferretti, and Gautam Maitra to found the Women's Brain Project. In her pro bono work with the Women's Brain Project, she contributes a psychosocial perspective to various WBP activities including educational events as well as publications, research, and other scientific events.

Today, she is employed at the University of Lucerne where she developed and is heading its programme of further education in Palliative Care and is currently President of Women's Brain Project.

Antonella Santuccione Chadha, MD
CEO pro bono and Co-founder Women's Brain Project, Guntershausen, Switzerland
Head of Stakeholder Engagement for Alzheimer's Disease, Biogen International.
Vice-President at Euresearch, Switzerland

Dr. Antonella Santuccione Chadha is a medical doctor with expertise in clinical pathology, neuroscience, and psychiatric disorders. She is head of stakeholder engagement for Alzheimer's disease at Biogen. She is cofounder and CEO of the nonprofit organization "Women's Brain Project," which is addressing the influence of sex and gender on mental and brain diseases. She is the Vice-president of Euresearch. As a medical doctor, Antonella has decades of experience in preclinical research, patient treatment, clinical development, medical affairs, and setting up the international regulatory framework for Alzheimer's disease.

Always focused on solving the puzzles related to Alzheimer's and other psychiatric diseases, she has worked with Swissmedic, the Bill and Melinda Gates Foundation, several European universities, the EU Commission Directorate for Health and Food Safety, the World Health Organization, the CEOi, and several Alzheimer's disease Organizations. Since 2018, she has been listed among the top 100 Women in Business in Switzerland, and in 2019, she was elected Woman of the Year in Switzerland by the magazine "Women in Business."

In 2020, she received the World Sustainability Award for her involvement in advancing precision medicine. She also received the award "Premio Medicina Italia" for her contribution to the management of the pandemic.

Dr. Santuccione Chadha is keenly interested in removing bias when developing solutions for mental and neurological diseases to achieve precision medicines.

Disclosure: Dr. A. Santuccione Chadha is currently an employee of Biogen Int. The opinion of the author expressed in this work are merely of the author and might not reflect the one of the organizations she is affiliated with. This work was conceived and produced before she joined Biogen Int.

Foreword

The Women's Brain Project is an initiative I fully support—this despite or precisely because I am a man. As a man, I'm in a minority in the context of this organization. Nevertheless, it is obvious why an initiative like this is important and needed. It is still the case in medical research today that women are given too little attention. Many research projects are androcentric and do not take sex and gender differences into account; for example, a medication that could be prescribed to both women and men has not even been researched on both genders.

It was in my hometown of Basel that the first cornerstone for gender-specific medicine was laid, hundreds of years ago. The famous medic Felix Platter was working in Basel as a physician and as professor of applied medicine when he published the oldest known illustration of a female skeleton in 1583, and described the differences between men and women. This was remarkable: it is generally assumed that thoughts on anatomical sex differences were characterized well into the 18th century by a "one-sex-model" assumption, which saw the male and female anatomy as more or less identical. However, Platter found that sex differences were at the very core of the body, in the skeleton.

Over 400 years have passed since Platter's observations, and yet parts of our bodies and especially our brain remain a source of mystery to us today. Or, as the German philosopher Immanuel Kant said: "If our brain were small enough for us to understand it, we would be so stupid that we still wouldn't understand it."

Research has shown that men's and women's brains function differently and also become diseased in different ways. It has been proven that vulnerability to brain and mental disease is affected by both sex and gender. I am sure that sex- and gender-specific medicine will become even more important in the future. Just like Felix Platter, we are still looking for answers. Answers that help us to understand ourselves, our bodies, and our brains better. This need is universal, regardless of which gender we identify with.

I will follow closely the initiatives that the Women's Brain Project adopts in the future and the discussion that it promotes. I hope that this book will provide insights not only into the tremendously important subject of Alzheimer's research but also into the passionate dedication the Women's Brain Project puts into its cause.

The Women's Brain Project team is currently in the process of taking their project into a larger dimension. Negotiations are ongoing to set up a foundation and a university institute in Basel. I very much hope that these plans will be successful. I wish the Women's Brain Project all the best for its future!

Lukas Engelberger
Head of the Public Health Department of the Canton Basel-Stadt

SECTION 1

Sex differences in fundamental neurobiological processes that are relevant to Alzheimer's disease

Maria Teresa Ferretti[a], Annemarie Schumacher Dimech[a,b], and Antonella Santuccione Chadha[a]

[a]*Women's Brain Project, Guntershausen, Switzerland*
[b]*Program Manager, Palliative Care, University of Lucerne, Lucerne, Switzerland*

As every cell has a sex, differences can be found in many fundamental cellular mechanisms throughout the body, as well as the brain. Such differences, which we are just starting to uncover, underlie the female- and male-specific presentation of diseases and deserve attention. For this reason, the book will start with three chapters that describe basic sex differences observed in the field of neurobiology and that could have an impact on the disease of Alzheimer's and dementia at large.

In Chapter 1, Ippati, Ittner and Ke provide an overview of sex differences in animal models widely used to study Alzheimer's disease; the knowledge of such differences is crucial, especially when using such models for drug development.

In Chapter 2, Lee, Puri and Galea describe the effects of sexual hormones on neurogenesis and synaptic plasticity. Sex differences in these fundamental processes are likely to impact the development of Alzheimer's pathology, especially during hormonal changes that characterize the menopausal/andropausal state.

Finally, in Chapter 3, Delage, Rendina, Malacon, Tremblay and Bilbo summarize the emerging field of sex differences in neuroimmunology, with a particular emphasis on microglial cells—the brain's resident immune cells.

These three chapters focus mostly on biological sex and only refer to gender-related aspects in specific cases.

CHAPTER 1

Sex differences in Alzheimer's disease animal models

Stefania Ippati[a], Lars Matthias Ittner[b], and Yazi Diana Ke[b]

[a]*San Raffaele Scientific Institute, San Raffaele Hospital, Milan, Italy*
[b]*Dementia Research Centre, Department of Biomedical Sciences, Faculty of Medicine Health and Human Sciences, Macquarie University, Sydney, NSW, Australia*

Overview of Alzheimer's disease

Alzheimer's disease (AD) is the most prevalent of all the neurodegenerative disorders characterized by a progressive loss of cognition. Distinct protein inclusions define most neurodegenerative diseases. In particular, the AD brain is characterized by two types of protein deposits, amyloid-β (Aβ) plaques and neurofibrillary tangles (NFTs), the latter formed by hyperphosphorylated forms of the microtubule-associated protein tau (Querfurth & LaFerla, 2010). Over recent decades, experiments on cellular and animal models have suggested that AD pathogenesis involves assemblies of Aβ peptides as a pathological trigger for what is commonly known as the "amyloid cascade hypothesis," which includes numerous pathological cellular events such as neuritic injury, inflammatory responses, oxidative stress, formation of neurofibrillary tangles via tau, neuronal dysfunction, and finally cell death (Hardy & Selkoe, 2002). Hence, clinical trials have focused on drug and vaccine development against Aβ or tau pathology as therapeutic approaches to AD (Panza, Lozupone, Logroscino, & Imbimbo, 2019). However, no clinical benefits by targeting Aβ or tau in humans have been obtained as yet (Imbimbo, Ippati, & Watling, 2020).

AD animal models

Animals are important models for Alzheimer's disease (AD) research. Over the past two decades, AD animal models have helped clarify the etiology of AD, testing therapeutic interventions, and validating hypotheses of mechanisms in the onset and progression of the disease. Mouse models are the most frequently used animal models of AD (Götz & Ittner, 2008). However, the pathophysiology observed in animal models may not necessarily reproduce all clinical findings observed in patients, which may explain why it is challenging to translate successful preclinical research in AD mouse models into clinical practice. The first transgenic mouse models for AD, established more than two decades ago, expressed human amyloid-β precursor protein (APP) carrying a single gene mutation associated with the inherited familial Alzheimer's disease (FAD) and recapitulated the histopathological lesions that are found in diseased human brains (Götz, Bodea, & Goedert, 2018). Since then, researchers have applied more precise gene-editing technologies to introduce pathogenic mutations in AD animal models and to accomplish endogenous gene expression levels rather than unphysiological overexpression (Scearce-Levie, Sanchez, & Lewcock, 2020). However, while most AD mouse models display histopathological features of AD (plaques and NFTs), they do not present the extensive neurodegeneration observed in the brains of AD patients. Moreover, the reproducibility of animal model research findings across laboratories is critical for the successful translation of experimental therapies to humans. The main mouse models that we will consider in this chapter are those most commonly used in preclinical studies

Mutant APP mouse models

The majority of AD models consist of transgenic mice expressing mutated human genes that result in the formation of amyloid plaques (by the expression of human APP alone or in combination with human presenilin 1 (PSEN1)) and neurofibrillary tangles (by the expression of human microtubule-associated protein tau (MAPT)) (Onos, Sukoff Rizzo, Howell, & Sasner, 2016). One of the earliest mouse models of Alzheimer's disease, the PDAPP line, expressing the human APP with the Indiana mutation V717F under control of the PDGF-β promoter, displayed human AD-like phenotype, including plaques in the hippocampus, gliosis, synaptic dysfunction, and cognitive impairment (Games et al., 1995). The Tg2576 line, one of the best-characterized and widely used mouse models of AD, expressing the human APP with the double Swedish mutation (APPK670N/M671L) driven by the hamster prion protein promoter (PrP), develops plaques in the frontal, temporal, and entorhinal cortices, hippocampus, and cerebellum. In addition, cerebral amyloid angiopathy (CAA), synaptic impairment, gliosis, and memory impairment are presented by this mouse model (Hsiao et al., 1996). APP23 mice also express K670N/M671L-mutant APP; however, they differ from Tg2576 mice by expressing the longer APP751 isoform driven by the neuronal Thy1 promoter. APP23 mice have more pronounced CAA, form compact plaques in comparison to the predominantly diffuse plaques found in Tg2576 mice, and have localized neurodegeneration that is not seen in the Tg2576 mice (Allué et al., 2016).

Mouse models with multiple FAD mutations

Transgenic mice with more severe pathology developed at a younger age have been developed by expressing multiple FAD-associated mutations together, such as the J20 line that expresses both the APP Swedish and Indiana mutations, and the APP/PS1 mouse, expressing both human APP (Swedish mutation) and PSEN1 (L166P mutation) transgenes under the control of the Thy1 promoter (Mucke et al., 2000). APP/

PS1 transgenic mice are widely used in AD research and have been developed with various specific FAD mutations and promoters. The APP/PS1 5xFAD mouse model expresses the Swedish (K670N/M671L), London (V717I), and Florida (I716V) APP mutations, M146L/L286V-mutant PSEN1 (Drummond & Wisniewski, 2017). The expression of five FAD mutations results in early intraneuronal Aβ accumulation at 6 weeks, followed by plaque formation at 2 months.

Mouse models of tau pathology

Mutant tau mice that showed NFTs formations expressed human tau containing mutations associated with frontotemporal lobar degeneration (FTLD). The first NFT-developing mouse was achieved by expressing the familial FTDP-17 MAPT mutation P301L under the control of the mouse PrP (Lewis et al., 2000). Another line, TAU58/2, expressing the P301S tau mutation under the control of the Thy1 promoter, presented early-onset motor deficits, progressively hyperphosphorylated tau resulting in NFT formation throughout the brain, increasing with age, and axonal pathology similar to human FTLD-tau and AD (van Eersel et al., 2015). Furthermore, mouse models that display both plaques and tangles have been reported. These models are characterized by the expression of mutated forms of APP and MAPT with or without PSEN1 or PSEN2 to drive plaque and tangle formation in the same model. The most commonly used model is the 3xTg-AD line, which develops intraneuronal Aβ at 3–4 months, followed by plaque development at approximately 6 months in the cortex and hippocampus. NFTs form at approximately 12 months, initially in CA1 and then in the cortex. To avoid transgene overexpression, gene targeting by homology-directed recombination (HDR) has been pursued to establish models, including ones in which AD-related genes are deleted (knockout (KO) models) or inserted (knock-in (KI) models) in endogenous murine gene loci. For example, in the APP^{NL-G-F} knock-in model, APP is not overexpressed, avoiding potential artifacts. In this model, levels of pathogenic Aβ are elevated due to the combined effects of three mutations associated with FAD (Saito et al., 2014). As these models are only emerging, potential sex differences have yet to be fully established.

Other AD mutant models

Over the past decade, neuroinflammation has been a focus of AD studies (see Chapter 3). Brain immune cells are associated with major AD risk factors, such as apolipoprotein E (APOE), a protein that is mainly produced by brain astrocytes, and TREM2, which is expressed by peripheral macrophages and brain microglial cells (Guerreiro et al., 2013; Liu, Kanekiyo, Xu, & Bu, 2013). In particular, in population-based studies, the epsilon-4 allele of APOE was reported to be a weaker predictor among African American (odds ratio (OR) 5.7) and Hispanic (OR 2.2) populations and instead a stronger predictor in Japanese people (OR 33.1) compared with white individuals (OR 12.5) (Farrer, 1997). The p.R47H variant of TREM2 was also found to confer a significant risk of AD in Iceland (OR 2.92) (Jonsson et al., 2013), and the same variant has been associated with both early and late-onset AD in the Spanish population (Benitez et al., 2013). Therefore, double/triple-mutant mouse lines have been generated by crossing FAD mice with APOE4 KI mice, which carry a humanized APOE4 gene, and with Trem2 KO or KI lines.

Transgenic rat models, overexpressing various FAD mutations, have been generated (Cohen et al., 2013; Leon et al., 2010). Basic neuropathological and behavioral characterization showed similar phenotypes in males and females McGill-R-Thy1-APP rats (Leon et al., 2010); minor differences in Morris Water Maze (Berkowitz, Harvey, Drake, Thompson, & Clark, 2018) and buried food task (Saré et al., 2020) performance have been described in the Tg-F344 model. Much less commonly used rat AD models include the use of vectors in which AD-related genes are selectively expressed in brain regions relevant to the disease and chemically induced models using intracranial streptozotocin administration. In the following chapter, we will discuss AD rodent models in which the phenotypic presentations have been extensively investigated in the light of sex differences. To our knowledge, mouse and rat models of Aβ infusions have not been characterized for sex differences.

Evidence for sex differences in AD animal models
The triple transgenic AD mouse model: 3xTg-AD
Age-dependent behavioral sex differences

Most animal studies that have addressed sex differences in AD have used transgenic mouse models. The widely used 3xTg-AD mouse, which expresses transgenes carrying three mutations associated with FAD (APP KM670/671NL, MAPT P301L, and PSEN1 M146V), has been extensively characterized for sex differences. One of the first studies conducted by LaFerla's laboratory investigated how sex influenced cognitive and neuropathological phenotypes and found that male and female 3xTg-AD mice show comparable behavioral impairments in the Morris water maze (MWM) inhibitory avoidance (IA) tests at 4 months (Clinton et al., 2007). Similarly, 3xTg-AD animals tested at 6 months of age for spatial cognition and memory displayed no sex differences (Giménez-Llort et al., 2010). However, Clinton and colleagues also found that female 3xTg-AD mice showed more significant deficits from 4 to 12 months than male 3xTg-AD mice in stressful behavioral tasks such as MWM, despite histological quantification of Aβ and tau brain pathology being comparable between sexes. Female 6-month-old 3xTg-AD mice were found to be impaired at spatial reorientation and at use of distal cues (Stimmell et al., 2019), while 6- and 12-month-old male 3xTg-AD mice were not impaired and presented with less brain pathology than females. Similarly, Yang et al. found that female 12-month-old 3xTg-AD mice displayed greater spatial cognitive deficits than males (Yang et al., 2018).

In the study from Clinton et al., sex differences were attributed to greater stress response in young female mice, also displayed by higher plasma corticosterone. Interestingly, the differential stress response between sexes was no longer apparent after 12 months of age, along with the disappearance of cognitive differences. In the same study, nonstressful conditions, such as the object recognition test, determined no behavioral sex differences across 3xTg-AD mice's lifespan. Old age has also been found to influence major sex-dependent changes in social behavior of 3xTg-AD mice (Bories et al., 2012) associated with a significant increase in prefrontal cortex synaptic activity (mIPSC and mEPSC frequencies). Moreover, 3xTg-AD females were more disinhibited than their male counterparts at 12 months of age, while the opposite was true at 18 months. Interestingly, increased Aβ42 concentrations in the brain were associated with disinhibition in male 3xTg-AD mice, while an inverse association was observed in females.

In summary, according to the studies mentioned earlier, it is evident that female 3xTg-AD mice from 6 to 12 months are more affected by AD pathology than are male 3xTg-ADs, and that these variabilities appeared to be no longer present in mice after 12 months.

Sex differences in glucose homeostasis and immune function
Concerning age, Giménez-Llort et al. have shown that at early stages of the disease, female 3xTg-AD mice showed a poorer ability to maintain weight and glucose homeostasis, while increased peak blood glucose was observed in both sexes. Total weights of the thymus were higher in female than in male 3xTg-AD mice, and this sex difference was more obvious when relative weights were considered, suggesting possible differences in immune function between the sexes. Amyloid deposits appeared slightly larger in females than in males, in agreement with other observations in this mouse line (Carroll et al., 2010; Yang et al., 2018), while male 3xTg-AD mice displayed increased lipid peroxidation and derangement of the glutathione system.

Olfaction and hormonal-related factors
It has been suggested that sex steroid hormones may influence sex differences in Aβ pathology in 3xTg-AD mice during development (Carroll et al., 2010), as male 3xTg-AD mice that were demasculinized during early development exhibited significantly increased Aβ accumulation in adulthood, while female mice defeminized during early development exhibited a less severe Aβ pathology in adulthood. Sex-dependent behavioral assessment of olfaction has been evaluated in 6-month-old 3xTg-AD mice, using an olfactory detection task with ethyl acetate as odorant (Roddick, Roberts, Schellinck, & Brown, 2016). At the highest odor concentration, male and female 3xTg-AD mice did not differ in accuracy from their wildtype controls, while only female 3xTg-AD animals showed impairment at the lowest concentration of the odorant. This study also analyzed 5XFAD mice, expressing the human APP and PSEN1 transgenes with a total of

five AD-linked mutations, and found that no olfactory deficits were present in either sex or compared to their wildtype controls.

Increased brain Aβ and tau pathology and neuroinflammation in female 3xTg-AD mice were associated with an altered PKA-CREB-MAPK signaling pathway, which is closely associated with synaptic plasticity and memory (Yang et al., 2018). In particular, expression levels of p-PKA and p-CREB in the hippocampus were markedly lower, and p38-MAPK was higher in 3xTg-AD mice, and especially in females. The authors suggested that impaired PKA-CREB-MAPK signaling might be induced by estrogen deficiency in 12-month-old female mice, and estrogen supplementation or gene therapy targeting PKA-CREB-MAPK signals could be beneficial in AD older females (see Chapter 2).

Lifespan

Studies have focused on sex differences in 3xTg-AD mice of various ages, underlining how age appears to have an appreciable role in determining sex differences in this mouse strain. It appears that female 3xTg-AD mice are generally more vulnerable to AD pathology from 4 up to 12 months, but on the contrary, and in line with a previous study (Rae & Brown, 2015), Kane and colleagues reported that male 3xTg-AD mice had a shorter lifespan than female 3xTg-AD mice (Kane et al., 2018). Moreover, male 3xTg-AD mice lived for a shorter time than male WT mice, but this genotype difference in lifespan was not seen in female mice. Additionally, both male 3xTg-AD and WT mice had higher frailty scores than the corresponding female groups, suggesting that these sex differences may be related to differences in genetic factors, epigenetic factors or immune system variables.

APP and PSEN1 transgenic mouse models: TgCRND8, APPswe/PSEN1dE9, APPPS1, and PS2APP/Trem2KO

In the TgCRND8 mouse line, an APP transgenic mouse model carrying the APP Swedish and Indiana mutations, male and female animals have been reported to exhibit adrenocortical hyperactivity, an endocrine hallmark of AD (Green, Billings, Roozendaal, McGaugh, & LaFerla, 2006), in a sex-specific manner (Touma et al., 2004). In 4-month-old TgCRND8 mice, the plasma corticosterone concentrations of both sexes were elevated; but whereas fecal corticosterone metabolites (CM) were present at 45 days in male mice, in females, they only appeared at 90 days, suggesting an involvement of adrenocortical activity in an age- and sex-dependent manner. However, adrenal tyrosine hydroxylase activity measured at 4 months showed no significant differences between the sexes. This study also found no sex differences in the number of amyloid plaques observed or in exploratory and anxiety-related behavior. Li and colleagues investigated sex differences in an APPswe/PSEN1dE9 mouse model containing the APP Swedish mutation and a knocked-in variant of the human PSEN1 (deltaE9) gene. They found that 6-month-old male APP/PS1 mice showed abnormal glucose and insulin tolerance and higher total cholesterol and triglyceride levels compared to female APP/PS1 mice. However, the amounts of Aβ in female APP/PS1 mice were significantly higher than in the males, and corresponded to reduced memory test performance of females as assessed in the MWM (Li et al., 2016). The authors concluded that, in this mouse model, Aβ deposits might affect cognitive function more than impaired insulin signaling and elevated plasma lipid levels.

Age- and sex-specific alterations in brain electrical network alterations have been described in APPswePS1dE9 mice (Papazoglou et al., 2016). Whereas male APPswePS1dE9 mice exhibit a reduction in theta waves during electroencephalography (EEG) recordings at the age of 14 weeks, which disappear as they age, female mice exhibit theta power reduction at 18 and 19 weeks of age. These findings are in line with a report from 2015 in which APPswePS1dE9 male and female mice showed significantly different brain deposition kinetics for Aβ (Ordóñez-Gutiérrez, Antón, & Wandosell, 2015). In particular, senile plaques in the cortex and hippocampus could be detected in 3-month-old male APPswePS1dE9 mice, but barely in females of the same age; however, starting from 9 months of age, amyloid levels in plasma increased among females but decreased among males. Aβ plaque deposition in the retina has been reported to appear earlier in aged female than male APPswePS1dE9 mice (Perez, Lumayag, Kovacs, Mufson, & Shunbin, 2009).

Another widely used AD mouse model is the APPPS1 line, expressing transgenes for both human APP bearing the Swedish mutation and human PSEN1 with an L166P mutation, both under the control of the murine neuronal Thy1 promoter (Radde et al., 2006). Several studies have focused on sex-dependent AD pathology using the APPPS1 line. Dodiya and colleagues investigated how antibiotic treatments resulted in microbiome changes in male and female APPPS1 mice (Dodiya et al., 2019). While postnatal antibiotic treatment determined similar changes in gut bacterial composition at 22 days of age in both sexes, long-term antibiotic cocktail treatment (ABX) resulted in sex-specific microbiome changes. Some bacterial clusters associated with gut tissue degradation and inflammatory activation (e.g., *Akkermansia muciniphila* and an *Allobaculum* spp.) were significantly enriched in females compared to males, along with proinflammatory pathway activation, such as the bacterial secretion system, bacterial toxins, lipopolysaccharide biosynthesis, and lipopolysaccharide synthesis protein. Moreover, ABX-treated male APPPS1 mice exhibited elevated levels of antiinflammatory/neuroprotective factors and, in contrast, ABX-treated female mice showed upregulation of proinflammatory cytokines/chemokines. Furthermore, long-term ABX treatment resulted in reduced Aβ deposition, neuroinflammation, and antiinflammatory transcriptional signatures only in male APPPS1 mice.

Various studies have found that the mood stabilizer valproic acid (VPA), traditionally used to treat bipolar disorder, may have therapeutic potential in other central nervous system diseases (Williams, Cheng, Mudge, & Harwood, 2002). Evidence indicates that there are neurotrophic and neuroprotective sex-related effects of VPA induced on AD pathology in APPPS1 mice. VPA treatment was found to relieve anxiety-related behavior in male APPPS1 mice, whereas no significant beneficial effects were found in female mice between the VPA- and saline-treated groups. The same results were obtained during MWM testing, where VPA-treated APPPS1 male mice exhibited reduced escape latency compared to treated females. Moreover, VPA modified the synaptic structure of male mice, while there was significantly reduced Aβ brain burden and neuronal cell death in both sexes. Genetic variants of TREM2, a gene with expression in brain microglia, have been shown to increase the risk of developing late-onset AD (Ulland & Colonna, 2018). Since human TREM2 variants were linked to a reduction of TREM2 function (Cheng-Hathaway et al., 2018), Trem2KO mice have been crossed with APP transgenic mice to study the effects of loss of TREM2 function in the context of amyloidosis and tauopathy. In a recent study, PSEN2APP/Trem2KO female mice have been reported to accumulate Aβ pathology more rapidly than males, while later, as the mice aged, plaque accumulation was reduced in both female and male PSEN2APP/Trem2KO mice compared to age-matched TREM2WT, and neuroinflammation was similar in both sexes (Meilandt et al., 2020).

ApoE transgenic mouse models: ApoE4/3xTg, 5xFAD/ApoE3, and 5xFAD/ApoE4

The ApoE KI strain of mice have been established to investigate the role of Apolipoprotein E4 (ApoE4), the most prevalent genetic risk factor of AD (Liu et al., 2013). Being a potential therapeutic target for AD, mechanisms involved in the interaction between ApoE4 and sex have been studied repeatedly. Hou and colleagues have evaluated sex-dependent ApoE4 effects on learning, memory, and AD histopathology using ApoE4/3xTg mice. Their findings from behavioral and spatial exploration testing support the hypothesis that ApoE4 contributes to learning and memory deficits in 10-month-old ApoE4/3xTg female mice, which may be associated with hormonal fluctuation starting around this time (Hou et al., 2015). Using mouse vaginal mucosa smears, it was confirmed that ApoE4/3xTg transgenic animals' cycle length became irregular and prolonged (> 5 days) compared to the normal cycle lasting 4–5 days. Moreover, female mice carrying ApoE4 displayed spatial and memory impairment earlier than their male counterparts and showed more prominent AD pathology in the hippocampus. Importantly, female ApoE4/3xTg mice showed increased BACE1 enzymatic activity and elevated expression of BACE1 and of its transcription factor SP1.

In a more recent report, microglial interactions with amyloid plaques have been investigated in 5xFAD/ApoE3 +/+ (E3FAD) and 5xFAD/ApoE4 +/+ (E4FAD) mice, and in particular, how ApoE genotypes and sex influence neuropathology in these mouse models (Stephen et al., 2019). The authors found that the ApoE genotype was a significant factor, with higher plaque coverage in E3FAD males than in E4FAD males. Further, there was a significant effect on microglial engulfment of plaques, which was twofold greater in male E3FAD than in female E3FAD mice. Moreover, in male E3FAD, microglial process interactions were increased and were associated with reduced plaque size. Using quantitative confocal analysis to check for plaque morphology, it has been found that TREM2 expression, microglial plaque coverage, and compaction, considered a beneficial consequence of microglial interactions with plaques, was diminished by ApoE4 and by female sex in E4FAD mice. Moreover, ApoE4 genotype and female sex were associated with the highest amyloid burden.

Tau mouse models: P301S, rTg4510, JNPL3

Tau P301S transgenic mice are one of the most widely used mouse models in AD research, and in recent years, have been considered for studies on sex- and age-related differences in neuropathology and behavior. Van Eersel and colleagues have investigated age and sex differences in the TAU58/2 line, a model of FTLD expressing the human 0N4R tau isoform with the P301S mutation, under the control of the murine Thy1.2 promoter. TAU58/2 mice presented early-onset motor deficits, axonal pathology, and NFT formation throughout the brain, with males displaying significantly more pronounced pathology than females (van Eersel et al., 2015). The authors found that the number of NFTs increased significantly in male TAU58/2 mice over time in the cortex, hippocampus, and brainstem. By 6 months of age, male TAU58/2 mice presented significant motor deficits, and at 10 months of age, both male and female TAU58/2 showed significant motor impairments. Furthermore, male TAU58/2 mice demonstrated greater amounts of phosphorylated tau-specific staining than female mice. Total soluble human tau levels in the cortex, hippocampus, and tau phosphorylated at Ser396/Ser404 (PHF-1) and Ser422 (pS422), and astrogliosis was significantly increased in male compared to female TAU58/2 mice. This corresponded to significantly higher amounts of insoluble tau in hippocampal extracts from male as compared to female TAU58/2 brains.

More recently, similar results have been obtained in P301S mice, although with a different background, and transgene driven by the murine prion protein instead (Sun et al., 2020). Male P301S mice undergo faster weight loss, more severe dyskinesia, and more severe memory dysfunction than female transgenic mice. Consistent with the sex differences in behavior and neuropathology, several plasma factors, including MIG, TNF-α, IL-10, and IL-13 exhibited specific changes in male P301S mice compared to females. In the same mouse line, microglial microRNA expression analysis showed that microRNA changes differ between male and female P301S mice, differently influencing tau pathology in each sex (Kodama et al., 2020). In this study, depletion of Dicer, an RNase III endonuclease (Song & Rossi, 2017) was used to determine the accumulation of miRNA precursors in P301S mice. Tau inclusions were more frequent in male P301S/Dicer KO mice than in their female counterparts in the cortex, amygdala, and piriform cortex. Consistently, male P301S/Dicer KO mice displayed more amoeboid-like microglia. Microglia bulk sequencing revealed that male microglia were enriched with genes involved in inflammation and phagocytosis, including Spp1, Ccl6, Lpl, Il1b, and Cst7. Single cell sequencing confirmed that sex-dependent microRNAs cluster enrichment supports the differential microglial response to tau pathology, as male P301S/Dicer KO exhibited increased disease-associated signatures and decreased homeostatic microglia compared to females. Conversely, in the rTg4510 mouse, expressing a repressible P301L tau transgene, female mice have been reported to show more severe cognitive impairment and higher levels of phosphorylated tau than male mice (Yue, Hanna, Wilson, Roder, & Janus, 2011). Sex differences have also been observed in the JNPL3 strain, which expresses mutant P301L tau driven by the mouse prion promoter, with higher numbers of NFTs and tau expression levels observed in female mice compared with males (Lewis et al., 2001). Whether different tau mutations used to generate these lines contribute to sex differences in tau-induced deficits remains to be determined.

Nontransgenic animals

To our knowledge, very few studies have used both sexes with nontransgenic animals, and most have used intracerebroventricular (ICV) injections of streptozotocin (STZ) to model AD-like phenotypes in rats and mice. Biasibetti and colleagues demonstrated that the behavioral effects and changes in neurochemical markers depended on sex and were more prominent in males (Biasibetti et al., 2017). In particular, in the object recognition test, a nonspatial memory test, a significant cognitive impairment was present in the male groups treated with STZ, whereas female rats were more resistant to STZ effects. Male STZ mice also displayed reduced choline acetyltransferase content, while in females, a significant decrease was present only 8 weeks after STZ infusion. Finally, in this model, male STZ mice showed reduced glucose metabolism, more activated hippocampal astrocytes, and oxidative imbalance in the hippocampus. Similarly, Bao and colleagues showed that females were more resistant to the learning and memory impairment induced by STZ administration (Bao et al., 2017). Moreover, male STZ mice had more tau hyperphosphorylation and Aβ40/42, and increased GSK-3β and BACE1 activities, with more pronounced loss of dendritic and synaptic plasticity.

Limitations

While AD is a strictly human disease, the generation of genetically modified mice expressing mutations in genes that cause AD has enabled progress in understanding its pathogenesis.

Most AD model studies show that females have more severe disease pathology and progression compared to males, which aligns with observations in humans. However, many factors should be considered when drawing conclusions on how sex influences AD pathology in preclinical models. As reviewed here, different mutations could worsen AD pathology in either male or female mice. Moreover, the type of promoter used might also have an impact on the outcome of behavioral and neuropathological tests. Yang et al., in 2006, reported a large-scale analysis of whole brains from more than 150 male and female mice, highlighting the degree of sex-dependent gene expression in the mammalian brain (Yang et al., 2006). Their study showed that gene expression levels in 14% of genes expressed in the brain were influenced by sex, with most of these genes being located on autosomal chromosomes. Such differences would be traditionally attributed to hormonal regulation, but in more recent studies, genetic and epigenetic effects have been associated with the inheritance of the X and Y chromosomes (Ratnu, Emami, & Bredy, 2017). Thus, sex-specific differences in epigenetic regulation may also influence promoters' expression, and hence mouse behavior and transgene pathology. Examples of this are the promoter for brain-derived neurotrophic factor (BDNF), which has been reported to be hypermethylated in female mice (Baker-Andresen, Flavell, Li, & Bredy, 2013), or the ERαpromoter, more methylated in male mice in the amygdala (Edelmann & Auger, 2011).

Taken together, the evidence suggests that different promoters may possess different activities in driving transgene expression in mice of different sexes. Moreover, what appears more challenging would be imitating the human reproductive decline in mouse models of AD, as mouse aging is not characterized by lowered gonadal steroid levels (Nelson, Felicio, Osterburg, & Finch, 1992; Nelson, Latham, & Finch, 1975), as occurs in men and, in particular, during menopause in women, during aging (Chakravarti et al., 1976; Ferrini & Barrett-Connor, 1998) (see Chapter 9). The other translation obstacle is represented by the difference in reproductive senescence, which is due to dysregulation of the neuroendocrine system in female rodents (Kermath & Gore, 2012), while in women, there is a decline of oocyte numbers and ovary function (Fitzgerald, Zimon, & Jones, 1998). Appropriate modeling could be accomplished by gonadectomy in rodents, recapitulating a critical aspect of human reproductive aging in males and females (Carroll et al., 2010). However, mouse studies on hormonal effects in AD have shown that gonadal steroids benefit cognition in the normal aging brain in both female and male mice (Dubal, Broestl, & Worden, 2012), raising several important questions about how to investigate the loss and replacement of hormones in models of AD.

Conclusion

Transgenic manipulation and mutations should be considered when interpreting and translating results from animal models to humans. Given that animal studies have helped to understand sex-dependent aspects in AD, sex differences should always be taken into account when examining the pathological characteristics of AD and related target molecules (Fig. 1). One should take sex differences in animals into account in both mechanism research and drug design—for example, the emerging role of novel sex-specific EEG fingerprints as potential early biomarkers of AD in the future, or highlighting the importance of considering sexes when

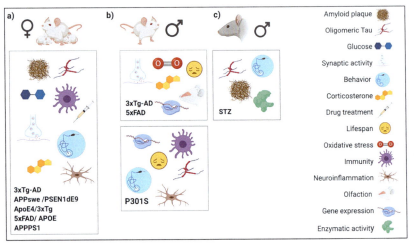

FIG. 1

The AD hallmarks displayed in (a) are worse in female compared to male mice in the listed mouse models; (b) worse in male mice compared to female mice in the listed mouse models; (c) worse in male rats compared to female rats in the STZ AD model.

evaluating the effect of long-term antibiotic treatment on the microbiome and peripheral inflammation. Moreover, treatment with VPA might not show the same beneficial results in male and female AD mice, as their sex may significantly influence AD. Thus, VPA may be a promising remedy for AD only if basic biological differences and sex specificity are taken into account. To develop potential therapeutic targets in postmenopausal female ApoE4 carriers, future studies with ovarian hormone manipulation in ApoE4 female rodents are necessary to probe the mechanisms underlying AD pathology. Moreover, further animal investigation will also be required to define the mechanisms driving APOE and sex differences in microglial function. Considering the sex differences existing in virtually all AD animal models in use (see Table 1), single sex-studies should be a thing of the past.

Chapter highlights

- Many AD mouse models present significant differences in phenotype between males and females, offering opportunities to understand sex-dependent disease mechanisms.
- Sex-biased studies in AD models should become obsolete, in particular for preclinical drug testing.
- Fundamental differences in reproductive senescence between mice and humans need to be taken into account when considering deficits in models of aging.

Table 1 Overview of AD features related to sexual differences in animal models.

AD animal model (mice)	Mutation	References	Features	Sex difference
3xTg-AD	APP KM670/671NL (Swedish), MAPT P301L, PSEN1 M146V	Clinton et al. (2007)	Behavioral impairment and corticosterone response	♀ > ♂ from 4 to 12 months
		Giménez-Llort et al. (2010)	Behavioral impairment	♀ = ♂
			Corticosterone response	♀ = ♂
			Brain amyloid pathology	♀ > ♂
			Glucose tolerance	♀ < ♂
			Oxidative stress	♀ < ♂
			Immune function	♀ > ♂
		Kane et al. (2018)	Frailty and lifespan	♀ > ♂
		Bories et al. (2012)	Disinhibition and increased cortical synaptic activity	♀ > ♂ at 12 months; ♀ < ♂ at 18 months
		Carroll et al. (2010)	Behavior and brain amyloid pathology	♀ > ♂
		Roddick et al. (2016)	Olfactory learning and detection abilities	♀ < ♂
		Stimmell et al. (2019)	Spatial memory impairment and brain amyloid pathology	♀ = ♂ at 3 months; ♀ > ♂ at 6 months
		Yang et al. (2018)	Brain amyloid and tau pathology, spatial memory impairment, neuroinflammation, and molecular factors dysregulation	♀ > ♂
5xFAD	APP KM670/671NL (Swedish), APP I716V (Florida), APP V717I (London), PSEN1 M146L (A>C), PSEN1 L286V	Roddick et al. (2016)	Olfactory learning and detection abilities	♀ = ♂
TgCRND8	APP KM670/671NL (Swedish), APP V717F (Indiana)	Touma et al. (2004)	Behavioral impairment and neuropathology	♀ = ♂
			Corticosterone response	♀ < ♂ at 1 month; ♀ = ♂ at 2 months

Continued

Table 1 Overview of AD features related to sexual differences in animal models—cont'd

AD animal model (mice)	Mutation	References	Features	Sex difference
APPswe/PSEN1dE9	APP KM670/671NL (Swedish), PSEN1: deltaE9	Li et al. (2016)	Glucose and insulin tolerance	♀ > ♂
			Total cholesterol and triglyceride levels	♀ < ♂
			Brain amyloid pathology	♀ > ♂
			Behavioral impairment	♀ > ♂
		Perez et al. (2009)	Retinal amyloid pathology	♀ > ♂
		Papazoglou et al. (2016)	EEG alterations	♀ < ♂ at 3.5 months; ♀ > ♂ at 4.5 months
APPPS1	APP KM670/671NL (Swedish), PSEN1 L166P	Dodiya et al. (2019)	Beneficial response to long-term antibiotic cocktail treatments	♀ < ♂
			Proinflammatory microbiome changes, brain amyloid pathology, and neuroinflammation	♀ > ♂
		Long, Zeng, Wang, Sharma, and He (2016)	Response to valproic acid on:	
			• behavioral impairment	♀ < ♂
			• synapse activity	♀ = ♂
			• neuronal cell loss	♀ = ♂
PSEN2APP/Trem2KO	APP KM670/671NL (Swedish), PSEN2 N141I (Volga German)/Trem2 KO	Meilandt et al. (2020)	Brain amyloid pathology	♀ > ♂ at 6 to 7 months ♀ = ♂ starting from 7 months
			Neuroinflammation	♀ = ♂
ApoE4/3xTg	hAPOE4 KI/APP KM670/671NL (Swedish), MAPT P301L, PSEN1 M146V	Hou et al. (2015)	Behavioral and memory impairment Brain amyloid pathology BACE1 and SP1 expression	♀ > ♂

5xFAD/ APOE3+/+	hAPOE3–4 Knock-in/APP KM670/671NL (Swedish), APP I716V (Florida), APP V717I (London), PSEN1 M146L (A>C), PSEN1 L286V	Stephen et al. (2019)	Brain amyloid pathology and TREM2 expression	♀ > ♂
5xFAD/ APOE4+/+			Microglia coverage and compaction	♀ < ♂
P301S	MAPT P301S	Kodama et al. (2020)	Pathological microglial transcriptome changes and tau pathology	♀ < ♂
		Sun et al. (2020)	Phenotype severity, brain tau pathology, behavior, neuroinflammation, and systemic inflammation	♀ < ♂
		van Eersel et al. (2015)	Phenotype severity, brain tau pathology, behavior and motor performance	♀ < ♂
rTg4510	MAPT P301L	Yue et al. (2011)	Brain tau pathology	♀ > ♂
JNPL3	MAPT P301L	Lewis et al. (2001)	Brain tau pathology and tau expression levels	♀ > ♂

AD animal model (rat)	Mutation	Reference	Features	Sex difference
STZ	N/A-sporadic	Biasibetti et al. (2017)	Behavioral and molecular factors impairment	♀ < ♂
		Bao et al. (2017)	Behavioral impairment; brain amyloid and tau pathology	♀ < ♂

References

Allué, J. A., Sarasa, L., Izco, M., Pérez-Grijalba, V., Fandos, N., Pascual-Lucas, M., et al. (2016). Outstanding phenotypic differences in the profile of amyloid-β between Tg2576 and APPswe/PS1dE9 transgenic mouse models of Alzheimer's disease. *Journal of Alzheimer's Disease, 53*(3), 773–785. https://doi.org/10.3233/JAD-160280.

Baker-Andresen, D., Flavell, C. R., Li, X., & Bredy, T. W. (2013). Activation of BDNF signaling prevents the return of fear in female mice. *Learning and Memory, 20*(5), 237–240. https://doi.org/10.1101/lm.029520.112.

Bao, J., Mahaman, Y. A. R., Liu, R., Wang, J. Z., Zhang, Z., Zhang, B., et al. (2017). Sex differences in the cognitive and hippocampal effects of streptozotocin in an animal model of sporadic AD. *Frontiers in Aging Neuroscience, 9*(OCT), 347. https://doi.org/10.3389/fnagi.2017.00347.

Benitez, B. A., Cooper, B., Pastor, P., Jin, S. C., Lorenzo, E., Cervantes, S., et al. (2013). TREM2 is associated with the risk of Alzheimer's disease in Spanish population. *Neurobiology of Aging, 34*(6). https://doi.org/10.1016/j.neurobiolaging.2012.12.018. 1711.e15–1711.e17.

Berkowitz, L. E., Harvey, R. E., Drake, E., Thompson, S. M., & Clark, B. J. (2018). Progressive impairment of directional and spatially precise trajectories by TgF344-Alzheimer's disease rats in the Morris Water Task. *Scientific Reports, 8*(1), 16153. https://doi.org/10.1038/s41598-018-34368-w.

Biasibetti, R., dos Santos, J. P. A., Rodrigues, L., Wartchow, K. M., Suardi, L. Z., Nardin, P., et al. (2017). Hippocampal changes in STZ-model of Alzheimer's disease are dependent on sex. *Behavioural Brain Research, 316*(January), 205–214. https://doi.org/10.1016/j.bbr.2016.08.057.

Bories, C., Guitton, M. J., Julien, C., Tremblay, C., Vandal, M., Msaid, M., et al. (2012). Sex-dependent alterations in social behaviour and cortical synaptic activity coincide at different ages in a model of Alzheimer's disease. Edited by David R. Borchelt *PLoS One, 7*(9), e46111. https://doi.org/10.1371/journal.pone.0046111.

Carroll, J. C., Rosario, E. R., Kreimer, S., Villamagna, A., Gentzschein, E., Stanczyk, F. Z., et al. (2010). Sex differences in β-amyloid accumulation in 3xTg-AD mice: Role of neonatal sex steroid hormone exposure. *Brain Research, 1366*, 233–245. https://doi.org/10.1016/j.brainres.2010.10.009.

Chakravarti, S., Collins, W. P., Forecast, J. D., Newton, T. R., Oram, D. H., & Studd, J. W. W. (1976). Hormonal profiles after the menopause. *British Medical Journal, 2*(6039), 784–787. https://doi.org/10.1136/bmj.2.6039.784.

Cheng-Hathaway, P. J., Reed-Geaghan, E. G., Jay, T. R., Casali, B. T., Bemiller, S. M., Puntambekar, S. S., et al. (2018). The Trem2 R47H variant confers loss-of-function-like phenotypes in Alzheimer's disease. *Molecular Neurodegeneration, 13*(1), 29. https://doi.org/10.1186/s13024-018-0262-8.

Clinton, L. K., Billings, L. M., Green, K. N., Caccamo, A., Ngo, J., Oddo, S., et al. (2007). Age-dependent sexual dimorphism in cognition and stress response in the 3xTg-AD mice. *Neurobiology of Disease, 28*(1), 76–82. https://doi.org/10.1016/j.nbd.2007.06.013.

Cohen, R. M., Rezai-Zadeh, K., Weitz, T. M., Rentsendorj, A., Gate, D., Spivak, I., … Town, T. (2013). A transgenic Alzheimer rat with plaques, tau pathology, behavioral impairment, oligomeric aβ, and frank neuronal loss. *The Journal of Neuroscience, 33*(15), 6245–6256. https://doi.org/10.1523/JNEUROSCI.3672-12.2013.

Dodiya, H. B., Kuntz, T., Shaik, S. M., Baufeld, C., Leibowitz, J., Zhang, X., et al. (2019). Sex-specific effects of microbiome perturbations on cerebral Aβ amyloidosis and microglia phenotypes. *Journal of Experimental Medicine, 216*(7), 1542–1560. https://doi.org/10.1084/jem.20182386.

Drummond, E., & Wisniewski, T. (2017). Alzheimer's disease: Experimental models and reality. *Acta Neuropathologica.* https://doi.org/10.1007/s00401-016-1662-x. Springer Verlag.

Dubal, D. B., Broestl, L., & Worden, K. (2012). Sex and gonadal hormones in mouse models of Alzheimer's disease: What is relevant to the human condition? *Biology of Sex Differences.* https://doi.org/10.1186/2042-6410-3-24. BioMed Central.

Edelmann, M. N., & Auger, A. P. (2011). Epigenetic impact of simulated maternal grooming on estrogen receptor alpha within the developing amygdala. *Brain, Behavior, and Immunity, 25*(7), 1299–1304. https://doi.org/10.1016/j.bbi.2011.02.009.

Farrer, L. A. (1997). Effects of age, sex, and ethnicity on the association between apolipoprotein E genotype and Alzheimer disease. *JAMA, 278*(16), 1349. https://doi.org/10.1001/jama.1997.03550160069041.

Ferrini, R. L., & Barrett-Connor, E. (1998). Sex hormones and age: A cross-sectional study of testosterone and estradiol and their bioavailable fractions in community-dwelling men. *American Journal of Epidemiology, 147*(8), 750–754. https://doi.org/10.1093/oxfordjournals.aje.a009519.

Fitzgerald, C., Zimon, A. E., & Jones, E. E. (1998). Aging and reproductive potential in women. *Yale Journal of Biology and Medicine, 71*(5), 367–381.

Games, D., Adams, D., Alessandrini, R., Barbour, R., Borthelette, P., Blackwell, C., et al. (1995). Alzheimer-type neuropathology in transgenic mice overexpressing V717F β-amyloid precursor protein. *Nature, 373*(6514), 523–527. https://doi.org/10.1038/373523a0.

Giménez-Llort, L., García, Y., Buccieri, K., Revilla, S., Suñol, C., Cristofol, R., et al. (2010). Gender-specific neuroimmunoendocrine response to treadmill exercise in 3xTg-AD mice. *International Journal of Alzheimer's Disease, 2010.* https://doi.org/10.4061/2010/128354.

Götz, J., & Ittner, L. M. (2008). Animal models of Alzheimer's disease and frontotemporal dementia. *Nature Reviews Neuroscience.* https://doi.org/10.1038/nrn2420. Nature Publishing Group.

Götz, J., Bodea, L. G., & Goedert, M. (2018). Rodent models for Alzheimer disease. *Nature Reviews Neuroscience.* https://doi.org/10.1038/s41583-018-0054-8. Nature Publishing Group.

Green, K. N., Billings, L. M., Roozendaal, B., McGaugh, J. L., & LaFerla, F. M. (2006). Glucocorticoids increase amyloid-β and tau pathology in a mouse model of Alzheimer's disease. *Journal of Neuroscience, 26*(35), 9047–9056. https://doi.org/10.1523/JNEUROSCI.2797-06.2006.

Guerreiro, R., Wojtas, A., Bras, J., Carrasquillo, M., Rogaeva, E., Majounie, E., et al. (2013). TREM2 variants in Alzheimer's disease. *New England Journal of Medicine, 368*(2), 117–127. https://doi.org/10.1056/nejmoa1211851.

Hardy, J., & Selkoe, D. J. (2002). The amyloid hypothesis of Alzheimer's disease: Progress and problems on the road to therapeutics. *Science.* https://doi.org/10.1126/science.1072994. Science.

Hou, X., Adeosun, S. O., Zhang, Q., Barlow, B., Brents, M., Zheng, B., et al. (2015). Differential contributions of ApoE4 and female sex to BACE1 activity and expression mediate Aβ deposition and learning and memory in mouse models of Alzheimer's disease. *Frontiers in Aging Neuroscience, 7*(OCT), 207. https://doi.org/10.3389/fnagi.2015.00207.

Hsiao, K., Chapman, P., Nilsen, S., Eckman, C., Harigaya, Y., Younkin, S., et al. (1996). Correlative memory deficits, Aβ elevation, and amyloid plaques in transgenic mice. *Science, 274*(5284), 99–102. https://doi.org/10.1126/science.274.5284.99.

Imbimbo, B. P., Ippati, S., & Watling, M. (2020). Should drug discovery scientists still embrace the amyloid hypothesis for Alzheimer's disease or should they be looking elsewhere? *Expert Opinion on Drug Discovery*, *15*(11), 1–11. https://doi.org/10.1080/17460441.2020.1793755.

Jonsson, T., Stefansson, H., Steinberg, S., Jonsdottir, I., Jonsson, P. V., Snaedal, J., et al. (2013). Variant of TREM2 associated with the risk of Alzheimer's disease. *New England Journal of Medicine*, *368*(2), 107–116. https://doi.org/10.1056/nejmoa1211103.

Kane, A. E., Shin, S., Wong, A. A., Fertan, E., Faustova, N. S., Howlett, S. E., et al. (2018). Sex differences in healthspan predict lifespan in the 3xTg-AD mouse model of Alzheimer's disease. *Frontiers in Aging Neuroscience*, *10*(JUN). https://doi.org/10.3389/fnagi.2018.00172.

Kermath, B. A., & Gore, A. C. (2012). Neuroendocrine control of the transition to reproductive senescence: Lessons learned from the female rodent model. *Neuroendocrinology*. https://doi.org/10.1159/000335994. NIH Public Access.

Kodama, L., Guzman, E., Etchegaray, J. I., Li, Y., Sayed, F. A., Zhou, L., et al. (2020). Microglial microRNAs mediate sex-specific responses to tau pathology. *Nature Neuroscience*, *23*(2), 167–171. https://doi.org/10.1038/s41593-019-0560-7.

Leon, W. C., Canneva, F., Partridge, V., Allard, S., Ferretti, M. T., DeWilde, A., … Cuello, A. C. (2010). A novel transgenic rat model with a full Alzheimer's-like amyloid pathology displays pre-plaque intracellular amyloid-beta-associated cognitive impairment. *Journal of Alzheimer's Disease*, *20*(1), 113–126. https://doi.org/10.3233/JAD-2010-1349.

Lewis, J., McGowan, E., Rockwood, J., Melrose, H., Nacharaju, P., Van Slegtenhorst, M., et al. (2000). Neurofibrillary tangles, amyotrophy and progressive motor disturbance in mice expressing mutant (P301L)tau protein. *Nature Genetics*, *25*(4), 402–405. https://doi.org/10.1038/78078.

Lewis, J., Dickson, D. W., Lin, W. L., Chisholm, L., Corral, A., Jones, G., et al. (2001). Enhanced neurofibrillary degeneration in transgenic mice expressing mutant tau and APP. *Science*, *293*(5534), 1487–1491. https://doi.org/10.1126/science.1058189.

Li, X., Feng, Y., Wu, W., Zhao, J., Fu, C., Li, Y., et al. (2016). Sex differences between APPswePS1dE9 mice in A-beta accumulation and pancreatic islet function during the development of Alzheimer's disease. *Laboratory Animals*, *50*(4), 275–285. https://doi.org/10.1177/0023677215615269.

Liu, C. C., Kanekiyo, T., Xu, H., & Bu, G. (2013). Apolipoprotein e and Alzheimer disease: Risk, mechanisms and therapy. *Nature Reviews Neurology*. https://doi.org/10.1038/nrneurol.2012.263. Nature Publishing Group.

Long, Z., Zeng, Q., Wang, K., Sharma, A., & He, G. (2016). Gender difference in valproic acid-induced neuroprotective effects on APP/PS1 double transgenic mice modeling Alzheimer's disease. *Acta Biochimica et Biophysica Sinica*, *48*(10). https://doi.org/10.1093/ABBS/GMW085.

Meilandt, W. J., Ngu, H., Gogineni, A., Lalehzadeh, G., Lee, S. H., Srinivasan, K., et al. (2020). TREM2 deletion reduces late-stage amyloid plaque accumulation, elevates the Aβ42:Aβ40 ratio, and exacerbates axonal dystrophy and dendritic spine loss in the PS2ApP Alzheimer's mouse model. *Journal of Neuroscience*, *40*(9), 1956–1974. https://doi.org/10.1523/JNEUROSCI.1871-19.2019.

Mucke, L., Masliah, E., Yu, G. Q., Mallory, M., Rockenstein, E. M., Tatsuno, G., et al. (2000). High-level neuronal expression of Aβ(1–42) in wild-type human amyloid protein precursor transgenic mice: Synaptotoxicity without plaque formation. *Journal of Neuroscience*, *20*(11), 4050–4058. https://doi.org/10.1523/jneurosci.20-11-04050.2000.

Nelson, J. F., Latham, K. R., & Finch, C. E. (1975). Plasma testosterone levels in C57BL/6J male mice: Effects of age and disease. *Acta Endocrinologica*, *80*(4), 744–752. https://doi.org/10.1530/acta.0.0800744.

Nelson, J. F., Felicio, L. S., Osterburg, H. H., & Finch, C. E. (1992). Differential contributions of ovarian and extraovarian factors to age-related reductions in plasma estradiol and progesterone during the estrous cycle of C57bl/6j mice. *Endocrinology*, *130*(2), 804–810. https://doi.org/10.1210/endo.130.2.1733727.

Onos, K. D., Sukoff Rizzo, S. J., Howell, G. R., & Sasner, M. (2016). Toward more predictive genetic mouse models of Alzheimer's disease. *Brain Research Bulletin*. https://doi.org/10.1016/j.brainresbull.2015.12.003. Elsevier Inc.

Ordóñez-Gutiérrez, L., Antón, M., & Wandosell, F. (2015). Peripheral amyloid levels present gender differences associated with aging in AβPP/PS1 mice. *Journal of Alzheimer's Disease*, *44*(4), 1063–1068. https://doi.org/10.3233/JAD-141158.

Panza, F., Lozupone, M., Logroscino, G., & Imbimbo, B. P. (2019). A critical appraisal of amyloid-β-targeting therapies for Alzheimer disease. *Nature Reviews Neurology*, *15*(2), 73–88. https://doi.org/10.1038/s41582-018-0116-6.

Papazoglou, A., Soos, J., Lundt, A., Wormuth, C., Ginde, V. R., Müller, R., et al. (2016). Gender-specific hippocampal dysrhythmia and aberrant hippocampal and cortical excitability in the APPswePS1dE9 model of Alzheimer's disease. *Neural Plasticity*, *2016*. https://doi.org/10.1155/2016/7167358.

Perez, S. E., Lumayag, S., Kovacs, B., Mufson, E. J., & Shunbin, X. (2009). β-Amyloid deposition and functional impairment in the retina of the APPswe/PS1ΔE9 transgenic mouse model of Alzheimer's disease. *Investigative Ophthalmology and Visual Science*, *50*(2), 793–800. https://doi.org/10.1167/iovs.08-2384.

Querfurth, H. W., & LaFerla, F. M. (2010). Alzheimer's disease. *New England Journal of Medicine*. https://doi.org/10.1056/NEJMra0909142. Massachussetts Medical Society.

Radde, R., Bolmont, T., Kaeser, S. A., Coomaraswamy, J., Lindau, D., Stoltze, L., et al. (2006). Aβ42-driven cerebral amyloidosis in transgenic mice reveals early and robust pathology. *EMBO Reports*, *7*(9), 940–946. https://doi.org/10.1038/sj.embor.7400784.

Rae, E. A., & Brown, R. E. (2015). The problem of genotype and sex differences in life expectancy in transgenic AD mice. *Neuroscience and Biobehavioral Reviews*. https://doi.org/10.1016/j.neubiorev.2015.09.002. Elsevier Ltd.

Ratnu, V. S., Emami, M. R., & Bredy, T. W. (2017). Genetic and epigenetic factors underlying sex differences in the regulation of gene expression in the brain. *Journal of Neuroscience Research*, *95*(1–2), 301–310. https://doi.org/10.1002/jnr.23886.

Roddick, K. M., Roberts, A. D., Schellinck, H. M., & Brown, R. E. (2016). Sex and genotype differences in odor detection in the 3× Tg-AD and 5XFAD mouse models of Alzheimer's disease at 6 months of age. *Chemical Senses*, *41*(5), 433–440. https://doi.org/10.1093/chemse/bjw018.

Saito, T., Matsuba, Y., Mihira, N., Takano, J., Nilsson, P., Itohara, S., et al. (2014). Single App knock-in mouse models of Alzheimer's disease. *Nature Neuroscience*, *17*(5), 661–663. https://doi.org/10.1038/nn.3697.

Saré, R. M., Cooke, S. K., Krych, L., Zerfas, P. M., Cohen, R. M., & Smith, C. B. (2020). Behavioral phenotype in the TgF344-AD rat model of Alzheimer's disease. *Frontiers in Neuroscience*, *14*, 601. https://doi.org/10.3389/fnins.2020.00601.

Scearce-Levie, K., Sanchez, P. E., & Lewcock, J. W. (2020). Leveraging preclinical models for the development of Alzheimer disease therapeutics. *Nature Reviews Drug Discovery*. https://doi.org/10.1038/s41573-020-0065-9. Nature Research.

Song, M. S., & Rossi, J. J. (2017). Molecular mechanisms of dicer: Endonuclease and enzymatic activity. *Biochemical Journal*. https://doi.org/10.1042/BCJ20160759. Portland Press Ltd.

Stephen, T. L., Cacciottolo, M., Balu, D., Morgan, T. E., Ladu, M. J., Finch, C. E., et al. (2019). APOE genotype and sex affect microglial interactions with plaques in Alzheimer's disease mice. *Acta Neuropathologica Communications*, *7*(1). https://doi.org/10.1186/s40478-019-0729-z.

Stimmell, A. C., Baglietto-Vargas, D., Moseley, S. C., Lapointe, V., Thompson, L. M., LaFerla, F. M., et al. (2019). Impaired spatial reorientation in the 3xTg-AD mouse model of Alzheimer's disease. *Scientific Reports*, *9*(1), 1–12. https://doi.org/10.1038/s41598-018-37151-z.

Sun, Y., Guo, Y., Feng, X., Jia, M., Ai, N., Dong, Y., et al. (2020). The behavioural and neuropathologic sexual dimorphism and absence of MIP-3α in tau P301S mouse model of Alzheimer's disease. *Journal of Neuroinflammation*, *17*(1). https://doi.org/10.1186/s12974-020-01749-w.

Touma, C., Ambrée, O., Görtz, N., Keyvani, K., Lewejohann, L., Palme, R., et al. (2004). Age- and sex-dependent development of adrenocortical hyperactivity in a transgenic mouse model of Alzheimer's disease. *Neurobiology of Aging*, *25*(7), 893–904. https://doi.org/10.1016/j.neurobiolaging.2003.09.004.

Ulland, T. K., & Colonna, M. (2018). TREM2—A key player in microglial biology and Alzheimer disease. *Nature Reviews Neurology*. https://doi.org/10.1038/s41582-018-0072-1.

van Eersel, J., Stevens, C. H., Przybyla, M., Gladbach, A., Stefanoska, K., Chan, C. K. X., et al. (2015). Early-onset axonal pathology in a novel P301S-tau transgenic mouse model of frontotemporal lobar degeneration. *Neuropathology and Applied Neurobiology*, *41*(7), 906–925. https://doi.org/10.1111/nan.12233.

Williams, R. S. B., Cheng, L., Mudge, A. W., & Harwood, A. J. (2002). A common mechanism of action for three mood-stabilizing drugs. *Nature*, *417*(6886), 292–295. https://doi.org/10.1038/417292a.

Yang, X., Schadt, E. E., Wang, S., Wang, H., Arnold, A. P., Ingram-Drake, L., et al. (2006). Tissue-specific expression and regulation of sexually dimorphic genes in mice. *Genome Research*, *16*(8), 995–1004. https://doi.org/10.1101/gr.5217506.

Yang, J. T., Wang, Z. J., Cai, H. Y., Yuan, L., Hu, M. M., Wu, M. N., et al. (2018). Sex differences in neuropathology and cognitive behavior in APP/PS1/tau triple-transgenic mouse model of Alzheimer's disease. *Neuroscience Bulletin*, *34*(5), 736–746. https://doi.org/10.1007/s12264-018-0268-9.

Yue, M., Hanna, A., Wilson, J., Roder, H., & Janus, C. (2011). Sex difference in pathology and memory decline in RTg4510 mouse model of tauopathy. *Neurobiology of Aging*, *32*(4), 590–603. https://doi.org/10.1016/j.neurobiolaging.2009.04.006.

CHAPTER 2

Sex and sex hormone differences in hippocampal neurogenesis and their relevance to Alzheimer's disease

Bonnie H. Lee[a,b,*], Tanvi A. Puri[a,b,*], and Liisa A.M. Galea[a,b,c]

[a]*Graduate Program in Neuroscience, University of British Columbia, Vancouver, BC, Canada*
[b]*Djavad Mowafaghian Centre for Brain Health, University of British Columbia, Vancouver, BC, Canada*
[c]*Department of Psychology, University of British Columbia, Vancouver, BC, Canada*

Introduction

Sex differences are apparent in the prevalence, manifestation, and treatment efficacy of a variety of neurological and neuropsychiatric disorders, including Alzheimer's Disease (AD) (Brookmeyer, Gray, & Kawas, 1998; Gutierrez-Lobos et al., 2002; Irvine et al., 2012; Khan et al., 2005; Koran et al., 2017; McLean et al., 2011; McPherson et al., 1999; Young et al., 2009). However, most studies do not investigate the effects of sex, and even when both sexes are used, over 80% of studies do not report their results by sex (Geller, Koch, Pelletieri, & Carnes, 2011; Mamlouk et al., 2020). Here, we emphasize the importance of examining sex differences in AD research to accelerate new knowledge and therapeutic discovery. AD is a progressive neurodegenerative brain disorder that involves impairments to hippocampal integrity and cognition (Allen et al., 2007; Demars et al., 2010; reviewed in Setti et al., 2017; Wilson et al., 2012). The CA1 area of the hippocampus and the entorhinal cortex, which provide afferent inputs into the dentate gyrus, are the first brain areas to be affected by AD (Adler et al., 2018; Devanand et al., 2012; Padurariu et al., 2012). The dentate gyrus of the hippocampus retains the ability to produce new neurons in adulthood (van Praag et al., 2002). These new neurons can modulate functions of the hippocampus, including various forms of learning and memory (Broadbent et al., 2004; Buzsaki and Moser, 2013; Scoville and Milner, 1957; Ofen et al., 2007). Indeed, impaired neurogenesis may have important implications for the cognitive

---

*Both authors contributed equally.

deficits seen in AD (Hollands et al., 2017). Sex differences in the morphology and function of the hippocampus are evident as well as sex differences in how the hippocampus is impacted in AD (Koutseff et al., 2014; Rijpma et al. 2013). Besides adult neurogenesis, the hippocampus demonstrates plasticity through changes in dendritic architecture, synapse density, synaptic plasticity, and adult neurogenesis, all of which are influenced by sex and sex hormones (reviewed in Leuner and Gould, 2010). In this chapter, we focus on the hippocampus because of its early involvement in AD and its profound plasticity, which make it an important area to target for early interventions (Apostolova et al., 2010; La Joie et al., 2013).

This chapter explores sex differences in hippocampal neurogenesis that influence hippocampal function which, in turn, may play a role in sex differences seen in the manifestation of AD. Importantly, we, using the terminology of others, make a distinction between sex differences, sex dimorphism, and sex divergent patterns (McCarthy et al., 2012). Sex dimorphism refers to absolute dimorphisms or opposites, sex divergent patterns may be revealed as consequences of experience or disease, and finally, sex differences are exhibited in a number of ways when males and females differ in a trait or in the underlying mechanisms of the trait (Becker and Koob, 2015). It is also imperative to acknowledge that sex differences in neurobiology may prevent sex differences in certain behaviours and disease outcomes, i.e., different mechanisms may underlie similar behaviors and symptoms in each sex (DeVries, 2004). Please note that the term "sex" is used to refer to the biological attributes that distinguish male from female. The term "gender", which refers to socially-constructed roles, identities, and behaviours for men and women, can certainly play an important role in the phenomena to be discussed, but it is beyond the scope of this chapter and the reader is directed to other reviews on the subject (Andrew and Tierney, 2018). This chapter considers hippocampal neurogenesis in the context of healthy aging and then in the context of AD. These discussions will highlight the important roles of sex hormones (estrogens and androgens) and female-specific experiences (pregnancy, parturition, and menopause) in influencing hippocampal function and neurogenesis in aging and AD.

Adult neurogenesis in the dentate gyrus

Neurogenesis is the process by which new neurons are created and consists of a series of stages, including proliferation, differentiation, migration, and survival of new neurons. Briefly, neural progenitor cells divide symmetrically or asymmetrically, migrate either short or long distances, and mature into neurons or glial cells, or remain as progenitor cells (Ihunwo, Tembo, & Dzamalala, 2016). Neurogenesis is crucial during embryonic development and continues in certain brain regions after birth and throughout the lifespan (Cameron, Woolley, McEwen, & Gould, 1993; Eriksson et al., 1998; Gould, Reeves, et al., 1999; Seki & Arai, 1995). The dentate gyrus of the hippocampus is a site of continual neurogenesis throughout adulthood (Altman, 1962; Altman & Das, 1965; Cameron et al., 1993). Each stage of neurogenesis is associated with different relative expressions of specific proteins, allowing researchers to identify different stages using immunohistochemistry (Fig. 1). In adults, new neurons project their axons to pyramidal neurons in the CA3 region, at which point the newborn neurons can become integrated into the hippocampal circuitry (van Praag et al., 2002). Toni et al. (2008) demonstrated that in female mice, adult-born neurons in the dentate gyrus form functional synapses with interneurons, mossy cells, and pyramidal cells in the CA3 region of the hippocampus to release glutamate (an excitatory neurotransmitter), similar to what is seen in mature granule neurons. However, young, new neurons in the adult dentate gyrus have different electrophysiological properties than older, mature neurons, in that new neurons are more efficient at converting synaptic stimulation into firing of action potentials, due to higher input resistance of ionic channels (Mongiat, Espósito, Lombardi, & Schinder, 2009; Schmidt-Hieber, Jonas, & Bischofberger, 2004). Because new neurons generated in adulthood that survive can become fully integrated, they can affect the function of the hippocampus. These new neurons are thought to play an important role in modulating functions of the hippocampus, such as certain forms of learning and

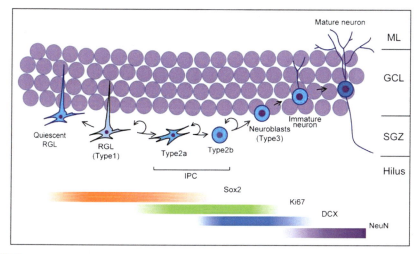

FIG. 1

Schematic illustration of the chronology of neural stem cell lineage with expression of stage-specific proteins. It is important to note that the timing and length of the progression vary depending on species (Snyder, Chloe, et al., 2009) and between sexes (Yagi, Splinter, Tai, Wong, & Galea, 2020). *DCX*, doublecortin; *GCL*, granule cell layer; *IPC*, intermediate proliferating cell; *Ki67*, antigen Ki-67; *ML*, molecular layer; *NeuN*, neuronal nuclei; *RGL*, radial glial cell; *SGZ*, subgranular zone; *Sox2*, SRY-box transcription factor 2.

Reprinted with permission from Yagi, S., Splinter, J. E. J., Tai, D., Wong, S., & Galea, L. A. M. (2020). Sex differences in maturation and attrition rate of adult born neurons in the hippocampus of rats. eNeuro, 7(4), 1–14.

memory (Broadbent et al., 2004; Buzsaki & Moser, 2013; Ofen et al., 2007; Scoville & Milner, 1957) and stress regulation (Anacker et al., 2018; Loi et al., 2017).

Adult hippocampal neurogenesis has been observed in all mammalian species, including rodents, nonhuman primates, and humans (Amrein, Isler, & Lipp, 2011; Miller et al., 2013). A recent paper suggested that there are no detectable levels of neurogenesis in the human adult hippocampus (Sorrells et al., 2018). However, there are many more studies using multiple methods which show that neurogenesis persists in the adult human hippocampus (Boldrini et al., 2018; Eriksson et al., 1998; Ernst et al., 2014; Gage, 2019; Kempermann et al., 2018; Knoth et al., 2010; Moreno-Jiménez et al., 2019; Sanai et al., 2011; Spalding et al., 2013; Tobin et al., 2019). Papers have outlined concerns regarding the negative findings of Sorrells et al.'s (2018) work, including the length of time for which postmortem brain tissues were processed, the type of fixative in which the tissues were stored, the number of brain sections analyzed, the lack of knowledge about neuropsychiatric or other chronic diseases among patients, and the inclusion of patients with epilepsy in their study (Kempermann et al., 2018; Moreno-Jiménez et al., 2019). Furthermore, Sorrells et al. (2018) used the rapid decline in neurogenesis levels from infants to adulthood to show that neurogenesis is present at much higher levels in the infant hippocampus than in that of adults (Altman & Bayer, 1990; Sanai et al., 2011; Sugiyama, Osumi, & Katsuyama, 2013). However, comparing the number of new neurons produced throughout the entire brain during development to those produced in the dentate gyrus of the adult hippocampus is problematic due to differences in scale, and because of the resulting dramatic reduction (~90%) in neurogenesis levels in the dentate gyrus in both humans and rodents from infancy to middle age (Kuhn, Dickinson-Anson, & Gage, 1996). The research supporting the argument that adult neurogenesis persists in humans conclusively shows not only that it persists, but also that these adult-born neurons are likely to make functional contributions (Boldrini et al., 2018; Eriksson et al., 1998; Ernst et al., 2014; Gage, 2019; Kempermann et al., 2018; Knoth et al., 2010; Moreno-Jiménez et al., 2019, Sanai et al., 2011; Spalding et al., 2013; Tobin et al., 2019).

The function of adult neurogenesis in the hippocampus

To examine the functionality of new adult-born neurons in the dentate gyrus, studies have employed a variety of methods—from correlational studies to optogenetic approaches (Saxe et al., 2006; Shors et al., 2001). Increasing proliferation of neural progenitor cells with pharmacological treatments like lithium (in males and females: Fiorentini, Rosi, Grossi, Luccarini, & Casamenti, 2010) or allopregnanolone (in males: Wang et al., 2010) reversed impairments in spatial learning and memory and associative learning and memory, respectively, in mouse models of AD. However, it should be noted that both lithium and allopregnanolone will alter other neuroplastic features besides neurogenesis that may impact learning and memory, and thus the changes in learning may not be limited to the effects on neurogenesis in the hippocampus (Chen et al., 2011; Gray & McEwen, 2013). Neurogenesis can also be enhanced genetically in vivo through single gene delivery of transcription factors known to target and accelerate different stages of neurogenesis (Beckervordersandforth, Zhang, & Liu, 2015). Female mice that received bilateral injections of the retroviral vector, *Neurod1,* into the dentate gyrus showed improved pattern separation performance (Richetin et al., 2015) and, as seen below, pattern separation relies on neurogenesis in the hippocampus (Clelland et al., 2009).

Using irradiation methods to focally inhibit neurogenesis in the dentate gyrus, studies found impaired contextual fear conditioning (Saxe et al., 2006) and long-term (but not short-term) spatial reference memory in male rats (Snyder, Hong, Mcdonald, & Wojtowicz, 2005), and impaired spatial pattern separation in female mice (Clelland et al., 2009). Employing a transgenic mouse model whereby adult-born hippocampal neurons are specifically ablated provided evidence for the role of adult neurogenesis in facilitating contextual discrimination ability in male mice (Tronel et al., 2012). Pharmacologically-induced inhibition of neurogenesis in male rats led to impaired associative learning (Shors et al., 2001). Importantly, when neurogenesis recovered to normal levels after the pharmacologically-induced inhibition was removed, the ability to acquire trace memories in the dentate gyrus also recovered (Shors et al., 2001). In summary, adult-born neurons in the dentate gyrus are functionally relevant to the hippocampus because they modulate various types of hippocampal-dependent cognitive functioning, including pattern separation, contextual discrimination, trace conditioning, and long-term spatial memory in both male and female rodents. However, to date, no work examining the influence of inhibiting neurogenesis on functional outcomes has been done to directly compare the sexes.

Other lines of research examining the function of adult-born dentate neurons have utilized optogenetic manipulations (reviewed in (Barnett, Perry, Dalrymple-Alford, & Parr-Brownlie, 2018)). Studies have shown that activating adult-born dentate neurons that had been active during fear learning induced freezing behavior, indicating that fear memory recall was encoded within these new neurons (sex not specified: Liu et al., 2012; Ramirez et al., 2013; Ryan, Roy, Pignatelli, Arons, & Tonegawa, 2015). Furthermore, silencing newborn neurons in the dentate gyrus of female mice via an optogenetic approach impaired performance in a hippocampal-dependent pattern separation task (Zhuo et al., 2016). Selective optogenetic inhibition of the pathway between the ventral hippocampus and the frontal cortex resulted in impaired spatial working memory performance in male mice (Spellman et al., 2015). Together, these optogenetic manipulations illustrate that functional integration of adult-born dentate neurons is necessary for fear memory, spatial working memory, and pattern separation; but again, to our knowledge, no studies have directly compared males and females. An exhaustive account of the literature surrounding neurogenesis and memory is beyond the scope of this chapter, and the reader is directed to reviews on the subject (Epp, Chow, & Galea, 2013; Kitabatake, Sailor, Ming, & Song, 2007; Yau, Li, & So, 2015).

Immediate early genes (IEGs) are transiently expressed in response to action potentials, indicating neuronal activation (Minatohara, Akiyoshi, & Okuno, 2016).

IEG expression in adult-born neurons in the dentate gyrus increases in response to spatial learning and memory retrieval in both male and female rodents (Chow, Epp, Lieblich, Barha, & Galea, 2013; Epp, Haack, & Galea, 2011; Jessberger & Kempermann, 2003; Kee, Teixeira, Wang, & Frankland, 2007; Ramirez-Amaya, Marrone, Gage, Worley, & Barnes, 2006; Snyder, Radik, Wojtowicz, & Cameron, 2009). Interestingly, positive correlations between memory performance and neuronal activation in new neurons have only been detected in female, and not male, rodents (Chow et al., 2013; Méndez-López, Méndez, López, & Arias, 2009). This will be examined in greater detail in Section "Sex differences in neurogenesis in the context of cognitive training."

The literature robustly shows that learning, exercise, enriched environments, and stress can modulate the different stages of adult neurogenesis in male rodents (Chow et al., 2013; van Praag, Kempermann, & Gage, 2000). For example, cognitive training in the Morris water maze 6–10 days after production or during the axon extension phase led to increased survival of adult-born neurons in the dentate gyrus of male rats (Chow et al., 2013; Epp et al., 2011; Gould, Beylin, Tanapat, Reeves, & Shors, 1999), but not in female rats (Chow et al., 2013). Furthermore, chronic stress decreased hippocampal neurogenesis and impaired hippocampal-dependent memory in male mice (Yun et al., 2010). Increasing neurogenesis in male mice resulted in a decrease in the activity of stress-responsive cells in the ventral dentate gyrus, thus conferring resilience to chronic stress (Anacker et al., 2018). The same study found that inhibiting neurogenesis in the ventral dentate gyrus of these male mice promoted stress-induced anxiety-like behavior (Anacker et al., 2018). As demonstrated, adult-born neurons play important roles in contextual learning, long-term spatial memory, and stress resilience. However, most studies were conducted in male rodents and very few studies examined sex differences in the contributions of new neurons to memory. To better understand adult neurogenesis, it is essential to consider possible sex differences in the function of adult neurogenesis in the hippocampus.

Neurogenesis and aging

Hippocampal neurogenesis is preserved in adulthood and throughout aging, although there is a large age-related decline in the number of newborn neurons in the dentate gyrus in both rodents and humans, with the largest decline occurring from young adulthood to middle-age in rodents, and perhaps humans as well (Boldrini et al., 2018; Epp et al., 2013; Knoth et al., 2010; Kuhn et al., 1996; Moreno-Jiménez et al., 2019). Knoth et al. (2010) detected expression of immature neurons (quantified via the endogenous marker doublecortin (DCX)) in the dentate gyrus in human individuals from birth to age 100. Importantly, qualitative analyses revealed that many of the DCX-expressing neurons in young individuals displayed the typical dendritic features of immature neurons, which were not identifiable in older individuals (Knoth et al., 2010). Nonetheless, DCX-expressing neurons with the morphology of maturing granule cells were present in both young and older individuals. Assessing the whole hippocampus postmortem from healthy human individuals, Boldrini et al. (2018) found stable numbers of immature neurons and mature neurons in the dentate gyrus, as well as stable volumes of the dentate gyrus, from ages 14 to 79. However, Boldrini et al. (2018) showed that with increasing age, there was a decrease in the number of quiescent neural stem cells (quantified via the endogenous marker SRY-box transcription factor 2 (Sox2)) in the anterior-mid dentate gyrus (equivalent to the rodent ventral region). Furthermore, there was an age-associated decline in neuroplasticity, quantified by cells labeled with the polysialylated neuronal cell adhesion molecule (PSA-NCAM), which is a marker of developing and migrating neurons and of NCAM-NCAM synaptic plasticity (Boldrini et al., 2018; Varbanov & Dityatev, 2017). This decline in neuroplasticity may be implicated in age-related changes in hippocampus-dependent cognitive function (Boldrini et al., 2018; reviewed in Murman, 2015; Ruffman, Henry, Livingstone, & Phillips, 2008).

Converging data from animals (Bizon et al., 2009; Robitsek, Fortin, Koh, Gallagher, & Eichenbaum, 2008) and humans (Stark, Yassa, & Stark, 2010; Toner, Pirogovsky, Kirwan, & Gilbert, 2009) reveal reduced ability to perform hippocampus-dependent tasks like pattern separation, episodic memory formation, and spatial learning and memory, with advancing age. Dillon et al. (2017) demonstrated age-related impairment of pattern separation ability in healthy older male participants, and further showed that the impairment was associated with an age-related reduction of dentate gyrus fractional volume. In middle-aged male rats, neurogenesis in the dentate gyrus positively correlated with learning and memory performance in the Morris water maze (Drapeau et al., 2003). Middle-aged animals with preserved spatial memory exhibited greater neurogenesis compared to those with impaired spatial memory (Drapeau et al., 2003). Curiously, the results of this study contrast with those obtained by Merrill, Karim, Darraq, Chiba, and Tuszynski (2003), which did not support a correlation between hippocampal neurogenesis and spatial learning ability in older female rats. Notably, the use of different sexes may, at least in part, explain the discrepancy between these studies. Further, the male rats in Drapeau et al.'s (2003) study were younger, at 10–11 months old, whereas the female rats in Merrill et al.'s (2003) study were 24 months old. Studies directly comparing the effects of aging on hippocampus-dependent cognition in both males and females remain scarce, but one such study conducted by Frick, Burlingame, Arters, and Berger-Sweeney (1999) used three age groups of male and female mice: 5-month-old (young adult mice), 17-month-old (middle-aged mice), and 25-month-old (aged mice). Both male and female aged mice exhibited impaired spatial reference memory relative to the middle-aged group and the young adult group (Frick et al., 1999). Although there were no sex differences in the young adult and aged groups, female middle-aged mice exhibited greater impairments in spatial reference memory relative to male middle-aged mice, suggesting that spatial reference memory decline may begin earlier in females compared to males (Frick et al., 1999). Markowska (1999) found similar results in middle-aged rats, where the onset of reference memory impairments occurred earlier in females compared to males. Additionally, analysis of estrous cycling in both studies show that loss of ovarian hormone cycling in middle-aged female rats may contribute to the earlier spatial cognitive decline seen in females (Frick et al., 1999; Markowska, 1999). It is thus suggested that ovarian hormone levels may contribute to the sex differences in how aging influences cognition. Further discussion of potential mechanisms driving these sex differences can be found in Section "Estrogens and aging."

In humans and rodents, sex differences in cognitive performance also exist at younger ages. Studies in humans report that females outperform males on certain cognitive tasks, including tasks that measure episodic memory performance (Finkel, Reynolds, McArdle, Gatz, & Pedersen, 2003) and verbal ability (Gerstorf & Ram, 2011), whereas males outperform females on visuospatial ability tasks (Voyer, Voyer, & Saint-Aubin, 2017). These sex differences need to be considered when measuring cognitive decline across time. Males show steeper rates of decline in verbal memory and attention, perceptuomotor speed and integration, and visuospatial ability (McCarrey, An, Kitner-Triolo, Ferrucci, & Resnick, 2016) (reviewed in Gur & Gur, 2002). These declines in different memory domains with age appear to mirror declines in testosterone levels in males with age (Moffat et al., 2002) and may be related to menopausal status in females (Epperson, Sammel, & Freeman, 2013; Weber, Rubin, & Maki, 2013). Collectively, these studies illustrate that age-related declines in hippocampus-dependent tasks, such as pattern separation, object recognition, and spatial memory, are associated with declines in hippocampal integrity and function that present differently in males and females and should be considered when examining age-related neurodegenerative diseases.

Sex differences in neurogenesis

There are prominent sex differences in the hippocampus and in the regulation of adult neurogenesis (reviewed in Galea et al., 2013; summarized in Fig. 2). Hippocampal volume is typically reported to be larger in males than in females (Liu, Seidlitz, Blumenthal, Clasen, & Raznahan, 2020; Ruigrok et al., 2014), although this finding depends on the method used to correct for total brain volume or intracranial volume, as sex differences either remain, reverse, or become no longer significant when different correction methods are used (Duarte-Guterman, Albert, Barha, & Galea, in press; Tan, Ma, Vira, Marwha, & Eliot, 2016). When using a regression method of correction, females have a smaller hippocampus than males (Duarte-Guterman et al., 2020; Mormino, Betensky, & Hedden, 2014; Tan et al., 2016) but this can reverse with females having a larger hippocampus than males when not using the ratio of hippocampal volume to intracranial volume (Duarte-Guterman et al., in press; Sohn et al., 2018; (Sundermann, Tran, Maki, & Bondi, 2018); Tan et al., 2016). There is also evidence for sex differences in the morphology of hippocampal neurons in both primates and rodents (Barrera, Jiménez, González, Monitle, & Aboitiz, 2001; Markham, McKian, Stroup, & Juraska, 2005; Mendell et al., 2017; reviewed in Scharfman & MacLusky, 2017). Males have greater dendritic complexity in dentate gyrus granule neurons (rats: Juraska, Fitch, & Washburne, 1989) and in CA1 pyramidal neurons

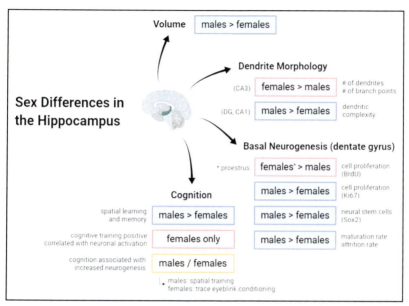

FIG. 2

Schematic summary of sex differences in hippocampal morphology, neurogenesis, and cognition. *BrdU*, bromodeoxyuridine; *CA*, Cornu Ammonis; *DG*, dentate gyrus; *Ki67*, antigen Ki-67; *Sox2*, SRY-box transcription factor 2.

(humans: Barrera et al., 2001; rats: Markham et al., 2005) compared to females. In the CA3 region of the hippocampus, Gould, Westlind-Danielsson, Frankfurt, and McEwen (1990) showed that female rats had more primary dendrites, and Galea et al. (1997) showed that female rats had greater branch points in the basal dendrites of CA3 pyramidal neurons, compared to male rats. Together, these results illustrate the presence of basal sex differences in the morphology of granule and pyramidal neurons in the hippocampus. The reader is directed to other reviews for a more comprehensive discussion on this topic (Choleris, Galea, Sohrabji, & Frick, 2018; Koss & Frick, 2017; Yagi & Galea, 2019).

Studies conducted in rats and meadow voles have shown sex differences in cell proliferation, depending on ovarian hormone levels in females (Galea & McEwen, 1999; Tanapat, Hastings, Reeves, & Gould, 1999). Comparing male and nonproestrus female rats, males had higher levels of cell proliferation, quantified by Ki67-expressing cells (Yagi et al., 2020), whereas Tanapat et al. (1999) found that proestrous females had higher levels of cell proliferation, quantified by bromodeoxyuridine (BrdU)-positive cells (using a 2h time point after the BrdU injection) compared to males and females in other phases of the estrous cycle. When considering this sex difference, it is pertinent to acknowledge the different markers used by the two studies to label proliferating cells. Ki67 is an endogenous marker that is expressed in actively dividing cells (in all stages of the cell cycle except for

G_0, the resting phase) whereas BrdU is an exogenous DNA synthesis marker that is incorporated into DNA only during the synthesis phase of the cell cycle (Kee, Sivalingam, Boonstra, & Wojtowicz, 2002). As such, Ki67 is expressed in a larger, and thus different, population of cells and will be expressed at higher levels than BrdU (Kee et al., 2002). Yagi et al. (2020) also quantified neural stem/progenitor cells (Sox2-expressing cells) and found a greater density of neural stem cells in the dorsal dentate gyrus in male rats compared to female rats. There were also remarkable sex differences in the maturation and attrition or survival rate of adult-born dentate neurons (Yagi et al., 2020). More specifically, Yagi et al. (2020) showed that adult-born neurons matured faster and had a greater attrition rate in male rats compared to female rats. Although this was the first study to directly compare basal maturation and survival rates in male and female rats, its findings are consistent with previous work that examined male (Snyder, Chloe, et al., 2009) or female (Brown et al., 2003) rats alone. In male rats, 65%–75% of BrdU-labeled cells matured in 2 weeks (i.e., expressed neuronal nuclei (NeuN), a neuronal nuclear protein) (Snyder, Chloe, et al., 2009), whereas only 10% of BrdU-labeled cells matured in 2 weeks in female rats (Brown et al., 2003). Given these sex differences in the trajectory of adult-born neurons, factors like stress exposure and cognitive training may modulate neurogenesis within each sex to different degrees because of existing differences in timing and maturation of new neurons (Yagi et al., 2020). Importantly, this also suggests that treatments targeting neurogenesis may need to be different for each sex.

The hippocampus contains sex hormone receptors, including estrogen receptors (ER), ERα, ERβ, and the G protein-coupled estrogen receptor (GPER), and an androgen receptor (AR). These receptors are expressed in both males and females to different degrees (Brailoiu et al., 2007; Cui, Shen, & Li, 2013; Duarte-Guterman, Yagi, Chow, & Galea, 2015; González et al., 2007; Hazell et al., 2009; Mitra et al., 2003). Perhaps predictably, sex hormones influence neurogenesis in the hippocampus differently in males and females (Barker & Galea, 2008; Duarte-Guterman, Lieblich, et al., 2019; Galea & McEwen, 1999; reviewed in Mahmoud, Wainwright, & Galea, 2016; Tanapat et al., 1999). Research has explored the mechanisms through which sex hormones like estrogens and androgens modulate neurogenesis, and these will be discussed in greater detail in Sections "Estrogens and neurogenesis" and "Testosterone and neurogenesis."

Sex differences in neurogenesis in the context of cognitive training

Meta-analyses have found sex differences in spatial learning and memory that favor males in both humans (Hyde, 2016) and rodents (Jonasson, 2005). Spatial training, either in the water maze or after a pattern separation task, increased hippocampal neurogenesis in the dentate gyrus in male but not female rats (Chow et al., 2013; Yagi & Galea, 2019). These findings coincided with better overall performance in males compared to females in both tasks. Intriguingly, spatial training was positively correlated with new neuronal activation in females, but not in males (Chow et al., 2013). However, another study found that females exhibited better cognitive performance (trace eyeblink conditioning) compared to males, which was linked to increased neurogenesis in the ventral hippocampus (Dalla, Papachristos, Whetstone, & Shors, 2009). This may be attributed to sex differences in the excitability of new neurons or in the timing of the recruitment of young new-born neurons during spatial learning and memory tasks (Méndez-López et al., 2009; Yagi, Chow, Lieblich, & Galea, 2016; Yagi et al., 2017). Méndez-López et al. (2009) found greater increase in c-Fos (an IEG) expression in the medial prefrontal cortex and dorsal hippocampus (in the CA3 and CA1) in adolescent female rats during spatial training relative to adolescent male rats. However, females exhibited greater zif268 (an IEG) expression than males after Morris water maze or pattern separation training (Yagi et al., 2016, 2017). New work by Yagi et al. (2020), as described above, suggests sex differences in maturation of new neurons, with new neurons in males maturing faster than in females, which has profound implications for sex differences in the function of new neurons and interpretation of current studies. Evidently, the nuances in the relationship between neurogenesis and cognition in the context of sex differences have yet to be fully understood.

Thus far, most studies examining activation of adult-born neurons after cognitive tasks have been conducted in male animals (Epp et al., 2011; Jessberger & Kempermann, 2003; Kee et al., 2007). Nonetheless, sex differences in hippocampal morphology, basal neurogenesis, as well as neurogenesis in response to cognitive training exist (summarized in Fig. 2) and future studies incorporating female animals and analyzing data with sex as a variable are necessary. Undeniably, this is especially important for understanding diseases and disorders that involve impairments to hippocampal integrity and cognition.

Alzheimer's disease

AD is a progressive neurodegenerative brain disorder that involves impairments to hippocampal integrity and cognition (Allen et al., 2007; Demars et al., 2010; reviewed in Setti et al., 2017; Wilson et al., 2012). Risk factors for AD include modifiable risk factors like obesity, diabetes, physical activity, sleep, and diet, as well as nonmodifiable risk factors like age, genetics, and female sex (Edwards, Gamez, Escobedo, Calderon, & Moreno-Gonzalez, 2019) (see also Chapter 10 and Chapter 12). When considering genotype, the apolipoprotein E (*APOE*) gene is compelling to examine because the human *APOE* isoform ε4 is the greatest genetic risk factor for late-onset sporadic AD (DiBattista, Heinsinger, & Rebeck, 2016). The *APOE*ε4 allele has a worldwide frequency of 13.7%, but the frequency dramatically increases to 40%–50% percent in AD patients (Farrer et al., 1997; Ward et al., 2012). Further, the presence of the *APOE*ε4 allele is associated with increased levels of amyloid-β (Aβ) and phosphorylated tau (ptau), which are two neuropathological hallmarks of AD (Tai et al., 2013). Examining postmortem brain tissue revealed that amyloid senile plaques were present in nearly 41% of *APOEε4* carriers, compared to only 8.2% of noncarriers in individuals who did not have AD (Kok et al., 2009). *APOEε4* carriers show decreased hippocampal volume and greater memory impairment in those with AD and mild cognitive impairment (MCI), compared to noncarriers (Manning et al., 2014; Wolk et al., 2010). Additionally, the possession of *APOEε4* alleles confers a greater risk of AD developing earlier in females compared to males (Altmann, Tian, Henderson, & Greicius, 2014; Neu et al., 2017), which will be discussed in greater detail below, along with other sex differences present in AD.

Sex differences in Alzheimer's disease

Lifetime risk for AD is greater in females than in males, even after taking into account their greater longevity (Andersen et al., 1999; Mielke, Vemuri, & Rocca, 2014). However, there is considerable debate on the sex differences in the incidence and prevalence of the disease: although AD incidence was found to be higher in females after age 80 in several European countries (Beam et al., 2018; Letenneur et al., 1999), other studies found no evidence for sex differences in AD incidence (Edland, Rocca, Petersen, Cha, & Kokmen, 2002) or prevalence in the United States (Edland et al., 2002; Jack et al., 2019). The reasons behind these discrepancies are unknown, but it is suggested that sex differences in incidence or prevalence of AD may depend on geographical region, which may point to cultural, dietary, social, genetic, and historical differences (Mielke et al., 2014). Regardless, there is evidence that the progression and symptom severity of AD are indeed different between the sexes, as females with AD show more severe symptoms (see Chapter 6 on neuropsychological symptoms, and Chapter 7 on psychiatric symptoms), greater neuropathology (Chapter 5), and faster cognitive decline, compared to males with AD (Barnes et al., 2005; reviewed in Ferretti et al., 2018; Holland, Desikan, Dale, & McEvoy, 2013). To illustrate this, Barnes et al. (2005) showed that each additional "unit" of AD pathology was associated with a 20-fold increase in the odds of being diagnosed with AD in females, compared to only a threefold increase in males. Irvine et al. (2012) carried out a meta-analysis of neurocognitive data from 15 studies involving individuals with AD that revealed a consistent and significant female disadvantage on verbal and visuospatial tasks and tests of episodic and semantic memory, which was independent of age, education level, and dementia severity (Irvine et al., 2012). The *APOEε4* allele also confers greater risk for AD in females compared to males, as there is a stronger association between carrying an *APOEε4* allele and developing AD at an earlier age in females compared to males (Altmann et al., 2014; Farrer et al., 1997). More recently, Neu et al. (2017) showed that females between 65 and 75 years old carrying one *APOEε4* allele had increased AD risk compared to males carrying one *APOEε4* allele. In addition, the association between *APOEε4* status and impaired verbal learning and memory performance in middle age is stronger in females compared to males (Beydoun et al., 2012; Sohn et al., 2018). Other studies have found that females with *APOEε4* are more likely to show greater ptau levels, whether they were cognitively normal (Damoiseaux et al., 2012), diagnosed with MCI, or diagnosed with AD (Altmann et al., 2014; Duarte-Guterman et al., 2020; Hohman, Dumitrescu, & Barnes, 2018) (see Chapter 4). Furthermore, females with *APOEε4* show a greater rate of hippocampal atrophy and executive function decline with AD neuropathology (ptau, Aβ) than do males with *APOEε4* (Koran et al., 2017). Taking these findings together, it becomes clear that female sex is associated with greater neuropathology, greater cognitive decline, and greater risk of developing AD when carrying the *APOEε4* allele.

Animal models for Alzheimer's disease and sex differences

Experimental models of AD are necessary for gaining a better understanding of the pathogenesis of the disease and to answer questions that are not yet possible to study in humans (Drummond & Wisniewski, 2017). The majority of AD cases are classified as sporadic, and the mechanisms underlying these cases remain largely unknown (reviewed in Chakrabarti et al., 2015; reviewed in Dorszewska, Prendecki, Oczkowska, Dezor, & Kozubski, 2016). However, the neuropathology and clinical phenotype of sporadic AD and early-onset familial AD have been suggested to be somewhat comparable (Duara et al., 1993; Holmes & Lovestone, 2002). As such, the majority of currently available animal models have applied genetic mutations associated with familial AD, like mutations or duplications in genes encoding for the amyloid precursor protein (APP), with the rationale that downstream events would be similar to that of sporadic AD (LaFerla & Green, 2012; Lanoiselee et al., 2017; Ohshima et al., 2018) (see also Chapter 1).

Most transgenic mouse models of AD involve expression of the human APP, which leads to the formation of amyloid plaques in brain regions typically rich in amyloid plaques in AD, such as the cortex and hippocampus (reviewed in Drummond & Wisniewski, 2017). Some common transgenic AD mouse models are PDAPP (Pasbakhsh, Mehdizadeh, & Omidi, 2005), Tg2576 (Westerman et al., 2002), APP23 (Sturchler-Pierrat & Staufenbiel, 2000), AβPP/PS/tau triple transgenic (3xTg-AD) (Hunter et al., 2011), 5xFAD (Jawhar, Trawicka, Jenneckens, Bayer, & Wirths, 2012), and APP/PS1 (Oakley et al., 2006). These mouse models show greater levels of age-dependent cognitive impairments compared to normal aging, particularly in spatial memory tasks (Drummond & Wisniewski, 2017). Furthermore, the amyloid plaques found in the brains of these transgenic mice are structurally similar to those found in the human brain (Yang, Ueda, Chen, Ashe, & Cole, 2000).

Although the causes of sporadic AD are unknown, it is well accepted that aging and possessing *APOEε4* alleles are strong risk factors for sporadic AD (Rebeck, Reiter, Strickland, & Hyman, 1993). As such, mouse models possessing human *APOE* isoforms have been generated to understand how *APOE* isoforms may affect AD-associated neuropathology. Expressing humanized (h) *APOEε3* (*hAPOEε3*) or *hAPOEε4* in the PDAPP mouse model resulted in development of fibrillar Aβ deposits and neuritic plaques by 15 months of age (sex not specified: Holtzman et al., 2000). PDAPP mice expressing *hAPOEε4* had higher levels of Aβ deposits, especially in the molecular layer of the dentate gyrus, relative to PDAPP mice expressing *hAPOEε3* (Holtzman et al., 2000). Although *ApoE*-deficient PDAPP mice also displayed significant levels of Aβ deposition, no plaque-associated neuritic dystrophy was detected (Holtzman et al., 2000). Castellano et al. (2011) showed that young (3–4 months) and old (20–21 months) male and female PDAPP mice expressing *hAPOEε4* had the greatest Aβ burden compared to mice expressing *hAPOEε2* or *hAPOEε3*. It is suggested that *APOE* isoform-dependent differences in soluble Aβ metabolism in young mice resulted in *APOE* isoform-dependent Aβ accumulation in later life (Castellano et al., 2011). Other studies employing similar *hAPOE* transgenic mouse models have replicated these findings of mice expressing *hAPOEε4* having the worst neuropathological outcomes relative to mice expressing other isoforms (Buttini et al., 2002; Carter et al., 2001; Dodart, Bales, Johnstone, Little, & Paul, 2002). To create true models of sporadic AD, researchers have developed *APOE*-targeted replacement mice lines by knocking-in *hAPOE* isoforms to wild-type mice instead of early-onset familial AD mouse models. Liraz, Boehm-Cagan, and Michaelson (2013) found higher levels of hyperphosphorylated tau and greater Aβ accumulation in hippocampal neurons in male mice with *hAPOEε4* compared to those with *hAPOEε3*. Additionally, *hAPOEε4* mice displayed worse spatial working memory compared to *hAPOEε3* mice in both males (Liraz et al., 2013) and females (Bour et al., 2008). Most AD mouse models that have been developed are representative of early-onset familial AD, and only more recently have studies incorporated mouse models that are representative of sporadic AD. Although it is argued that early-onset familial AD mouse models can be used to study sporadic AD, research using these mouse models must be cautiously interpreted, as the type of model used will have implications on the findings. More work dedicated to further developing and studying sporadic mouse models is needed as they will undoubtedly allow greater understanding of the nuances of sporadic AD.

Sex differences are seen in some AD animal models (Chapter 1), with either greater levels or earlier expression of neuropathology in female compared to male mice. For example, in Tg2576 mice, Aβ was detected earlier in females, at 6 months old, compared to 12 months old in males (Allué et al., 2016). In APP/PS1, APP23, 3xTg and 3xTg mice expressing *hAPOEε4*, female mice exhibited either higher levels of Aβ or more rapid amyloid plaque deposition compared to males (Allué et al., 2016; Hirata-Fukae et al., 2008; Hou et al., 2015; Sturchler-Pierrat & Staufenbiel, 2000). Furthermore, female *hAPOEε4* 3xTg mice had impaired spatial learning and memory performance compared to male *hAPOEε4* 3xTg mice (Hou et al., 2015). Thus, although there has been some significant progress in developing experimental mouse models of AD, sex differences within these models still need to be thoroughly assessed.

As transgenic technology has advanced, the generation of transgenic rat models has become more reliable and accessible. This is advantageous because rats are physiologically, genetically, and morphologically closer to humans than mice (Gibbs et al., 2004; Jacob & Kwitek, 2002). One transgenic rat line, coded McGill

R-Thy1-APP, reliably produces extracellular Aβ deposits and amyloid plaques equally in both sexes (Leon et al., 2010; Petrasek et al., 2018). These rats display spatial cognitive impairment that becomes more prominent in older age and performance correlates with cortical levels of soluble Aβ in both males and females (Leon et al., 2010). More recently, a transgenic rat model (TgF344-AD) developed by Cohen et al. (2013) showed age-dependent cerebral Aβ accumulation that precedes development of amyloid plaques, apoptotic loss of neurons in the cerebral cortex and hippocampus, and cognitive impairments—closely embodying the progression of AD neurodegeneration—in both sexes. However, as noted, these models do not reflect the sex differences in pathology that are seen in humans (Altmann et al., 2014; Hohman et al., 2018). One explanation may be that these transgenic rats only model early-onset familial AD, and not the more commonly diagnosed sporadic AD. Future rat models that represent sporadic AD will be immensely valuable in moving the field forward.

Neurogenesis in Alzheimer's disease

Individuals diagnosed with amnestic MCI (aMCI) transition to AD at a rate of 10%–30% annually compared to a rate of about 1% in the general population; thus, aMCI could be considered a prodromal state to AD (Busse, Hensel, Gühne, Angermeyer, & Riedel-Heller, 2006). MCI can present as different clinical subtypes, and further discussion about MCI can be found in other reviews (Boyle, Wilson, Aggarwal, Tang, & Bennett, 2006; Edmonds et al., 2019; Langa & Levine, 2014). People with aMCI have reduced CA1 and entorhinal cortex volumes, but CA3 and dentate gyrus volumes are spared (Mueller et al., 2010). As AD begins to develop, neural hallmarks of the disease, primarily neurofibrillary tangles, aggregated hyperphosphorylated tau, and aggregated Aβ depositions, become evident in and around neurons in the entorhinal-hippocampal circuit (Thal et al., 2000). However, there is considerable debate over whether the neuropathology within this circuit correlates significantly with the degree of dementia as the disease progresses (Thal et al., 2000). Furthermore, the literature indicates a lack of correlation between amyloid pathology and severity of dementia, duration of dementia, and cognitive decline (Giannakopoulos et al., 2003; Ingelsson et al., 2004; Nelson et al., 2012; reviewed in Kametani & Hasegawa, 2018). It will be important for future studies to examine sex differences in these relationships (Duarte-Guterman et al., 2020). The hippocampus is particularly vulnerable to changes early in the pathogenesis of AD, in part because many of the key molecular players in AD are also modulators of neurogenesis.

In humans, there is evidence that neurogenesis is impaired in AD (Ekonomou et al., 2015; Moreno-Jiménez et al., 2019). In AD patients (data not analyzed by sex), the number of immature cells in the dentate gyrus is consistently lower than healthy age-matched individuals (Moreno-Jiménez et al., 2019). Moreover, the number and maturation of neurons in the dentate gyrus progressively declines as AD advances, suggesting that the extent of neurogenesis depletion is associated with disease progression (Moreno-Jiménez et al., 2019). Alterations in adult neurogenesis are detected even before the presence of neurofibrillary tangles or senile plaques in the dentate gyrus (Moreno-Jiménez et al., 2019). Consistent with these findings, a study showed a significant association between the number of proliferating neuroblasts in the hippocampus and cognitive diagnosis, where patients with MCI had fewer proliferating neuroblasts than cognitively normal males and females (Tobin et al., 2019). Intriguingly, there is literature suggesting that neurogenesis may actually be increased in AD patients (Jin et al., 2004). Specifically, Jin et al. (2004) found increased numbers of immature neurons in the hippocampus of AD individuals (sex not analyzed) compared to healthy controls. Increased neurogenesis may be a compensatory mechanism, allowing for replacement of "lost" or damaged neurons from AD neuropathology (Jin et al., 2004). Despite neurogenesis appearing to be increased in AD patients, progressive cell loss was still observed in the dentate gyrus (Jin et al., 2004), which may be due to the failure of the newborn neurons to develop into mature neurons or integrate into brain circuitry (Jin et al., 2004).

Another critical factor to contemplate in terms of the effects of AD on neurogenesis is disease severity. Using validated stage-specific and type-specific markers in autopsied human tissue to examine neurogenesis levels in male and female AD patients, Ekonomou et al. (2015) found that the number of newborn neurons significantly declined in the dentate gyrus, but only in patients with severe tau pathology. Together, the human and animal literature suggests that although there may be an early compensatory phenomenon of increased neurogenesis during the early stages of AD, impaired neurogenesis is observed in AD perhaps at later stages and altered neurogenesis may underlie the pathogenesis and cognitive deficits of the disease. However, much of the research in this area has either not included both sexes or has failed to analyze for sex differences. Researchers are encouraged to examine sex as a variable to further the current understanding of the nuanced relationship between Alzheimer's disease and neurogenesis.

Neurogenesis in models of Alzheimer's disease

ApoE expression is widespread in the dentate gyrus of the hippocampus, particularly in neural stem and progenitor cells (Tensaouti, Stephanz, Yu, & Kernie, 2018). Thus, it is not surprising that *ApoE*-deficient male and female mice show decreased numbers of neural stem and progenitor cells in the dentate gyrus (Tensaouti et al., 2018). Furthermore, *ApoE* deficiency, as well as *hAPOEε4* expression, are associated with less complexity in newborn neurons in the dentate gyrus of both male and female mice (Tensaouti et al., 2018). *ApoE*-deficient mice have deficient levels of cell proliferation (Tensaouti et al., 2018; Yang, Gilley, Zhang, & Kernie, 2011), but no changes in cell survival and differentiation, compared to wildtype mice (Tensaouti et al., 2018). Together, these findings demonstrate that *ApoE*-deficiency influences neuroplasticity by impairing the development of the neural progenitor pool but leaving the survival of new neurons and differentiation unaffected. However, in these studies, new neurons were created in adolescence and not adulthood, and given that sporadic AD is not a disease seen in adolescence, it is imperative to further investigate differences in neurogenesis in such mouse models in midlife.

Considering the link between *APOEε4* expression and the development of AD (Hartman et al., 2001; Manning et al., 2014; Tai et al., 2013; Wolk et al., 2010), one might expect *APOEε4* expression to impair neurogenesis and hippocampal function. Indeed, studies suggest this is true with increasing age, as *hAPOEε4* expression decreases hippocampal cell proliferation in middle-aged (12 months) male and female mice, with a greater degree of effect in females (Koutseff et al., 2014). In adult (6–7 months) female mice, there is an association between *hAPOEε4* expression and an impairment in maturation and dendritic development of newborn hippocampal neurons (Li et al., 2009), which is not seen in young adult (2 months) male and female mice (Tensaouti et al., 2018). Interestingly, some studies show that a compensatory increase in proliferation occurs during early stages of the disease, and decreased proliferation and survival of new neurons occurs during more advanced stages of pathology in APP/PS1 mice (Biscaro, Lindvall, Hock, Ekdahi, & Nitsch, 2009) and transgenic (pPDGF-APPSw, Ind) mice (Gan et al., 2008). Besides neurogenesis, Rijpma et al. (2013) found decreased presynaptic density in the dentate gyrus of middle-aged female, but not male *hAPOEε4* mice, compared to wildtype mice. These findings demonstrate that the effects of *hAPOEε4* on hippocampal neurogenesis are dependent on age and sex and may be dependent on disease and pathology severity.

Research of familial AD in mouse models shows that the induced AD neuropathology is linked to impaired hippocampal neurogenesis (Demars et al., 2010; Haughey et al., 2002; Scopa et al., 2019). One study in APP/PS1 male mice found that proliferation and differentiation of neural precursor cells were impaired in the hippocampus of young adult mice as early as 2 months of age, and this was linked to APP misprocessing in the hippocampus induced by the model (Demars et al., 2010). Decreases in neurogenesis seen in 2- and 6-month-old male and female double transgenic (TgCRND8) AD mice were accompanied by deficits in the performance of spatial (Morris Water Maze) and nonspatial ("step down" inhibitory avoidance test) cognitive tasks, which worsened with age and pathology severity (Fiorentini et al., 2010). Complementing these studies, cognitive performance and neurogenesis levels were improved along with reduced Aβ load in both male and female APP/PS1 AD mice via a combination of exercise and pharmacological methods, indicating some therapeutic potential of these interventions (Choi et al., 2018). These studies demonstrate that AD neuropathology and the hippocampus are closely related, and that changes in neurogenesis in the context of AD have important implications for cognitive function.

Estrogens and aging

Estrogens are related to cognitive function and neuroplasticity, primarily in females (reviewed in Galea, Frick, Hampson, Sohrabji, & Choleris, 2017) (see also Chapter 9). There are three types of estrogens: estrone, estradiol, and estriol. Of these, estradiol (17β-estradiol) is both the most potent and abundant during the reproductive years in females (Nugent et al., 2012; Perez-Martin et al., 2005). 17β-Estradiol levels change over the course of the menstrual cycle in primates (or estrous cycle in rodents) and across the lifespan (Nugent et al., 2012). At menopause, there is a significant drop in both 17β-estradiol and estrone levels; however, unlike premenopause, postmenopause results in estrone levels that are comparatively higher than 17β-estradiol levels (Rannevik et al., 2008). Estrogens can bind with the two "classic" estrogen receptors ERα and ERβ (Jensen et al., 1968; Kuiper, Enmark, Pelto-Huikko, Nilsson, & Gustafsson, 1996; Matthews, Celius, Halgren, & Zacharewski, 2000) or GPER (Prossnitz, Sklar, Oprea, & Arterburn, 2008; Revankar, Cimino, Sklar, Arterburn, & Prossnitz, 2005; Thomas, Pang, Filardo, & Dong, 2005; Waters et al., 2015). Significant changes in levels of estrogens across the lifespan can affect hippocampal neuroplasticity (reviewed in Sheppard, Choleris, & Galea, 2019), cognition (reviewed in Albert & Newhouse, 2019), and brain volume (reviewed in Russell, Jones, & Newhouse, 2019), depending on the amount of lifetime estrogen exposure, aging, and the type and duration of hormone therapy (HT). These factors are discussed in greater detail below.

Rodents do not undergo typical menopause, such as that seen in humans, but like humans, they show a decrease in ovarian follicle levels, irregular cycling, elevated levels of FSH, and lowered fertility in older age (Finch & Gosden, 1986; Rubin, 2000; Van Kempen, Milner, & Waters, 2011; Williams, 2005; for detailed review, see Maffucci & Gore, 2006). In middle age, rodents transition to "estropause," a state where they exhibit irregular cycling, and during which most animals enter a state of acyclic persistent estrus that is eventually followed by persistent diestrus and cessation of ovulation (Lefevre & Mcclintock, 1988; Rousseau, 2006). Therefore, estropause shares many characteristics of menopause and can be considered an appropriate model for normal ovarian aging in humans.

Menopause can be modeled in a variety of ways in rodents, including normal aging, ovariectomy, and drug-induced paradigms. The aging model may be best at mimicking natural age-related changes because there is no external manipulation of hormone levels (Baeza, De Castro, Giménez-Llort, & De la Fuente, 2010). Surgical menopause is best modeled in rodents through ovariectomy because it results in the sudden and significant reduction of ovarian hormones postsurgery, and this model is relevant because approximately 16% of human females undergo surgical removal of both the uterus and ovaries before the onset of menopause (Flaws, Doerr, Sipes, & Hoyer, 1994; Mayer et al., 2002). However, it is important to note that ovariectomy may have different effects than hysterectomy or both ovariectomy and hysterectomy combined (Koebele et al., 2019). Another menopause model uses the drug 4-vinylcyclohexene diepoxide (VCD) to destroy ovarian follicles and lower levels of ovarian hormones to model perimenopausal and menopausal transition in females (Koebele & Bimonte-Nelson, 2016; Mayer et al., 2002). Although VCD lowers FSH, progesterone, and anti-Müllerian hormone levels successfully (Koebele & Bimonte-Nelson, 2016; Mayer et al., 2002), it leaves 17β-estradiol levels unchanged or increased, unlike natural menopause (Carolino, Barros, Kalil, &

Anselmo-Franci, 2019). Furthermore, this model is generally initiated in immature prepubescent rodents (28-day-old rats) and thus disrupts puberty, which will have implications on brain maturation. Lastly, VCD has toxic and carcinogenic effects on other organs besides ovaries (Mayer et al., 2002; Koebele & Bimonte-Nelson, 2016). Therefore, VCD must be used with caution and careful attention must be paid to these side effects when interpreting its effects. Even though none of these models can perfectly model human menopause, they each allow researchers to investigate specific characteristics of the menopausal transition.

Estrogens and neurogenesis

Estrogens can increase or decrease various stages of neurogenesis in the hippocampus of adult rodents, depending on several parameters including sex, age, type, dose, and duration of estrogens. In adult female rodents, short-term (1 week) ovariectomy decreases cell proliferation (Banasr, Hery, Brezun, & Daszuta, 2001; Ormerod, Falconer, & Galea, 2003; Ormerod & Galea, 2001; Tanapat et al., 1999) compared to intact female rodents, and this effect is rescued by 17β-estradiol administration (Banasr et al., 2001; Ormerod & Galea, 2003; Tanapat et al., 1999). The length of time following ovariectomy in adult rodents is also linked to how effective 17β-estradiol is at increasing neurogenesis. For instance, in young adult female rats, 17β-estradiol increases cell proliferation 7 days, but not 28 days, following ovariectomy (Barker & Galea, 2008; Tanapat, Hastings, & Gould, 2005). Most estrogens (17β-estradiol, 17α-estradiol, and estrone) increase cell proliferation rapidly in young adult rats (within 30 min) in a dose-dependent manner (Barha, Lieblich, & Galea, 2009). Moreover, acute activation of ERα or ERβ with selective agonists can increase cell proliferation (Mazzucco et al., 2006), but activation of the membrane estrogen receptor GPER (via a GPER agonist) decreases cell proliferation in the hippocampus (Duarte-Guterman et al., 2015). This indicates that estrogens might be acting through nongenomic pathways to increase cell proliferation.

Both sex and duration of 17β-estradiol exposure can affect the ability of estrogens to modulate neuroplasticity. Depending on when BrdU is administered relative to hormone treatment, one can see different effects on neurogenesis (Fig. 3). For example, chronic administration (15 days) of 17β-estradiol benzoate (EB) led to a decrease in neurogenesis, independent of its early effects on cell proliferation (as BrdU was administered prior to EB) in female but not male rats (Barker & Galea, 2008). However, if BrdU is administered after 17β-estradiol (labeling cells that are initially increased due to estrogen's ability to enhance cell proliferation), chronic 17β-estradiol increases neurogenesis in adult female rats and mice (Eid et al., 2020; McClure, Barha, & Galea, 2013). Surprisingly, unlike what is seen after acute doses, chronic doses of ERα or ERβ agonists do not increase neurogenesis in adult female mice (Eid et al., 2020). Male rats show increased neurogenesis after 5 days of EB exposure that positively corresponds with spatial memory performance (Ormerod, Lee, & Galea, 2004). Interestingly, this effect was only seen when EB was administered

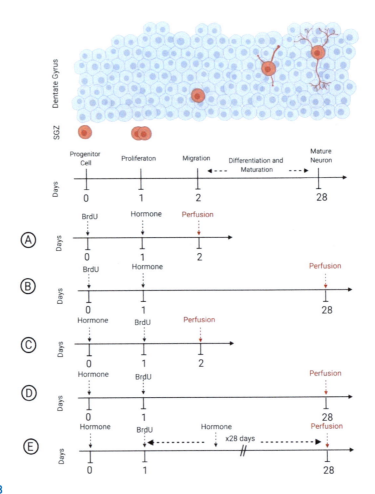

FIG. 3

A timeline of proliferation and maturation of adult-born hippocampal neurons in the dentate gyrus of the rat. The time of BrdU injection relative to hormone can affect results and conclusions drawn from data (A-E). If BrdU is injected >2h before the hormone, any effects observed are independent of cell proliferation. The timelines show: (A) the effect of the hormone in the short term; (B) long-term survival of new cells independent of the effects of hormones on cell proliferation; (C) the effects of hormones on cell proliferation; (D) the long-term survival of cells that proliferated after exposure to the hormone; and (E) effects of chronic hormone treatment on long-term survival of cells and initial proliferation. *BrdU*, bromodeoxyuridine; *SGZ*, subgranular zone.

Created with BioRender.com.

in the "axon extension" window (6–10 days) after BrdU, indicating a critical period during which EB can influence neurogenesis in males (Ormerod et al., 2004). Moreover, male rats show no significant changes in the survival of new neurons after chronic (30 days) EB administration but do show changes after testosterone exposure (Spritzer & Galea, 2007), as reviewed below in Section "Testosterone and neurogenesis in the context of aging and Alzheimer's disease." Taken together, these data show that the effect of estradiol administration on hippocampal plasticity is affected by sex and that the length of exposure to estradiol can influence its efficacy in modulating neuroplasticity.

Estrogens and neurogenesis in the context of aging

As noted earlier, adult hippocampal neurogenesis persists in middle and older age although it is decreased from young adulthood, and this lower rate of neurogenesis is maintained into older age for both sexes (Driscoll et al., 2006; Hattiangady, Rao, Shetty, & Shetty, 2005; Kuhn et al., 1996; Nacher, Alonso-Llosa, Rosell, & McEwen, 2003; Rao, Hattiangady, Abdel-Rahman, Stanley, & Shetty, 2005; Rao & Shetty, 2004). The efficacy of 17β-estradiol treatment on neurogenesis is dependent on age. Acute administration of 17β-estradiol dose-dependently increased cell proliferation in ovariectomized young-adult, but not middle-aged (12-month-old) nulliparous (i.e., having no previous reproductive experience) female rats (Barha & Galea, 2011; Barha et al., 2009; Chiba, Suzuki, Yamanouchi, & Nishihara, 2007; Tanapat et al., 2005). However, the impact of 17β-estradiol on cell proliferation can also be dependent on the length of exposure. Long term 17β-estradiol treatment (10 weeks) increased cell proliferation in older (22-month-old) nulliparous ovariectomized female rats (Perez-Martin et al., 2005) and chronic administration of 17β-estradiol (either 10 days or 2 months) increased cell proliferation in middle-aged (10- to 12-month-old) female mice, but did not affect survival of new neurons (Saravia, Beauquis, Pietranera, & De Nicola, 2007). Thus, acute administration of 17β-estradiol leads to increased cell proliferation in young adult, but not middle-aged, female rats, which may be overcome with longer exposure to 17β-estradiol and/or with reproductive experience (described below in Section "Parity and neurogenesis").

To our knowledge, no studies have directly examined the influence of estrogens on neurogenesis in humans, but a number of studies have measured hippocampal volume, which has been shown to positively correlate with increased neurogenesis (Boldrini et al., 2018). In females, hippocampal volume increases during the late follicular phase of the menstrual cycle (when 17β-estradiol and progesterone levels are high) compared to other stages (Barth et al., 2016; Lisofsky et al., 2015; Taylor et al., 2020). There is evidence that females receiving HT in middle age have larger hippocampal volume than females who did not report HT use (Eberling et al., 2003; Pintzka & Håberg, 2015). Studies in postmenopausal females given 17β-estradiol-based HT in both the short and longer term showed larger hippocampal volume compared to those who did not take HT (Hu et al., 2006). These effects are seen in a dose-dependent manner, as chronic (3 months) 17β-estradiol treatment with a 2 mg dose, but not 1 mg dose, showed increased gray matter volume in the posterior hippocampus (Albert et al., 2017). Conversely, the Women's Health Initiative Memory Study found that the use of estrone-based HT in females between the ages of 71 and 89 leads to a decrease in hippocampal volume (Resnick et al., 2009). Estradiol- and progesterone-based HT correlate with larger hippocampal volume, whereas estrone-based HT is linked to smaller hippocampal volume (Albert et al., 2017; Hu et al., 2006; Resnick et al., 2009). Thus, exposure to estrogens over the lifespan can differentially alter hippocampal volume in middle and old age depending on dose and estrogen type, and this suggests that the same relationships seen with estrogens and rodents on neurogenesis may also be seen in human females.

Estrogens, aging, and cognition

Studies have found that earlier age of menopause onset in females (whether naturally occurring or surgically induced) is associated with an increased risk of developing AD (Fox, Berzuini, & Knapp, 2013a; Rocca, Mielke, Vemuri, & Miller, 2014; Ryan et al., 2014) (see also Chapter 9). Surgically induced menopause is associated with faster decline in verbal and episodic memory task performance compared to naturally occurring menopause (Bove et al., 2014; Gervais et al., 2018; Rocca et al., 2007). Lower cumulative exposure to estrogens and changes in hormone levels (particularly sudden changes) negatively affect cognitive function in females, but a full account of this literature is beyond the scope of this review and the reader is directed to other reviews on the subject (Georgakis, Beskou-Kontou, Theodoridis, Skalkidou, & Petridou, 2019).

HT has been suggested as a potential treatment to ameliorate cognitive decline with menopause. Studies investigating the effect of HT on cognition in older females have shown inconsistent results, mostly due to the type of HT, duration of HT, and age given postmenopause varying between experiments (Espeland et al., 2013; Henderson et al., 2000). A large study indicated that females prescribed with combined equine estrogens (CEE) and medroxyprogesterone acetate (MPA, a progestin-based HT) had reduced performance on the Mini-Mental State Exam and increased risk of dementia (Espeland et al., 2004). However, this study has been widely criticized for a number of factors, including time since menopause and type of HT given (Craig et al., 2005; Espeland et al., 2004; Henderson et al., 2000). It is important to note that CEEs contain 50%–70% estrone sulfate but only 0.1%–1% estradiol sulfate (Rapp et al., 2003; Shumaker et al., 2003). This is crucial because, although estrone can be converted to estradiol, the preferential pathway is from estradiol to estrone, and estrone has a lower affinity for the ER (Anstead, Carlson, & Katzenellenbogen, 1997; Brzozowski et al., 1997; Hu & Aizawa, 2003). Treatment with 17β-estradiol-based HT can improve cognition in both healthy females and females with AD (Wharton et al., 2011), whereas treatment with estrone-based therapies has fewer positive effects on cognition (Hogervorst et al., 2000). Indeed, meta-analyses confirm that the type of HT (estrone versus 17β-estradiol-based), duration of HT use, and age at initiation of HT can impact how HT affects cognition (Hogervorst, Williams, Budge, Riedel, & Jolles, 2000; Ryan, Scali, Carriere, Ritchie, & Ancelin, 2008).

Several studies suggest that, in order to be effective, HT must be initiated within a "critical window" after declines in gonadal hormones in both males and females (see also Section "Testosterone and neurogenesis"). The critical window hypothesis states that the efficacy of HT depends on the time window in which treatment is started relative to menopause (Henderson & Rocca, 2012; Rocca, Grossardt, & Shuster, 2011; Sherwin, 2007, 2009). For example, females who started HT within 5 years of menopause onset were 30% less likely to develop late-onset AD compared to those who started HT more than 5 years after menopause onset or those who did not receive HT at all (Matyi, Rattinger, Schwartz, Buhusi, & Tschanz, 2019; Shao et al., 2012). These findings suggest that if HT is started long after menopause onset, it is no longer effective and may even be detrimental to cognition (Henderson & Rocca, 2012; Sherwin, 2009; Whitmer, Quesenberry, Zhou, & Yaffe, 2011).

The critical window hypothesis is supported by the animal literature (Bohacek & Daniel, 2010). Hippocampus-dependent cognition is improved and ER-α levels in the hippocampus are increased when middle-aged rats are treated with 17β-estradiol shortly but not long after estropause or ovariectomy (Bohacek & Daniel, 2009; Daniel & Bohacek, 2010; Gibbs, 2010; Vedder, Bredemann, & McMahon, 2014). This shows that the hippocampus is not as sensitive to acute 17β-estradiol administration after long-term ovariectomy or deprivation from ovarian hormones. Therefore, any study examining the effect of HT on neuroplasticity and cognition would need to carefully account for time of treatment onset relative to ovariectomy. Although we know that estrogens modulate both hippocampal neurogenesis and hippocampus-dependent learning and memory, there is an urgent need to investigate the role of the critical period (Resnick & Henderson, 2002; Sherwin, 2005), genotype (Brown, Choi, Xu, Vitek, & Colton, 2008; Burkhardt et al., 2004; Heikkinen et al., 1999; Kang & Grodstein, 2012; Kunzler, Youmans, Yu, LaDu, & Tai, 2014; Rippon et al., 2006; Yaffe, Haan, Byers, Tangen, & Kuller, 2000), reproductive experience (reviewed in Section "Parity and neurogenesis"), HT type (Hogervorst et al., 2000; Luine, Jacome, & MacLusky, 2003; Ryan et al., 2008), and dose of HT (Barha, Dalton, & Galea, 2010; Barha et al., 2009; Galea, Spritzer, Barker, & Pawluski, 2006; Tanapat et al., 2005, 1999) before we can conclude whether HT is beneficial as a treatment or prophylactic for AD by modulating neuroplasticity and cognition.

Estrogens and neurogenesis in the context of Alzheimer's disease

17β-Estradiol regulates hippocampal neuropathology, neuroplasticity, and cognitive function in animal models of AD (Li et al., 2019; Rodríguez & Verkhratsky, 2011; Shohayeb, Diab, Ahmed, & Ng, 2018; Vaucher et al., 2002). In both sexes and in a variety of animal models of AD, 17β-estradiol reduces AD pathology, neurodegeneration, and consequently, cognitive deficits (Chen, Nilsen, & Brinton, 2006; Kong et al., 2019; Tschiffely, Schuh, Prokai-Tatrai, Ottinger, & Prokai, 2018; Wang et al., 2017; Ramsden, Shin, & Pike, 2003; Wang, Gu, Masters, & Wang, 2017; Zheng et al., 2017). Reminiscent of the healthy brain bias, administration of 17β-estradiol at an early (but not late) stage of AD pathology in females led to increased hippocampal neurogenesis (which was positively correlated with performance on the Morris water maze test in an $A\beta_{1-42}$ mouse model of AD (Zheng et al., 2017)). 17β-Estradiol affects more than just neuropathology and neurogenesis, however, a thorough discussion of this is beyond the scope of this chapter (see Galea et al., 2017). One possible downstream mechanism underlying the effects of 17β-estradiol may be through brain-derived neurotrophic factor (BDNF), as in female rats, 17β-estradiol leads to increased production of BDNF in young, adult, and middle-aged animals and this increase correlates with improved cognitive performance on a spatial memory task in adult and middle-aged rats (Kiss et al., 2012). Collectively, these data show that in middle age, and in animal models of AD, 17β-estradiol can positively influence hippocampal neurogenesis and improve performance on cognitive tasks in both males and females.

The efficacy of 17β-estradiol on modulating cognition and neuroplasticity may also be modulated by *APOE* genotype (de Lange et al., 2020; Kunzler et al., 2014). Numerous studies in humans have shown that, across different cohorts and ethnicities, 17β-estradiol has beneficial effects in non-*APOE*ε4 subjects, but 17β-estradiol has either detrimental or no effects on cognition and AD pathology in females carrying the *APOE*ε4 allele (Burkhardt et al., 2004; Heikkinen et al., 1999; Kang & Grodstein, 2012; Rippon et al., 2006; Yaffe et al., 2000). A similar relationship between 17β-estradiol and *APOE* status is seen in mouse models, where 17β-estradiol decreased AD pathology in *APOE*ε2 and *APOE*ε3 carriers, but increased AD pathology in *APOE*ε4 carriers (Brown et al., 2008; Kunzler et al., 2014). Thus, both the human and animal literature show that the efficacy of 17β-estradiol as a treatment for cognitive decline in middle age is mediated by *APOE* genotype, such that *APOE*ε2 or ε3 carriers benefit from 17β-estradiol treatment, but carriers of *APOE*ε4 show either detrimental or no effect on cognitive performance.

Parity and neurogenesis

Parity (i.e., pregnancy and parturition) and the postpartum period are characterized by major and unique changes in steroid and peptide hormone levels (Heidrich et al., 1994; Schock et al., 2016), brain plasticity, and function (Kinsley et al., 2006; Lambert, 2012; Woodside, 2006). In humans, one study found that overall brain volume decreases over the course of pregnancy, which then rebounds to preconception levels 6 months after parturition (Oatridge et al., 2002). In 2018, Luders et al. used a "BrainAGE index" to identify anatomical correlates of brain age using cortical volume and cortical thickness as key markers and found that female brains were significantly "younger" 4–6 weeks after giving birth compared to the immediate postpartum (1–2 days) (Luders et al., 2018). This aligns with Oatridge et al.'s (2002) findings showing an increase in total volume from parturition to 6 months postpartum. Consistent with the Luders et al. (2018) study, Kim et al. (2010) found that compared to 2–3 weeks postpartum, total gray matter volume increased during the first 3–4 months. Kim, Dufford, and Tribble (2018) also found that for the first 6 months after parturition, cortical thickness increased with time since birth. During late gestation and the postpartum period, mice show a transient increase in gray matter volume in several brain regions, including the hippocampus and amygdala (Barrière et al., 2020). Another study investigating long-term effects of pregnancy found that that gray matter reductions (compared to preconception levels) in several regions, including the hippocampus, anterior cingulate cortex, and the inferior prefrontal gyri could be seen 2 years after birth (Hoekzema et al., 2017). Long-term (>2 years) changes with parity are seen using the same BrainAGE index as de Lange et al. (2019), such that middle-aged parous females had "younger" brains compared to nulliparous females, and this effect was independent of common genetic variations. Although both BrainAGE studies found that long-term changes in the brain persist after giving birth, they do not provide clear information as to exactly what those changes are, although the algorithm does consider cortical structure and volume. A very recent study shows that the largest effects of the long-term effects of parity on "BrainAGE" are seen in the limbic and striatal regions, including the hippocampus and nucleus accumbens (de Lange et al., 2020). Therefore, although overall brain volume returns to preconception levels 6 months after giving birth, there are many changes in the weeks following birth, and the long-term effects of parity on gray matter volume in specific areas including the hippocampus persist well after parturition and weaning.

Reproductive experience directly influences neurogenesis in the hippocampus (for a detailed review, see Duarte-Guterman, Leuner, & Galea, 2019). Primiparous (having one previous reproductive experience) rats and biparous (having two previous reproductive experiences) rats have decreased cell proliferation in the hippocampus in the early postpartum compared to nulliparous age-matched controls (Darnaudéry et al., 2007; Eid et al., 2019; Leuner, Mirescu, Noiman, & Gould, 2007; Pawluski & Galea, 2007). This reduced neurogenesis in the early postpartum can be attributed to adrenal steroids, as both adrenalectomy and the removal of pups eliminated this effect (Leuner et al., 2007). Furthermore, this postpartum-induced reduction in neurogenesis was due to pregnancy alone, as "mothering" or exposure of nulliparous rats to pups led to increased cell proliferation in the dentate gyrus (Pawluski & Galea, 2007; Ruscio et al., 2008). Indeed, withdrawal from a hormone-simulated pregnancy decreased levels of proliferation compared to vehicle-treated female rats (Green & Galea, 2008). Different stages of pregnancy can also have varying effects on neurogenesis, as there is decreased cell proliferation in the hippocampus in mid to late pregnancy (Eid et al., 2019; Pawluski et al., 2020; Rolls, Schori, London, & Schwartz, 2008) but there is no such change in the early stages of pregnancy. Notably, unlike in the dentate gyrus, there is increased cell proliferation in the subventricular zone in both early and late gestation in rodents (Furuta &

Bridges, 2005; Shingo et al., 2003). These findings show that pregnancy and mothering decrease hippocampal neurogenesis, and these effects can vary based on the stage of pregnancy.

Parity influences the survival of new neurons in an age-dependent manner. Across the postpartum, rats show reduced survival of new neurons in the hippocampus compared to age-matched controls (Eid et al., 2019; Hillerer, Jacobs, Fischer, & Aigner, 2014; Pawluski & Galea, 2007). However, primiparous and multiparous (having more than two reproductive experiences) rats had greater density of immature neurons (as expressed by doublecortin) in middle age compared to nulliparous rats (Barha, Lieblich, Chow, & Galea, 2015; Eid et al., 2019; Galea, Qiu, & Duarte-Guterman, 2018). Curiously, administration of estrogens led to increased hippocampal cell proliferation in multiparous middle-aged rats but not in nulliparous rats (Barha & Galea, 2011). However, treatment with chronic estrogens or Premarin, an estrone-based HT, led to decreased immature neurons in the dentate gyrus regardless of parity in rats (Barha et al., 2015; Galea, Qiu, & Duarte-Guterman, 2018), although this depended on the region of the dentate gyrus. Therefore, estrogens influence neurogenesis in older age, dependent on parity.

Pregnant rats in late gestation demonstrate impaired hippocampal-dependent spatial reference memory compared to controls (Darnaudéry et al., 2007; Galea et al., 2000). Following pregnancy, after pups are weaned, primiparous rats show enhanced hippocampal-dependent learning and memory relative to nulliparous rats (Gatewood et al., 2005; Kinsley et al., 1999; Love et al., 2005; Pawluski, Walker, & Galea, 2006). These changes are not due to pregnancy or mothering alone, as neither pregnant-only nor foster mothers showed these same enhancing effects on working or reference memory (Pawluski & Galea, 2007; but see Kinsley et al., 1999). In middle and older age, primiparous and multiparous rats also show increased performance on working or reference memory tasks (Barha et al., 2015; Galea, Qiu, & Duarte-Guterman, 2018; Gatewood et al., 2005; Love et al., 2005; Zimberknopf, Xavier, Kinsley, & Felicio, 2011). Indeed, although data is scarce, parity is also associated with enhanced episodic memory in older females (Orchard et al., 2020). Collectively, these studies indicate that reproductive experience significantly influences hippocampal plasticity and cognition in middle and older age in rodents and humans.

Parity and Alzheimer's disease

When considering female sex as a risk factor for AD, it is necessary to acknowledge that experiences unique to females, like parity, may play a role in this increased risk. Indeed, parity results in long-term repercussions to health, including increased risk for AD (Prince et al., 2018; Ptok, Barkow, & Heun, 2002; reviewed in Galea et al., 2018). A higher proportion of females who have experienced more than three pregnancies are diagnosed with AD compared to females who have experienced no pregnancies (Colucci et al., 2006). This is supported by a recent study conducted by Jang et al. (2018), which reported a 1.7-fold higher risk of developing AD for grand multiparous (five or more pregnancies) females relative to those who experienced four or fewer. Bae et al. (2020) found that increased dementia risk for grand multiparous females was only observed in Europe and Latin America, whereas in Asia, nulliparous females showed a higher dementia risk compared to parous females, suggesting that parity-associated dementia risk may not be uniform across geographical regions. These findings are reminiscent of the geographical influences on whether sex differences are seen in the prevalence of AD (Mielke et al., 2014). Interestingly, females who experienced incomplete pregnancies (i.e., no childbirth) had half the level of AD risk compared to those with complete pregnancies, suggesting that besides pregnancy-induced hormonal changes, motherhood experiences may also influence AD risk (Jang et al., 2018). Indeed, there is evidence showing that longer breastfeeding duration corresponds to reduced AD risk (Fox, Berzuini, & Knapp, 2013b). Besides increased risk, parous females (two or more children) also show greater AD neuropathology, measured by higher concentrations of neuritic plaque in the brain, relative to females with fewer or no children and males with children (Beeri et al., 2009). However, these findings do not align with those from the BrainAGE studies, which show that parity is associated with a more "youthful" brain (de Lange et al., 2020, 2019). These data can be reconciled with the idea of the healthy cell bias (Brinton, 2008) such that parity may be beneficial in a healthy brain, but be detrimental in AD. In a study using an AD mouse model (APP23), multiparity increased the number of amyloid plaques in the hippocampus and decreased spatial memory performance of AD (APP24) middle-aged female mice (Cui et al., 2014). However, multiparity improved performance on spatial memory task in wild-type female mice at middle age (Cui et al., 2014). Furthermore, aged (24 months) primiparous and multiparous rats also showed lower levels of APP (Gatewood et al., 2005). These changes may be detected early, as in an AD mouse model (5xFAD) early postpartum mice showed more amyloid plaques in the hippocampus when examined on gestation day 10, and less neurogenesis (quantified by Ki67 and DCX) in the early postpartum (day 20) compared to wild-type mice (Ziegler-Waldkirch et al., 2018). To summarize, these studies demonstrate that multiple pregnancies may be neuroprotective in healthy individuals, but may increase neuropathology and symptoms in individuals with AD. Furthermore, parity can affect neuroplasticity and cognition depending on genotype in both animal models and humans.

Testosterone and neurogenesis

Testosterone is a sex hormone primarily secreted by the testes and, to a lesser extent, by the ovaries. Testosterone can be converted to 17β-estradiol via aromatase or to a more potent androgen, dihydrotestosterone (DHT), via 5-α reductase (Ishikawa, Glidewell-Kenney, & Jameson, 2006). In healthy human males, circulating testosterone levels in the blood decrease with age, starting from the age of 30 (Harman et al., 2001; Vermeulen, Goemaere, & Kaufman, 1999). In both males and females, testosterone and DHT can circulate and bind to ARs. AR efficacy varies by a polymorphism of the AR gene that codes for cytosine-adenine-guanine (CAG) repeats, which varies from 8 to 35 repeats in humans (Buchanan et al., 2004; Lanz, 1995). Fewer CAG repeats are associated with increased sensitivity to testosterone due to greater AR gene expression and functionality (Buchanan et al., 2004; Tirabassi et al., 2015). Thus, although studies have examined the influence of plasma levels of testosterone on neuroplasticity and cognition, future studies should examine these changes in the context of this AR polymorphism.

Adult hippocampal neurogenesis is increased with androgens in young adult males but not in young adult females (Duarte-Guterman, Lieblich, et al., 2019; Hamson et al., 2013; Spritzer & Galea, 2007). Male meadow voles with higher levels of testosterone levels show increased survival of new neurons in the dentate gyrus compared to meadow voles with lower levels of testosterone (Ormerod & Galea, 2003). In adult male rats, castration decreases neurogenesis in the dentate gyrus via a decrease in survival of new neurons but not via any changes in cell proliferation (Spritzer & Galea, 2005, 2007). Chronic (30 days) administration of testosterone and dihydrotestosterone, but not 17β-estradiol, increased the survival of new neurons in male rats, indicating that testosterone is acting through an AR-dependent mechanism to increase neurogenesis in the hippocampus (Hamson et al., 2013; Spritzer & Galea, 2007; Spritzer, Ibler, Inglis, & Curtis, 2011). Indeed, pharmacological or genetic manipulations of the AR resulted in a failure of testosterone or DHT to increase neurogenesis in the hippocampus of male rats or mice (Hamson et al., 2013; Swift-Gallant et al., 2018). Furthermore, androgens increase neurogenesis in young adult male rats but not in young adult female rats, despite the fact that ARs are present in the female hippocampus (Duarte-Guterman, Lieblich, et al., 2019), although, curiously, there are few ARs in the dentate gyrus (Duarte-Guterman, Lieblich, et al., 2019; Hamson et al., 2013; Swift-Gallant et al., 2018). This is intriguing given that androgens directly stimulate neurogenesis in the dentate gyrus via AR (Hamson et al., 2013) and suggests that the ability of androgens to increase neurogenesis via AR is dependent on AR located in other regions of the hippocampus, such as in the CA3 region. Indeed, ARs are found more frequently in the stratum lucidum of the CA3 region, where mossy fibers from the dentate gyrus terminate (Tabori et al., 2005). These studies show that androgens differently affect the survival of new neurons in the hippocampus, and that these effects are mediated through the AR.

Duration and dose of exposure to androgens are known to affect neurogenesis. Studies generally show that 30 days of treatment with androgens dose-dependently increases hippocampal neurogenesis, but shorter duration of treatment with androgens (15–21 days) does not (Buwalda et al., 2010; Carrier & Kabbaj, 2012; Spritzer, Ibler, et al., 2011; Spritzer, Daviu, et al., 2011; Wainwright et al., 2016). Why 21 days of treatment is insufficient to lead to lasting neuroplastic changes is not yet known. Moreover, higher but not lower doses of testosterone increase neurogenesis in the hippocampus of adult male rats (Spritzer & Galea, 2007), though supraphysiological doses of anabolic steroids decrease neurogenesis in the hippocampus (Novaes Gomes et al., 2014). One study has shown that long-term castration (14 days) in rats is associated with neuronal loss in the dentate gyrus (Ramsden et al., 2004), which can be rescued with chronic (21 days) administration of DHT if the treatment is initiated 2 weeks after castration, but not longer than that (Ramsden et al., 2004). This is suggestive of a critical window of androgens to influence neuroplasticity in males, similar to the effects of estrogens in females (Bohacek and Daniel, 2010; Sherwin, 2007). Overall, testosterone can dose-dependently increase neurogenesis with long exposures in males but not in females, via an AR-dependent mechanism.

Testosterone and neurogenesis in the context of aging and Alzheimer's disease

There are very few studies investigating aging and testosterone in the hippocampus. Unlike females, males do not undergo a dramatic menopause-like transition in gonadal hormone levels, but instead experience a gradual reduction in testosterone with age (Vermeulen, 1999). In older men, peripheral testosterone levels positively correlate with hippocampal volume in individuals with MCI, but not in males with normal cognitive aging (Lee et al., 2017). Chronic (30 days) testosterone or dihydrotestosterone increases adult hippocampal neurogenesis in young-adult male rats, but fails to alter neurogenesis in middle-aged male or female rats (Duarte-Guterman, Lieblich, et al., 2019; Moser et al., 2019). This is surprising as ARs are still present in middle age, and in fact may increase in expression in middle-aged, compared to young, adults (Duarte-Guterman, Lieblich, et al., 2019). As mentioned earlier, AR responsivity to testosterone can be dependent on the number of CAG repeats in the AR (Fischbeck et al., 2001; Kumar et al., 2011), and an increased number of CAG repeats is correlated with increased neurodegeneration (Kumar et al., 2011; Piccioni et al., 2001). Taken together, these point to a role for androgens in modulating hippocampal neuroplasticity in middle age, and the idea that androgens are acting through other pathways, perhaps not directly involving ARs, to affect neuroplasticity in the hippocampus. How different factors (including age and length of treatment) mediate these effects remain to be investigated thoroughly.

In humans, low circulating levels of testosterone is an independent risk factor for AD (Hogervorst, Bandelow, Combrinck, & Smith, 2004; Hogervorst, Combrinck, & Smith, 2003). Older males, but not females, with AD show lower levels of serum testosterone than age-matched controls (Carcaillon et al., 2014; Mora et al., 2012; Pfankuch et al., 2005), and testosterone affects cognitive performance in older adults. Briefly, in healthy older men, administration of exogenous testosterone led to a significant improvement on the Mini-Mental State Exam (Wahjoepramono et al., 2016) and spatial cognitive function, but did not affect any other type of cognitive domain tested (Janowsky et al., 1994). In human male patients suffering from AD, increasing serum total testosterone levels to $>2.5\times$ baseline levels leads to a significant improvement in spatial and verbal memory, but to no significant changes in selective and divided attention or language-based tasks (Cherrier et al., 2005). Additionally, males with AD or MCI have lower brain testosterone and DHT levels compared to age-matched controls (Rosario et al., 2004, 2011). Furthermore, lower testosterone levels were inversely associated with AD neuropathology among *APOEε4* carriers in the ADNI database in both males and females (Sundermann et al., 2020). There is a clear correlation between the lower levels of circulating testosterone and impaired performance on cognitive tasks in healthy individuals, and treatment with testosterone may lead to improved performance on cognitive tasks in patients with cognitive impairment.

Conclusion

There are striking sex differences in AD, with females having a greater lifetime risk, greater neuropathology, and more severe cognitive symptoms compared to males. Sex differences also exist in adult hippocampal neurogenesis and cognition that are affected by age, hormone exposure, cognitive training, and genetics, among other factors. Understanding the mechanisms underlying sex differences in neurogenesis and cognition could help explain the increased AD-related lifetime risk, neuropathology, and cognitive decline faced by females. The development and severity of AD are related to steroid hormones in both females and males, with lower levels of 17β-estradiol and testosterone in middle age correlating with greater cognitive decline. Estrogens and androgens modulate adult hippocampus neurogenesis in females and males, respectively. These hormones can also improve performance across different cognitive domains in both sexes in humans and rodents. However, the efficacy of these hormones in improving cognition and neurogenesis is dependent on hormone type, dose, and genotype. Furthermore, the efficacy of these hormones follows the critical window hypothesis and the healthy cell bias. In females, past reproductive experience, length of reproductive period, and the time of HT onset relative to menopause also affect the efficacy of HT to influence neuroplasticity and cognition. Future research should work to understand differences in aging trajectories between males and females to help build better precision medicine frameworks for timely intervention in AD and related dementias. Understanding the basic biological mechanisms underlying sex differences in neuroplasticity within the hippocampus will provide insight on the etiology and treatment of diseases such as AD that affect hippocampal integrity.

Chapter highlights

- Neurogenesis in the hippocampus is necessary for some forms of cognition, including pattern separation, and levels of hippocampal neurogenesis are reduced with aging and Alzheimer's disease in both humans and in mouse models, with some notable sex differences in all of these effects.
- Sex differences exist in hippocampal neurogenesis, with males showing greater proliferation and faster maturation than females and in response to hormone therapy which may be related to aging differences.

- Androgens enhance neurogenesis in adult, but not middle-aged, males or in females, whereas estrogens can enhance neurogenesis in females but not in males. The ability of estrogens to enhance neurogenesis in middle-aged females is related to reproductive experience.
- Understanding the role of sex and sex hormones on hippocampal plasticity and their underlying mechanisms may lead to new therapeutic targets to combat cognitive decline and neuropathology related to AD.

References

Adler, D. H., Wisse, L. E. M., Ittyerah, R., Pluta, J. B., Ding, S. L., Xie, L., … Yushkevich, P. A. (2018). Characterizing the human hippocampus in aging and Alzheimer's disease using a computational atlas derived from ex vivo MRI and histology. *Proceedings of the National Academy of Sciences of the United States of America, 115*(16).

Albert, K., Hiscox, J., Boyd, B., Dumas, J., Taylor, W., & Newhouse, P. (2017). Estrogen enhances hippocampal gray-matter volume in young and older postmenopausal women: A prospective dose-response study. *Neurobiology of Aging, 56*, 1–6.

Albert, K. M., & Newhouse, P. A. (2019). Estrogen, stress, and depression: Cognitive and biological interactions. *Annual Review of Clinical Psychology, 15*(1), 399–423.

Allen, G., Barnard, H., McColl, R., Hester, A. L., Fields, J. A., Weiner, M. F., & Cullum, C. M. (2007). Reduced hippocampal functional connectivity in Alzheimer's disease. *Archives of Neurology, 64*(10), 1482–1487.

Allué, J. A., Leticia, S., Maria, I., Virginia, P. G., Noelia, F., Pascual-Lucas, M., … Sarasa, M. (2016). Outstanding phenotypic differences in the profile of amyloid-β between Tg2576 and APPswe/PS1dE9 transgenic mouse models of Alzheimer's disease. *Journal of Alzheimer's Disease, 53*(3), 773–785.

Altman, J. (1962). Are new neurons formed in the brains of adult mammals? *Science, 135*(3509), 1127–1128.

Altman, J., & Bayer, S. A. (1990). Mosaic organization of the hippocampal neuroepithelium and the multiple germinal sources of dentate granule cells. *Journal of Comparative Neurology, 301*(3), 325–342.

Altman, J., & Das, G. D. (1965). Autoradiographic and histological evidence of postnatal hippocampal neurogenesis in rats. *Journal of Comparative Neurology, 124*(3), 319–335.

Altmann, A., Tian, L., Henderson, V. W., & Greicius, M. D. (2014). Sex modifies the APOE-related risk, of developing Alzheimer's disease. *Annals of Neurology, 75*(4), 563–573.

Amrein, I., Isler, K., & Lipp, H. P. (2011). Comparing adult hippocampal neurogenesis in mammalian species and others: Influence of chronological age and life history stage. *European Journal of Neuroscience, 34*(6), 978–987.

Anacker, C., Luna, V. M., Stevens, G. S., Millette, A., Shores, R., Jimenez, J., … Hen, R. (2018). Hippocampal neurogenesis confers stress resilience by inhibiting the ventral dentate gyrus. *Nature, 559*(7712), 98–102.

Andersen, K., Launer, L. J., Dewey, M. E., Letenneur, L., Otta, A., Copeland, J. R., … Hofman, A. (1999). Gender differences in the incidence of AD and vascular dementia: The EURODEM studies. EURODEM Incidence Research Group. *Neurology, 53*(9), 1992–1997.

Andrew, M. K., & Tierney, M. C. (2018). The puzzle of sex, gender and Alzheimer's disease: Why are women more often affected than men? *Women's Health (London, England), 14*, 1745506518817995.

Anstead, G. M., Carlson, K. E., & Katzenellenbogen, J. A. (1997). The estradiol pharmacophore: Ligand structure-estrogen receptor binding affinity relationships and a model for the receptor binding site. *Steroids, 62*, 268–303.

Apostolova, L. G., Mosconi, L., Thompson, P. M., Green, A. E., Hwang, K. S., Ramirez, A., … de Leon, M. J. (2010). Subregional hippocampal atrophy predicts Alzheimer's dementia in the cognitively normal. *Neurobiology of Aging, 31*(7), 1077–1088.

Bae, J. B., Lipnicki, D. M., Han, J. W., Sachdev, P. S., Kim, T. H., Kwak, K. P., … Cohort Studies of Memory in an International Consortium (COSMIC). (2020). Does parity matter in women's risk of dementia? A COSMIC collaboration cohort study. *BMC Medicine, 18*(210). https://doi.org/10.1186/s12916-020-01671-1.

Baeza, I., De Castro, N. M., Giménez-Llort, L., & De la Fuente, M. (2010). Ovariectomy, a model of menopause in rodents, causes a premature aging of the nervous and immune systems. *Journal of Neuroimmunology, 219*(1–2), 90–99.

Banasr, M., Hery, M., Brezun, J. M., & Daszuta, A. (2001). Serotonin mediates oestrogen stimulation of cell proliferation in the adult dentate gyrus. *European Journal of Neuroscience, 14*(9), 1417–1424.

Barha, C. K., Dalton, G. L., & Galea, L. A. M. (2010). Low doses of 17alpha-estradiol and 17beta-estradiol facilitate, whereas higher doses of estrone and 17alpha- and 17beta-estradiol impair, contextual fear conditioning in adult female rats. *Neuropsychopharmacology: Official Publication of the American College of Neuropsychopharmacology, 35*(2), 547–559.

Barha, C. K., & Galea, L. A. M. (2011). Motherhood alters the cellular response to estrogens in the hippocampus later in life. *Neurobiology of Aging, 32*(11), 2091–2095.

Barha, C. K., Lieblich, S. E., Chow, C., & Galea, L. A. M. (2015). Multiparity-induced enhancement of hippocampal neurogenesis and spatial memory depends on ovarian hormone status in middle age. *Neurobiology of Aging, 36*(8), 2391–2405.

Barha, C. K., Lieblich, S. E., & Galea, L. A. M. (2009). Different forms of oestrogen rapidly upregulate cell proliferation in the dentate gyrus of adult female Rats. *Journal of Neuroendocrinology, 21*(3), 155–166.

Barker, J. M., & Galea, L. A. M. (2008). Repeated estradiol administration alters different aspects of neurogenesis and cell death in the hippocampus of female, but not male, rats. *Neuroscience, 152*(4), 888–902.

Barnes, L. L., Wilson, R. S., Bienias, J. L., Schneider, J. A., Evans, D. A., & Bennett, D. A. (2005). Sex differences in the clinical manifestations of Alzheimer disease pathology. *Archives of General Psychiatry, 62*(6), 685–691.

Barnett, S. C., Perry, B. A. L., Dalrymple-Alford, J. C., & Parr-Brownlie, L. C. (2018). Optogenetic stimulation: Understanding memory and treating deficits. *Hippocampus, 28*(7), 457–479.

Barrera, Á., Jiménez, L., González, G. M., Monitle, J., & Aboitiz, F. (2001). Dendritic structure of single hippocampal neurons according to sex and hemisphere of origin in middle-aged and elderly human subjects. *Brain Research, 906*(1–2), 31–37.

Barrière, A. D., Ella, A., Szeremeta, F., Adriaensen, H., Même, W., Chaillou, E., … Keller, M. (2020). Brain orchestration of pregnancy and maternal behavior in mice. *bioRxiv, 2020*.05.23.112045.

Barth, C., Steele, C. J., Mueller, K., Rekkas, V. P., Arélin, K., Pampel, A., ... Sacher, J. (2016). In-vivo dynamics of the human hippocampus across the menstrual cycle. *Scientific Reports*, *6*(1), 1–9.

Beam, C. R., Kaneshiro, C., Jang, J. Y., Reynolds, C. A., Pedersen, N. L., & Gatz, M. (2018). Differences between women and men in incidence rates of dementia and Alzheimer's disease. *Journal of Alzheimer's Disease*, *64*(4), 1077–1083.

Becker, J. B., & Koob, G. F. (2016). Sex differences in animal models: Focus on addiction. *Pharmacological Reviews*, *68*(2), 242–263.

Beckervordersandforth, R., Zhang, C. L., & Liu, D. C. (2015). Transcription-factor-dependent control of adult hippocampal neurogenesis. *Cold Spring Harbor Perspectives in Biology*, *7*(10), a018879.

Beeri, M. S., Rapp, M., Schmeidler, J., Reichenberg, A., Purohit, D. P., Perl, D. P., ... Silverman, J. M. (2009). Number of children is associated with neuropathology of Alzheimer's disease in women. *Neurobiology of Aging*, *30*(8), 1184–1191.

Beydoun, M. A., Boueiz, A., Abougergi, M. S., Kitner-Triolo, M. H., Beyduon, H. A., Resnick, S. M., ... Zonderman, A. B. (2012). Sex differences in the association of the apolipoprotein E epsilon 4 allele with incidence of dementia, cognitive impairment, and decline. *Neurobiology of Aging*, *33*(4), 720–731.

Biscaro, B., Lindvall, O., Hock, C., Ekdahi, C. T., & Nitsch, R. M. (2009). Abeta immunotherapy protects morphology and survival of adult-born neurons in doubly transgenic APP/PS1 mice. *Journal of Neuroscience*, *29*(45), 14108–14119.

Bizon, J. L., LaSarge, C. L., Montgomery, K. S., McDermott, A. N., Setlow, B., & Griffith, W. H. (2009). Spatial reference and working memory across the lifespan of male Fischer 344 rats. *Neurobiology of Aging*, *30*(4), 646–655.

Bohacek, J., & Daniel, J. M. (2009). The ability of oestradiol administration to regulate protein levels of oestrogen receptor alpha in the hippocampus and prefrontal cortex of middle-aged rats is altered following long-term ovarian hormone deprivation. *Journal of Neuroendocrinology*, *21*(7), 640–647.

Bohacek, J., & Daniel, J. M. (2010). The beneficial effects of estradiol on attentional processes are dependent on timing of treatment initiation following ovariectomy in middle-aged rats. *Psychoneuroendocrinology*, *35*(5), 694–705.

Boldrini, M., Fulmore, C. A., Tartt, A. N., Simeon, L. R., Pavlova, I., Poposka, V., ... Mann, J. J. (2018). Human hippocampal neurogenesis persists throughout aging. *Cell Stem Cell*, *22*(4), 589–599.e5.

Bour, A., Grootendorst, J., Vogel, E., Kelche, C., Dodart, J. C., Bales, K., ... Mathis, C. (2008). Middle-aged human apoE4 targeted-replacement mice show retention deficits on a wide range of spatial memory tasks. *Behavioural Brain Research*, *193*(2), 174–182.

Bove, R., Secor, E., Chibnik, L. B., Barnes, L. L., Schneider, J. A., Bennett, D. A., & De Jager, P. L. (2014). Age at surgical menopause influences cognitive decline and Alzheimer pathology in older women. *Neurology*, *82*(3), 222–229.

Boyle, P. A., Wilson, R. S., Aggarwal, N. T., Tang, Y., & Bennett, D. A. (2006). Mild cognitive impairment. *Neurology*, *67*(3).

Brailoiu, E., Dun, S. L., Brailoiu, G. C., Mizuo, K., Sklar, L. A., Opera, T. I., ... Dun, N. J. (2007). Distribution and characterization of estrogen receptor G protein-coupled receptor 30 in the rat central nervous system. *Journal of Endocrinology*, *193*(2), 311–321.

Brinton, R. D. (2008). The healthy cell bias of estrogen action: Mitochondrial bioenergetics and neurological implications. *Trends in Neurosciences*, *31*(10), 529–537.

Broadbent, N. J., Squire, L. R., & Clark, R. E. (2004). Spatial memory, recognition memory, and the hippocampus. *Proceedings of the National Academy of Sciences of the United States of America, 101*(40), 14515–14520.

Brookmeyer, R., Gray, S., & Kawas, C. (1998). Projections of Alzheimer's disease in the United States and the public health impact of delaying disease onset. *American Journal of Public Health, 88*(9), 1337–1342.

Brown, C. M., Choi, E., Xu, Q., Vitek, M. P., & Colton, C. A. (2008). The APOE4 genotype alters the response of microglia and macrophages to 17β-estradiol. *Neurobiology of Aging, 29*(12), 1783–1794.

Brown, J. P., Couillard-Després, S., Cooper-Kuhn, C. M., Winkler, J., Aigner, L., & Kuhn, H. G. (2003). Transient expression of doublecortin during adult neurogenesis. *Journal of Comparative Neurology, 467*(1), 1–10.

Brzozowski, A. M., Pike, A. C. W., Dauter, Z., Hubbard, R. E., Bonn, T., Engström, O., … Carlquist, M. (1997). Molecular basis of agonism and antagonism in the oestrogen receptor. *Nature, 389*(6652), 753–758.

Buchanan, G., Yang, M., Cheong, A., Harris, J. M., Irvine, R. A., Lambert, P. F., … Tilley, W. D. (2004). Structural and functional consequences of glutamine tract variation in the androgen receptor. *Human Molecular Genetics, 13*(16), 1677–1692.

Burkhardt, M. S., Foster, J. K., Laws, S. M., Baker, L. D., Craft, S., Gandy, S. E., … Martins, R. N. (2004). Oestrogen replacement therapy may improve memory functioning in the absence of APOE ε4. *Journal of Alzheimer's Disease, 6*(3), 221–228.

Busse, A., Hensel, A., Gühne, U., Angermeyer, M. C., & Riedel-Heller, S. G. (2006). Mild cognitive impairment: Long-term course of four clinical subtypes. *Neurology, 67*(12), 2176–2185.

Buttini, M., Yu, G. Q., Shockley, K., Huang, Y., Jones, B., Masliah, E., … Mucke, L. (2002). Modulation of Alzheimer-like synaptic and cholinergic deficits in transgenic mice by human apolipoprotein E depends on isoform, aging, and overexpression of amyloid beta peptides but not on plaque formation. *Journal of Neuroscience, 22*(24), 10539–10548.

Buwalda, B., van der Borght, K., Koolhaas, J. M., & McEwen, B. S. (2010). Testosterone decrease does not play a major role in the suppression of hippocampal cell proliferation following social defeat stress in rats. *Physiology and Behavior, 101*(5), 719–725.

Buzsaki, G., & Moser, E. I. (2013). Memory, navigation, and theta rhythm in the hippocampal-entorhinal system. *Nature Neuroscience, 16*, 130–138.

Cameron, H. A., Woolley, C. S., McEwen, B. S., & Gould, E. (1993). Differentiation of newly born neurons and glia in the dentate gyrus of the adult rat. *Neuroscience, 56*(2), 337–344.

Carcaillon, L., Brailly-Tabard, S., Ancelin, M., Tzourio, C., Foubert-Samier, A, Dartigues, JF, et al. (2014). Low testosterone and the risk of dementia in elderly men: Impact of age and education. *Alzheimer's & Dementia, 10*, 306–314 (in Spanish).

Carolino, R. O. G., Barros, P. T., Kalil, B., & Anselmo-Franci, J. (2019). Endocrine profile of the VCD-induced perimenopausal model rat. *PLoS One, 14*(12), e0226874.

Carrier, N., & Kabbaj, M. (2012). Testosterone and imipramine have antidepressant effects in socially isolated male but not female rats. *Hormones and Behavior, 61*(5), 678–685.

Carter, D. B., Dunn, E., McKinley, D. D., Stratman, N. C., Boyle, T. P., Kuiper, S. L., … Gurney, M. E. (2001). Human apolipoprotein E4 accelerates beta-amyloid deposition in APPsw transgenic mouse brain. *Annals of Neurology, 50*(4), 468–475.

Castellano, J. M., Kim, J., Stewart, F. R., Jiang, H., DeMattos, R. B., Patterson, B. W., … Holtzman, D. M. (2011). Human apoE isoforms differentially regulate brain amyloid-β peptide clearance. *Science Translational Medicine, 3*(89), 89ra57.

References

Chakrabarti, S., Khemka, V. K., Banerjee, A., Chatterjee, G., Ganguly, A., & Biswas, A. (2015). Metabolic risk factors of sporadic Alzheimer's disease: Implications in the pathology, pathogenesis, and treatment. *Aging and Disease, 6*(4), 282–299.

Chen, S., Nilsen, J., & Brinton, R. D. (2006). Dose and temporal pattern of estrogen exposure determines neuroprotective outcome in hippocampal neurons: Therapeutic implications. *Endocrinology, 147*(11), 5303–5313.

Chen, S., Wang, J. M., Irwin, R. W., Yao, J., Liu, L., & Brinton, R. D. (2011). Allopregnanolone promotes regeneration and reduces B-amyloid burden in a preclinical model of Alzheimer's disease. *PLoS One, 6*(8), e24293.

Cherrier, M. M., Matsumoto, A. M., Amory, J. K., Asthana, S., Bremner, W., Peskind, E. R., … Craft, S. (2005). Testosterone improves spatial memory in men with Alzheimer disease and mild cognitive impairment. *Neurology, 64*(12), 2063–2068.

Chiba, S., Suzuki, M., Yamanouchi, K., & Nishihara, M. (2007). Involvement of granulin in estrogen-induced neurogenesis in the adult rat hippocampus. *Journal of Reproduction and Development, 53*(2), 297–307.

Choi, S. H., Bylykbashi, E., Chatila, Z. K., Lee, S. W., Pulli, B., Clemenson, G. D., … Tanzi, R. E. (2018). Combined adult neurogenesis and BDNF mimic exercise effects on cognition in an Alzheimer's mouse model. *Science, 361*(6406).

Choleris, E., Galea, L. A. M., Sohrabji, F., & Frick, K. M. (2018). Sex differences in the brain: Implications for behavioural and biomedical research. *Neuroscience and Biobehavioural Reviews, 85*, 126–145.

Chow, C., Epp, J. R., Lieblich, S. E., Barha, C. K., & Galea, L. A. M. (2013). Sex difference in neurogenesis and activation of new neurons in response to spatial learning and memory. *Psychoneuroendocrinology, 38*, 1236–1250.

Clelland, C. D., Choi, M., Romberg, C., Clemenson, G. D., Jr., Fragniere, A., Tyers, P., … Bussey, T. J. (2009). A functional role for adult hippocampal neurogenesis in spatial pattern separation. *Science, 325*(5937), 210–213.

Cohen, R. M., Rezai-Zadeh, K., Weitz, T. M., Rentsendorj, A., Gate, D., Spivak, I., … Town, T. (2013). A transgenic Alzheimer rat with plaques, tau pathology, behavioural impairment, oligomeric aβ, and frank neuronal loss. *Journal of Neuroscience, 33*(15), 6245–6256.

Colucci, M., Cammarata, S., Assini, A., Croce, R., Clerici, F., Novello, C., … Tanganelli, P. (2006). The number of pregnancies is a risk factor for Alzheimer's disease. *European Journal of Neurology, 13*(12), 1374–1377.

Craig, M. C., Maki, P. M., & Murphy, D. G. (2005). The women's health initiative memory study: Findings and implications for treatment. *The Lancet Neurology, 4*(3), 190–194.

Cui, J., Jothishankar, B., He, P., Staufenbiel, M., Shen, Y., & Li, R. (2014). Amyloid precursor protein mutation disrupts reproductive experience-enhanced normal cognitive development in a mouse model of Alzheimer's disease. *Molecular Neurobiology, 49*(1), 102–112.

Cui, J., Shen, Y., & Li, R. (2013). Estrogen synthesis and signaling pathways during aging: From periphery to brain. *Trends in Molecular Medicine, 19*(3), 197–209.

Dalla, C., Papachristos, E. F., Whetstone, A. S., & Shors, T. J. (2009). Female rats learn trace memories better than male rats and consequently retain a greater proportion of new neurons in their hippocampi. *Proceedings of the National Academy of Sciences of the United States of America, 106*(8), 2927–2932.

Damoiseaux, J. S., Seeley, W. W., Zhou, J., Shirer, W. R., Coppola, G., Karydas, A., … ADNI. (2012). Gender modulates the APOE ε4 effect in healthy older adults: Convergent evidence from functional brain connectivity and spinal fluid tau levels. *The Journal of Neuroscience, 32*(24), 8254–8262.

Daniel, J. M., & Bohacek, J. (2010). The critical period hypothesis of estrogen effects on cognition: Insights from basic research. *Biochimica et Biophysica Acta (BBA)—General Subjects*, *1800*(10), 1068–1076.

Darnaudéry, M., Perez-Martin, M., Del Favero, F., Gomez-Roldan, C., Garcia-Segura, L. M., & Maccari, S. (2007). Early motherhood in rats is associated with a modification of hippocampal function. *Psychoneuroendocrinology*, *32*(7), 803–812.

de Lange, A.-M. G., Barth, C., Kaufmann, T., Anatürk, M., Suri, S., Ebmeier, K. P., & Westlye, L. T. (2020). The maternal brain: Region-specific patterns of brain aging are traceable decades after childbirth. *Human Brain Mapping*, *41*(16), 4718–4729. https://doi.org/10.1002/hbm.25152.

de Lange, A.-M. G., Barth, C., Kaufmann, T., Maximov, I. I., van der Meer, D., Agartz, I., & Westlye, L. T. (2020). Women's brain aging: Effects of sex-hormone exposure, pregnancies, and genetic risk for Alzheimer's disease. *Human Brain Mapping*, *41*, 5141–5150.

de Lange, A. M. G., Kaufmann, T., van der Meer, D., Maglanoc, L. A., Alnæs, D., Moberget, T., ... Westlye, L. T. (2019). Population-based neuroimaging reveals traces of childbirth in the maternal brain. *Proceedings of the National Academy of Sciences of the United States of America*, *116*(44), 22341–22346.

Demars, M., Hu, Y., Gadadhar, A., & Lazarov, O. (2010). Impaired neurogenesis is an early event in the etiology of familial Alzheimer's disease in transgenic mice. *Journal of Neuroscience Research*, *88*(1), 2103–2117.

Devanand, D. P., Bansal, B., Liu, J., Hao, X., Pradhaban, G., & Peterson, B. S. (2012). MRI hippocampal and entorhinal cortex mapping in predicting conversion to Alzheimer's disease. *NeuroImage*, *60*(3), 1622–1629.

DeVries, G. J. (2004). Minireview: Sex differences in adult and developing brains: Compensation, compensation, compensation. *Endocrinology*, *145*(3), 1063–1068.

DiBattista, A. M., Heinsinger, N. M., & Rebeck, G. W. (2016). Alzheimer's disease genetic risk factor APOE-ε4 also affects normal brain function. *Current Alzheimer Research*, *13*(11), 1200–1207.

Dillon, S. E., Tsivos, D., Knight, M., McCann, B., Pennington, C., Shiel, A. I., ... Coulthard, E. J. (2017). The impact of ageing reveals distinct roles for human dentate gyrus and CA3 in pattern separation and object recognition memory. *Scientific Reports*, *7*(14069), 1–13.

Dodart, J. C., Bales, K. R., Johnstone, E. M., Little, S. P., & Paul, S. M. (2002). Apolipoprotein E alters the processing of the beta-amyloid precursor protein in APP (V717F) transgenic mice. *Brain Research*, *955*(1-2), 191–199.

Dorszewska, J., Prendecki, M., Oczkowska, A., Dezor, M., & Kozubski, W. (2016). Molecular basis of familial and sporadic Alzheimer's disease. *Current Alzheimer Research*, *13*(9), 952–963.

Drapeau, E., Mayo, W., Aurousseau, C., Moal, M. L., Piazza, P. V., & Abrous, D. N. (2003). Spatial memory performances of aged rats in the water maze predict levels of hippocampal neurogenesis. *Proceedings of the National Academy of Sciences of the United States of America*, *100*(24), 14385–14390.

Driscoll, I., Howard, S. R., Stone, J. C., Monfils, M. H., Tomanek, B., Brooks, W. M., & Sutherland, R. J. (2006). The aging hippocampus: A multi-level analysis in the rat. *Neuroscience*, *139*(4), 1173–1185.

Drummond, E., & Wisniewski, T. (2017). Alzheimer's disease: Experimental models and reality. *Acta Neuropathology*, *133*(2), 155–175.

Duara, R., Lopez-Alberola, R. F., Barker, W. W., Loewenstein, D. A., Zatinsky, M., Eisdorfer, C. E., & Weinberg, G. B. (1993). A comparison of familial and sporadic Alzheimer's disease. *Neurology, 43*(7), 1377–1384.

Duarte-Guterman, P., Albert, A. Y., Barha, C. K., & Galea, L. A. M. (in press). Sex influences the effects of APOE genotype and Alzheimer's diagnosis on neuropathology and memory. Psychoneuroendocrinology.

Duarte-Guterman, P., Leuner, B., & Galea, L. A. M. (2019). The long and short term effects of motherhood on the brain. *Frontiers in Neuroendocrinology, 53*, 100740.

Duarte-Guterman, P., Lieblich, S. E., Wainwright, S. R., Chow, C., Chaiton, J. A., Watson, N. V., & Galea, L. A. M. (2019). Androgens enhance adult hippocampal neurogenesis in males but not females in an age-dependent manner. *Endocrinology, 160*(9), 2128–2136.

Duarte-Guterman, P., Yagi, S., Chow, C., & Galea, L. A. M. (2015). Hippocampal learning, memory, and neurogenesis: Effects of sex and estrogens across the lifespan in adults. *Hormones and Behavior, 74*, 37–52.

Eberling, J. L., Wu, C., Haan, M. N., Mungas, D., Buonocore, M., & Jagust, W. J. (2003). Preliminary evidence that estrogen protects against age-related hippocampal atrophy. *Neurobiology of Aging, 24*(5), 725–732.

Edland, S. D., Rocca, W. A., Petersen, R. C., Cha, R. H., & Kokmen, E. (2002). Dementia and Alzheimer's disease incidence rates do not vary by sex in Rochester, Minn. *Archives in Neurology, 59*(1), 1589–1593.

Edmonds, E. C., McDonald, C. R., Marshall, A., Thomas, K. R., Eppig, J., Weigand, A. J., … Alzheimer's Disease Neuroimaging Initiative. (2019). Early versus late MCI: Improved MCI staging using a neuropsychological approach. *Alzheimer's & Dementia, 15*(5), 699–708.

Edwards, G. A., Gamez, N., Escobedo, G., Calderon, O., & Moreno-Gonzalez, I. (2019). Modifiable risk factors for Alzheimer's disease. *Frontiers in Aging Neuroscience, 11*(146), 1–18.

Eid, R. S., Chaiton, J. A., Lieblich, S. E., Bodnar, T. S., Weinberg, J., & Galea, L. A. M. (2019). Early and late effects of maternal experience on hippocampal neurogenesis, microglia, and the circulating cytokine milieu. *Neurobiology of Aging, 78*, 1–17.

Eid, R. S., Lieblich, S. E., Duarte-Guterman, P., Chaiton, J. A., Mah, A. G., Wong, S. J., … Galea, L. A. M. (2020). Selective activation of estrogen receptors α and β: Implications for depressive-like phenotypes in female mice exposed to chronic unpredictable stress. *Hormones and Behavior, 119*, 104651.

Ekonomou, A., Savva, G. M., Brayne, C., Forster, G., Francis, P. T., Johnson, M., … Ballard, C. G. (2015). Stage-specific changes in neurogenic and glial markers in Alzheimer's disease. *Biological Psychiatry, 77*, 711–719.

Epp, J. R., Chow, C., & Galea, L. A. M. (2013). Hippocampus-dependent learning influences hippocampal neurogenesis. *Frontiers in Neuroscience, 7*(57).

Epp, J. R., Haack, A. K., & Galea, L. A. M. (2011). Activation and survival of immature neurons in the dentate gyrus with spatial memory is dependent on time of exposure to spatial learning and age of cells at examination. *Neurobiology of Learning and Memory, 95*(2011), 316–325.

Epperson, C. N., Sammel, M. D., & Freeman, E. W. (2013). Menopause effects on verbal memory: Findings from a longitudinal community cohort. *Journal of Clinical Endocrinology and Metabolism, 98*(9), 3829–3838.

Eriksson, P. S., Perfilieva, E., Bjork-Eriksson, T., Alborn, A. M., Nordborg, C., Peterson, D. A., & Gage, F. H. (1998). Neurogenesis in the adult human hippocampus. *Nature Medicine, 4*(11), 1313–1317.

Ernst, A., Alkass, K., Bernard, S., Salehpour, M., Perl, S., Tisdale, J., … Frisen, J. (2014). Neurogenesis in the striatum of the adult human brain. *Cell*, *156*(5), 1072–1083.

Espeland, M. A., Rapp, S. R., Shumaker, S. A., Brunner, R., Manson, J. A. E., Sherwin, B. B., … Hays, J. (2004). Conjugated equine estrogens and global cognitive funtion in postmenopausal women: Women's health initiative memory study. *Journal of the American Medical Association*, *291*(24), 2959–2968.

Espeland, M., Shumaker, S., Leng, I., Manson, J., Brown, C., LeBlanc, E., … Resnick, S. (2013). Long-term effects on cognitive function of postmenopausal hormone therapy prescribed to women aged 50-54 years: Results from the women's health initiative memory study of younger women (WHIMSY). *Alzheimer's & Dementia*, *9*, 529–530.

Farrer, L. A., Cupples, L. A., Haines, J. L., Hyman, B., Kukull, W. A., Mayeux, R., … van Duijn, C. M. (1997). Effects of age, sex, and ethnicity on the association between apolipoprotein E genotype and Alzheimer's disease. A meta-analysis. APOE and Alzheimer Disease Meta Analysis Consortium. *JAMA*, *278*(16), 1349–1356.

Ferretti, M. T., Iulita, M. F., Cavedo, E., Chiesa, P. A., Schumacher Dimech, A., Chadha, A., … Hampel, H. (2018). Sex differences in Alzheimer's disease—The gateway to precision medicine. *Nature Reviews. Neurology*, *14*(8), 457–469.

Finch, C. E., & Gosden, R. G. (1986). Animal models for the human menopause. In L. Mastroianni, & C. A. Paulsen (Eds.), *Aging, reproduction, and the climacteric* (pp. 3–34). Boston, MA: Springer.

Finkel, D., Reynolds, C. A., McArdle, J. J., Gatz, M., & Pedersen, N. L. (2003). Latent growth curve analyses of accelerating decline in cognitive abilities in late adulthood. *Developmental Psychology*, *38*(3), 535–550.

Fiorentini, A., Rosi, M. C., Grossi, C., Luccarini, I., & Casamenti, F. (2010). Lithium improves hippocampal neurogenesis, neuropathology and cognitive functions in APP mutant mice. *PLoS One*, *5*(12), e14382.

Fischbeck, K. H. (2001). Polyglutamine expansion neurodegenerative disease. *Brain Research Bulletin*, *56*(3–4), 161–163.

Flaws, J. A., Doerr, J. K., Sipes, I. G., & Hoyer, P. B. (1994). Destruction of preantral follicles in adult rats by 4-vinyl-1-cyclohexene diepoxide. *Reproductive Toxicology*, *8*(6), 509–514.

Fox, M., Berzuini, C., & Knapp, L. A. (2013a). Cumulative estrogen exposure, number of menstrual cycles, and Alzheimer's risk in a cohort of British women. *Psychoneuroendocrinology*, *38*(12), 2973–2982.

Fox, M., Berzuini, C., & Knapp, L. A. (2013b). Maternal breastfeeding history and Alzheimer's disease risk. *Journal of Alzheimer's Disease*, *37*(4), 809–821.

Frick, K. M., Burlingame, L. A., Arters, J. A., & Berger-Sweeney, J. (1999). Reference memory, anxiety and estrous cyclicity in 57BL/6NIA mice are affected by age and sex. *Neuroscience*, *95*(1), 293–307.

Furuta, M., & Bridges, R. S. (2005). Gestation-induced cell proliferation in the rat brain. *Developmental Brain Research*, *156*(1), 61–66.

Gage, F. H. (2019). Adult neurogenesis in mammals. *Science*, *364*(6443), 827–828.

Galea, L. A., Frick, K. M., Hampson, E., Sohrabji, F., & Choleris, E. (2017). Why estrogens matter for behavior and brain health. *Neuroscience & Biobehavioral Reviews*, *76*, 363–379.

Galea, L. A. M., & McEwen, B. S. (1999). Sex and seasonal differences in the rate of cell proliferation in the dentate gyrus of adult wild meadow voles. *Neuroscience*, *89*(3), 955–964.

Galea, L. A. M., McEwen, B. S., Tanapat, P., Deak, T., Spencer, R. L., & Dhabhar, F. S. (1997). Sex differences in dendritic atrophy of CA3 pyramidal neurons in response to chronic restraint stress. *Neuroscience*, *81*(3), 689–697.

Galea, L. A. M., Ormerod, B. K., Sampath, S., Kostaras, X., Wilkie, D. M., & Phelps, M. T. (2000). Spatial working memory and hippocampal size across pregnancy in rats. *Hormones and Behavior*, *37*, 86–95.

Galea, L. A., Qiu, W., & Duarte-Guterman, P. (2018). Beyond sex differences: Short and long-term implications of motherhood on women's health. *Current Opinion in Physiology*, *6*, 82–88.

Galea, L. A. M., Roes, M. M., Dimech, C. J., Chow, C., Mahmoud, R., Lieblich, S. E., & Duarte-Guterman, P. (2018). Premarin has opposing effects on spatial learning, neural activation, and serum cytokine levels in middle-aged female rats depending on reproductive history. *Neurobiology of Aging*, *70*, 291–307.

Galea, L. A. M., Spritzer, M. D., Barker, J. M., & Pawluski, J. L. (2006). Gonadal hormone modulation of hippocampal neurogenesis in the adult. *Hippocampus*, *16*(3), 225–232.

Galea, L. A. M., Wainwright, S. R., Roes, M. M., Duarte-Guterman, P., Chow, C., & Hamson, D. K. (2013). Sex, hormones and neurogenesis in the hippocampus: Hormonal modulation of neurogenesis and potential functional implications. *Journal of Neuroendocrinology*, *25*(11), 1039–1061.

Gan, L., Qiao, S., Lan, X., Chi, L., Luo, C., Lien, L., … Liu, R. (2008). Neurogenic responses to amyloid-beta plaques in the brain of Alzheimer's disease-like transgenic (pPDGF-APPSw,Ind) mice. *Neurobiology of Disease*, *29*(1), 71–80.

Gatewood, J. D., Morgan, M. D., Eaton, M., McNamara, I. M., Stevens, L. F., MacBeth, A. H., … Kinsley, C. H. (2005). Motherhood mitigates aging-related decrements in learning and memory and positively affects brain aging in the rat. *Brain Research Bulletin*, *66*(2), 91–98.

Geller, S. E., Koch, A., Pelletieri, B., & Carnes, M. (2011). Inclusion, analysis, and reporting of sex and race/ethnicity in clinical trials: Have we made progress? *Journal of Women's Health*, *20*(3), 315–320.

Georgakis, M. K., Beskou-Kontou, T., Theodoridis, I., Skalkidou, A., & Petridou, E. T. (2019). Surgical menopause in association with cognitive function and risk of dementia: A systematic review and meta-analysis. *Psychoneuroendocrinology*, *106*, 9–19.

Gerstorf, D., & Ram, N. (2011). Cohort differences in cognitive aging and terminal decline in the Seattle longitudinal study. *Developmental Psychology*, *47*(4), 1026–1041.

Gervais, N. J., Baker-Sullivan, E., Grady, C., Olsen, R., Gravelsins, L., Reuben, R. B., & Einstein, G. (2018). P3-373: Structural integrity of the medial temporal lobe and recognition memory following natural and surgical menopause. *Alzheimer's & Dementia*, *14*(7S_Part_23), P1234.

Giannakopoulos, P., Hermann, F. R., Bussière, T., Bouras, C., Kövari, E., Perl, D. P., … Hof, P. R. (2003). Tangle and neuron numbers, but not amyloid load, predict cognitive status in Alzheimer's disease. *Neurology*, *60*(9), 1495–1500.

Gibbs, R. A., Weinstock, G. M., Metzker, M. L., Muzny, D. M., Sodergren, E. J., Scherer, S., … Collins, R. (2004). Genome sequence of the Brown Norway rat yields insights into mammalian evolution. *Nature*, *428*(6982), 493–521.

Gibbs, R. B. (2010). Estrogen therapy and cognition: A review of the cholinergic hypothesis. *Endocrine Reviews*, *21*(2), 224–253. https://doi.org/10.1210/er.2009-0036.

González, M., Cabrera-Socorro, A., Pérez-Garcia, C. G., Fraser, J. D., López, F. J., Alonso, R., & Meyer, G. (2007). Distribution patterns of estrogen receptor alpha and beta in the human cortex and hippocampus during development and adulthood. *Journal of Comparative Neurology*, *503*(6), 790–802.

Gould, E., Beylin, A., Tanapat, P., Reeves, A., & Shors, T. J. (1999). Learning enhances adult neurogenesis in the hippocampal formation. *Nature Neuroscience*, *2*(3), 260–265.

Gould, E., Reeves, A. J., Fallah, M., Tanapat, P., Gross, C. G., & Fuchs, E. (1999). Hippocampal neurogenesis in adult Old World primates. *Proceedings of the National Academy of Sciences of the United States of America*, *96*, 5263–5267.

Gould, E., Westlind-Danielsson, A., Frankfurt, M., & McEwen, B. S. (1990). Sex differences and thyroid hormone sensitivity of hippocampal pyramidal cells. *Journal of Neuroscience*, *10*(3), 996–1003.

Gray, J. D., & McEwen, B. S. (2013). Lithium's role in neural plasticity and its implications for mood disorders. *Acta Psychiatrica Scandinavica*, *128*(5), 347–361.

Green, A. D., & Galea, L. A. M. (2008). Adult hippocampal cell proliferation is suppressed with estrogen withdrawal after a hormone-simulated pregnancy. *Hormones and Behavior*, *54*(1), 203–211.

Gur, R. E., & Gur, R. C. (2002). Gender differences in aging: Cognition, emotions, and neuroimaging studies. *Dialogues in Clinical Neuroscience*, *4*(2), 197–210.

Gutierrez-Lobos, K., Scherer, M., Anderer, P., & Katschnig, H. (2002). The influence of age on the female/male ratio of treated incidence rates in depression. *BMC Psychiatry*, *2*(3).

Hamson, D. K., Wainwright, S. R., Taylor, J. R., Jones, B. A., Watson, N. V., & Galea, L. A. M. (2013). Androgens increase survival of adult-born neurons in the dentate gyrus by an androgen receptor-dependent mechanism in male rats. *Endocrinology*, *154*(9), 3294–3304.

Harman, S. M., Metter, E. J., Tobin, J. D., Pearson, J., Blackman, M. R., & Baltimore Longitudinal Study of Aging. (2001). Longitudinal effects of aging on serum total and free testosterone levels in healthy men. Baltimore Longitudinal Study of Aging. *Journal of Clinical Endocrinology and Metabolism*, *88*(2), 724–731.

Hartman, R. E., Wozniak, D. F., Nardi, A., Olney, J. W., Sartorius, L., & Holtzman, D. M. (2001). Behavioural phenotyping of GFAP-apoE3 and -apoE4 transgenic mice: ApoE4 mice show profound working memory impairments in the absence of Alzheimer's-like neuropathology. *Experimental Neurology*, *170*(2), 326–344.

Hattiangady, B., Rao, M. S., Shetty, G. A., & Shetty, A. K. (2005). Brain-derived neurotrophic factor, phosphorylated cyclic AMP response element binding protein and neuropeptide Y decline as early as middle age in the dentate gyrus and CA1 and CA3 subfields of the hippocampus. *Experimental Neurology*, *195*(2), 353–371.

Haughey, N. J., Nath, A., Chan, S. L., Borchard, A. C., Rao, M. S., & Mattson, M. P. (2002). Disruption of neurogenesis by amyloid β-peptide, and perturbed neural progenitor cell homeostasis, in models of Alzheimer's disease. *Journal of Neurochemistry*, *83*(6), 1509–1524.

Hazell, G. G., Yao, S. T., Roper, J. A., Prossnitz, E. R., O'Carroll, A. M., & Lolait, S. J. (2009). Localisation of GPR30, a novel G protein-coupled oestrogen receptor, suggests multiple functions in rodent brain and peripheral tissues. *Journal of Endocrinology*, *202*(2), 223–236.

Heidrich, A., Schleyer, M., Spingler, H., Albert, P., Knoche, M., Fritze, J., & Lanczik, M. (1994). Postpartum blues: Relationship between non-protein bound steroid hormones in plasma and postpartum mood changes. *Journal of Affective Disorders*, *30*(2), 94–98.

Heikkinen, A. M., Niskanen, L., Ryynänen, M., Komulainen, M. H., Tuppurainen, M. T., Parviainen, M., & Saarikoski, S. (1999). Is the response of serum lipids and lipoproteins to postmenopausal hormone replacement therapy modified by apoE genotype? *Arteriosclerosis, Thrombosis, and Vascular Biology*, *19*(2), 402–407.

Henderson, V. W., Paganini-Hill, A., Miller, B. L., Elble, R. J., Reyes, P. F., Shoupe, D., … Farlow, M. R. (2000). Estrogen for Alzheimer's disease in women. *Neurology*, *48*(6), 1517–1521.

Henderson, V. W., & Rocca, W. A. (2012). Estrogens and Alzheimer disease risk: Is there a window of opportunity? *Neurology*, *79*(18), 1840–1841.

Hillerer, K. M., Jacobs, V. R., Fischer, T., & Aigner, L. (2014). The maternal brain: An organ with peripartal plasticity. *Neural Plasticity*, *2014*, 1–20. https://doi.org/10.1155/2014/574159.

Hirata-Fukae, C., Li, H. F., Hoe, H. S., Gray, A. J., Miniami, S. S., Hamada, K., ... Matsuoka, Y. (2008). Female exhibit more extensive amyloid, but not tau, pathology in an Alzheimer transgenic model. *Brain Research*, *24*(1216), 92–103.

Hoekzema, E., Barba-Müller, E., Pozzobon, C., Picado, M., Lucco, F., García-García, D., ... Ballesteros, A. (2017). Pregnancy leads to long-lasting changes in human brain structure. *Nature Neuroscience*, *20*(2), 287–296.

Hogervorst, E., Bandelow, S., Combrinck, M., & Smith, A. D. (2004). Low free testosterone is an independent risk factor for Alzheimer's disease. *Experimental Gerontology*, *39*(11–12 Spec. Iss), 1633–1639.

Hogervorst, E., Combrinck, M., & Smith, A. D. (2003). Testosterone and gonadotropin levels in men with dementia. *Neuroendocrinology Letters*, *24*(3–4), 203–208.

Hogervorst, E., Williams, J., Budge, M., Riedel, W., & Jolles, J. (2000). The nature of the effect of female gonadal hormone replacement therapy on cognitive function in post-menopausal women: A meta-analysis. *Neuroscience*, *101*(3), 485–512.

Hohman, T. J., Dumitrescu, L., & Barnes, L. L. (2018). Sex-specific association of apolipoprotein E with cerebrospinal fluid levels of tau. *JAMA Neurology*, *75*(8), 989–998.

Holland, D., Desikan, R. S., Dale, A. M., & McEvoy, L. K. (2013). Higher rates of decline for women and APOE ε4 carriers. *AJNR. American Journal of Neuroradiology*, *34*(12), 2287–2293.

Hollands, C., Tobin, M. K., Hsu, M., Musaraca, K., Yu, T., Mishra, R., ... Lazarov, O. (2017). Depletion of adult neurogenesis exacerbates cognitive deficits in Alzheimer's disease by compromising hippocampal inhibition. *Molecular Neurodegeneration*, *12*(64), 1–13.

Holmes, C., & Lovestone, S. (2002). The clinical phenotype of familial and sporadic late onset Alzheimer's disease. *International Journal of Geriatric Psychiatry*, *17*(2), 146–149.

Holtzman, D. M., Bales, K. R., Tenkova, T., Fagan, A. M., Parsadanian, M., Sartorius, L. J., ... Paul, S. M. (2000). Apolipoprotein E isoform-dependent amyloid deposition and neuritic degeneration in a mouse model of Alzheimer's disease. *Proceedings of the National Academy of Sciences of the United States of America*, *97*(6), 2892–2897.

Hou, X., Adeosun, S. O., Zhang, Q., Barlow, B., Brents, M., Zheng, B., & Wang, J. (2015). Differential contributions of ApoE4 and female sex to BACE1 activity and expression mediate Aβ deposition and learning and memory in mouse models of Alzheimer's disease. *Frontiers in Aging Neuroscience*, *31*(7).

Hu, J. Y., & Aizawa, T. (2003). Quantitative structure-activity relationships for estrogen receptor binding affinity of phenolic chemicals. *Water Research*, *37*(6), 1213–1222.

Hu, L., Yue, Y., Zuo, P. P., Jin, Z. Y., Feng, F., You, H., ... Ge, Q. S. (2006). Evaluation of neuroprotective effects of long-term low dose hormone replacement therapy on postmenopausal women brain hippocampus using magnetic resonance scanner. *Chinese Medical Sciences Journal*, *21*(4), 214–218.

Hunter, J. M., Bowers, W. J., Maarouf, C. L., Mastrangelo, M. A., Daugs, I. D., Kokjohn, T. A., ... Roher, A. E. (2011). Biochemical and morphological characterization of the AβPP/PS/tau triple transgenic mouse model and its relevance to sporadic Alzheimer's disease. *Journal of Alzheimer's Disease*, *27*(2), 361–376.

Hyde, J. S. (2016). Sex and cognition: Gender and cognitive functions. *Current Opinion in Neurobiology*, *38*, 53–56.

Ihunwo, A. O., Tembo, L. H., & Dzamalala, C. (2016). The dynamics of adult neurogenesis in human hippocampus. *Neural Regeneration Research*, *11*(12), 1869–1883.

Ingelsson, M., Fukumoto, H., Newell, K. L., Growdon, J. H., Hedley-Whyte, E. T., Frosch, M. P., ... Irizarry, M. C. (2004). Early Abeta accumulation and progressive synaptic loss, gliosis, and tangle formation in AD brain. *Neurology, 62*(6), 925–931.

Irvine, K., Laws, K. R., Gale, T. M., & Kondel, T. K. (2012). Grater cognitive deterioration in women than men with Alzheimer's disease: A meta analysis. *Journal of Clinical and Experimental Neuropsychology, 34*(9), 989–998.

Ishikawa, T., Glidewell-Kenney, C., & Jameson, J. L. (2006). Aromatase-independent testosterone conversion into estrogenic steroids is inhibited by a 5α-reductase inhibitor. *Journal of Steroid Biochemistry and Molecular Biology, 98*(2–3), 133–138.

Jack, C. R. J., Therneu, T. M., Weigand, S. D., Wiste, H. J., Knopman, D. S., Vemuri, P., ... Petersen, R. C. (2019). Prevalence of biologically vs clinically defined Alzheimer spectrum entities using the National Institute on Aging-Alzheimer's Association Research Framework. *JAMA Neurology, 76*(10), 1174–1183.

Jacob, H. J., & Kwitek, A. E. (2002). Rat genetics: Attaching physiology and pharmacology to the genome. *Nature Reviews. Genetics, 3*(1), 33–42.

Jang, H., Bae, J. B., Dardiotis, E., Scarmeas, N., Sachdev, P. S., Lipnicki, D. M., ... Kim, K. W. (2018). Differential effects of completed and incomplete pregnancies on the risk of Alzheimer disease. *Neurology, 91*(7), e643–e651.

Janowsky, J. S., Oviatt, S. K., & Orwoll, E. S. (1994). Testosterone influences spatial cognition in older men. *Behavioral Neuroscience, 108*(2), 325–332.

Jawhar, S., Trawicka, A., Jenneckens, C., Bayer, T. A., & Wirths, O. (2012). Motor deficits, neuron loss, and reduced anxiety coinciding with axonal degeneration and intraneuronal Aβ aggregation in the 5XFAD mouse model of Alzheimer's disease. *Neurobiology of Aging, 33*(1), 196.e29–196.e40.

Jensen, E. V., Suzuki, T., Kawashima, T., Stumpf, W. E., Jungblut, P. W., & DeSombre, E. R. (1968). A two-step mechanism for the interaction of estradiol with rat uterus. *Proceedings of the National Academy of Sciences of the United States of America, 59*(2), 632–638.

Jessberger, S., & Kempermann, G. (2003). Adult-born hippocampal neurons mature into activity-dependent responsiveness. *European Journal of Neuroscience, 18*(10), 2707–2712.

Jin, K., Peel, A. L., Mao, X. O., Xie, L., Cottrell, B. A., Henshall, D. C., & Greenberg, D. A. (2004). Increased hippocampal neurogenesis in Alzheimer's disease. *Proceedings of the National Academy of Sciences of the United States of America, 101*(1), 343–347.

Jonasson, Z. (2005). Meta-analysis of sex differences in rodent models of learning and memory: A review of behavioral and biological data. *Neuroscience and Biobehavioral Reviews, 28*(8), 811–825.

Juraska, J. M., Fitch, J. M., & Washburne, D. L. (1989). The dendritic morphology of pyramidal neurons in the rat hippocampal CA3 area. II. Effects of gender and the environment. *Brain Research, 479*(1), 115–119.

Kametani, F., & Hasegawa, M. (2018). Reconsideration of amyloid hypothesis and tau hypothesis in Alzheimer's disease. *Frontiers in Neuroscience, 21*, 25.

Kang, J. H., & Grodstein, F. (2012). Postmenopausal hormone therapy, timing of initiation, APOE and cognitive decline. *Neurobiology of Aging, 33*(7), 1129–1137.

Kee, N., Sivalingam, S., Boonstra, R., & Wojtowicz, J. M. (2002). The utility of Ki-67 and BrdU as proliferative markers of adult neurogenesis. *Journal of Neuroscience Methods, 115*(1), 97–105.

Kee, N., Teixeira, C. M., Wang, A. H., & Frankland, P. W. (2007). Preferential incorporation of adult-generated granule cells into spatial memory networks in the dentate gyrus. *Nature Neuroscience, 10*(3), 355–362.

Kempermann, G., Gage, F. H., Aigner, L., Song, H., Curtis, M., Thuret, S., … Frisen, J. (2018). Human adult neurogenesis: Evidence and remaining questions. *Cell Stem Cell*, *23*(1), 25–30.

Khan, A., Brodhead, A. E., Schwartz, K. A., Kolts, R. L., & Brown, W. A. (2005). Sex differences in antidepressant response in recent antidepressant clinical trials. *Journal of Clinical Psychopharmacology*, *25*(4), 318–324.

Kim, P., Dufford, A. J., & Tribble, R. C. (2018). Cortical thickness variation of the maternal brain in the first 6months postpartum: Associations with parental self-efficacy. *Brain Structure and Function*, *223*(7), 3267–3277.

Kim, P., Leckman, J. F., Mayes, L. C., Feldman, R., Wang, X., & Swain, J. E. (2010). The plasticity of human maternal brain: Longitudinal changes in brain anatomy during the early postpartum period. *Behavioral Neuroscience*, *124*(5), 695–700.

Kinsley, C. H., Madonia, L., Gifford, G. W., Tureski, K., Griffin, G. R., Lowry, C., … Lambert, K. G. (1999). Motherhood improves learning and memory. *Nature*, *402*(6758), 137–138.

Kinsley, C. H., Trainer, R., Stafisso-Sandoz, G., Quadros, P., Marcus, L. K., Hearon, C., … Lambert, K. G. (2006). Motherhood and the hormones of pregnancy modify concentrations of hippocampal neuronal dendritic spines. *Hormones and Behavior*, *49*(2), 131–142.

Kiss, Á., Delattre, A. M., Pereira, S. I. R., Carolino, R. G., Szawka, R. E., Anselmo-Franci, J. A., … Ferraz, A. C. (2012). 17β-Estradiol replacement in young, adult and middle-aged female ovariectomized rats promotes improvement of spatial reference memory and an antidepressant effect and alters monoamines and BDNF levels in memory- and depression-related brain areas. *Behavioural Brain Research*, *227*(1), 100–108.

Kitabatake, Y., Sailor, K. A., Ming, G. L., & Song, H. (2007). Adult neurogenesis and hippocampal memory function: New cells, more plasticity, new memories? *Neurosurgery Clinics of North America*, *18*(1), 105–113.

Knoth, R., Singec, I., Ditter, M., Pantazis, G., Capetian, P., Meyer, R. P., … Kempermann, G. (2010). Murine features of neurogenesis in the human hippocampus across the lifespan from 0 to 100 years. *PLoS One*, *591*, e8809.

Koebele, S. V., & Bimonte-Nelson, H. A. (2016). Modeling menopause: The utility of rodents in translational behavioral endocrinology research. *Maturitas*, *87*, 5–17.

Koebele, S. V., Palmer, J. M., Hadder, B., Melikian, R., Fox, C., Strouse, I. M., … Bimonte-Nelson, H. A. (2019). Hysterectomy uniquely impacts spatial memory in a rat model: A role for the nonpregnant uterus in cognitive processes. *Endocrinology*, *160*(1), 1–19.

Kok, E., Haikonen, S., Luoto, T., Huhtala, H., Goebeler, S., Haapasalo, H., & Karhunen, P. J. (2009). Apolipoprotein E-dependent accumulation of Alzheimer disease-related lesions begins in middle age. *Annals of Neurology*, *65*(6), 650–657.

Kong, D., Yan, Y., He, X. Y., Yang, H., Liang, B., Wang, J., … Yu, H. (2019). Effects of resveratrol on the mechanisms of antioxidants and estrogen in Alzheimer's disease. *BioMed Research International*, *2019*.

Koran, M. E. I., Wagener, M., Hohman, T. J., & ADNI. (2017). Sex differences in the association between AD biomarkers and cognitive decline. *Brain Imagining and Behaviour*, *11*(1), 205–213.

Koss, W. A., & Frick, K. M. (2017). Sex differences in hippocampus function. *Journal of Neuroscience Research*, *95*, 539–562.

Koutseff, A., Mittelhaeuser, C., Essabri, K., Auwerx, J., & Meziane, H. (2014). Impact of the apolipoprotein E polymorphism, age, and sex on neurogenesis in mice: Pathophysiological relevance for Alzheimer's disease? *Brain Research*, *1542*, 32–40.

Kuhn, H. G., Dickinson-Anson, H., & Gage, F. H. (1996). Neurogenesis in the dentate gyrus of the adult rat: Age-related decrease of neuronal progenitor proliferation. *Journal of Neuroscience*, *16*(6), 2027–2033.

Kuiper, G. G. J. M., Enmark, E., Pelto-Huikko, M., Nilsson, S., & Gustafsson, J.Å. (1996). Cloning of a novel estrogen receptor expressed in rat prostate and ovary. *Proceedings of the National Academy of Sciences of the United States of America*, *93*(12), 5925–5930.

Kumar, R., Atamna, H., Zakharov, M. N., Bhasin, S., Khan, S. H., & Jasuja, R. (2011). Role of the androgen receptor CAG repeat polymorphism in prostate cancer, and spinal and bulbar muscular atrophy. *Life Sciences*, *88*, 565–571.

Kunzler, J., Youmans, K. L., Yu, C., LaDu, M. J., & Tai, L. M. (2014). APOE modulates the effect of estrogen therapy on Aβ accumulation EFAD-Tg mice. *Neuroscience Letters*, *560*, 131–136.

La Joie, R., Perrotin, A., de La Sayette, V., Egret, S., Doeuvre, L., Belliard, S., … Chételat, G. (2013). Hippocampal subfield volumetry in mild cognitive impairment, Alzheimer's disease and semantic dementia. *NeuroImage Clinical*, *14*(3), 155–162.

LaFerla, F. M., & Green, K. N. (2012). Animal models of Alzheimer's disease. *Cold Spring Harbor Perspectives in Medicine*, *2*(11), a006320.

Lambert, K. G. (2012). The parental brain: Transformations and adaptations. *Physiology and Behavior*, *107*(5), 792–800.

Langa, K. M., & Levine, D. A. (2014). The diagnosis and management of mild cognitive impairment: A clinical review. *The Journal of the American Medical Association*, *313*(23), 255–2561.

Lanoiselee, H. M., Nicolas, G., Wallon, D., Rovelet-Lecrux, A., Lacour, M., Rousseau, S., … Campion, D. (2017). *APP*, *PSEN1*, and *PSEN2* mutations in early-onset Alzheimer's disease: A genetic screening study of familial and sporadic cases. *PLoS Medicine*, *14*(3), e1002270.

Lanz, R. (1995). Translation of a Trinucleotide Repeat. *Nucleic Acids Research*, *23*(1), 138–145.

Lee, J. H., Byun, M. S., Yi, D., Choe, Y. M., Choi, H. J., Baek, H., … KBASE Research Group. (2017). Sex-specific association of sex hormones and gonadotropins, with brain amyloid and hippocampal neurodegeneration. *Neurobiology of Aging*, *58*, 34–40.

Lefevre, J., & Mcclintock, M. K. (1988). Reproductive senescence in female rats: A longitudinal study of individual differences in estrous cycles and behavior1. *Biology of Reproduction*, *38*(4), 780–789.

Leon, W. C., Canneva, F., Partridge, V., Allard, S., Ferretti, M. T., DeWilde, A., … Cuello, A. C. (2010). A novel transgenic rat model with a full Alzheimer's-like amyloid pathology displays pre-plaque intracellular amyloid-beta-associated cognitive impairment. *Journal of Alzheimer's Disease*, *20*(1), 113–125.

Letenneur, L., Gilleron, V., Comenges, D., Helmer, C., Orgogozo, J. M., & Dartigues, J. F. (1999). Are sex and educational level independent predictors of dementia and Alzheimer's disease? Incidence data from the PAQUID project. *Journal of Neurology, Neurosurgery, and Psychiatry*, *66*(2), 177–183.

Leuner, B., & Gould, E. (2010). Structural plasticity and hippocampal function. *Annual Review of Psychology*, *61*, 111–140.

Leuner, B., Mirescu, C., Noiman, L., & Gould, E. (2007). Maternal experience inhibits the production of immature neurons in the hippocampus during the postpartum period through elevations in adrenal steroids. *Hippocampus*, *17*(6), 434–442.

Li, G., Bien-Ly, N., Andrews-Zwilling, Y., Xu, Q., Bernado, A., Ring, K., … Huang, Y. (2009). GABAergic Interneuron dysfunction impairs hippocampal neurogenesis in adult apolipoprotein E4 knock-in mice. *Cell Stem Cell*, *5*(6), 634–645. https://doi.org/10.1016/j.stem.2009.10.015.

Li, W., Li, H., Wei, H., Lu, Y., Lei, S., Zheng, J., … Zhang, P. (2019). 17β-Estradiol treatment attenuates neurogenesis damage and improves behavior performance after ketamine exposure in neonatal rats. *Frontiers in Cellular Neuroscience, 13*, 251.

Liraz, O., Boehm-Cagan, A., & Michaelson, D. M. (2013). ApoE4 induces Aβ42, tau, and neuronal pathology in the hippocampus of young targeted replacement apoE4 mice. *Molecular Neurodegeneration, 8*, 16.

Lisofsky, N., Mårtensson, J., Eckert, A., Lindenberger, U., Gallinat, J., & Kühn, S. (2015). Hippocampal volume and functional connectivity changes during the female menstrual cycle ☆. *NeuroImage, 118*, 154–162.

Liu, X., Ramirez, S., Pang, P. T., Puryear, C. B., Govindarajan, A., Deisseroth, K., & Tonegawa, S. (2012). Optogenetic stimulation of a hippocampal engram activates fear memory recall. *Nature, 484*(7394), 381–385.

Liu, S., Seidlitz, J., Blumenthal, J. D., Clasen, L. S., & Raznahan, A. (2020). Integrative structural, functional, and transcriptomic analyses of sex-biased brain organization in humans. *Proceedings of the National Academy of Sciences of the United States of America, 117*(31), 18788–18798. https://doi.org/10.1073/pnas.1919091117.

Loi, M., Mossink, J. C., Meerhoff, G. F., Den Blaauwen, J. L., Lucassen, P. J., & Joels, M. (2017). Effects of early-life stress on cognitive function and hippocampal structure in female rodents. *Neuroscience, 342*, 101–119.

Love, G., Torrey, N., McNamara, I., Morgan, M., Banks, M., Hester, N. W., … Lambert, K. G. (2005). Maternal experience produces long-lasting behavioral modifications in the rat. *Behavioral Neuroscience, 119*(4), 1084–1096.

Luders, E., Gingnell, M., Poromaa, I. S., Engman, J., Kurth, F., & Gaser, C. (2018). Potential brain age reversal after pregnancy: Younger brains at 4–6weeks postpartum. *Neuroscience, 386*, 309–314.

Luine, V. N., Jacome, L. F., & MacLusky, N. J. (2003). Rapid enhancement of visual and place memory by estrogens in rats. *Endocrinology, 144*(7), 2836–2844.

Maffucci, J. A., & Gore, A. C. (2006). Age-related changes in hormones and their receptors in animal models of female reproductive senescence. *Handbook of models for human aging* (pp. 533–552). Academic Press.

Mahmoud, R., Wainwright, S. R., & Galea, L. A. M. (2016). Sex hormones and adult hippocampal neurogenesis: Regulation, implications, and potential mechanisms. *Frontiers in Neuroendocrinology, 51*, 129–152.

Mamlouk, G. M., Dorris, D., Barrett, L. R., & Meitzen, J. (2020). Sex bias and omission in neuroscience research is influenced by research model and journal, but not reported NIH funding. *Frontiers in Neuroendocrinology, 57*(100835).

Manning, E. N., Barnes, J., Cash, D. M., Bartlett, J. W., Leung, K. K., Ourselin, S., & Fox, N. C. (2014). APOE ε4 is associated with disproportionate progressive hippocampal atrophy in AD. *PLoS One, 9*(5), e97608.

Markham, J. A., McKian, K. P., Stroup, T. S., & Juraska, J. M. (2005). Sexually dimorphic aging of dendritic morphology in CA1 of hippocampus. *Hippocampus, 15*(1), 97–103.

Markowska, A. L. (1999). Sex dimorphisms in the rate of age-related decline in spatial memory: Relevance to alterations in the estrous cycle. *Journal of Neuroscience, 19*(18), 8122–8133.

Matthews, J., Celius, T., Halgren, R., & Zacharewski, T. (2000). Differential estrogen receptor binding of estrogenic substances: A species comparison. *Journal of Steroid Biochemistry and Molecular Biology, 74*(4), 223–234.

Matyi, J. M., Rattinger, G. B., Schwartz, S., Buhusi, M., & Tschanz, J. T. (2019). Lifetime estrogen exposure and cognition in late life. *Menopause, 26*(12), 1366–1374.

Mayer, L. P., Pearsall, N. A., Christian, P. J., Devine, P. J., Payne, C. M., McCuskey, M. K., ... Hoyer, P. B. (2002). Long-term effects of ovarian follicular depletion in rats by 4-vinylcyclohexene diepoxide. *Reproductive Toxicology*, *16*(6), 775–781.

Mazzucco, C. A., Lieblich, S. E., Bingham, B. I., Williamson, M. A., Viau, V., & Galea, L. A. M. (2006). Both estrogen receptor α and estrogen receptor β agonists enhance cell proliferation in the dentate gyrus of adult female rats. *Neuroscience*, *141*(4), 1793–1800.

McCarrey, A. C., An, Y., Kitner-Triolo, M. H., Ferrucci, L., & Resnick, S. M. (2016). Sex differences in cognitive trajectories in clinically normal older adults. *Psychology and Aging*, *31*(2), 166–175.

McCarthy, M. M., Arnold, A. P., Ball, G. F., Blaustein, J. D., & De Vries, G. J. (2012). Sex differences in the brain: The not so inconvenient truth. *Journal of Neuroscience*, *32*(7), 2241–2247.

McClure, R. E. S., Barha, C. K., & Galea, L. A. M. (2013). 17β-Estradiol, but not estrone, increases the survival and activation of new neurons in the hippocampus in response to spatial memory in adult female rats. *Hormones and Behavior*, *63*(1), 144–157.

McLean, C. P., Asnaani, A., Litz, B. T., & Hofmann, S. G. (2011). Gender differences in anxiety disorders: Prevalence, course of illness, comorbidity and burden of illness. *Journal of Psychiatric Research*, *45*(8), 1027–1035.

McPherson, S., Back, C., Buckwalter, J. G., & Cummings, J. L. (1999). Gender-related cognitive deficits in Alzheimer's disease. *International Psychogeriatrics*, *11*(2), 117–122.

Mendell, A. L., Atwi, S., Bailey, C. D., McCloskey, D., Scharfman, H. E., & MacLusky, N. J. (2017). Expansion of mossy fibers and CA3 apical dendritic length accompanies the fall in dendritic spine density after gonadectomy in male, but not female, rats. *Brain Structure and Function*, *222*(1), 587–601.

Méndez-López, M., Méndez, M., López, L., & Arias, J. L. (2009). Sexually dimorphic c-Fos expression following spatial working memory in young and adult rats. *Physiology & Behavior*, *98*, 307–317.

Merrill, D. A., Karim, R., Darraq, M., Chiba, A. A., & Tuszynski, M. H. (2003). Hippocampal cell genesis does not correlate with spatial learning ability in aged rats. *The Journal of Comparative Neurology*, *259*(2), 201–207.

Mielke, M. M., Vemuri, P., & Rocca, W. A. (2014). Clinical epidemiology of Alzheimer's disease: Assessing sex and gender differences. *Clinical Epidemiology*, *6*, 37–48.

Miller, J. A., Nathanson, J., Franjic, D., Shim, S., Dalley, R. A., Shapouri, S., ... Lein, E. S. (2013). Conserved molecular signatures of neurogenesis in the hippocampal subgranular zone of rodents and primates. *Development*, *140*, 4633–4644.

Minatohara, K., Akiyoshi, M., & Okuno, H. (2016). Role of immediate-early genes in synaptic plasticity and neuronal ensembles underlying the memory trace. *Frontiers in Molecular Neuroscience*, *8*(78), 1–11.

Mitra, S. W., Hoskin, E., Yudkovitz, J., Pear, L., Wilkinson, H. A., Hayashi, S., & Alves, S. E. (2003). Immunolocalization of estrogen receptor beta in the mouse brain: Comparison with estrogen receptor alpha. *Endocrinology*, *144*(5), 2055–2067.

Moffat, S. D., Zonderman, A. B., Metter, E. J., Blackman, M. R., Harman, S. M., & Resnick, S. M. (2002). Longitudinal assessment of serum free testosterone concentration predicts memory performance and cognitive status in elderly men. *Journal of Clinical Endocrinology and Metabolism*, *87*(11), 5001–5007.

Mongiat, L. A., Espósito, M. S., Lombardi, G., & Schinder, A. F. (2009). Reliable activation of immature neurons in the adult hippocampus. *PLoS One*, *4*(4), e5320.

Mora, M., Sánchez, L., Serra-Prat, M., Palomera, E., Blanco, J., Aranda, G., … Puig-Domingo, M. (2012). Hormonal determinants and effect of ER22/23EK glucocorticoid receptor gene polymorphism on health status deterioration in the participants of the Mataró Ageing Study. *Age, 34*(3), 553–561.

Moreno-Jiménez, E. P., Flor-García, M., Terreros-Roncal, J., Rábano, A., Cafini, F., Pallas-Bazarra, N., … Llorens-Martín, M. (2019). Adult hippocampal neurogenesis is abundant in neurologically healthy subjects and drops sharply in patients with Alzheimer's disease. *Nature Medicine, 25*(4), 554–560.

Mormino, E. C., Betensky, R. A., Hedden, T., et al. (2014). Synergistic effect of beta-amyloid and neurodegeneration on cognitive decline in clinically normal individuals. *JAMA Neurology, 71*(11), 1379–1385. https://doi.org/10.1001/jamaneurol.2014.2031.

Moser, V. A., Christensen, A., Liu, J., Zhou, A., Yagi, S., Beam, C. R., … Pike, C. J. (2019). Effects of aging, high-fat diet, and testosterone treatment on neural and metabolic outcomes in male brown Norway rats. *Neurobiology of Aging, 73*, 145–160.

Mueller, S. G., Schuff, N., Yaffe, K., Madison, C., Miller, B., & Weiner, M. W. (2010). Hippocampal atrophy patterns in mild cognitive impairment and Alzheimer's disease. *Human Brain Mapping, 31*(9), 1339–1347.

Murman, D. S. (2015). The impact of age on cognition. *Seminars in Hearing, 36*(3), 111–121.

Nacher, J., Alonso-Llosa, G., Rosell, D. R., & McEwen, B. S. (2003). NMDA receptor antagonist treatment increases the production of new neurons in the aged rat hippocampus. *Neurobiology of Aging, 24*(2), 273–284.

Nelson, P. T., Alafuzoff, I., Bigio, E. H., Bouras, C., Braak, H., Cairns, N. J., … Beach, T.G. (2012). Correlation of Alzheimer disease neuropathologic changes with cognitive status: A review of the literature. *Journal of Neuropathology and Experimental Neurology, 71*(5), 362–381.

Neu, S. C., Pa, J., Kukull, W., Beekly, D., Kuzma, A., Gangadharan, P., … Toga, A.W. (2017). Apolipoprotein E genotype and sex risk factors for Alzheimer's disease. *JAMA Neurology, 74*(10), 1178–1189.

Novaes Gomes, F. G., Fernandes, J., Vannucci Campos, D., Cassilhas, R. C., Viana, G. M., D'Almeida, V., … Arida, R. M. (2014). The beneficial effects of strength exercise on hippocampal cell proliferation and apoptotic signaling is impaired by anabolic androgenic steroids. *Psychoneuroendocrinology, 50*, 106–117.

Nugent, B. M., Tobet, S. A., Lara, H. E., Lucion, A. B., Wilson, M. E., Recabarren, S. E., & Paredes, A. H. (2012). Hormonal programming across the lifespan. *Hormone and Metabolic Research, 44*, 577–586.

Oakley, H., Cole, S. L., Logan, S., Maus, E., Shao, P., Craft, J., … Vassar, R. (2006). Intraneuronal beta-amyloid aggregates, neurodegeneration, and neuron loss in transgenic mice with five familial Alzheimer's disease mutations: Potential factors in amyloid plaque formation. *Journal of Neuroscience, 26*(4), 10129–10140.

Oatridge, A., Holdcroft, A., Saeed, N., Hajnal, J. V., Puri, B. K., Fusi, L., & Bydder, G. M. (2002). Change in brain size during and after pregnancy: Study in healthy women and women with preeclampsia. *American Journal of Neuroradiology, 23*(1), 19–26.

Ofen, N., Kao, Y. C., Sokol-Hessner, P., Kim, H., Whitfield-Gabrieli, S., & Gabrieli, J. D. (2007). Development of the declarative memory system in the human brain. *Nature Neuroscience, 10*(9), 1198–1205.

Ohshima, Y., Taguchi, K., Mizuta, I., Tanaka, M., Tomiyama, T., Kametani, F., … Tokuda, T. (2018). Mutations in the β-amyloid precursor protein in familial Alzheimer's disease increase Aβ oligomer production in cellular models. *Heliyon, 4*(1), e00511.

Orchard, E. R., Ward, P. G., Sforazzini, F., Storey, E., Egan, G. F., & Jamadar, S. D. (2020). Relationship between parenthood and cortical thickness in late adulthood. *PLoS One*, *15*(7), e0236031.

Ormerod, B. K., Falconer, E. M., & Galea, L. A. M. (2003). N-Methyl-D-aspartate receptor activity and estradiol: Separate regulation of cell proliferation in the dentate gyrus of adult female meadow vole. *Journal of Endocrinology*, *179*(2), 155–164.

Ormerod, B. K., & Galea, L. A. M. (2001). Reproductive status inclueces cell proliferation and cell survival in the dentate gyrus of adult female meadow voles: A possible regulatory role for estradiol. *Neuroscience*, *102*(2), 369–379.

Ormerod, B. K., & Galea, L. A. M. (2003). Reproductive status influences the survival of new cells in the dentate gyrus of adult male meadow voles. *Neuroscience Letters*, *346*(1–2), 25–28.

Ormerod, B. K., Lee, T. T. Y., & Galea, L. A. M. (2004). Estradiol enhances neurogenesis in the dentate gyri of adult male meadow voles by increasing the survival of young granule neurons. *Neuroscience*, *128*(3), 645–654.

Padurariu, M., Ciobica, A., Mavroudis, I., Fotiou, D., & Baloyannis, S. (2012). Hippocampal neuronal loss in the CA1 and CA3 areas of Alzheimer's disease patients. *Psychiatria Danubina*, *24*(2), 152–158.

Pasbakhsh, P., Mehdizadeh, M., & Omidi, N. (2005). Neuropathological changes in the PDAPP transgenic mouse model of Alzheimer's disease. *Acta Medica Iranica*, *43*(3), 161–168.

Pawluski, J. L., & Galea, L. A. M. (2007). Reproductive experience alters hippocampal neurogenesis during the postpartum period in the dam. *Neuroscience*, *149*(1), 53–67.

Pawluski, J. L., Paravatou, R., Even, A., Cobraiville, G., Fillet, M., Kokras, N., … Charlier, T. D. (2020). Effect of sertraline on central serotonin and hippocampal plasticity in pregnant and non-pregnant rats. *Neuropharmacology*, *166*.

Pawluski, J. L., Walker, S. K., & Galea, L. A. M. (2006). Reproductive experience differentially affects spatial reference and working memory performance in the mother. *Hormones and Behavior*, *49*(2), 143–149.

Perez-Martin, M., Salazar, V., Castillo, C., Ariznavarreta, C., Azcoitia, I., Garcia-Segura, L. M., & Tresguerres, J. A. F. (2005). Estradiol and soy extract increase the production of new cells in the dentate gyrus of old rats. *Experimental Gerontology*, *40*(5), 450–453.

Petrasek, T., Vojtechova, I., Lobellova, V., Popelikova, A., Janikova, M., Brozka, H., … Stuchlik, A. (2018). The McGill transgenic rat model of Alzheimer's disease displays cognitive and motor impairments, changes in anxiety and social behaviour, and altered circadian activity. *Frontiers in Aging Neuroscience*, *10*(25).

Pfankuch, T., Rizk, A., Olsen, R., Poage, C., & Raber, J. (2005). Role of circulating androgen levels in effects of apoE4 on cognitive function. *Brain Research*, *1053*(1–2), 88–96.

Piccioni, F., Simeoni, S., Andriola, I., Armatura, E., Bassanini, S., Pozzi, P., & Poletti, A. (2001). Polyglutamine tract expansion of the androgen receptor in a motoneuronal model of spinal and bulbar muscular atrophy. *Brain Research Bulletin*, *56*(3–4), 215–220.

Pintzka, C. W. S., & Håberg, A. K. (2015). Perimenopausal hormone therapy is associated with regional sparing of the CA1 subfield: A HUNT MRI study. *Neurobiology of Aging*, *36*(9), 2555–2562.

Prince, M. J., Acosta, D., Guerra, M., Huang, Y., Jimenez-Velazquez, I. Z., Llibre Rodriguez, J. J., … Valhuerdi, A. (2018). Reproductive period, endogenous estrogen exposure and dementia incidence among women in Latin America and China; A 10/66 population-based cohort study. *PLoS One*, *13*(2), e0192889.

Prossnitz, E. R., Sklar, L. A., Oprea, T. I., & Arterburn, J. B. (2008). GPR30: A novel therapeutic target in estrogen-related disease. *Trends in Pharmacological Sciences, 29*(3), 116–123.

Ptok, U., Barkow, K., & Heun, R. (2002). Fertility and number of children in patients with Alzheimer's disease. *Archives of Women's Mental Health, 5*(2), 83–86.

Ramirez, S., Liu, X., Lin, P. A., Suh, J., Pignatelli, M., Redondo, R. L., … Tonegawa, S. (2013). Creating a false memory in the hippocampus. *Science, 341*(6144), 387–391.

Ramirez-Amaya, V., Marrone, D. F., Gage, F. H., Worley, P. F., & Barnes, C. A. (2006). Integration of new neurons into functional neural networks. *The Journal of Neuroscience, 26*(47), 12237–12241.

Ramsden, M., Nyborg, A. C., Murphy, M. P., Chang, L., Stanczyk, F. Z., Golde, T. E., & Pike, C. J. (2004). Androgens modulate β-amyloid levels in male rat brain. *Journal of Neurochemistry, 87*(4), 1052–1055.

Ramsden, M., Shin, T. M., & Pike, C. J. (2003). Androgens modulate neuronal vulnerability to kainate lesion. *Neuroscience, 122*(3), 573–578.

Rannevik, G., Jeppsson, S., Johnell, O., Bjerre, B., Laurell-Borulf, Y., & Svanberg, L. (2008). A longitudinal study of the perimenopausal transition: Altered profiles of steroid and pituitary hormones, SHBG and bone mineral density. *Maturitas, 61*(1–2), 67–77.

Rao, M. S., Hattiangady, B., Abdel-Rahman, A., Stanley, D. P., & Shetty, A. K. (2005). Newly born cells in the ageing dentate gyrus display normal migration, survival and neuronal fate choice but endure retarded early maturation. *European Journal of Neuroscience, 21*(2), 464–476.

Rao, M. S., & Shetty, A. K. (2004). Efficacy of doublecortin as a marker to analyse the absolute number and dendritic growth of newly generated neurons in the adult dentate gyrus. *European Journal of Neuroscience, 19*(2), 234–246.

Rapp, S. R., Espeland, M. A., Shumaker, S. A., Henderson, V. W., Brunner, R. L., Manson, J. A. E., … Bowen, D. (2003). Effect of estrogen plus progestin on global cognitive function in postmenopausal women—The women's health initiative memory study: A randomized controlled trial. *Journal of the American Medical Association, 289*(20), 2663–2672.

Rebeck, G. W., Reiter, J. S., Strickland, D. K., & Hyman, B. T. (1993). Apolipoprotein E in sporadic Alzheimer's disease: Allelic variation and receptor interactions. *Neuron, 11*(4), 575–580.

Resnick, S. M., Espeland, M. A., Jaramillo, S. A., Hirsch, C., Stefanick, M. L., Murray, A. M., … Davatzikos, C. (2009). Postmenopausal hormone therapy and regional brain volumes: The WHIMS-MRI Study. *Neurology, 72*(2), 135–142.

Resnick, S. M., & Henderson, V. W. (2002). Hormone therapy and risk of Alzheimer disease: A critical time. *JAMA, 288*(17), 2170–2172.

Revankar, C. M., Cimino, D. F., Sklar, L. A., Arterburn, J. B., & Prossnitz, E. R. (2005). A transmembrane intracellular estrogen receptor mediates rapid cell signaling. *Science, 307*(5715), 1625–1630.

Richetin, K., Leclerc, C., Toni, N., Gallopin, T., Pech, S., Roybon, L., & Rampon, C. (2015). Genetic manipulation of adult-born hippocampal neurons rescues memory in a mouse model of Alzheimer's disease. *Brain, 138*(2), 440–455.

Rijpma, A., Jansen, D., Arnoldussen, I. A. C., Fang, X. T., Wiesmann, M., Mutsaers, M. P. C., … Kiliaan, A. J. (2013). Sex differences in presynaptic density and neurogenesis in middle-aged ApoE4 and ApoE knockout mice. *Journal of Neurodegenerative Diseases, 2013*.

Rippon, G. A., Tang, M. X., Lee, J. H., Lantigua, R., Medrano, M., & Mayeux, R. (2006). Familial Alzheimer disease in Latinos: Interaction between APOE, stroke, and estrogen replacement. *Neurology, 66*(1), 35–40.

Robitsek, R. J., Fortin, N. J., Koh, M. T., Gallagher, M., & Eichenbaum, H. (2008). Cognitive aging: A common decline of episodic recollection and spatial memory in rats. *The Journal of Neuroscience, 28*(36), 8945–8954.

Rocca, W. A., Bower, J. H., Maraganore, D. M., Ahlskog, J. E., Grossardt, B. R., De Andrade, M., & Melton, L. J. (2007). Increased risk of cognitive impairment or dementia in women who underwent oophorectomy before menopause. *Neurology, 69*(11), 1074–1083.

Rocca, W. A., Grossardt, B. R., & Shuster, L. T. (2011). Oophorectomy, menopause, estrogen treatment, and cognitive aging: Clinical evidence for a window of opportunity. *Brain Research, 1379*, 188–198.

Rocca, W. A., Mielke, M. M., Vemuri, P., & Miller, V. M. (2014). Sex and gender differences in the causes of dementia: A narrative review. *Maturitas, 79*, 196–201.

Rodríguez, J. J., & Verkhratsky, A. (2011). Neurogenesis in Alzheimer's disease. *Journal of Anatomy, 219*(1), 78–89.

Rolls, A., Schori, H., London, A., & Schwartz, M. (2008). Decrease in hippocampal neurogenesis during pregnancy: A link to immunity. *Molecular Psychiatry, 13*, 468–469.

Rosario, E. R., Chang, L., Head, E. H., Stanczyk, F. Z., & Pike, C. J. (2011). Brain levels of sex steroid hormones in men and women during normal aging and in Alzheimer's disease. *Neurobiology of Aging, 32*(4), 604–613.

Rosario, E. R., Chang, L., Stanczyk, F. Z., & Pike, C. J. (2004). Age-related testosterone depletion and the development of Alzheimer disease. *JAMA, 292*(12), 1431–1432.

Rousseau, M. E. (2006). Managing menopausal symptoms. *Handbooks of models for human aging* (pp. 873–879). Academic Press.

Rubin, B. S. (2000). Hypothalamic alterations and reproductive aging in female rats: Evidence of altered luteinizing hormone-releasing hormone neuronal function[1]. *Biology of Reproduction, 63*(4), 968–976.

Ruffman, T., Henry, J. D., Livingstone, V., & Phillips, L. H. (2008). A meta-analytic review of emotion recognition and aging: Implications for neuropsychological models of aging. *Neuroscience and Biobehavioural Reviews, 32*(4), 863–881.

Ruigrok, A. N., Salimi-Khorshidi, G., Lai, M. C., Baron-Cohen, S., Lombardo, M. V., Tait, R. J., & Suckling, J. (2014). A meta-analysis of sex differences in human brain structure. *Neuroscience and Biobehavioral Reviews, 39*, 34–50.

Ruscio, M. G., Sweeny, T. D., Hazelton, J. L., Suppatkul, P., Boothe, E., & Carter, C. S. (2008). Pup exposure elicits hippocampal cell proliferation in the prairie vole. *Behavioural Brain Research, 187*, 9–16.

Russell, J. K., Jones, C. K., & Newhouse, P. A. (2019). The role of estrogen in brain and cognitive aging. *Neurotherapeutics*, 1–17.

Ryan, T. J., Roy, D. S., Pignatelli, M., Arons, A., & Tonegawa, S. (2015). Engram cells retain memory under retrograde amnesia. *Science, 348*(6238), 1007–1013.

Ryan, J., Scali, J., Carrière, I., Amieva, H., Rouaud, O., Berr, C., ... Ancelin, M.-L. (2014). Impact of a premature menopause on cognitive function in later life. *BJOG: An International Journal of Obstetrics & Gynaecology, 121*(13), 1729–1739.

Ryan, J., Scali, J., Carriere, I., Ritchie, K., & Ancelin, M. L. (2008). Hormonal treatment, mild cognitive impairment and Alzheimer's disease. *International Psychogeriatrics, 20*(1), 47–56.

Sanai, N., Nguyen, T., Ihrie, R. A., Mirzadeh, Z., Tsai, H. H., Wong, M., ... Alvarez-Buylla, A. (2011). Corridors of migrating neurons in human brain and their decline during infancy. *Nature, 478*(7369), 382–386.

Saravia, F., Beauquis, J., Pietranera, L., & De Nicola, A. F. (2007). Neuroprotective effects of estradiol in hippocampal neurons and glia of middle age mice. *Psychoneuroendocrinology*, *32*(5), 480–492.

Saxe, M. D., Battaglia, F., Wang, J. W., Malleret, G., David, D. J., Monckton, J. E., ... Drew, M. R. (2006). Ablation of hippocampal neurogenesis impairs contextual fear conditioning and synaptic plasticity in the dentate gyrus. *Proceedings of the National Academy of Sciences of the United States of America*, *103*(46), 17501–17506.

Scharfman, H. E., & MacLusky, N. J. (2017). Sex differences in hippocampal area CA3 pyramidal cells. *Journal of Neuroscience Research*, *95*(1–2), 563–575.

Schmidt-Hieber, C., Jonas, P., & Bischofberger, J. (2004). Enhanced synaptic plasticity in newly generated granule cells of the adult hippocampus. *Nature*, *429*(6988), 184–187.

Schock, H., Zeleniuch-Jacquotte, A., Lundin, E., Grankvist, K., Lakso, H.Å., Idahl, A., ... Fortner, R. T. (2016). Hormone concentrations throughout uncomplicated pregnancies: A longitudinal study. *BMC Pregnancy and Childbirth*, *16*(1), 146.

Scopa, C., Marrocco, F., Latina, V., Ruggeri, F., Corvaglia, V., Regina, F. L., ... Cattaneo, A. (2019). Impaired adult neurogenesis is an early event in Alzheimer's disease neurodegeneration, mediated by intracellular Aβ oligomers. *Cell Death and Differentiation*, *27*(3), 934–948.

Scoville, W. B., & Milner, B. (1957). Loss of recent memory after bilateral hippocampal loss. *Journal of Neurology, Neurosurgery, and Psychiatry*, *20*(1), 11–21.

Seki, T., & Arai, Y. (1995). Age-related production of new granule cells in the adult dentate gyrus. *Neuroreport*, *6*(18), 2479–2482.

Setti, S. E., Hunsberger, H. C., & Reed, M. N. (2017). Alterations in hippocampal activity and Alzheimer's disease. *Translational Issues in Psychological Science*, *3*(4), 348–356.

Shao, H., Breitner, J. C. S., Whitmer, R. A., Wang, J., Hayden, K., Wengreen, H., ... Zandi, P. P. (2012). Hormone therapy and Alzheimer disease dementia: New findings from the cache county study. *Neurology*, *79*(18), 1846–1852.

Sheppard, P. A., Choleris, E., & Galea, L. A. (2019). Structural plasticity of the hippocampus in response to estrogens in female rodents. *Molecular Brain*, *12*(1), 22.

Sherwin, B. B. (2005). Estrogen and memory in women: How can we reconcile the findings? *Hormones and Behavior*, *47*(3), 371–375.

Sherwin, B. B. (2007). The critical period hypothesis: Can it explain discrepancies in the oestrogen-cognition literature? *Journal of Neuroendocrinology*, *19*(2), 77–81.

Sherwin, B. B. (2009). Estrogen therapy: Is time of initiation critical for neuroprotection? *Nature Reviews Endocrinology*, *5*(11), 620–627.

Shingo, T., Gregg, C., Enwere, E., Fujikawa, H., Hassam, R., Geary, C., ... Weiss, S. (2003). Pregnancy-stimulated neurogenesis in the adult female forebrain mediated by prolactin. *Science*, *299*(5603), 117–120.

Shohayeb, B., Diab, M., Ahmed, M., & Ng, D. C. H. (2018). Factors that influence adult neurogenesis as potential therapy. *Translational Neurodegeneration*, *7*(1), 1–19.

Shors, T. J., Miesegaes, G., Beylin, A., Zhao, M., Rydel, T., & Gould, E. (2001). Neurogenesis in the adult is involved in the formation of trace memories. *Nature*, *410*(6826), 372–376.

Shumaker, S. A., Legault, C., Rapp, S. R., Thal, L., Wallace, R. B., Ockene, J. K., ... Wactawski-Wende, J. (2003). Estrogen plus progestin and the incidence of dementia and mild cognitive impairment in postmenopausal women—The women's health initiative memory study: A randomized controlled trial. *Journal of the American Medical Association*, *289*(20), 2651–2662.

Snyder, J. S., Chloe, J. S., Clifford, M. A., Jeurling, S. I., Hurley, P., Brown, A., ... Cameron, H. A. (2009). Adult-born hippocampal neurons are more numerous, faster maturing, and more involved in behaviour in rats than in mice. *Journal of Neuroscience, 29*(46), 14484–14495.

Snyder, J. S., Hong, N. S., Mcdonald, R. J., & Wojtowicz, J. M. (2005). A role for adult neurogenesis in spatial long-term memory. *Neuroscience, 130*(2005), 843–852.

Snyder, J. S., Radik, R., Wojtowicz, M., & Cameron, H. A. (2009). Anatomical gradients of adult neurogenesis and activity: Young neurons in the ventral dentate gyrus are activated by water maze training. *Hippocampus, 19*, 360–370.

Sohn, D., Shpanskaya, K., Lucas, J. E., Petrella, J. R., Saykin, A. J., Tanzi, R. E., ... Doraiswamy, P. M. (2018). Sex differences in cognitive decline in subjects with high likelihood of milt cognitive impairment due to Alzheimer's disease. *Scientific Reports, 8*(1), 7490.

Sorrells, S. F., Paredes, M. F., Cebrian-Silla, A., Sandoval, K., Qi, D., Kelley, K. W., ... Alvarez-Buylla, A. (2018). Human hippocampal neurogenesis drops sharply in children to undetectable levels in adults. *Nature, 555*(7696), 377–381.

Spalding, K. L., Bergmann, O., Alkass, K., Bernard, S., Salehpour, M., Huttner, H. B., ... Buchholz, B. A. (2013). Dynamics of hippocampal neurogenesis in adult humans. *Cell, 153*(6), 1219–1227.

Spellman, T., Rigotti, M., Ahmari, S. E., Fusi, S., Gogos, J. A., & Gordon, J. A. (2015). Hippocampal-prefrontal input supports spatial encoding in working memory. *Nature, 522*(7556), 309–314.

Spritzer, M. D., Daviau, E. D., Coneeny, M. K., Engelman, S. M., Prince, W. T., & Rodriguez-Wisdom, K. N. (2011). Effects of testosterone on spatial learning and memory in adult male rats. *Hormones and Behavior, 59*(4), 484–496.

Spritzer, M. D., & Galea, L. A. M. (2005). Androgens enhance cell survival but not cell proliferation in adult male rats. *Hormones and Behavior, 48*(1).

Spritzer, M. D., & Galea, L. A. M. (2007). Testosterone and dihydrotestosterone, but not estradiol, enhance survival of new hippocampal neurons in adult male rats. *Developmental Neurobiology, 67*(10), 1321–1333.

Spritzer, M. D., Ibler, E., Inglis, W., & Curtis, M. G. (2011). Testosterone and social isolation influence adult neurogenesis in the dentate gyrus of male rats. *Neuroscience, 195*, 180–190.

Stark, S. M., Yassa, M. A., & Stark, C. E. L. (2010). Individual differences in spatial pattern separation performance associated with healthy aging in humans. *Learning and Memory, 17*, 284–288.

Sturchler-Pierrat, C., & Staufenbiel, M. (2000). Pathogenic mechanisms of Alzheimer's disease analyzed in the APP23 transgenic mouse model. *Annals of the New York Academy of Sciences, 920*, 134–139.

Sugiyama, T., Osumi, N., & Katsuyama, Y. (2013). The germinal matrices in the developing dentate gyrus are composed of neuronal progenitors at distinct differentiation stages. *Developmental Dynamics, 242*(12), 1442–1453.

Sundermann, E., Panizzon, M. S., Chen, X., Andrews, M., Galasko, D., & Banks, S. J. (2020). *Sex differences in Alzheimer's-related Tau biomarkers and a mediating effect of testosterone*. ORCiD https://orcid.org/0000-0001-5821-8035.

Sundermann, E. E., Tran, M., Maki, P. M., & Bondi, M. W. (2018). Sex differences in the association between apolipoprotein E e4 allele and Alzheimer's disease markers. *Alzheimer's & Dementia (Amsterdam Netherlands), 10*, 438–447.

Swift-Gallant, A., Duarte-Guterman, P., Hamson, D. K., Ibrahim, M., Monks, D. A., & Galea, L. A. M. (2018). Neural androgen receptors affect the number of surviving new neurones in the adult dentate gyrus of male mice. *Journal of Neuroendocrinology, 30*(4), e12578.

Tabori, N. E., Stewart, L. S., Znamensky, V., Romeo, R. D., Alves, S. E., McEwen, B. S., & Milner, T. A. (2005). Ultrastructural evidence that androgen receptors are located at extranuclear sites in the rat hippocampal formation. *Neuroscience*, *130*(1), 151–163.

Tai, L. M., Bilousova, T., Jungbauer, L., Roeske, S. K., Youmans, K. L., Yu, C., ... LaDu, M. J. (2013). Levels of soluble apolipoprotein E/amyloid-beta (Abeta) complex are reduced and oligomeric Abeta increased with APOE4 and Alzheimer disease in a transgenic mouse model and human samples. *The Journal of Biological Chemistry*, *288*(8), 5914–5926.

Tan, A., Ma, W., Vira, A., Marwha, D., & Eliot, L. (2016). The human hippocampus is not sexually-dimorphic: Meta-analysis of structural MRI volumes. *NeuroImage*, *1*(124), 350–366.

Tanapat, P., Hastings, N. B., & Gould, E. (2005). Ovarian steroids influence cell proliferation in the dentate gyrus of the adult female rat in a dose- and time-dependent manner. *Journal of Comparative Neurology*, *481*(3), 252–265.

Tanapat, P., Hastings, N. B., Reeves, A. J., & Gould, E. (1999). Estrogen stimulates a transient increase in the number of new neurons in the dentate gyrus of the adult female rat. *Journal of Neuroscience*, *19*(14), 5792–5801.

Taylor, C. M., Pritchet, L., Olsen, R., Layher, E., Santander, T., Grafton, S. T., & Jacobs, E. G. (2020). Progesterone shapes medial temporal lobe volume across the human menstrual cycle. *NeuroImage*, *220*, 117–125.

Tensaouti, Y., Stephanz, E. P., Yu, T. S., & Kernie, S. G. (2018). ApoE regulates the development of adult newborn hippocampal neurons. *eNeuro*, *5*(4), 1–15.

Thal, D. R., Holzer, M., Rub, U., Waldmann, G., Gunzel, S., Zedlick, D., & Schober, R. (2000). Alzheimer-related τ-pathology in the preforant path target zone and in the hippocampal stratum oriens and radiatum correlates with onset and degree of dementia. *Experimental Neurology*, *163*(1), 98–110.

Thomas, P., Pang, Y., Filardo, E. J., & Dong, J. (2005). Identity of an estrogen membrane receptor coupled to a G protein in human breast cancer cells. *Endocrinology*, *146*(2), 624–632.

Tirabassi, G., Cignarelli, A., Perrini, S., Furlani, G., Gallo, M., Pallotti, F., ... Lenzi, A. (2015). Influence of CAG repeat polymorphism on the targets of testosterone action. *International Journal of Endocrinology*, *2015*.

Tobin, M. K., Musaraca, K., Disouky, A., Shetti, A., Bheri, A., Honer, W. G., ... Lazarov, O. (2019). Human hippocampal neurogenesis persists in aged adults and Alzheimer's disease patients. *Cell Stem Cell*, *24*, 974–982.

Toner, C. K., Pirogovsky, E., Kirwan, C. B., & Gilbert, P. E. (2009). Visual object pattern separation deficits in nondemented older adults. *Learning and Memory*, *16*, 338–342.

Toni, N., Laplagne, D. A., Zhao, C., Lombardi, G., Ribak, C. E., Gage, F. G., & Schinder, A. F. (2008). Neurons born in the adult dentate gyrus form functional synapses with target cells. *Nature Neuroscience*, *11*(8), 901–907.

Tronel, S., Belnoue, L., Grosjean, N., Revest, J. M., Piazza, P. V., Koehl, M., & Abrous, D. N. (2012). Adult-born neurons are necessary for extended contextual discrimination. *Hippocampus*, *22*(2), 292–298.

Tschiffely, A. E., Schuh, R. A., Prokai-Tatrai, K., Ottinger, M. A., & Prokai, L. (2018). An exploratory investigation of brain-selective estrogen treatment in males using a mouse model of Alzheimer's disease. *Hormones and Behavior*, *98*, 16–21.

Van Kempen, T. A., Milner, T. A., & Waters, E. M. (2011). Accelerated ovarian failure: A novel, chemically induced animal model of menopause. *Brain Research*, *1379*, 176–187.

van Praag, H., Kempermann, G., & Gage, F. H. (2000). Neural consequences of environmental enrichment. *Nature Reviews Neuroscience*, *1*, 191–198.

van Praag, H., Schinder, A. F., Christie, B. R., Toni, N., Palmer, T. D., & Gage, F. H. (2002). Functional neurogenesis in the adult hippocampus. *Nature*, *415*(6875), 1030–1034.

Varbanov, H., & Dityatev, A. (2017). Regulation of extrasynaptic signaling by polysialylated NCAM: Impact for synaptic plasticity and cognitive functions. *Molecular and Cellular Neurosciences*, *81*, 12–21.

Vaucher, E., Reymond, I., Najaffe, R., Kar, S., Quirion, R., Miller, M. M., & Franklin, K. B. J. (2002). Estrogen effects on object memory and cholinergic receptors in young and old female mice. *Neurobiology of Aging*, *23*(1), 87–95.

Vedder, L. C., Bredemann, T. M., & McMahon, L. L. (2014). Estradiol replacement extends the window of opportunity for hippocampal function. *Neurobiology of Aging*, *35*(10), 2183–2192.

Vermeulen, A., Goemaere, S., & Kaufman, J. M. (1999). Testosterone, body composition and aging. *Journal of Endocrinological Investigation*, *22*(5 Suppl), 110–116.

Voyer, D., Voyer, S., & Saint-Aubin, J. (2017). Sex differences in visual-spatial working memory: A meta-anaysis. *Psychonomic Bulletin and Review*, *24*(2), 307–334.

Waters, E.M., Thompson, L.I., Patel, P., Gonzales, A.D., Ye, H.Z., Filardo, E.J., ...Milner, T.A. (2015). G-protein-coupled Estrogen receptor 1 is anatomically positioned to modulate synaptic plasticity in the mouse hippocampus *Journal of Neuroscience* 35(6), 2384–2397.

Wahjoepramono, E. J., Asih, P. R., Aniwiyanti, V., Taddei, K., Dhaliwal, S. S., Fuller, S. J., … Martins, R. N. (2016). The effects of testosterone supplementation on cognitive functioning in older men. *CNS & Neurological Disorders - Drug Targets*, *15*(3), 337–343.

Wainwright, S. R., Workman, J. L., Tehrani, A., Hamson, D. K., Chow, C., Lieblich, S. E., & Galea, L. A. M. (2016). Testosterone has antidepressant-like efficacy and facilitates imipramine-induced neuroplasticity in male rats exposed to chronic unpredictable stress. *Hormones and Behavior*, *79*, 58–69.

Wang, J., Gu, B. J., Masters, C. L., & Wang, Y. J. (2017). A systemic view of Alzheimer disease—Insights from amyloid-β metabolism beyond the brain. *Nature Reviews Neurology*, *13*(10), 612.

Wang, J. M., Singh, C., Liu, L., Irwin, R. W., Chen, S., Chung, E. J., … Brinton, R. B. (2010). Allopregnanolone reverses neurogenic and cognitive deficits in mouse model of Alzheimer's disease. *Proceedings of the National Academy of Sciences of the United States of America*, *107*(14), 6498–6503.

Ward, A., Crean, S., Mercaldi, C. J., Collins, J. M., Boyd, D., Cook, M. N., & Arrighi, H. M. (2012). Prevalence of Apolipoprotein E4 genotype and homozygotes (APOE e4/4) among patients diagnosed with Alzheimer's disease: A systematic review and meta-analysis. *Neuroepidemiology*, *38*(1), 1–17.

Weber, M. R., Rubin, L. H., & Maki, P. M. (2013). Cognition in perimenopause: The effect of transition stage. *Menopause*, *20*(5).

Westerman, M. A., Cooper-Blacketer, D., Mariash, A., Kotilinek, L., Kawarabayashi, T., Younkin, L. H., … Ashe, K. H. (2002). The relationship between Aβ and memory in the Tg2576 mouse model of Alzheimer's disease. *Journal of Neuroscience*, *22*(5), 1858–1867.

Wharton, W., Baker, L. D., Gleason, C. E., Dowling, M., Barnet, J. H., Johnson, S., … Asthana, S. (2011). Short-term hormone therapy with transdermal estradiol improves cognition for postmenopausal women with Alzheimer's disease: Results of a randomized controlled trial. *Journal of Alzheimer's Disease*, *26*(3), 495–505.

Whitmer, R. A., Quesenberry, C. P., Zhou, J., & Yaffe, K. (2011). Timing of hormone therapy and dementia: The critical window theory revisited. *Annals of Neurology*, *69*(1), 163–169.

Williams, J. K. (2005). A mouse model of the perimenopausal transition: Importance for cardiovascular research. *Arteriosclerosis, Thrombosis, and Vascular Biology*, *25*(9), 1765–1766.

Wilson, R. S., Segawa, E., Boyle, P. A., Anagnos, S. E., Hizel, L. P., & Bennett, D. A. (2012). The natural history of cognitive decline in Alzheimer's disease. *Psychology and Aging*, *27*(4), 1008–1017.

Wolk, D. A., Dickerson, B. C., & Alzheimer's Disease Neuroimaging Initiative. (2010). Apolipoprotein E (APOE) genotype has dissociable effects on memory and attentional-executive network function in Alzheimer's disease. *Proceedings of the National Academy of Sciences of the United States of America*, *107*(22), 10256–10261.

Woodside, B. (2006). Morphological plasticity in the maternal brain: Comment on Kinsley et al.; motherhood and the hormones of pregnancy modify concentrations of hippocampal neuronal dendritic spines. *Hormones and Behavior*, *49*, 129–130.

Yaffe, K., Haan, M., Byers, A., Tangen, C., & Kuller, L. (2000). Estrogen use, APOE, and cognitive decline: Evidence of gene-environment interaction. *Neurology*, *54*(10), 1949–1953.

Yagi, S., Chow, C., Lieblich, S. E., & Galea, L. A. (2016). Sex and strategy use matters for pattern separation, adult neurogenesis, and immediate early gene expression in the hippocampus. *Hippocampus*, *26*(1), 87–101.

Yagi, S., Drewczynski, C., Wainwright, S. R., Barha, C. K., Hershorn, O., & Galea, L. A. M. (2017). Sex and estrous cycle differences in immediate early gene activation in the hippocampus and the dorsal striatum after the cue competition task. *Hormones and Behavior*, *87*, 69–79.

Yagi, S., & Galea, L. A. M. (2019). Sex differences in hippocampal cognition and neurogenesis. *Neuropsychopharmacology*, *44*(1), 200–213.

Yagi, S., Splinter, J. E. J., Tai, D., Wong, S., & Galea, L. A. M. (2020). Sex differences in maturation and attrition rate of adult born neurons in the hippocampus of rats. *eNeuro*, *7*(4), 1–14.

Yang, C. P., Gilley, J. A., Zhang, G., & Kernie, S. G. (2011). ApoE is required for maintenance of the dentate gyrus neural progenitor pool. *Development*, *138*(2), 4351–4362.

Yang, F., Ueda, K., Chen, P. P., Ashe, K. H., & Cole, G. M. (2000). Plaque-associated alpha-synuclein (NACP) pathology in aged transgenic mice expressing amyloid precursor protein. *Brain Research*, *853*(2), 381–383.

Yau, S. Y., Li, A., & So, K. F. (2015). Involvement of adult hippocampal neurogenesis in learning and forgetting. *Neural Plasticity*, *2015*. 717958.

Young, E. A., Kornstein, S. G., Marcus, S. M., Harvey, A. T., Warden, D., Wisniewski, S. R., … John Rush, A. (2009). Sex differences in response to citalopram: A STAR*D report. *Journal of Psychiatric Research*, *43*(5), 503–511.

Yun, J., Koike, H., Ibi, D., Toth, E., Mizoguchi, H., Nitta, A., … Yamada, K. (2010). Chronic restraint stress impairs neurogenesis and hippocampus-dependent fear memory in mice: Possible involvement of a brain-specific transcription factor Npas4. *Journal of Neurochemistry*, *114*(6), 1840–1851.

Zheng, J. Y., Liang, K. S., Wang, X. J., Zhou, X. Y., Sun, J., & Zhou, S. N. (2017). Chronic estradiol administration during the early stage of Alzheimer's disease pathology rescues adult hippocampal neurogenesis and ameliorates cognitive deficits in Aβ1-42 mice. *Molecular Neurobiology*, *54*(10), 7656–7669.

Zhuo, J. M., Tseng, H. A., Desai, M., Bucklin, M., Mohammed, A. I., Robinson, N. T. M., … Jasanoff, A. P. (2016). Young adult born neurons enhance hippocampal dependent performance via influences on bilateral networks. *eLife*, *5*, e22429.

Ziegler-Waldkirch, S., Marksteiner, K., Stoll, J., d'Errico, P., Friesen, M., Eiler, D., … Meyer-Luehmann, M. (2018). Environmental enrichment reverses Aβ pathology during pregnancy in a mouse model of Alzheimer's disease. *Acta Neuropathologica Communications*, *6*. https://doi.org/10.1186/s40478-018-0549-6, 44.

Zimberknopf, E., Xavier, G. F., Kinsley, C. H., & Felicio, L. F. (2011). Prior parity positively regulates learning and memory in young and middle-aged rats. *Comparative Medicine*, *61*(4), 336–377.

CHAPTER

Sex differences in microglia as a risk factor for Alzheimer's disease

3

Charlotte Delage[a,*], Danielle N. Rendina[b,*], Karen E. Malacon[b], Marie-Ève Tremblay[a], and Staci D. Bilbo[b,c]

[a]*Division of Medical Sciences, University of Victoria, Victoria, BC, Canada*
[b]*Department of Psychology and Neuroscience, Duke University, Durham, NC, United States*
[c]*Department of Neurobiology, Duke University, Durham, NC, United States*

Introduction

Alzheimer's disease (AD) is the leading cause of dementia and affects 50 million people worldwide, the majority of whom are women (Alzheimer's Association, 2020). The pathological features of this neurodegenerative disease include extracellular neurotoxic amyloid-β (Aβ) plaques and intracellular neurofibrillary tangles that result from the aggregation of hyperphosphorylated tau (Holtzman, 2001). Hallmarks of disease progression include synaptic and neuronal loss, as well as elevated levels of inflammatory cytokines and an increase in reactive gliosis (Gallardo & Holtzman, 2019; Spires-Jones & Hyman, 2014). Genomic and transcriptomic studies identifying the enrichment of immune pathways in AD (Efthymiou & Goate, 2017) highlight the importance of the immune system in understanding the pathophysiology of the disease.

Of particular interest are microglia, the resident immune cells of the central nervous system (CNS). These cells survey the local environment and engage in tissue defense and repair through phagocytosis and cytokine secretion, among other functions (Bilbo & Schwarz, 2012). Under homeostatic conditions, microglia are characterized by a small soma with motile, ramified processes covered in protrusions that continuously survey their microenvironment (Hanisch & Kettenmann, 2007; Nimmerjahn, Kirchhoff, & Helmchen, 2005). Following the detection of parenchymal injury or infection, microglia undergo morphological and functional transformations, for instance, becoming more amoeboid in shape and adopting a neuroprotective role through the phagocytosis of necrotic cells, removal of apoptotic cells, and release of cytotoxic signaling factors (Arcuri, Mecca, Bianchi, Giambanco, & Donato, 2017).

---

[*] Delage and Rendina share first authorship.

In addition to their canonical immune roles, microglia are key regulators of synaptic pruning and the organization of neural circuits during development (Paolicelli et al., 2011; Wake, Moorhouse, Miyamoto, & Nabekura, 2013), and help regulate learning-induced synapse formation in adulthood (Parkhurst et al., 2013). Microglia are increasingly known to play a critical role in disorders of the central nervous system such as AD (Salter & Stevens, 2017). Whether microglial reactivity is detrimental or protective in neurodegeneration remains unclear, although current evidence suggests a dual role for microglia that transforms as the disease progresses.

Gene network analyses from genome-wide association studies (GWAS) reveal the enrichment of immune pathways (Efthymiou & Goate, 2017), and many of these risk genes are enriched or exclusively expressed in microglia or myeloid cells (including triggering receptor expressed on myeloid cells-2 (TREM2)) (Karch & Goate, 2015), supporting a role for microglia as key players in the pathogenesis of AD. The identification of the enrichment of pathways involved in microglial function has propelled research of these immune cells in the context of AD in animal models (see also Chapter 1). It is important to note, however, that although there are known sex and gender differences in AD, the majority of studies have ignored sex or failed to report it, revealing a gap in the field and an avenue for improvement.

Microglia: Protection and pathology in Alzheimer's disease

The generation and accumulation of Aβ peptides and amyloid deposition are believed to play a critical role in AD pathogenesis. Mutations in amyloid precursor protein (APP), presenilin-1 (PSEN1), and presenilin-2 (PSEN2) cause autosomal forms of early-onset familial AD and result in increased production of amyloidogenic Aβ (Selkoe & Hardy, 2016). While it has long been known that microglia interact with and surround Aβ plaques—an observation made by Alois Alzheimer in 1911 (Möller & Graeber, 1998)—many questions remain on whether microglia are protective or detrimental in disease progression. These cells appear to behave in opposing manners, with evidence suggesting that they are protective during earlier stages of AD but assume a more harmful role during late stages of the disease.

Protective functions of microglia in Alzheimer's disease
TREM2 and Aβ plaques

TREM2, which codes for a transmembrane protein expressed by microglia and other myeloid cells, is one of the most well-studied risk genes in the context of microglia. The R47H variant of TREM2 is a strong genetic risk factor for AD (Jonsson et al., 2013) and confers a loss-of-function phenotype while increasing plaque-associated neuritic dystrophy (Cheng-Hathaway et al., 2018). The receptor signals through its binding partner DAP12 to bind anionic ligands, including phospholipids, lipopolysaccharide (LPS), and Aβ oligomers (Kawabori et al., 2015; Wang et al., 2015; Zhao et al., 2018). Furthermore, TREM2 plays a crucial role in maintaining microglial cell survival (Wang et al., 2015), while Aβ-induced microglial cytokine expression, proliferation, migration, and morphological changes are all dependent on TREM2 signaling (Zhao et al., 2018). Levels of TREM2 are elevated in the cerebrospinal fluid (CSF) of individuals with an inherited form of AD, prior to symptom onset but after the elevation of markers for amyloidosis and neuronal injury (Suárez-Calvet et al., 2016), which may reflect microglial reactivity at an early stage of the disease.

Microglia prevent outward Aβ plaque expansion and subsequent neuritic dystrophy by forming barriers that enclose the plaques in compact microregions (Condello, Yuan, Schain, & Grutzendler, 2015). TREM2 has been shown to modulate the ability of microglia to form this barrier and alter plaque structure, as mice deficient in TREM2 accumulate greater amounts of Aβ due to a dysfunctional response of microglia, which fail to cluster around the plaques and become apoptotic (Wang et al., 2015, 2016). In line with these studies, genetically increasing the expression of TREM2 results in a reduction of amyloid burden and a shift toward more phagocytic microglia in both early and late disease progression (Lee et al., 2018). Additionally, injecting macrophage colony-stimulating factor (M-CSF) into a mouse model of AD prevents cognitive decline, decreases the number of plaques, and results in the proliferation of microglia (Boissonneault et al., 2009). The authors propose that the decrease in Aβ was a direct result of the proliferation of bone marrow-derived microglia, suggesting that different populations of microglia could interact with plaques in functionally diverse ways. Not only do microglia compact plaques, but they could play an integral role in their formation in the first place. Long-term microglial depletion prior to the onset of amyloid plaques reduces both intraneuronal amyloid and neuritic plaque deposition (Spangenberg et al., 2019). TREM2 signaling plays a role in the initial formation of plaques, as plaque seeding is accelerated in TREM2 knockout mice (Parhizkar et al., 2019). However, studies found that microglia ablation in advanced stages of amyloidosis did not affect plaque number and size (Grathwohl et al., 2009). In fact, microglia envelopment was most prominent at the early stages of fibrillar amyloid deposition, indicating that microglia are perhaps less effective at modulating plaques as they grow in size (Condello et al., 2015).

While studies have demonstrated more severe disease-related phenotypes, such as amyloid plaque pathology, in female compared to male mice (Oakley et al., 2006), most have failed to look at sex differences in AD in the context of microglia or TREM2. One of the few studies to investigate sex differences in the transcriptomic effects of the 5xFAD mouse model of AD found that transcriptomic changes occur earlier and more robustly in female than in male 5xFAD mice, and that increased TREM2 gene dosage in 5xFAD mice similarly results in a larger transcriptomic change in females compared to males (Lee et al., 2018). Recently, two studies have examined microglial molecular signals that are associated with the course of disease progression in neurodegenerative disease, including AD. These overlapping sets contain a critical group of microglia genes that are dependent on TREM2 for their disease-associated upregulation (Keren-Shaul et al., 2017; Krasemann et al., 2017). The disease-associated microglia (DAM) genes, as termed by one study, reveal elevated levels of phagocytic-related genes and an enhancement of several known protective risk factors in AD, including TREM2, raising the possibility that this microglial subtype could be protective (Keren-Shaul et al., 2017). In addition, other studies have identified an ultrastructurally distinct microglia subset, "dark" microglia, that is primarily associated with pathological states, revealing heterogeneity within the microglial community (St-Pierre et al., 2020). It is yet to be determined whether neuronal loss initiates transformation of homeostatic microglia into this microglia subtype or is a result of the activation of these molecular signatures.

TREM2's role in amyloid pathogenesis appears to evolve dynamically and temporally with the disease state, with evidence demonstrating that TREM2 deficiency ameliorates amyloid pathology early in disease progression but exacerbates it late in AD (Jay et al., 2017). Such disparate findings could be the result of using different AD mouse models or different TREM2 knockout methods. They could alternatively suggest a model in which the role of microglia in AD shifts as the disease progresses, perhaps playing a more beneficial role early on while exacerbating damage late in the disease.

TREM2 and tau

Tau, a microtubule-associated protein, helps maintain microtubule assembly and stabilization in neurons. Abnormal tau phosphorylation leads to the accumulation of neurofibrillary fibers, which is a major neuropathological hallmark of AD (Goedert & Spillantini, 2006). Tau protein aggregation and neurofibrillary tangle pathology correlate with AD-associated cognitive decline (Arriagada, Growdon, Hedley-Whyte, & Hyman, 1992). As a result, tau protein aggregation and neurofibrillary lesions are considered to be critical in AD pathogenicity. While microglia have been shown to take up tau (Bolós et al., 2015), there is debate as to whether microglia are able to degrade tau efficiently (Hopp et al., 2018). In fact, evidence suggests that microglia themselves may contribute to tau pathology and that microglial reactivity, rather than tau-induced direct neurotoxicity, is a main contributor to neurodegeneration in tauopathy (Maphis et al., 2015). TREM2 also plays a role in tau pathology, with TREM2 deficiency resulting in accelerated tau aggregation and dysregulation of neuronal stress kinase pathways in one tauopathy mouse model (Bemiller et al., 2017), but significantly less brain atrophy and reduced microgliosis in a different model (Leyns et al., 2017). Such disparate findings may be explained by the use of different tauopathy mouse models or in differences in the brain regions and time points that were investigated. It is also possible that, as with Aβ pathology, TREM2's role in tau pathology evolves and changes with disease progression.

Detrimental roles of microglia in Alzheimer's disease

Although proper microglial function protects against AD, there is also evidence that altered microglial activity can mediate synaptic loss in AD and exacerbate tau pathology.

In their canonical immune cell role, microglia release a host of inflammatory factors that can directly injure neurons or indirectly cause damage through the activation of astrocytes.

Complement and synapse elimination

Synaptic loss is an early hallmark of AD and is associated with cognitive decline (Terry et al., 1991), and an increasing number of studies demonstrate the importance of the complement system in microglial synaptic pruning (Salter & Stevens, 2017; Schafer et al., 2012). The complement system consists of a large number of distinct plasma proteins (e.g., C1, C2, C3) that react together to induce a series of inflammatory reactions to help fight infection (Dunkelberger & Song, 2010). Complement factors are highly expressed in AD brains (Efthymiou & Goate, 2017; Yasojima, Schwab, McGeer, & McGeer, 1999), and the level of complement immunoreactivity is positively correlated with Alzheimer's disease severity (Zanjani et al., 2005). Interestingly, there is a connection between amyloid plaques and complement, as Aβ oligomers, which cause synapse degeneration (Wilcox, Lacor, Pitt, & Klein, 2011), activate the classical arm of the complement cascade when Aβ binds to C1q (Sim, Kishore, Villiers, Marche, & Mitchell, 2007).

While complement and microglia have been shown to mediate synapse loss in mouse models early in AD-like amyloid pathology (Hong, Beja-Glasser, et al., 2016), evidence on whether complement is detrimental to AD pathology throughout all disease stages remains controversial. A study investigating normal aging found that knocking out complement component C3 results in less synaptic loss and enhances cognition in aged mice (Shi et al., 2015). Since this suggests that complement is detrimental in normal aging, the authors tested whether knocking out C3 in a mouse model of AD improves neuropathology at later stages of disease. They found that, despite having more plaques, the C3-deficient mice perform better on a learning and memory task, are protected against age-dependent loss of synapses and neurons, and display a reduction in several proinflammatory cytokines (Shi et al., 2017). Complement exacerbates tau pathology, with decreased levels of tau pathology following complement inhibition (Fonseca et al., 2009). However, this decrease in tau pathology is correlated to the level of microglial reactivity, suggesting that complement inhibition could be affecting tau pathology by modulating microglial activity.

There are other studies, however, that provide evidence of a more protective role of complement in later stages of AD pathology. Knocking out C3 in different AD mouse models results in increased Aβ and amyloid plaque burden, along with increased neuronal loss in late stages of the disease (Maier et al., 2008). In line with these studies, knocking out or blocking other complement components, including C1q and C5a, results in an increase in plaque burden and in the accumulation of degenerating neurons (Fonseca, 2004; Fonseca et al., 2009). The increase in amyloid plaque burden, however, is in line with previous work mentioned and is not by itself indicative of negative cognitive or behavioral outcomes.

Neuroinflammation

Neuroinflammation is a central feature of AD, and polymorphisms in inflammation-related genes have been shown to be associated with AD. Polymorphisms in canonically proinflammatory interleukin 1 alpha (IL-1α), IL-1β, IL-6, and tumor necrosis factor alpha (TNFα) have been associated with AD, with higher levels of IL-1 and IL-6 found in the brains of individuals with AD (Su, Bai, & Zhang, 2016). Antiinflammatory cytokines have also been found to be associated with AD. Transforming growth factor beta (TGF-β) signaling has been reported to be insufficient in the brains of AD patients (Tesseur et al., 2006). Polymorphisms in IL-10 and IL-4 have also been found to be associated with AD risk, although discrepancies exist depending on the population studied (Li, Qian, Teng, Ding, & Zhang, 2014; Ribizzi, Fiordoro, Barocci, Ferrari, & Megna, 2010; Zhang et al., 2011).

In addition to damaging synapses through complement-dependent pruning and worsening tau pathology, microglia can also release inflammatory mediators that wreak havoc on neurons. Some protein aggregates present in AD can even activate microglial signaling pathways. Aβ aggregates can act as disease-associated molecular patterns to activate Toll-like receptors (TLRs) and the NRLP3 inflammasome, an innate immune system sensor that regulates the activation of caspase-1 and induces inflammation in response to pathogens or sterile inflammatory factors (Heneka, Golenbock, & Latz, 2015), resulting in the microglial production of inflammatory cytokines such as tumor necrosis factor alpha (TNFα) and interleukin 1 beta (IL-1β). In support of the idea that classical inflammation exacerbates AD pathogenesis, genetic deletion of NLRP3, caspase-1, and TLRs have been shown to decrease Aβ deposition and ameliorate cognitive deficits in AD mouse models (Heneka et al., 2015). However, the role of TLR signaling in mouse models of AD remains unclear. In contrast to TLRs' detrimental role in disease progression, other studies found that TLR inhibition or reduced expression of myeloid differentiation factor 88 (MyD88) adaptor protein impedes microglia ability to detect Aβ and exacerbates disease pathology (Michaud et al., 2013; Michaud, Richard, & Rivest, 2011).

The e4 allele of apolipoprotein E (APOE) is a major genetic risk factor for AD. The human APOE protein is expressed highly in the brain and functions as a ligand in receptor-mediated endocytosis of lipoprotein particles. In the brain, nonneuronal cells, namely astrocytes and microglia, are the major cell types that express APOE (Kim, Basak, & Holtzman, 2009). Knocking-in human apoE4 in a tau mouse model results in significantly higher tau levels, brain atrophy, and neuroinflammation compared with other APOE isoforms and APOE knockout. In the context of tau pathology, the detrimental effects of apoE4 are associated with increased TNFα production by microglia in vitro (Shi et al., 2017). Another study found that IL-1 antagonists blocked the exacerbation of tau pathology in Cx3cr1 deficient mice (Maphis et al., 2015).

Microglia were also shown to act in conjunction with astrocytes to promote neuronal damage. The release of IL-1α, TNFα, and C1q induces a neurotoxic astrocytes subtype that subsequently causes neuronal death (Liddelow et al., 2017). These reactive astrocytes are found in CNS tissue from patients with AD (Liddelow et al., 2017)

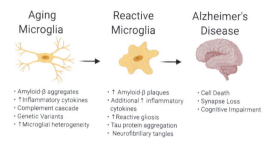

FIG. 1

Role of aging microglia in the development of Alzheimer's disease. Original illustration created with BioRender.com.

and are present in tau transgenic mice expressing human apoE4 (Shi et al., 2017). Notably, microglial-astrocyte cross-talk via C3 and C3R worsens Aβ pathology, through a cycle in which Aβ activates astroglial NF-κβ, which then elicits C3 release. C3 in turn interacts with neuronal and microglial CR3 to impair Aβ phagocytosis and alter cognitive function (Lian et al., 2016). Thus, in the presence of inflammatory mediators, astrocytes could cooperate with microglia to modulate complement-dependent neurotoxicity and contribute to AD pathogenesis (Fig. 1).

Sex differences in the immune system

Given that neuroinflammation is strongly associated with the pathophysiology of AD, it is significant that there are evolutionarily conserved differences in immune function between the sexes. Females of many species, including humans, mount more vigorous innate and adaptive immune responses than males (Gaillard & Spinedi, 1998; Jaillon, Berthenet, & Garlanda, 2019). These differences in the nature and strength of immune responses result in sex-specific differences in the manifestation and prevalence of malignancies and must be acknowledged when considering disparities in health vulnerability. For instance, the stronger immune responses observed in females result in a lower burden of viral, bacterial, and parasitic infections and better vaccine responsiveness (Klein & Flanagan, 2016); however, they also contribute to greater susceptibility to inflammatory and autoimmune diseases. Systemic lupus erythematosus, multiple sclerosis, autoimmune myocarditis, and rheumatoid arthritis are all more prevalent in females (Schurz et al., 2019), as is AD, which has been characterized by some as an autoimmune disease (Lehrer & Rheinstein, 2015).

Since the immune system regulates neuronal development and synaptic refinement (Thion & Garel, 2017), sex differences in immune response during critical stages of CNS development may program mental health throughout the individual's lifespan. Consequently, disruption of immune functionality or microglial reactivity in response to early life perturbations may have far-reaching ramifications on neuroimmune function and behavior later in life (Schwarz & Bilbo, 2012). This is evidenced by the observation that many mental health disorders exhibit a distinct etiology in the development and dysregulation of the immune system (Giefing-Kröll, Berger, Lepperdinger, & Grubeck-Loebenstein, 2015). Sex differences in both neurodevelopment and immune function may contribute to the sex and gender bias observed in the prevalence and severity of developmental and neurodegenerative conditions (Hanamsagar et al., 2017). Specifically, more males than females are diagnosed with early onset or developmental neurological disorders such as autism spectrum disorder (ASD) and attention deficit/hyperactivity disorder (ADHD), whereas more females are diagnosed with conditions manifesting later in life such as AD (Hanamsagar & Bilbo, 2016). These sex-specific immune phenotypes are thought to arise from the chromosomal differences between the sexes set at conception and differences in the immunomodulatory actions of sex steroids that develop over ontogeny.

A higher susceptibility to infection is observed in males from birth to adulthood, suggesting that sexually dimorphic functioning of the innate immune system is germline encoded (Jaillon et al., 2019). In humans, sex chromosomes are homologous in females (XX) and heterologous in males (XY). During embryonic development in females, one X chromosome in each cell is randomly transcriptionally inactivated, resulting in about half the cells expressing genes derived from the maternal X chromosome and half expressing genes from the paternal X chromosome (Libert, Dejager, & Pinheiro, 2010). Female mammals thus have greater diversity in immune-relevant genes relative to males, potentially amplifying their capacity to respond to the onslaught of diverse pathogens (Marais et al., 2018), and are less susceptible to damaging X-linked gene mutations. Additionally, while the human Y chromosome contains approximately 100 genes, the human X chromosome contains more than 1000 genes, including a significant number of genes known to regulate immune function, which may further amplify this effect (Libert et al., 2010). TLR7 and TLR8, for example, are encoded by genes on the X chromosome (Schurz et al., 2019). Sex differences are additionally present in posttranscriptional mechanisms. The X chromosome contains 10% of the ~800 microRNAs (miRNAs) in the human genome, whereas only two miRNAs are observed on the Y chromosome (Bianchi, Lleo, Gershwin, & Invernizzi, 2012). miRNAs are noncoding RNAs involved in posttranscriptional gene regulation, and there is compelling evidence that they are key regulators of inflammatory pathways. Notably, miRNAs are present on macrophages with increased expression levels found to induce an activated phenotype (Pinheiro, Dejager, & Libert, 2011). Due to incomplete X inactivation, the high density of miRNAs on the X chromosome suggests females express more miRNAs, further contributing to sex-specific differences in immune function.

Sex steroids also have immunomodulatory actions, and receptors for estradiol, progesterone, and androgen are expressed on neurons (see also Chapter 2) and immunocompetent cells, including microglia and astrocytes in the CNS (Nelson, Saulsbery, & Lenz, 2019). In females, reproductive steroids are dynamic and change considerably during reproductive periods, as well as over the lifespan. In general, progesterone inhibits innate immune responses, favoring regulatory T cell (Treg) differentiation and exerting an inhibitory effect on natural killer (NK) cells. Conversely, estradiol generally has immune-enhancing effects; however, actions on cell-mediated immunity are dependent on its concentration (Metcalf, Roth, & Graham, 2020). At lower concentrations (e.g., during the follicular stage of the reproductive cycle), estradiol stimulates TNF, interferon (IFN)-γ, IL-1β, and NK cells, whereas high concentrations (e.g., during the luteal phase of the reproductive cycle or during pregnancy) suppress NK cell activity and reduce cytokine production, in particular type-I IFN (Pazos, Kraus, Muñoz-Fontela, & Moran, 2012; Robinson & Klein, 2012; Slominski et al., 2013). In line with these hormone functions, it has been observed that, with the exception of pregnancy, antibody production in response to vaccinations is most evident during women's reproductive years (Giefing-Kröll et al., 2015). The rapid age-related loss of the activational effects of steroid hormones that is characteristic of menopause is believed to be a contributor to sex differences in vulnerability to AD (Vest & Pike, 2013) (see Chapter 9 on hormones and dementia).

Testosterone has the potential to suppress immune defenses and was traditionally believed to be the main factor explaining the weaker immune response in males (Roberts & Peters, 2009). However, more recent research suggests that, while androgens can diminish aspects of immunity such as glial activation or the expression of TLR4 on macrophages (Klein & Flanagan, 2016), the effects of testosterone may be more immunomodulatory than strictly immunosuppressive. Testosterone may also enhance immunity indirectly through the complement cascade (Churchill, Weintraub, Borsos, & Rapp, 1967) and is central in orchestrating inflammatory responses (Da Costa et al., 2018). Studies in rodents have shown that castration of males results in a reduction of peripheral complement activity, and supplementing female mice with androgens increases late-acting complement activity (Churchill et al., 1967; Tanaka, Suzuki, & Nishioka, 1986). Taken together, these studies demonstrate the complex role of sex steroids in the regulation of immune responses.

Immune responses generally become less robust with age, and elderly individuals are more susceptible to infection and display diminished vaccine efficacy (Giefing-Kröll et al., 2015). However, most studies of sex differences in immune function utilize young adults and there is no clear consensus on whether sex-specific immune phenotypes are maintained in advanced age. That said, the available data in humans suggest that adaptive immune traits decline at a lower rate in women than in men, and the innate immune system of aged females may be more inflammatory, which is known to contribute to the pathogenesis of AD and other neurodegenerative disorders (Bupp, Potluri, Fink, & Klein, 2018).

Sex differences in microglia

Along with their roles in immunity, microglia are increasingly recognized for their role in shaping many aspects of brain development, including sexual differentiation. Among their many proposed functions throughout ontogeny, microglia regulate neurogenesis and oligodendrogenesis, support myelination, promote dendritic spine formation, prune and refine spurious synaptic connections, and phagocytose necrotic and apoptotic cells (Hong, Dissing-Olesen, et al., 2016; Menassa & Gomez-Nicola, 2018; Ransohoff & El Khoury, 2016; Reemst, Noctor, Lucassen, & Hol, 2016; Thion & Garel, 2017). These neural processes follow sexually dimorphic developmental trajectories and robust sex differences are seen in microglial density, morphology, and functional phenotype. In rodents, sex differences in microglial maturation are apparent in the early postnatal stages. At PN2–4, males have more microglia than females within the parietal cortex, the amygdala, and the CA1, CA3, and dentate gyrus (DG) regions of the hippocampus (Schwarz, Sholar, & Bilbo, 2012). Male-derived cells are also denser and exhibit more amoeboid morphologies (indicative of reactivity) in the preoptic area (POA), a brain region critical to the manifestation of masculinized copulatory behavior in adulthood (Lenz, Nugent, Haliyur, & McCarthy, 2013), suggesting that the microglia involved in the early-life sex-specific organization of the brain can influence later behavior.

Sex differences in microglial and neuroimmune signaling during the peripubertal period and adulthood have received markedly less attention than these relationships in early development (Nelson et al., 2019). However, it is known that sex differences in microglia morphology and density reverse in juveniles and in early adulthood (P30–60). Female rats have significantly more microglia with an amoeboid morphology and thicker, longer processes in the amygdala and parietal cortex and in regions of the hippocampus (Schwarz et al., 2012). Consistently, a recent transcriptome analysis revealed that microglia-specific gene expression (a proxy for maturation) is enriched in the hippocampus of P60 females relative to males, and female-derived microglia display higher expression of genes associated with inflammatory processes, apoptosis, and in response to LPS (Hanamsagar et al., 2017). This suggests that microglia derived from mature females adopt a more immune-activated phenotype, congruent with the observation that female-mounted innate and adaptive immune responses are stronger than those of males (Gaillard & Spinedi, 1998; Jaillon et al., 2019), and also suggests that females are more sensitive to immune dysregulation later in life.

Microglia express receptors for sex hormones and it has been demonstrated that the roles of microglia and sex hormones in neural development are interwoven (Nelson et al., 2019). For instance, following the prenatal testosterone surge, microglia in the neonatal hippocampus of females phagocytose a greater number of cells than microglia in male neonates. This sex difference is hormone-driven; treating female neonates with estradiol was shown to reduce the phagocytic activity of microglia to male-typical levels (Nelson, Warden, & Lenz, 2017). In line with the increases in phagocytic activity, expression of CD68, a marker of phagolysosomal activity, was enriched in female-derived microglia across the first 4 postnatal weeks (Weinhard et al., 2018). The aforementioned sex-specific differences in the number and morphology of microglia in the POA are also organized by exposure to sex hormones. Estradiol aromatized from testosterone upregulates the microglial production of prostaglandin E2 (PGE2), a proinflammatory lipid, which in turn is responsible for the masculinization of the dendritic spine phenotype in neurons and subsequent male-typical sexual behavior (Lenz et al., 2013). In this pathway, microglial reactivity is necessary for sexual differentiation of the brain and behavior. There was no induction of the male-typical dendritic spine patterning that underlies masculine copulatory behavior in pups treated with minocycline, a nonspecific microglial reactivity inhibitor.

Taken together, microglia and their sexually dependent roles in healthy brain development may partially mediate the establishment and maintenance of sex differences in immune response and behavioral outcomes in later life. Subsequently, aberrant immune signaling and disruption of microglial function during critical windows in brain development may confer sex-biased susceptibility for neurodevelopmental and neurodegenerative disorders in later life (Hanamsagar & Bilbo, 2016). Such windows may occur at early developmental time points, when male offspring have greater quantities of amoeboid microglia and are reported to be more sensitive to inflammatory insults than females (Bilbo et al., 2008; Schwarz et al., 2012). These early perturbations of immune function during ontogeny may reprogram the course of microglial maturation in males, priming microglia to be more susceptible to a heightened proinflammatory phenotype in response to subsequent perturbations in adulthood (Bilbo, Smith, & Schwarz, 2012). However, research into sensitive windows of microglial development has largely been limited to early life, and further studies at time points later in the lifespan—including aging—may identify periods of vulnerability specific to females.

Aging microglia

In both the healthy and diseased aging brain, microglia assume primed phenotypes, which are defined by an exaggerated inflammatory response in presence of a pathogen or other immune stimuli (Perry & Holmes, 2014). Priming is known to be associated with several changes in microglial characteristics with age, such as density, distribution, morphology, cell body mobility, process motility, proliferation, and gene expression, as well as intercellular communication and phagocytosis.

Overall, the microglial population seems to become more diverse and heterogeneous in both humans and rodents as aging goes on, although the overlap in the genes they regulate during this process is limited between the two groups (Galatro et al., 2017). While this suggests that microglial cells age differently in rodents and humans (Galatro et al., 2017), both of their aging microglia exhibit a dystrophic morphology (rodents: Chan et al., 2018; Sierra, Gottfried-Blackmore, McEwen, & Bulloch, 2007; Miller & Streit, 2007; Shaerzadeh et al., 2020; humans: Streit, Sammons, Kuhns, & Sparks, 2004), transcriptomically distinct subtypes (humans: Olah et al., 2018; rodents: Hammond et al., 2019; both: see (Stratoulias, Venero, Tremblay, & Joseph, 2019) for review), and an increase in an ultrastructural subset named "dark microglia," which is characterized by signs of cellular stress along with a condensed cytoplasm and nucleoplasm (Bisht et al., 2016; St-Pierre, Simoncicova, Bogi, & Tremblay, 2020). However, beyond dark microglia, whether these transcriptomic subtypes would display a specific morphology or ultrastructure is still unclear.

Microglial cells in the aging brain might also showcase enhanced numbers (rodents: visual and auditory cortices, Tremblay, Zettel, Ison, Allen, & Majewska, 2012; corpus callosum, Hua, Schindler, McQuail, Forbes, & Riddle, 2012) as well as an increased inflammatory and phagocytic profile (rodents: Rahimian, Cordeau, & Kriz, 2019; Frank, Barrientos, Watkins, & Maier, 2011; Mosher & Wyss-Coray, 2014; Ye & Johnson, 2001; humans and rodents: Nissen, 2017; Niraula, Sheridan, & Godbout, 2017), thus keeping them in a constant "ready to fight" instead of surveillance state. Strikingly, their abilities to efficiently protect the brain and maintain homeostasis are conversely decreased. In rodents, microglia downregulate homeostatic markers such as CD200 (Frank et al., 2006), take longer to scan the tissue following injury or an immune challenge (Damani et al., 2011; Hefendehl et al., 2014), accumulate phagocytic inclusions, which can eventually lead to compromised phagocytic degradation and reduced uptake (Sierra et al., 2007; Streit & Xue, 2010), and aggregate in injured or inflamed zones long after the issue has been resolved (Damani et al., 2011; Tremblay et al., 2012). These time-dependent changes seem, overall, to render aging microglial cells hazardous to the nervous system as they upregulate proinflammatory cytokines, which are known to nefariously affect neurons and cognition (Norden & Godbout, 2014). Furthermore, microglia have been shown to be involved in synaptic loss and subsequent cognitive decline in neurodegenerative diseases including AD (Hammond et al., 2020; Hong, Beja-Glasser, et al., 2016; Wilton, Dissing-Olesen, & Stevens, 2019). It is also worth noting that microglial priming could partly stem from the aged neuroenvironment itself, as the near constant inflammatory state of both the brain and rest of the body (Niraula et al., 2017) might affect microglia and their reactivity (Heneka et al., 2018).

While few studies focus on the sex differences in aging microglia, there is evidence that these cells age differently and use different strategies to resolve inflammation in the aging brain of both sexes. First, evidence suggests that in rodents, aged females may have more microglial cells than age-matched males in the hippocampus, dentate gyrus, and field CA1 of Ammon's horn (Mouton et al., 2002). Furthermore, microglia may specifically accumulate in the bed nucleus of the stria terminalis (BNST), which is involved in social recognition, of aged female rats compared to their younger adult counterparts (Perkins, Piazza, & Deak, 2018). Exercising also seems to modulate microglial reactivity in a sex-dependent manner, as having access to a running wheel decreased the expression of antigen presenting receptors (MHC II, CD86) in the hippocampus of aged female mice, whereas CD86 expression diminished but MHC II increased in the whole brain of aged males that were housed under the same conditions (Kohman, Bhattacharya, Wojcik, & Rhodes, 2013). At the basal level and under inflammatory conditions, it has further been shown in vitro that microglial cells from male rats had a higher migratory activity compared to age-matched females, but that microglial cells from females were characterized by enhanced phagocytosis, as measured by the quantification of fluorescent beads and neural debris engulfed by the cells (Yanguas-Casás et al., 2018; Yanguas-Casás, Crespo-Castrillo, Arevalo, & Garcia-Segura, 2020).

Regarding transcriptomic sex differences, expression of neuroinflammatory genes in mice was enriched both in the cortex and hippocampus of the aged female genome, specifically, complement pathway components such as C1q (Mangold et al., 2017). Interestingly, these findings correlate with the observed increase in female microglia phagocytic activity described earlier. Aging-related changes in the transcriptome were also characterized by heightened interanimal gene expression variability in aged male mice but not females (Mangold et al., 2017).

In humans, similar findings were observed in the gene expression profiles of the hippocampus, entorhinal cortex, superior frontal gyrus, and postcentral gyrus, with aged males undergoing more gene change than females in all regions analyzed and females being characterized by a greater immune activation (Berchtold et al., 2008). Prominent change in cellular processes such as energy production, RNA processing, and ribosome-related processes also occurred in the cortical area of males between 60 and 70, thus suggesting that a critical transition in the aging process transpires during this period in this sex (Berchtold et al., 2008). A recent study assessing sex differences in peripheral blood mononuclear cells also uncovered greater genomic changes in older men, who were characterized by a decline in B-cell specific loci compared to females (Márquez et al., 2020).

Therefore, data consistently show that aging affects both male and female brains in a similar yet distinctive manner. Moreover, exercise seems to induce sex-specific changes in the expression of antigen-presenting receptors (Kohman et al., 2013). Strikingly, exposing female mice to outdoor living was further shown to decrease microglial phagocytosis, just like exercising did, and further reduced microglial numbers in both healthy and infected animals, which was correlated with an increase in juvenile neurons (Cope et al., 2019). Experiences with nature thus seem to cause beneficial microglial changes in mice and have further been linked to improved cognition and stress relief in humans (Savage & Tremblay, 2019). These results overall suggest that aging male microglia might be better at maintaining homeostasis and resolving inflammation than females and that both sexes use alternative strategies to keep the aging brain relatively healthy.

Interactions between AD, sex, and inflammation in the aged brain

Sex differences in microglial properties and aging could influence the way a given sex fights neurodegenerative diseases such as AD, in which microglia plays a prevalent role. AD is known to prevalently affect females in an age-dependent and more severe manner (Neu et al., 2017), but the exact mechanisms driving this sex and gender difference have remained elusive. As briefly described in previous sections, over the past few years, many studies have uncovered sexually differentiated biological factors (such as APOE, protein tau levels, Aβ plaques, metabolic processes, neurotrophins, inflammation, and microglia) that could explain the mechanisms leading to the increased incidence of AD in females.

The APOE gene encodes a protein playing a major role in cholesterol metabolism that is also a potent genetic factor for AD. Expression of the ε4 allele increases risk of developing the disease and diminishes age at onset in a dose-dependent manner in humans (Corder et al., 1993). Human studies showed that, while ε4 carriers are more likely to exhibit cognitive decline, this effect seems stronger in women (Altmann, Tian, Henderson, & Greicius, 2014; Beydoun et al., 2012; Damoiseaux et al., 2012; Farrer et al., 1997; Fleisher et al., 2005; Payami et al., 1994) and that female ε4 carriers displayed reduced default connectivity in the precuneus compared to female ε3 homozygotes and male ε4 carriers (Damoiseaux et al., 2012).

Moreover, APOE genotype has, to some extent, been linked with sex/gender and cerebrospinal fluid (CSF) tau levels, tau being a protein binding and stabilizing component of neurons in the brain and whose accumulation leads to the formation of neurofibrillary tangles in AD. Some studies showed that human female ε4 carriers display increased CSF tau levels (Altmann et al., 2014; Damoiseaux et al., 2012; Hohman et al., 2018), a sex and gender difference that was either accompanied by a matching difference in amyloid burden and cognitive decline (Koran, Wagener, & Hohman, 2017) or was only present in amyloid-positive subjects (Hohman et al., 2018). A recent study uncovered similar results, with women carrying the ε4 allele possessing higher CSF tau levels, a difference associated with early disease stages (Mofrad et al., 2020). The APOE genotype is thought to influence tau phosphorylation and amyloid burden in AD and, even though the exact mechanisms are still unclear (Bu, 2009), these results suggest that this interaction may affect females more strongly as well as accelerating and aggravating AD pathogenesis.

Independently of the APOE genotype, sex and gender differences in tau levels and Aβ plaques have also been studied in the literature. In rodents, tau/APP females (a crossing of JNPL3 and Tg2576 parents) seem to develop neurofibrillary tangles at an earlier age and also express higher tau levels (Lewis et al., 2001) (see Chapter 1 on animal models). Similar findings have been found in humans, where women with higher amyloid burden showed greater entorhinal cortical tau levels compared to men with higher amyloid content (Buckley et al., 2019). Another human study further observed comparable results, with women suffering from AD displaying increased levels of tau tangle density (Oveisgharan et al., 2018). Overall, tau accumulation may thus be accelerated in females while males might be more protected against neurofibrillary tangle formation. Regarding Aβ plaques, some studies seem to show a female-biased sex and gender difference (Fisher, Bennett, & Dong, 2018), hinting that females might also accumulate soluble and insoluble Aβ (Tg2576 mice with the Swedish mutation APP695SWE; Callahan et al., 2001), amyloid plaques (Tg2576 mice, Callahan et al., 2001; EFAD mice, Stephen et al., 2019), plasma Aβ (AβPP/PS1 mice; Ordóñez-Gutiérrez, Antón, & Wandosell, 2015), and CSF Aβ (human patients; Koran et al., 2017) faster than males.

In addition, sex differences were observed for genes related to metabolic processes in the 129/C57BL/6 mouse hippocampus, with females downregulating genes involved in glycolysis and upregulating genes related to amyloid metabolism (Zhao, Mao, Woody, & Brinton, 2016). Conversely, gene changes were of lesser magnitude in males, occurred later in life, and mostly consisted of an upregulation of genes involved in metabolic processes and apoptosis. These results suggest a potential adaptive response to the aging process in males, while females display a hypometabolic phenotype, putting them at risk of AD (Zhao et al., 2016). In humans, metabolic alterations hint at a greater impairment of mitochondrial energy in women, a difference that seems to rely on the APOE genotype (Arnold et al., 2020). Human studies further uncovered another potential sexually differentiated biomarker, the brain-derived neurotrophic factor (BDNF), which plays a crucial role in the control of dendritic spine formation notably exerted by microglia (Parkhurst et al., 2013). As was the case with the APOE gene, some BDNF polymorphisms were revealed to affect cognitive decline and AD risk, an effect that was stronger in female carriers (Chen, Liang, Li, Jiang, & Xu, 2014; Fukumoto et al., 2010; Li et al., 2017).

Although the mechanisms driving these sexually differentiated effects are still unclear, AD pathogenesis seems to stem from numerous deficiencies associated with the exposure to various environmental risk factors across life and not solely from Aβ accumulation, as the amyloid cascade hypothesis would suggest (Herrup, 2015). Strikingly, AD pathogenesis is also associated with neuroinflammation and increased reactivity of the immune system. Indeed, systemic and brain inflammation in aging subjects is likely to stimulate neuroimmunological processes involving microglia and promote disease progression (Heneka et al., 2018; Perry, Cunningham, & Holmes, 2007). Reciprocally, AD seems to modulate innate immunity through immune receptor genes that have been linked with the disease (CD33, TREM2; Griciuc et al., 2013, 2019) as well as upholding neuroinflammation and microglial priming with the accumulation of amyloid plaques and neuronal debris (Heneka et al., 2018; Tuppo & Arias, 2005). There also exists a hypothesis proposing that the progressive accumulation of Aβ triggers early plaque-independent neuroinflammation, constituting a "disease-aggravating" process (Cuello, 2017).

Both inflammation in the aged brain and microglia are sexually differentiated and could thus further explain AD prevalence in women. It is likely that these sex differences would have consequences in regards to how each sex responds to neurodegenerative diseases like AD, as well as their risk factors. For instance, transcriptomic changes in the cerebral hippocampus and cortex of mice (APP/PS1-Apoe^{null}, App^{NL-G-F}) and humans were observed with normal aging and led to two reactive microglial states: activated response microglia (ARMs) and interferon response microglia (IRMs), with the former state progressing faster in females (Frigerio et al., 2019). ARMs were characterized by expression of genes involved in inflammatory processes and MHC II presentation, whereas IRMs displayed high expression of genes related to innate immune response and interferon response type I pathways (Frigerio et al., 2019). Both microglial states were enhanced following Aβ accumulation, and ARMs were found to be enriched with genes associated with AD, such as APOE.

In another study, transgenic mice (EFAD; homozygotes for the human APOE ε4 or ε3 allele) showed a significant reduction of Aβ plaque coverage and/or compaction by microglial cells in the hippocampus of ε4 carriers as well as females as a whole (Stephen et al., 2019). This reduction was correlated with a decrease in TREM2 expression, a marker present on the surface of microglia (including the dark microglia subset) that affects their survival, proliferation, phagocytosis, chemokine receptor expression, metabolism, clustering around Aβ plaques, and motility (Klesney-Tait, Turnbull, & Colonna, 2006; Yeh, Hansen, & Sheng, 2017). By contrast, plaque coverage and compaction were enhanced in male ε3 carriers, together with TREM2 expression (Stephen et al., 2019). These data suggest that the APOE genotype might influence microglial phagocytosis and further hint at the fact that male microglia may be more efficient at getting rid of plaques than females. In a human study focusing on patients with autosomal dominant AD, TREM2 ectodomain released by proteolysis as a soluble variant was also found to be more concentrated in the CSF of men (Suárez-Calvet et al., 2016).

Furthermore, Kodama and colleagues observed that depletion of microglial microRNAs in Dicer knockout (KO) mice specifically induced transcriptomic changes in males with tau pathology (Kodama et al., 2020). Loss of mature microRNAs, via depletion of the microRNA-processing enzyme Dicer, thus resulted in male microglial cells displaying enrichment of genes involved in inflammation and phagocytosis characteristic of disease-associated microglia (DAM), a subset associated with AD-like pathology in mice (Keren-Shaul et al., 2017). Moreover, these KO mice demonstrated more amoeboid and decreased homeostatic microglia in males compared to females, an effect accompanied by higher tau levels in KO males (Kodama et al., 2020). These results both support a differential microglial response to tau pathology in both sexes and highlight the importance of microglial microRNAs in driving this differential response (Kodama et al., 2020).

Conclusion

Overall, there are many factors that may interact and contribute to the enhanced sensitivity of females with regards to the development of AD. Specifically, microglia are an important factor that might explain AD susceptibility, as they are sexually differentiated. While aged microglial cells of both sexes demonstrate an overall reactive profile, microglia may be more homeostatic and neuroprotective in aged males. Conversely, age-matched females may be characterized by dystrophic microglial cells that fail to clean the brain properly, thus allowing the accumulation of tangles and Aβ plaques and ultimately leading to poor neuronal survival and synaptic integrity (Frigerio et al., 2019; Kodama et al., 2020). Therefore, sex differences in microglial properties and aging described previously most certainly warrant a deeper investigation of the sexually differentiated mechanisms and functions of aging microglia as well as their response to environmental cues. Further research is thus necessary to definitively characterize these sex differences and to provide insight into the female-biased susceptibility to neurodegenerative disorders.

Chapter highlights

- Female brains seem to showcase increased neuroinflammation, microglial reactivity, and microglial numbers compared to males during normal aging and under neurodegenerative conditions.

- Microglia may be more homeostatic and effective in aged males compared to age-matched females.
- Enhanced microglial reactivity and neuroinflammation in older females might ultimately lead to failure to clean the brain properly, hence resulting in accumulation of both tangles and Aβ plaques in Alzheimer's disease.

References

Altmann, A., Tian, L., Henderson, V. W., & Greicius, M. D. (2014). Sex modifies the APOE-related risk of developing Alzheimer disease. *Annals of Neurology*, *75*(4), 563–573.

Alzheimer's Association. (2020). *Alzheimer's Association 2020 facts and figures report* (p. 1). Alzheimer's Association. https://www.alz.org/alzheimers-dementia/facts-figures.

Arcuri, C., Mecca, C., Bianchi, R., Giambanco, I., & Donato, R. (2017). The pathophysiological role of microglia in dynamic surveillance, phagocytosis and structural remodeling of the developing CNS. *Frontiers in Molecular Neuroscience*, *10*(June), 1–22.

Arnold, M., Nho, K., Kueider-Paisley, A., Massaro, T., Huynh, K., Brauner, B., … Kastenmüller, G. (2020). Sex and APOE ε4 genotype modify the Alzheimer's disease serum metabolome. *Nature Communications*, *11*(1), 1–12.

Arriagada, P. V., Growdon, J. H., Hedley-Whyte, E. T., & Hyman, B. T. (1992). Neurofibrillary tangles but not senile plaques parallel duration and severity of Alzheimer's disease. *Neurology*, *42*(3), 631–639.

Bemiller, S. M., McCray, T. J., Allan, K., Formica, S. V., Xu, G., Wilson, G., … Lamb, B. T. (2017). TREM2 deficiency exacerbates tau pathology through dysregulated kinase signaling in a mouse model of tauopathy. *Molecular Neurodegeneration*, *12*(1), 74.

Berchtold, N. C., Cribbs, D. H., Coleman, P. D., Rogers, J., Head, E., Kim, R., … Cotman, C. W. (2008). Gene expression changes in the course of normal brain aging are sexually dimorphic. *Proceedings of the National Academy of Sciences of the United States of America*, *105*(40), 15605–15610.

Beydoun, M. A., Boueiz, A., Abougergi, M. S., Kitner-Triolo, M. H., Beydoun, H. A., Resnick, S. M., … Zonderman, A. B. (2012). Sex differences in the association of the apolipoprotein E epsilon 4 allele with incidence of dementia, cognitive impairment, and decline. *Neurobiology of Aging*, *33*(4), 720–731. e4.

Bianchi, I., Lleo, A., Gershwin, M. E., & Invernizzi, P. (2012). The X chromosome and immune associated genes. *Journal of Autoimmunity*, *38*(2), J187–J192.

Bilbo, S. D., Barrientos, R. M., Eads, A. S., Northcutt, A., Watkins, L. R., Rudy, J. W., & Maier, S. F. (2008). Early-life infection leads to altered BDNF and IL-1β mRNA expression in rat hippocampus following learning in adulthood. *Brain, Behavior, and Immunity*, *22*(4), 451–455.

Bilbo, S. D., & Schwarz, J. M. (2012). The immune system and developmental programming of brain and behavior. *Frontiers in Neuroendocrinology*, *33*(3), 267–286.

Bilbo, S. D., Smith, S. H., & Schwarz, J. M. (2012). A lifespan approach to neuroinflammatory and cognitive disorders: A critical role for glia. *Journal of Neuroimmune Pharmacology*, *7*(1), 24–41.

Bisht, K., Sharma, K. P., Lecours, C., Gabriela Sánchez, M., El Hajj, H., Milior, G., … Tremblay, M.È. (2016). Dark microglia: A new phenotype predominantly associated with pathological states. *Glia*, *64*(5), 826–839.

Boissonneault, V., Filali, M., Lessard, M., Relton, J., Wong, G., & Rivest, S. (2009). Powerful beneficial effects of macrophage colony-stimulating factor on -amyloid deposition and cognitive impairment in Alzheimer's disease. *Brain*, *132*(4), 1078–1092.

Bolós, M., Llorens-Martín, M., Jurado-Arjona, J., Hernández, F., Rábano, A., & Avila, J. (2015). Direct evidence of internalization of tau by microglia in vitro and in vivo. *Journal of Alzheimer's Disease*, *50*(1), 77–87.

Bu, G. (2009). Apolipoprotein E and its receptors in Alzheimer's disease: Pathways, pathogenesis and therapy. *Nature Reviews Neuroscience*, *10*(5), 333–344.

Buckley, R. F., Mormino, E. C., Rabin, J. S., Hohman, T. J., Landau, S., Hanseeuw, B. J., … Sperling, R.A. (2019). Sex differences in the association of global amyloid and regional tau deposition measured by positron emission tomography in clinically normal older adults. *JAMA Neurology*, *76*(5), 542–551.

Bupp, M. R. G., Potluri, T., Fink, A. L., & Klein, S. L. (2018). The confluence of sex hormones and aging on immunity. *Frontiers in Immunology*, *9*(JUN), 1269.

Callahan, M. J., Lipinski, W. J., Bian, F., Durham, R. A., Pack, A., & Walker, L. C. (2001). Augmented senile plaque load in aged female β-amyloid precursor protein-transgenic mice. *American Journal of Pathology*, *158*(3), 1173–1177.

Chan, T. E., Grossman, Y. S., Bloss, E. B., Janssen, W. G., Lou, W., McEwen, B. S., … Morrison, J. H. (2018). Cell-type specific changes in glial morphology and glucocorticoid expression during stress and aging in the medial prefrontal cortex. *Frontiers in Aging Neuroscience*, *10*, 146.

Chen, J., Liang, X., Li, B., Jiang, X., & Xu, Z. (2014). Gender-related association of brain-derived neurotrophic factor gene 196A/G polymorphism with Alzheimer's disease—A meta-analysis including 6854 cases and 6868 controls. *International Journal of Neuroscience*, *124*(10), 724–733.

Cheng-Hathaway, P. J., Reed-Geaghan, E. G., Jay, T. R., Casali, B. T., Bemiller, S. M., Puntambekar, S. S., … Landreth, G. E. (2018). The Trem2 R47H variant confers loss-of-function-like phenotypes in Alzheimer's disease. *Molecular Neurodegeneration*, *13*(1), 29.

Churchill, W. H., Weintraub, R. M., Borsos, T., & Rapp, H. J. (1967). Mouse complement: The effect of sex hormones and castration on two of the late-acting components. *Journal of Experimental Medicine*, *125*(4), 657–672.

Condello, C., Yuan, P., Schain, A., & Grutzendler, J. (2015). Microglia constitute a barrier that prevents neurotoxic protofibrillar Aβ42 hotspots around plaques. *Nature Communications*, *6*(1), 6176.

Cope, E., Opendak, M., LaMarca, E., Murthy, S., Park, C., Olson, L., … Gould, E. (2019). The effects of living in an outdoor enclosure on hippocampal plasticity and anxiety-like behavior in response to nematode infection. *Hippocampus*, *29*(4), 366–377.

Corder, E. H., Saunders, A. M., Strittmatter, W. J., Schmechel, D. E., Gaskell, P. C., Small, G. W., … Pericak-Vance, M. A. (1993). Gene dose of Apolipoprotein E type 4 allele and the risk of Alzheimer's disease in late onset families. *Science*, *261*(14), 41–43.

Cuello, A. C. (2017). Early and late CNS inflammation in Alzheimer's disease: Two extremes of a continuum? *Trends in Pharmacological Sciences*, *38*(11), 956–966.

Da Costa, M. G., Poppelaars, F., Van Kooten, C., Mollnes, T. E., Tedesco, F., Würzner, R., … Seelen, M. A. (2018). Age and sex-associated changes of complement activity and complement levels in a healthy caucasian population. *Frontiers in Immunology*, *9*(NOV), 1–14.

Damani, M. R., Zhao, L., Fontainhas, A. M., Amaral, J., Fariss, R. N., & Wong, W. T. (2011). Age-related alterations in the dynamic behavior of microglia. *Aging Cell*, *10*(2), 263–276.

Damoiseaux, J. S., Seeley, W. W., Zhou, J., Shirer, W. R., Coppola, G., Karydas, A., … Greicius, M. D. (2012). Gender modulates the APOE ε4 effect in healthy older adults: Convergent evidence from functional brain connectivity and spinal fluid tau levels. *Journal of Neuroscience*, *32*(24), 8254–8262.

Dunkelberger, J. R., & Song, W.-C. (2010). Complement and its role in innate and adaptive immune responses. *Cell Research*, *20*(1), 34–50.

Efthymiou, A. G., & Goate, A. M. (2017). Late onset Alzheimer's disease genetics implicates microglial pathways in disease risk. *Molecular Neurodegeneration*, *12*(1), 43.

Farrer, L. A., Cupples, L. A., Haines, J. L., Hyman, B., Kukull, W. A., Mayeux, R., … Van Duijn, C. M. (1997). Effects of age, sex, and ethnicity on the association between apolipoprotein E genotype and Alzheimer disease: A meta-analysis. *Journal of the American Medical Association*, *278*(16), 1349–1356.

Fisher, D. W., Bennett, D. A., & Dong, H. (2018). Sexual dimorphism in predisposition to Alzheimer's disease. *Neurobiology of Aging*, *70*, 308–324.

Fleisher, A., Grundman, M., Jack, C. R., Petersen, R. C., Taylor, C., Kim, H. T., … Thal, L. J. (2005). Sex, apolipoprotein E ε4 status, and hippocampal volume in mild cognitive impairment. *Archives of Neurology*, *62*(6), 953–957.

Fonseca, M. I. (2004). Absence of C1q leads to less neuropathology in transgenic mouse models of Alzheimer's disease. *Journal of Neuroscience*, *24*(29), 6457–6465.

Fonseca, M. I., Ager, R. R., Chu, S.-H., Yazan, O., Sanderson, S. D., LaFerla, F. M., … Tenner, A. J. (2009). Treatment with a C5aR antagonist decreases pathology and enhances behavioral performance in murine models of Alzheimer's disease. *Journal of Immunology*, *183*(2), 1375–1383.

Frank, M. G., Barrientos, R. M., Biedenkapp, J. C., Rudy, J. W., Watkins, L. R., & Maier, S. F. (2006). mRNA up-regulation of MHC II and pivotal pro-inflammatory genes in normal brain aging. *Neurobiology of Aging*, *27*(5), 717–722.

Frank, M. G., Barrientos, R. M., Watkins, L. R., & Maier, S. F. (2011). Aging sensitizes rapidly isolated hippocampal microglia to LPS ex vivo. *Journal of Neuroimmunology*, *226*(1–2), 181–184.

Frigerio, C. S., Wolfs, L., Fattorelli, N., Thrupp, N., Voytyuk, I., Schmidt, I., … De Strooper, B. (2019). The major risk factors for Alzheimer's disease: Age, sex, and genes modulate the microglia response to Aβ plaques. *Cell Reports*, *27*(4), 1293–1306.

Fukumoto, N., Fujii, T., Combarros, O., Kamboh, M. I., Tsai, S. J., Matsushita, S., … Kunugi, H. (2010). Sexually dimorphic effect of the Val66Met polymorphism of BDNF on susceptibility to Alzheimer's disease: New data and meta-analysis. *American Journal of Medical Genetics, Part B: Neuropsychiatric Genetics*, *153*(1), 235–242.

Gaillard, R. C., & Spinedi, E. (1998). Sex- and stress-steroids interactions and the immune system: Evidence for a neuroendocrine-immunological sexual dimorphism. *Domestic Animal Endocrinology*, *15*(5), 345–352.

Galatro, T. F., Holtman, I. R., Lerario, A. M., Vainchtein, I. D., Brouwer, N., Sola, P. R., … Eggen, B. J. L. (2017). Transcriptomic analysis of purified human cortical microglia reveals age-associated changes. *Nature Neuroscience*, *20*(8), 1162–1171.

Gallardo, G., & Holtzman, D. M. (2019). Amyloid-β and Tau at the crossroads of Alzheimer's disease. *Advances in Experimental Medicine and Biology*, *1184*, 187–203.

Giefing-Kröll, C., Berger, P., Lepperdinger, G., & Grubeck-Loebenstein, B. (2015). How sex and age affect immune responses, susceptibility to infections, and response to vaccination. *Aging Cell*, *14*(3), 309–321.

Goedert, M., & Spillantini, M. G. (2006). A century of Alzheimer's disease. *Science*, *314*(5800), 777–781.

Grathwohl, S. A., Kälin, R. E., Bolmont, T., Prokop, S., Winkelmann, G., Kaeser, S. A., … Jucker, M. (2009). Formation and maintenance of Alzheimer's disease β-amyloid plaques in the absence of microglia. *Nature Neuroscience*, *12*(11), 1361–1363.

Griciuc, A., Patel, S., Federico, A. N., Choi, S. H., Innes, B. J., Oram, M. K., ... Tanzi, R. E. (2019). TREM2 acts downstream of CD33 in modulating microglial pathology in Alzheimer's disease. *Neuron, 103*(5), 820–835.

Griciuc, A., Serrano-Pozo, A., Parrado, A. R., Lesinski, A. N., Asselin, C. N., Mullin, K., ... Tanzi, R. E. (2013). Alzheimer's disease risk gene CD33 inhibits microglial uptake of amyloid beta. *Neuron, 78*(4), 631–643.

Hammond, J. W., Bellizzi, M. J., Ware, C., Qiu, W. Q., Saminathan, P., Li, H., ... Gelbard, H. A. (2020). Complement-dependent synapse loss and microgliosis in a mouse model of multiple sclerosis. *Brain, Behavior, and Immunity, 87*, 739–750.

Hammond, T. R., Dufort, C., Dissing-Olesen, L., Giera, S., Young, A., Wysoker, A., ... Stevens, B. (2019). Single-cell RNA sequencing of microglia throughout the mouse lifespan and in the injured brain reveals complex cell-state changes. *Immunity, 50*(1), 253–271.

Hanamsagar, R., Alter, M. D., Block, C. S., Sullivan, H., Bolton, J. L., & Bilbo, S. D. (2017). Generation of a microglial developmental index in mice and in humans reveals a sex difference in maturation and immune reactivity. *Glia, 65*(9), 1504–1520.

Hanamsagar, R., & Bilbo, S. D. (2016). Sex differences in neurodevelopmental and neurodegenerative disorders: Focus on microglial function and neuroinflammation during development. *Journal of Steroid Biochemistry and Molecular Biology, 160*, 127–133.

Hanisch, U. K., & Kettenmann, H. (2007). Microglia: Active sensor and versatile effector cells in the normal and pathologic brain. *Nature Neuroscience, 10*(11), 1387–1394.

Hefendehl, J. K., Neher, J. J., Sühs, R. B., Kohsaka, S., Skodras, A., & Jucker, M. (2014). Homeostatic and injury-induced microglia behavior in the aging brain. *Aging Cell, 13*(1), 60–69.

Heneka, M. T., Carson, M. J., El Khoury, J., Gary, E., Brosseron, F., Feinstein, D. L., ... Ransohoff, R. M. (2018). Neuroinflammation in Alzheimer's disease. *Lancet Neurology, 14*(4), 388–405.

Heneka, M. T., Golenbock, D. T., & Latz, E. (2015). Innate immunity in Alzheimer's disease. *Nature Immunology, 16*(3), 229–236.

Herrup, K. (2015). The case for rejecting the amyloid cascade hypothesis. *Nature Neuroscience, 18*(6), 794–799.

Hohman, T. J., Dumitrescu, L., Barnes, L. L., Thambisetty, M., Beecham, G., Kunkle, B., ... Zhao, Y. (2018). Sex-specific association of apolipoprotein e with cerebrospinal fluid levels of tau. *JAMA Neurology, 75*(8), 989–998.

Holtzman, D. M. (2001). Role of apoE/Aβ interactions in the pathogenesis of Alzheimer's disease and cerebral amyloid angiopathy. *Journal of Molecular Neuroscience, 17*, 9.

Hong, S., Beja-Glasser, V. F., Nfonoyim, B. M., Frouin, A., Li, S., Ramakrishnan, S., ... Stevens, B. (2016). Complement and microglia mediate early synapse loss in Alzheimer mouse models. *Science, 352*(6286), 712–716.

Hong, S., Dissing-Olesen, L., & Stevens, B. (2016). New insights on the role of microglia in synaptic pruning in health and disease. *Current Opinion in Neurobiology, 36*(11), 128–134.

Hopp, S. C., Lin, Y., Oakley, D., Roe, A. D., DeVos, S. L., Hanlon, D., & Hyman, B. T. (2018). The role of microglia in processing and spreading of bioactive tau seeds in Alzheimer's disease. *Journal of Neuroinflammation, 15*(1), 269.

Hua, K., Schindler, M. K., McQuail, J. A., Forbes, M. E., & Riddle, D. R. (2012). Regionally distinct responses of microglia and glial progenitor cells to whole brain irradiation in adult and aging rats. *PLoS One, 7*(12), e52728.

Jaillon, S., Berthenet, K., & Garlanda, C. (2019). Sexual dimorphism in innate immunity. *Clinical Reviews in Allergy and Immunology, 56*(3), 308–321.

Jay, T. R., Hirsch, A. M., Broihier, M. L., Miller, C. M., Neilson, L. E., Ransohoff, R. M., … Landreth, G. E. (2017). Disease progression-dependent effects of TREM2 deficiency in a mouse model of Alzheimer's disease. *Journal of Neuroscience*, *37*(3), 637–647.

Jonsson, T., Stefansson, H., Steinberg, S., Jonsdottir, I., Jonsson, P. V., Snaedal, J., … Stefansson, K. (2013). Variant of *TREM2* associated with the risk of Alzheimer's disease. *New England Journal of Medicine*, *368*(2), 107–116.

Karch, C. M., & Goate, A. M. (2015). Alzheimer's disease risk genes and mechanisms of disease pathogenesis. *Biological Psychiatry*, *77*(1), 43–51.

Kawabori, M., Kacimi, R., Kauppinen, T., Calosing, C., Kim, J. Y., Hsieh, C. L., … Yenari, M. A. (2015). Triggering receptor expressed on myeloid cells 2 (TREM2) deficiency attenuates phagocytic activities of microglia and exacerbates ischemic damage in experimental stroke. *Journal of Neuroscience*, *35*(8), 3384–3396.

Keren-Shaul, H., Spinrad, A., Weiner, A., Matcovitch-Natan, O., Dvir-Szternfeld, R., Ulland, T. K., … Amit, I. (2017). A unique microglia type associated with restricting development of Alzheimer's disease. *Cell*, *169*(7), 1276–1290. e17.

Kim, J., Basak, J. M., & Holtzman, D. M. (2009). The role of apolipoprotein E in Alzheimer's disease. *Neuron*, *63*(3), 287–303.

Klein, S. L., & Flanagan, K. L. (2016). Sex differences in immune responses. *Nature Reviews Immunology*, *16*(10), 626–638.

Klesney-Tait, J., Turnbull, I. R., & Colonna, M. (2006). The TREM receptor family and signal integration. *Nature Immunology*, *7*(12), 1266–1273.

Kodama, L., Guzman, E., Etchegaray, J. I., Li, Y., Sayed, F. A., Zhou, L., … Gan, L. (2020). Microglial microRNAs mediate sex-specific responses to tau pathology. *Nature Neuroscience*, *23*(2), 167–171.

Kohman, R. A., Bhattacharya, T. K., Wojcik, E., & Rhodes, J. S. (2013). Exercise reduces activation of microglia isolated from hippocampus and brain of aged mice. *Journal of Neuroinflammation*, *10*(114), 1–9.

Koran, M. E. I., Wagener, M., & Hohman, T. J. (2017). Sex differences in the association between AD biomarkers and cognitive decline. *Brain Imaging and Behavior*, *11*(1), 205–213.

Krasemann, S., Madore, C., Cialic, R., Baufeld, C., Calcagno, N., El Fatimy, R., … Butovsky, O. (2017). The TREM2-APOE pathway drives the transcriptional phenotype of dysfunctional microglia in neurodegenerative diseases. *Immunity*, *47*(3), 566–581. e9.

Lee, C. Y. D., Daggett, A., Gu, X., Jiang, L.-L., Langfelder, P., Li, X., … Yang, X. W. (2018). Elevated TREM2 gene dosage reprograms microglia responsivity and ameliorates pathological phenotypes in Alzheimer's disease models. *Neuron*, *97*(5), 1032–1048. e5.

Lehrer, S., & Rheinstein, P. H. (2015). Is Alzheimer's disease autoimmune inflammation of the brain that can be treated with nasal nonsteroidal anti-inflammatory drugs? *American Journal of Alzheimer's Disease and Other Dementias*, *30*(3), 225–227.

Lenz, K. M., Nugent, B. M., Haliyur, R., & McCarthy, M. M. (2013). Microglia are essential to masculinization of brain and behavior. *Journal of Neuroscience*, *33*(7), 2761–2772.

Lewis, J., Dickson, D. W., Lin, W. L., Chisholm, L., Corral, A., Jones, G., … McGowan, E. (2001). Enhanced neurofibrillary degeneration in transgenic mice expressing mutant tau and APP. *Science*, *293*(5534), 1487–1491.

Leyns, C. E. G., Ulrich, J. D., Finn, M. B., Stewart, F. R., Koscal, L. J., Remolina Serrano, J., … Holtzman, D. M. (2017). TREM2 deficiency attenuates neuroinflammation and protects against neurodegeneration in a mouse model of tauopathy. *Proceedings of the National Academy of Sciences*, *114*(43), 11524–11529.

Li, G. D., Bi, R., Zhang, D. F., Xu, M., Luo, R., Wang, D., ... Yao, Y. G. (2017). Female-specific effect of the BDNF gene on Alzheimer's disease. *Neurobiology of Aging*, *53*. 192.e11–192.e19.

Li, W., Qian, X., Teng, H., Ding, Y., & Zhang, L. (2014). Association of interleukin-4 genetic polymorphisms with sporadic Alzheimer's disease in Chinese Han population. *Neuroscience Letters*, *563*, 17–21.

Lian, H., Litvinchuk, A., Chiang, A. C.-A., Aithmitti, N., Jankowsky, J. L., & Zheng, H. (2016). Astrocyte-microglia cross talk through complement activation modulates amyloid pathology in mouse models of Alzheimer's disease. *Journal of Neuroscience*, *36*(2), 577–589.

Libert, C., Dejager, L., & Pinheiro, I. (2010). The X chromosome in immune functions: When a chromosome makes the difference. *Nature Reviews Immunology*, *10*(8), 594–604.

Liddelow, S. A., Guttenplan, K. A., Clarke, L. E., Bennett, F. C., Bohlen, C. J., Schirmer, L., ... Barres, B.A. (2017). Neurotoxic reactive astrocytes are induced by activated microglia. *Nature*, *541*(7638), 481–487.

Maier, M., Peng, Y., Jiang, L., Seabrook, T. J., Carroll, M. C., & Lemere, C. A. (2008). Complement C3 deficiency leads to accelerated amyloid plaque deposition and neurodegeneration and modulation of the microglia/macrophage phenotype in amyloid precursor protein transgenic mice. *Journal of Neuroscience*, *28*(25), 6333–6341.

Mangold, C. A., Wronowski, B., Du, M., Masser, D. R., Hadad, N., Bixler, G. V., ... Freeman, W. M. (2017). Sexually divergent induction of microglial-associated neuroinflammation with hippocampal aging. *Journal of Neuroinflammation*, *14*(1), 1–19.

Maphis, N., Xu, G., Kokiko-Cochran, O. N., Jiang, S., Cardona, A., Ransohoff, R. M., ... Bhaskar, K. (2015). Reactive microglia drive tau pathology and contribute to the spreading of pathological tau in the brain. *Brain*, *138*(6), 1738–1755.

Marais, G. A. B., Gaillard, J. M., Vieira, C., Plotton, I., Sanlaville, D., Gueyffier, F., & Lemaitre, J. F. (2018). Sex gap in aging and longevity: Can sex chromosomes play a role? *Biology of Sex Differences*, *9*(1), 1–14.

Márquez, E. J., Chung, C. H., Marches, R., Rossi, R. J., Nehar-Belaid, D., Eroglu, A., ... Ucar, D. (2020). Sexual-dimorphism in human immune system aging. *Nature Communications*, *11*(1), 751.

Menassa, D. A., & Gomez-Nicola, D. (2018). Microglial dynamics during human brain development. *Frontiers in Immunology*, *9*(MAY), 1014.

Metcalf, C. J. E., Roth, O., & Graham, A. L. (2020). Why leveraging sex differences in immune trade-offs may illuminate the evolution of senescence. *Functional Ecology*, *34*(1), 129–140.

Michaud, J.-P., Halle, M., Lampron, A., Theriault, P., Prefontaine, P., Filali, M., ... Rivest, S. (2013). Toll-like receptor 4 stimulation with the detoxified ligand monophosphoryl lipid A improves Alzheimer's disease-related pathology. *Proceedings of the National Academy of Sciences*, *110*(5), 1941–1946.

Michaud, J.-P., Richard, K. L., & Rivest, S. (2011). MyD88-adaptor protein acts as a preventive mechanism for memory deficits in a mouse model of Alzheimer's disease. *Molecular Neurodegeneration*, *6*(1), 5.

Miller, K. R., & Streit, W. J. (2007). The effects of aging, injury and disease on microglial function: A case for cellular senescence. *Neuron Glia Biology*, *3*(3), 245–253.

Mofrad, B. R., Tijms, B. M., Scheltens, P., Barkhof, F., van der Flier, W. M., Sikkes, S. A. M., & Teunissen, C. E. (2020). Sex differences in CSF biomarkers vary by Alzheimer disease stage and APOE ε4 genotype. *Neurology*, *95*(17), e2378–e2388.

Möller, H.-J., & Graeber, M. B. (1998). The case described by Alois Alzheimer in 1911. *European Archives of Psychiatry and Clinical Neuroscience, 248*(3), 111–122.

Mosher, K. I., & Wyss-Coray, T. (2014). Microglial dysfunction in brain aging and Alzheimer's disease. *Biochemical Pharmacology, 88*(4), 594–604.

Mouton, P. R., Long, J. M., Lei, D. L., Howard, V., Jucker, M., Calhoun, M. E., & Ingram, D. K. (2002). Age and gender effects on microglia and astrocyte numbers in brains of mice. *Brain Research, 956*(1), 30–35.

Nelson, L. H., Saulsbery, A. I., & Lenz, K. M. (2019). Small cells with big implications: Microglia and sex differences in brain development, plasticity and behavioral health. *Progress in Neurobiology, 176*(September), 103–119.

Nelson, L. H., Warden, S., & Lenz, K. M. (2017). Sex differences in microglial phagocytosis in the neonatal hippocampus. *Brain, Behavior, and Immunity, 64*(1), 11–22.

Neu, S. C., Pa, J., Kukull, W., Beekly, D., Kuzma, A., Gangadharan, P., ... Toga, A. W. (2017). Apolipoprotein E genotype and sex risk factors for Alzheimer's disease. *JAMA Neurology, 74*(10), 1178.

Nimmerjahn, A., Kirchhoff, F., & Helmchen, F. (2005). Resting microglial cells are highly dynamic surveillants of brain parenchyma in vivo. *Science, 308*(5726), 1314–1318.

Niraula, A., Sheridan, J. F., & Godbout, J. P. (2017). Microglia priming with aging and stress. *Neuropsychopharmacology, 42*(1), 318–333.

Nissen, J. C. (2017). Microglial function across the spectrum of age and gender. *International Journal of Molecular Sciences, 18*(561), 1–13.

Norden, D. M., & Godbout, J. P. (2014). Microglia of the aged brain: Primed to be activated and resistant to regulation. *Neuropathology and Applied Neurobiology, 39*(1), 19–34.

Oakley, H., Cole, S. L., Logan, S., Maus, E., Shao, P., Craft, J., ... Vassar, R. (2006). Intraneuronal beta-amyloid aggregates, neurodegeneration, and neuron loss in transgenic mice with five familial Alzheimer's disease mutations: Potential factors in amyloid plaque formation. *Journal of Neuroscience, 26*(40), 10129–10140.

Olah, M., Patrick, E., Villani, A. C., Xu, J., White, C. C., Ryan, K. J., ... Bradshaw, E. M. (2018). A transcriptomic atlas of aged human microglia. *Nature Communications, 9*(1), 1–8.

Ordóñez-Gutiérrez, L., Antón, M., & Wandosell, F. (2015). Peripheral amyloid levels present gender differences associated with aging in AβPP/PS1 mice. *Journal of Alzheimer's Disease, 44*(4), 1063–1068.

Oveisgharan, S., Arvanitakis, Z., Yu, L., Farfel, J., Schneider, J. A., & Bennett, D. A. (2018). Sex differences in Alzheimer's disease and common neuropathologies of aging. *Acta Neuropathologica, 136*(6), 887–900.

Paolicelli, R. C., Bolasco, G., Pagani, F., Maggi, L., Scianni, M., Panzanelli, P., ... Gross, C. T. (2011). Synaptic pruning by microglia is necessary for normal brain development. *Science, 333*(6048), 1456–1458.

Parhizkar, S., Arzberger, T., Brendel, M., Kleinberger, G., Deussing, M., Focke, C., ... Haass, C. (2019). Loss of TREM2 function increases amyloid seeding but reduces plaque-associated ApoE. *Nature Neuroscience, 22*(2), 191–204.

Parkhurst, C. N., Yang, G., Ninan, I., Savas, J. N., Yates, J. R., Lafaille, J. J., ... Gan, W. B. (2013). Microglia promote learning-dependent synapse formation through brain-derived neurotrophic factor. *Cell, 155*(7), 1596–1609.

Payami, H., Montee, K. R., Kaye, J. A., Bird, T. D., Yu, C. E., Wijsman, E. M., & Schellenberg, G. D. (1994). Alzheimer's disease, apolipoprotein E4, and gender. *Journal of the American Medical Association, 271*(17), 1316–1317.

Pazos, M. A., Kraus, T. A., Muñoz-Fontela, C., & Moran, T. M. (2012). Estrogen mediates innate and adaptive immune alterations to influenza infection in pregnant mice. *PLoS One*, *7*(7), e40502.

Perkins, A. E., Piazza, M. K., & Deak, T. (2018). Stereological analysis of microglia in aged male and female Fischer 344 rats in socially-relevant brain regions. *Neuroscience*, *377*, 40–52.

Perry, V. H., Cunningham, C., & Holmes, C. (2007). Systemic infections and inflammation affect chronic neurodegeneration. *Nature Reviews Immunology*, *7*(2), 161–167.

Perry, V. H., & Holmes, C. (2014). Microglial priming in neurodegenerative disease. *Nature Reviews Neurology*, *10*(4), 217–224.

Pinheiro, I., Dejager, L., & Libert, C. (2011). X-chromosome-located microRNAs in immunity: Might they explain male/female differences? The X chromosome-genomic context may affect X-located miRNAs and downstream signaling, thereby contributing to the enhanced immune response of females. *BioEssays: News and Reviews in Molecular, Cellular and Developmental Biology*, *33*(11), 791–802.

Rahimian, R., Cordeau, P., & Kriz, J. (2019). Brain response to injuries: When microglia go sexist. *Neuroscience*, *405*, 14–23.

Ransohoff, R. M., & El Khoury, J. (2016). Microglia in health and disease. *Cold Spring Harbor Perspectives in Biology*, *8*(1), 1–15.

Reemst, K., Noctor, S. C., Lucassen, P. J., & Hol, E. M. (2016). The indispensable roles of microglia and astrocytes during brain development. *Frontiers in Human Neuroscience*, *10*(NOV2016), 1–28.

Ribizzi, G., Fiordoro, S., Barocci, S., Ferrari, E., & Megna, M. (2010). Cytokine polymorphisms and Alzheimer disease: Possible associations. *Neurological Sciences*, *31*(3), 321–325.

Roberts, M., & Peters, A. (2009). Is testosterone immunosuppressive in a condition-dependent manner? An experimental test in blue tits. *Journal of Experimental Biology*, *212*(12), 1811–1818.

Robinson, D. P., & Klein, S. L. (2012). Pregnancy and pregnancy-associated hormones alter immune responses and disease pathogenesis. *Hormones and Behavior*, *62*(3), 263–271.

Salter, M. W., & Stevens, B. (2017). Microglia emerge as central players in brain disease. *Nature Medicine*, *23*(9), 1018–1027.

Savage, J. C., & Tremblay, M.È. (2019). Studying laboratory mice – Into the wild. *Trends in Neurosciences*, *42*(9), 566–568.

Schafer, D. P., Lehrman, E. K., Kautzman, A. G., Koyama, R., Mardinly, A. R., Yamasaki, R., … Stevens, B. (2012). Microglia Sculpt postnatal neural circuits in an activity and complement-dependent manner. *Neuron*, *74*(4), 691–705.

Schurz, H., Salie, M., Tromp, G., Hoal, E. G., Kinnear, C. J., & Möller, M. (2019). The X chromosome and sex-specific effects in infectious disease susceptibility. *Human Genomics*, *13*(1), 2.

Schwarz, J. M., & Bilbo, S. D. (2012). Sex, glia, and development: Interactions in health and disease. *Hormones and Behavior*, *62*(3), 243–253.

Schwarz, J. M., Sholar, P. W., & Bilbo, S. D. (2012). Sex differences in microglial colonization of the developing rat brain. *Journal of Neurochemistry*, *120*(6), 948–963.

Selkoe, D. J., & Hardy, J. (2016). The amyloid hypothesis of Alzheimer's disease at 25 years. *EMBO Molecular Medicine*, *8*(6), 595–608.

Shaerzadeh, F., Phan, L., Miller, D., Dacquel, M., Hachmeister, W., Hansen, C., … Khoshbouei, H. (2020). Microglia senescence occurs in both substantia nigra and ventral tegmental area. *Glia*, *68*(11), 2228–2245.

Shi, Q., Chowdhury, S., Ma, R., Le, K. X., Hong, S., Caldarone, B. J., ... Lemere, C. A. (2017). Complement C3 deficiency protects against neurodegeneration in aged plaque-rich APP/PS1 mice. *Science Translational Medicine*, *9*(392). eaaf6295.

Shi, Q., Colodner, K. J., Matousek, S. B., Merry, K., Hong, S., Kenison, J. E., ... Lemere, C. A. (2015). Complement C3-deficient mice fail to display age-related hippocampal decline. *Journal of Neuroscience*, *35*(38), 13029–13042.

Sierra, A., Gottfried-Blackmore, A. C., McEwen, B., & Bulloch, K. (2007). Microglia derived from aging mice exhibit an altered inflammatory profile. *Glia*, *55*(4), 412–424.

Sim, R. B., Kishore, U., Villiers, C. L., Marche, P. N., & Mitchell, D. A. (2007). C1q binding and complement activation by prions and amyloids. *Immunobiology*, *212*(4–5), 355–362.

Slominski, A., Zbytek, B., Nikolakis, G., Manna, P. R., Skobowiat, C., Zmijewski, M., ... Tuckey, R. C. (2013). Steroidogenesis in the skin: Implications for local immune functions. *Journal of Steroid Biochemistry and Molecular Biology*, *137*, 107–123.

Spangenberg, E., Severson, P. L., Hohsfield, L. A., Crapser, J., Zhang, J., Burton, E. A., ... Green, K.N. (2019). Sustained microglial depletion with CSF1R inhibitor impairs parenchymal plaque development in an Alzheimer's disease model. *Nature Communications*, *10*(1), 3758.

Spires-Jones, T. L., & Hyman, B. T. (2014). The intersection of amyloid beta and tau at synapses in Alzheimer's disease. *Neuron*, *82*(4), 756–771.

Stephen, T. L., Cacciottolo, M., Balu, D., Morgan, T. E., Ladu, M. J., Finch, C. E., & Pike, C. J. (2019). APOE genotype and sex affect microglial interactions with plaques in Alzheimer's disease mice. *Acta Neuropathologica Communications*, *7*(1), 1–11.

St-Pierre, M.-K., Simoncicova, E., Bogi, E., & Tremblay, M. E. (2020). Shedding light on the dark side of microglia. *ASN Nero*, *12*. American Society for Neurochemistry. 1759091420925335.

Stratoulias, V., Venero, J. L., Tremblay, M.È., & Joseph, B. (2019). Microglial subtypes: Diversity within the microglial community. *EMBO Journal*, *38*(17), 1–18.

Streit, W. J., Sammons, N. W., Kuhns, A. J., & Sparks, D. L. (2004). Dystrophic microglia in the aging human brain. *Glia*, *45*(2), 208–212.

Streit, W. J., & Xue, Q. (2010). The brain's aging immune system. *Aging and Disease*, *1*(3), 254–261.

Su, F., Bai, F., & Zhang, Z. (2016). Inflammatory cytokines and Alzheimer's disease: A review from the perspective of genetic polymorphisms. *Neuroscience Bulletin*, *32*(5), 469–480.

Suárez-Calvet, M., Caballero, M.Á. A., Kleinberger, G., Bateman, R. J., Fagan, A. M., Morris, J. C., ... Haass, C. (2016). Early changes in CSF sTREM2 in dominantly inherited Alzheimer's disease occur after amyloid deposition and neuronal injury. *Science Translational Medicine*, *8*(369), 34–38.

Tanaka, S., Suzuki, T., & Nishioka, K. (1986). Assay of classical and alternative pathway activities of murine complement using antibody-sensitized rabbit erythrocytes. *Journal of Immunological Methods*, *86*(2), 161–170.

Terry, R. D., Masliah, E., Salmon, D. P., Butters, N., DeTeresa, R., Hill, R., ... Katzman, R. (1991). Physical basis of cognitive alterations in Alzheimer's disease: Synapse loss is the major correlate of cognitive impairment. *Annals of Neurology*, *30*(4), 572–580.

Tesseur, I., Zou, K., Esposito, L., Bard, F., Berber, E., Can, J. V., ... Wyss-Coray, T. (2006). Deficiency in neuronal TGF-β signaling promotes neurodegeneration and Alzheimer's pathology. *Journal of Clinical Investigation*, *116*(11), 3060–3069.

Thion, M. S., & Garel, S. (2017). On place and time: Microglia in embryonic and perinatal brain development. *Current Opinion in Neurobiology*, *47*, 121–130.

Tremblay, M. E., Zettel, M. L., Ison, J. R., Allen, P. D., & Majewska, A. K. (2012). Effects of aging and sensory loss on glial cells in mouse visual and auditory cortices. *Glia*, *60*(4), 541–558.

Tuppo, E. E., & Arias, H. R. (2005). The role of inflammation in Alzheimer's disease. *International Journal of Biochemistry and Cell Biology*, *37*(2), 289–305.

Vest, R. S., & Pike, C. J. (2013). Gender, sex steroid hormones, and Alzheimer's disease. *Hormones and Behavior*, *63*(2), 301–307.

Wake, H., Moorhouse, A. J., Miyamoto, A., & Nabekura, J. (2013). Microglia: Actively surveying and shaping neuronal circuit structure and function. *Trends in Neurosciences*, *36*(4), 209–217.

Wang, Y., Cella, M., Mallinson, K., Ulrich, J. D., Young, K. L., Robinette, M. L., … Colonna, M. (2015). TREM2 lipid sensing sustains the microglial response in an Alzheimer's disease model. *Cell*, *160*(6), 1061–1071.

Wang, Y., Ulland, T. K., Ulrich, J. D., Song, W., Tzaferis, J. A., Hole, J. T., … Colonna, M. (2016). TREM2-mediated early microglial response limits diffusion and toxicity of amyloid plaques. *Journal of Experimental Medicine*, *213*(5), 667–675.

Weinhard, L., Neniskyte, U., Vadisiute, A., di Bartolomei, G., Aygün, N., Riviere, L., … Gross, C. (2018). Sexual dimorphism of microglia and synapses during mouse postnatal development. *Developmental Neurobiology*, *78*(6), 618–626.

Wilcox, K. C., Lacor, P. N., Pitt, J., & Klein, W. L. (2011). Aβ oligomer-induced synapse degeneration in Alzheimer's disease. *Cellular and Molecular Neurobiology*, *31*(6), 939–948.

Wilton, D. K., Dissing-Olesen, L., & Stevens, B. (2019). Neuron-glia signaling in synapse elimination. *Annual Review of Neuroscience*, *42*(1), 107–127.

Yanguas-Casás, N., Crespo-Castrillo, A., Arevalo, M. A., & Garcia-Segura, L. M. (2020). Aging and sex: Impact on microglia phagocytosis. *Aging Cell*, *19*(8), 1–13.

Yanguas-Casás, N., Crespo-Castrillo, A., de Ceballos, M. L., Chowen, J. A., Azcoitia, I., Arevalo, M. A., & Garcia-Segura, L. M. (2018). Sex differences in the phagocytic and migratory activity of microglia and their impairment by palmitic acid. *Glia*, *66*(3), 522–537.

Yasojima, K., Schwab, C., McGeer, E. G., & McGeer, P. L. (1999). Up-regulated production and activation of the complement system in Alzheimer's disease brain. *American Journal of Pathology*, *154*(3), 927–936.

Ye, S. M., & Johnson, R. W. (2001). An age-related decline in interleukin-10 may contribute to the increased expression of interleukin-6 in the brain of aged mice. *Neuroimmunomodulation*, *9*(4), 183–192.

Yeh, F. L., Hansen, D. V., & Sheng, M. (2017). TREM2, microglia, and neurodegenerative diseases. *Trends in Molecular Medicine*, *23*(6), 512–533.

Zanjani, H., Finch, C. E., Kemper, C., Atkinson, J., McKeel, D., Morris, J. C., & Price, J. L. (2005). Complement activation in very early Alzheimer disease. *Alzheimer Disease & Associated Disorders*, *19*(2), 55–66.

Zhang, Y., Zhang, J., Tian, C., Xiao, Y., Li, X., He, C., … Fan, H. (2011). The −1082G/A polymorphism in IL-10 gene is associated with risk of Alzheimer's disease: A meta-analysis. *Journal of the Neurological Sciences*, *303*(1–2), 133–138.

Zhao, L., Mao, Z., Woody, S., & Brinton, R. D. (2016). Sex differences in metabolic aging of the brain: insights into female susceptibility to Alzheimer's disease. *Neurobiology of Aging*, *42*(2), 69–79.

Zhao, Y., Wu, X., Li, X., Jiang, L.-L., Gui, X., Liu, Y., … Xu, H. (2018). TREM2 is a receptor for β-amyloid that mediates microglial function. *Neuron*, *97*(5), 1023–1031. e7.

SECTION 2

Sex and gender differences in clinical aspects of Alzheimer's disease

Maria Teresa Ferretti[a], Annemarie Schumacher Dimech[a,b], and Antonella Santuccione Chadha[a]

[a]*Women's Brain Project, Guntershausen, Switzerland*
[b]*Program Manager, Palliative Care, University of Lucerne, Lucerne, Switzerland*

A growing body of evidence has emerged in recent years indicating the occurrence of important differences in the clinical manifestation of Alzheimer's disease, from biomarker profile to response to treatments. In this section, leading scientists in the field describe the current state of the art of sex and gender differences in clinical aspects of Alzheimer's and potential implications for clinical practice.

In Chapter 4, Mielke provides an overview of established sex differences in fluid biomarkers for Alzheimer's with a focus on CSF biomarkers; such differences are relevant for individual-level assessment of biomarker prognostic value.

Chapter 5 by Massa and colleagues focuses on imaging biomarkers (covering a variety of modalities, from structural MRI to FDG-PET). In this chapter, not only are the main differences between men and women highlighted, but also current limitations and potential caveats that will need to be considered in future studies.

In Chapter 6, Gammada, Au and Foldi describe sex differences in neuropsychological symptoms pertaining to executive memory, language, and executive function, highlighting their potential implications for clinical diagnosis of early impairments in men and women.

In Chapter 7, Biskup, Jordan, Nasta and Rauen describe the role of psychiatric symptoms, in particular depression, in Alzheimer's and the important sex and gender differences that occur in their presentation and response to treatment.

In Chapter 8, Nasta, Hill-Strathy, Biskup and Rauen examine another aspect related to Alzheimer's, namely sleep disturbances, under a sex and gender lens.

The complex interaction between sexual hormones and dementia, with a special focus on hormonal replacement therapy, will be examined by Szoeke, Downie, Phillips and Campbell in Chapter 9.

As it is becoming increasingly clear that genetic and lifestyle factors have an impact on risk of Alzheimer's, and as many of them are different in men and women, we invited Sindi and colleagues in Chapter 10 to share the current understanding in this field, focusing on the physiological impact of lifestyle factors and on the role of the apolipoprotein E gene. The impact of socioeconomic factors on risk of Alzheimer's and related gender differences are discussed in the third section of the book.

Finally, in Chapter 11, Rosende-Roca and colleagues examine the importance of sex and gender differences in clinical trials for Alzheimer's disease and how better consideration of such factors might improve clinical trial design.

These chapters mostly focus on differences between men and women driven by biological sex; gender aspects are discussed whenever relevant and in more depth in section 3.

CHAPTER 4

Sex differences in CSF biomarkers of Alzheimer's disease

Michelle M. Mielke

Departments of Health Sciences Research and Neurology, Mayo Clinic, Rochester, MN, United States

Introduction

Alzheimer's disease (AD) dementia is a progressive neurodegenerative disease that results in cognitive decline, especially in memory, behavioral changes, and functional loss. AD dementia is the most common form of dementia, comprising 60%–70% of all cases. With the aging of the population, the burden of AD dementia is growing to epidemic proportions. More than 6 million Americans are currently diagnosed with AD dementia and it is estimated that this number will grow to 15 million by 2050 unless new treatments or interventions to prevent or delay the onset of AD are identified (Brookmeyer, Abdalla, Kawas, & Corrada, 2018).

About two thirds of persons with a clinical diagnosis of AD dementia are women. Age is the greatest risk factor for AD dementia and the life expectancy for women is longer than for men (Alzheimer's Association, 2017). As a result, and similar to other aging-related diseases, the lifetime risk of AD dementia is greater for women than men (Plassman et al., 2007; Seshadri et al., 1997). Although the frequency, or count, of AD dementia is higher in women, the age-adjusted prevalence was not found to differ by sex/gender in a metaanalysis of 45 studies (Fiest et al., 2016). Sex and gender differences in the incidence of AD dementia are less clear and may vary across countries and over time (Mielke, Vemuri, & Rocca, 2014; Rocca, 2017). However, even if the prevalence or incidence of AD dementia does not differ by sex/gender in a specific region, sex and gender differences are still important. As evidenced from the cardiovascular field, there are sex and gender differences in the presentation of symptoms, risk factors, treatment response, and mortality. Thus, assessing sex and gender differences in the development and progression of AD, especially in understanding underlying mechanisms and treatment response, is critical (Mielke et al., 2014; Mielke, Ferretti, Iulita, Hayden, & Khachaturian, 2018; Nebel et al., 2018).

A complication of the many epidemiological and clinic studies assessing sex and gender differences in the prevalence or incidence of AD dementia is that they are almost always based on a clinical diagnosis, with no information about underlying pathology. This is problematic because 10%–30% of clinically defined AD dementia patients do not have AD pathology at autopsy (Nelson et al., 2011; Salloway et al., 2014). Moreover, approximately 30%–40% of the population who are cognitively unimpaired and aged 70 and older have elevated brain amyloid (Knopman et al., 2003; Roberts et al., 2018; Rowe et al., 2010). Therefore, incorporating a biological definition for AD provides a more accurate clinical diagnosis (e.g., separating AD dementia from other dementia types). The use of a biological definition also provides the opportunity to incorporate the preclinical phase of AD (i.e., the presence of pathology before clinical symptoms are apparent), when interventions are most likely to be beneficial in slowing or halting disease progression.

The hallmark pathologies of AD include the presence of amyloid-beta (Aβ) plaques, neurofibrillary tangles, and neurodegeneration (Jack et al., 2013). As part of the new National Institutes of Health-Alzheimer's Association (NIA-AA) research framework, several biomarkers have been proposed for amyloid-beta (Aβ) plaques, neurofibrillary tangles, and neurodegeneration (Jack et al., 2018) with the opportunity to include additional biomarkers as they become available and validated. Biomarkers of Aβ plaques included amyloid PET, CSF Aβ42, or the CSF Aβ42/Aβ40 ratio. Biomarkers of neurofibrillary tangles included tau PET or CSF phosphorylated tau (P-tau). Lastly, biomarkers of neurodegeneration included fluorodeoxyglucose (FDG)-PET hypometabolism, magnetic resonance imaging (MRI)-based measures of cortical thickness in specific brain regions or hippocampal atrophy, and CSF measures of total tau (T-tau). However, recent evidence since the NIA-AA research framework was published suggests that CSF or blood neurofilament light chain (NfL) and CSF neurogranin (Ng) may also be included as biomarkers of neurodegeneration.

The overarching goal of this chapter is to provide an impetus to consider biological sex differences in the measurement and interpretation of AD-related CSF biomarkers. In some countries, CSF Aβ42, P-tau, and T-tau are already being used clinically for the differential diagnosis or prognosis of AD dementia. Rapid technological advances are leading to the enhancement of existing assays, and to the development of other CSF biomarkers of AD pathophysiology. Thus, it is a critical time to consider what factors, such as sex, might affect the clinical interpretation of AD-related biomarker concentrations. There are multiple ways by which sex can affect the measurement or interpretation of CSF biomarkers. For some CSF markers, the biomarker concentrations may vary by sex. For other CSF biomarkers, the concentrations might not vary by sex, but the impact or interpretation may vary by sex depending on the context of use (e.g., diagnostic vs prognostic). Finally, for others, there will be no sex differences in concentrations or in their interpretation.

This chapter will address a series of topics. First, to provide a basis for sex differences, brain structural and functional differences will be described and the means by which these differences could contribute to sex differences in CSF concentrations will be discussed. Second, the current state of sex differences in the core AD-related CSF biomarkers (i.e., Aβ, P-tau, T-tau, NfL, and neurogranin (Ng)) will be reviewed. Third, sex differences in CSF markers of other molecular pathways that may be involved in the development and/or progression of AD pathology will be discussed. Finally, factors that can lead to the misinterpretation of observed or unobserved sex differences in CSF biomarkers will be considered. Throughout, sex is defined as the biological and physiological differences between women and men, with sex chromosomes (XX vs XY) and gonadal hormones primarily contributing to these differences (Institute of Medicine, 2001).

Sex differences in brain structure and function

Several differences in the brain of men and women have been reported, some of which start before birth and others that emerge around puberty. However, many of them remain controversial. The most obvious difference is that men have a larger head size and cerebral brain volume, about 10% larger, compared to women (Giedd, Raznahan, Mills, & Lenroot, 2012; Gur et al., 1991). As a result, men have greater CSF and sulcal volumes and larger lateral ventricles compared to women (Grant et al., 1987; Gur et al., 1991, 1999). Another difference is that men have a higher percentage of white matter while women have a higher percentage of gray matter (Lotze et al., 2019; Witte, Savli, Holik, Kasper, & Lanzenberger, 2010). In contrast, women have a higher cerebral blood flow at rest and during cognitive activities (Gur et al., 1982). The exact mechanisms for many of these differences are not well known but are largely impacted by sex hormones and sex chromosomes (van Amelsvoort, Compton, & Murphy, 2001; Witte et al., 2010).

These sex differences in brain structure and function could contribute to important sex differences in CSF biomarker levels and/or to their interpretation. For example, because men have a higher percentage of white matter, a CSF biomarker of white matter integrity might be naturally higher in men compared to women. Thus, sex-specific intervals may be needed for clinical use. In addition, sex differences in brain structure and function could contribute to differences in the susceptibility to specific brain pathologies. For example, women have greater white matter hyperintensity volumes than men after adjusting for age, hypertension, and diabetes, whereas men have a higher prevalence of cerebral microbleeds and cortical infarctions (Fatemi et al., 2018). CSF biomarkers of these vascular pathologies may also warrant sex-specific cut points for diagnostic and/or prognostic use.

Autopsy studies have also demonstrated sex differences in AD pathology, with women having more neurofibrillary tangles, but not Aβ plaques, then men (Barnes et al., 2005; Filon et al., 2016; Liesinger et al., 2018). More specifically, one study showed that women had a more pronounced increase in neurofibrillary tangle burden in the hippocampus with age, but not other regions, compared to men (Liesinger et al., 2018). This finding suggests a sex-specific neuroanatomic susceptibility. In addition, for the same amount of AD pathology, women are more likely to express clinical symptoms than men (Barnes et al., 2005; Filon et al., 2016; Liesinger et al., 2018). Thus, a biomarker of AD pathology could have sex-specific cut points to enhance diagnosis, either because of differences in the quantity of pathology or because of differences in susceptibility. When translating these sex differences at autopsy to the development and utility of in vivo biomarkers of AD neuropathology, it is important to note that there can be multiple biomarkers of each pathology that provide different information. For example, amyloid PET is a measure of aggregated amyloid plaque burden that accumulates over time. In contrast, CSF Aβ40 and Aβ42 reflect the rates of both amyloid production and clearance. Thus, CSF Aβ is a biomarker of an AD pathologic state associated with plaque burden, but it is not a measure of amyloid plaque load (Jack et al., 2018). As a result, sex differences may be observed in some modalities for assessing biomarkers of AD pathology but not in others. (For a thorough discussion on sex differences in imaging biomarkers, see Chapter 5)

Sex differences in the core AD-related biomarkers

The overwhelming majority of studies that have examined CSF biomarkers of Aβ, tau, and neurodegeneration have adjusted for sex. This is problematic because adjusting for sex (i.e., including it as a covariate in a model) treats it as a nuisance variable (i.e., an unwanted variable that influences the relationship between the independent and dependent variable). Instead, in order to determine whether there are sex differences in CSF biomarkers, either the results need to be stratified by sex or an interaction term with the biomarker and sex is needed. A study developing MCI and dementia risk models of CSF biomarkers found that models that stratified the markers by sex were more predictive than those that did not (van Maurik et al., 2019), suggesting the importance of sex differences in precision medicine approaches (Ferretti et al., 2018). Unfortunately, few studies of CSF AD biomarkers have adequately assessed sex differences. Below is an overview of studies that have assessed sex differences in CSF biomarkers of Aβ, tau, and neurodegeneration. Table 1 is a brief summary of the literature.

Amyloid-beta

Low CSF concentrations of Aβ42 or the Aβ42/Aβ40 ratio are indicative of elevated brain amyloid pathology. This may seem counterintuitive, but the low levels are thought to be due to the increased brain amyloid deposited in plaques in the brain, so that less is available for secretion to the CSF. Although controversial, some studies suggest that the CSF P-tau/Aβ42 or T-tau/Aβ42 ratios are better indicators of elevated brain amyloid deposition compared to either Aβ42 alone or the Aβ42/40 ratio (Palmqvist et al., 2015; Wang et al., 2016).

Cross-sectional studies have not found sex differences in the concentrations of CSF Aβ42, Aβ40, or in the Aβ42/40 ratio for individuals who are cognitively unimpaired, have mild cognitive impairment (MCI), or have AD dementia (Bouter, Vogelgsang, & Wiltfang, 2019; Buckley et al., 2019; Hohman et al., 2018; Li et al., 2017; Mattsson, Lonneborg, et al., 2017; Schoonenboom et al., 2004; Wolfsgruber et al., 2019). Interestingly, one study reported that CSF Aβ42 levels increased with age among AD patients who were women, but not men (Dumurgier et al., 2013). One longitudinal study also did not find a sex difference in the change of CSF Aβ42 over a specified period of time (Li et al., 2017). However, some studies have found that,

Table 1 Overview of sex differences in Alzheimer's disease-related CSF biomarkers.

CSF marker	Sex differences	Notes
Amyloid-beta40 (Aβ40)	–	
Amyloid-beta42 (Aβ42)	–	For a given CSF Aβ42, women may have greater subsequent declines in memory and hippocampal volume
Amyloid-beta42/40 ratio (Aβ42/Aβ40)	–	
Phosphorylated tau (P-tau)	–	Although levels do not differ by sex overall, there may be a sex difference once APOE and clinical diagnosis are considered
Total tau (P-tau)	–	Although levels do not differ by sex overall, there may be a sex difference once APOE and clinical diagnosis are considered
Neurofilament light (NfL)	↑ Men	There is enough evidence that it has been suggested that there may be sex-specific reference intervals
Neurogranin (Ng)	↑ Women	The evidence is mixed. One study reported higher levels in women but two other studies found no sex differences

for a given CSF Aβ42 concentration, women have greater subsequent declines in hippocampal atrophy and memory performance, and a greater increase in CSF tau levels than men (Buckley et al., 2019; Koran et al., 2017). These sex differences were more pronounced among APOE ε4 allele carriers. These results suggest that sex-specific cut points are not needed for diagnostic purposes. However, if additional studies determine that, for a given level of amyloid, women are more likely to develop neurodegeneration and cognitive decline, then sex-specific cutoffs might be considered for prognostic purposes.

Phosphorylated tau and total tau

High levels of CSF P-tau and T-tau are indicative of abnormal hyperphosphorylation of the microtubule-associated protein tau, and neurodegeneration, respectively. Similar to CSF Aβ42, cross-sectional studies of CSF P-tau and T-tau concentrations generally have not found differences in levels among women compared to men (Bouter et al., 2019; Buckley et al., 2019; Mielke et al., 2019a; Schoonenboom et al., 2004). In addition, one study examining longitudinal change in CSF P-tau or T-tau did not find a sex difference (Li et al., 2017). However, despite the lack of sex differences in levels of P-tau and T-tau, some studies have reported three-way interactions of sex, APOE genotype, and either CSF P-tau or T-tau. These studies are described later, under the section "Genetic factors."

Neurofilament light chain

Neurofilament light chain (NfL) is a biomarker of subcortical large-caliber axonal degeneration (Hoffman et al., 1987; Norgren, Rosengren, & Stigbrand, 2003). Multiple studies of patients with neurodegenerative diseases, including AD dementia, and of cognitively unimpaired individuals have reported higher CSF NfL concentrations in men compared to women (Bridel et al., 2019; Mattsson, Insel, et al., 2016; Mielke et al., 2019a). As a result, it has been suggested that reference intervals for CSF NfL should be sex-specific (Bridel et al., 2019; Mielke et al., 2019a). Although the underlying mechanism for this sex difference is not completely known, one potential explanation for the higher CSF NfL concentrations is the greater proportion of brain white matter in men versus women.

Neurogranin

Neurogranin (Ng) is a neural-specific postsynaptic protein that is highly enriched in dendrites, is regulated by synaptic activity, and promotes synaptogenesis (Garrido-Garcia et al., 2019). Although Ng is a marker of neurodegeneration, it is more specific to AD dementia compared to other neurodegenerative diseases (Kvartsberg et al., 2019; Wellington et al., 2016). One large community-based study reported higher CSF Ng levels in women compared to men (Mielke et al., 2019a). However, two other studies did not find a sex difference in CSF Ng concentrations (Casaletto et al., 2017; Tarawneh et al., 2016).

Sex differences in CSF biomarkers of other mechanisms related to the development and progression of AD pathology and clinical symptoms

There are multiple mechanisms and pathways that may contribute to the development and progression of AD pathology and clinical symptoms including inflammation, lipids, mitochondrial dysfunction, insulin resistance, synaptogenesis, and neurovascular dysfunction (Nebel et al., 2018). For many of these pathways, sex differences have been observed at the animal and/or human level, but sex differences in CSF levels have not been examined. Although some blood-based vascular-related markers differ by sex (e.g., Ekblad et al., 2015; Mielke et al., 2015a, 2015b) or show sex differences in relation to risk of AD or AD pathology (e.g., (Geijselaers et al., 2018; Mielke, Haughey, et al., 2017)), it cannot be assumed that the same relationships will be observed for CSF markers. Some CSF markers do not readily cross the blood-brain barrier and sex differences in blood-brain barrier function have been observed (see next section). Unlike many pathways, sex differences in inflammatory markers have been examined, so these results are reviewed below.

Inflammatory markers

Inflammation has been proposed to be a major contributor to the initiation and progression of AD pathology and the development of clinical symptoms (Brosseron et al., 2018; Calsolaro & Edison, 2016). Amyloid-beta plaques and neurofibrillary tangles can activate microglia and astrocytes (McGeer, Itagaki, Tago, & McGeer, 1987; Rogers, Luber-Narod, Styren, & Civin, 1988). This activation can affect Aβ clearance, the development of tau pathology and propagation, and increase neurodegeneration and the emergence of clinical symptoms (Asai et al., 2015; Block, Zecca, & Hong, 2007; Calsolaro & Edison, 2016; Hickman, Allison, & El Khoury, 2008; Liu et al., 2017). Although there is a growing body of literature suggesting sex differences in microglial number, morphology, and transcriptome (see Kodama and Gan (2019) for review and Chapter 3 in this book), studies of CSF inflammatory biomarkers are conflicting. One analysis consisting of participants across the AD clinical spectrum found that five of 21 CSF inflammatory markers were higher in men than in women, including chitinase-3-like protein 1 (YKL-40), complement 4, factor B, factor H, and properdin (Brosseron et al., 2020). Another study of cognitively unimpaired, MCI, and AD patients found that CSF levels of IL-6 and MCP-1 were also higher in men compared to women, but there were no sex differences in the concentrations of YKL-40, IL-7, IL-8, IL-15, or IP-10 (Janelidze et al., 2018). A third study also did not find a sex difference in CSF YKL-40 or triggering receptor expressed on myeloid cells 2 (TREM2) levels (Nordengen et al., 2019). A possible explanation for these relatively inconsistent results is that none of the studies stratified by APOE status. Indeed, a study using ADNI data reported that female APOE ε4 noncarriers had lower CSF IL-16 and IL-8 levels compared to males (Duarte-Guterman, Albert, Inkster, Barha, & Galea, 2020). Among APOE ε4 carriers, females similarly had lower levels of CSF IL-8 and IL-16, but also had lower levels of ICAM1 and IgA. Future studies are needed to examine whether inflammatory markers differ by both sex and APOE across the AD clinical spectrum. In addition, studies have not yet examined whether associations between inflammatory markers and longitudinal change in AD pathophysiology or clinical progression differ by sex.

Examples of sex-related factors that can influence the interpretation of AD-related biofluid biomarker results

The anatomy and physiology of men and women differ in multiple ways across systems, organs, tissues, and cells. These differences can be caused by sex hormones (e.g., testosterone, estrogen), sex chromosomes (e.g., presence of X and Y genes), and/or physical and social environments that contribute to social determinants of health. These differences can have marked effects on the measurement and interpretation of CSF-related AD biomarkers. A few examples are provided below.

Genetic factors
APOE genotype
The ε4 allele of the apolipoprotein ε gene (APOE) is the strongest known genetic risk factor for late-onset AD dementia (Corder et al., 1993; Strittmatter et al., 1993). The ε4 allele codes for the apoE4 protein, which contributes to reduced brain Aβ clearance and a reduced neuronal injury response (Mahley & Huang, 2012; Verghese et al., 2013). Several studies have found that the effects of the ε4 allele for AD risk and progression are stronger in women compared to men, and that these effects are age-dependent (e.g., Altmann, Tian, Henderson, & Greicius, 2014; Corder et al., 2004; Damoiseaux et al., 2012; Farrer et al., 1997; Liu et al., 2010; Payami et al., 1996). As an example, an analysis comprised of almost 60,000 people from several AD studies showed that the risk of AD dementia for women with the APOE ε3/ε4 genotype was fourfold higher compared to men with the same genotype, but only among those aged 65–75. The sex difference disappeared at older ages (Neu et al., 2017). In addition, although studies have generally not found sex differences in levels of CSF P-tau and T-tau, as mentioned earlier, sex differences have been observed in these CSF markers after consideration of APOE. Among MCI participants who were APOE ε4 carriers, women had higher CSF T-tau levels compared to men (Altmann et al., 2014). This finding has been replicated in other studies of participants across the AD clinical spectrum (Buckley et al., 2019; Damoiseaux et al., 2012; Hohman et al., 2018). Babapour Mofrad et al. (2020) extended this research to show three-way interactions between sex, disease stage, and APOE. Among APOE ε4 carriers, women had higher CSF P-tau and T-tau concentrations than men among those diagnosed with subjective cognitive decline or MCI, but not AD dementia. In contrast, among APOE ε4 noncarriers, women had higher CSF P-tau and T-tau concentrations for those diagnosed with MCI and AD dementia, but not subjective cognitive decline. These results suggest a difference in the neuropathological trajectory for women and men that is dependent on APOE genotype. Future research is needed to determine the mechanism by which these sex differences occur and how to interpret these differences for clinical purposes.

Other genetic factors
Sex differences in other genetic predictors of AD dementia and AD pathology are now being identified. In an autopsy study of more than 5700 individuals, the minor allele of intergenic SNP on chr7p21.1 (rs34331204) was associated with a lower risk of neurofibrillary tangles in men, but not women (Dumitrescu et al., 2019). This same SNP was also associated with greater hippocampal volume and better executive function among men. It will be important for future research to determine whether this SNP relates to CSF P-tau or T-tau levels. Another analysis that included multiple cohorts reported a female-specific association of SERPINB1 gene expression levels

on CSF Aβ, and associations between OSTN or CLDN16 expression on CSF T-tau levels (Deming et al., 2018). Additional studies are needed to confirm these findings and to examine other sex-specific genetic effects on CSF AD biomarkers.

The development of polygenic risk scores for AD dementia clinical diagnosis, AD pathology, and risk stratification has historically not considered sex differences. Considering sex in the development of AD risk scores will lead to less bias and a more accurate prognosis. Indeed, one study that developed a sex-stratified genome-wide association study on one cohort and then tested it on two others determined that the sex-stratified polygenic hazard scores showed significantly stronger prognostic value for age-at-disease-onset, clinical progression, amyloid deposition, neurofibrillary tangles, and composite neuropathological scores (Fan et al., 2020). Moreover, these findings were independent of APOE genotype. Future studies will need to consider if and how such genetic information should be incorporated into the clinical interpretation of the CSF biomarkers for the diagnosis and prognosis of AD.

Sex differences in the permeability of the blood-brain barrier

The blood-brain barrier (BBB) selectively regulates the transfer of molecules between the blood, brain parenchyma, and CSF. Permeability of the BBB increases with age and in the preclinical stages of many neurodegenerative diseases. This leads to the accumulation of various molecules in the brain from the periphery and an increase of brain molecules in the blood (Zlokovic, 2011). A standard way of measuring BBB permeability is the CSF/serum albumin ratio (Q_{ALB}) (Tibbling, Link, & Ohman, 1977). Because albumin is almost exclusively produced in the liver, an increased Q_{ALB} is indicative of higher permeability and a higher potential for the transfer of proteins from the blood to the brain. Notably, there are sex differences in the Q_{ALB}. A study of more than 20,000 patients and volunteers, aged 1–90 years, found higher Q_{ALB} in men compared to women, which started around the age of 6 years and continued throughout the lifespan (Parrado-Fernandez et al., 2018). Because the sex difference was not markedly changed at puberty or menopause, this observation cannot be explained by sex hormones. One proposed explanation was that sex differences in CSF drainage or production could contribute to higher concentrations in men, but these mechanisms remain to be examined (Blennow et al., 1993; Reiber, 1994; Seyfert, Kunzmann, Schwertfeger, Koch, & Faulstich, 2002). The sex difference in Q_{ALB} is important because it could result in higher concentrations of blood-specific isoforms in the CSF, and higher concentrations of CSF-specific isoforms in the blood, among men. This aspect will need to be considered when examining sex differences in the concentrations of both blood and CSF AD-related biomarkers.

Consideration of study design

When designing studies to assess sex differences or critically reviewing and interpreting studies that report on sex differences, it is important to consider the demographics (i.e., age) and other characteristics of the women and men enrolled. For example, the effect of menopause and subsequent use of menopausal hormone therapy for women, and the use of testosterone for men, on CSF biomarkers have not been adequately assessed (for a discussion on the role of hormones, see Chapter 9). Differences in comorbidities by sex could also influence CSF biomarker levels. For example, many cardiovascular risk factors are more prevalent in men compared to women, due to the protective effects of estrogen, until the age of about 75 years when women catch up to and even exceed the prevalence among men (sex differences in comorbidities and risk factors are discussed later in this book: Chapter 10). Thus, study design issues could either hide or enhance potential sex differences in biomarkers levels and need to be considered when interpreting the results.

Future potential of blood-based biomarkers

Compared to CSF markers, blood-based biomarkers are less invasive, less costly, and more feasible for serial assessments. Concentrations of blood Aβ42, Aβ40, P-tau, T-tau, and NfL are lower than that of CSF, so it has been historically difficult to accurately measure levels of these biomarkers in blood. However, ultrasensitive technologies provide new opportunities for the development of blood-based biomarkers of AD pathology including plasma or serum Aβ42 (Nakamura et al., 2018; Ovod et al., 2017; Vergallo et al., 2019), P-tau181 (Barthelemy et al., 2020; Janelidze et al., 2020; Karikari et al., 2020; Mielke, Hagen, et al., 2018), total tau (Dage et al., 2016; Mattsson, Zetterberg, et al., 2016; Mielke, Hagen, et al., 2017; Pase et al., 2019), and NfL (Gaetani et al., 2019; Mattsson, Andreasson, Zetterberg, & Blennow, 2017; Mielke et al., 2019b). Although few studies have assessed sex differences in these blood-based biomarkers, studies of plasma or serum NfL have reported that levels do not vary by sex. This is notable because CSF NfL levels are consistently higher in men than women. The reason for this disparity is not yet understood. As future research determines the clinical utility of these AD-related blood-based biomarkers for diagnostic and prognostic purposes, the assessment of sex differences must be integrated to enhance precision medicine.

Conclusion

Even though there is a current shift and focus on "precision" or "individualized" medicine, it is astonishing how few studies assess sex differences in CSF biomarkers of AD-related pathology and contributing pathways. There appear to be sex differences in many mechanisms contributing to the development and progression of AD pathology and clinical symptoms. As the development of CSF biomarkers of these pathways continue, it is critical to understand whether sex differences exist and how to interpret them in order to enhance the prevention, care, and treatment of both women and men. Even if no sex difference is observed, it is essential to state this in each manuscript to prevent a bias of studies that are only published if they show higher CSF levels in one sex or if the effect on disease progression appears to be stronger for one sex.

Chapter highlights

- Although concentrations of CSF Aβ42, Aβ40, or in the Aβ42/40 ratio do not differ in a cross-sectional way by sex, for a given CSF Aβ42 concentration, women have greater subsequent declines in hippocampal atrophy and memory performance, and a greater increase in CSF tau levels than men.
- There are sex differences in CSF levels of phosphorylated tau, total tau, and neurofilament light, some of which vary by APOE genotype and stage of clinical diagnosis.
- There can be misinterpretations of sex differences in AD-related CSF biomarkers when sex differences in genetics or blood-brain barrier permeability are not considered, or as a result of biases in the study design.

References

Altmann, A., Tian, L., Henderson, V. W., & Greicius, M. D. (2014). Sex modifies the APOE-related risk of developing Alzheimer disease. *Annals of Neurology, 75*, 563–573.

Alzheimer's Association. (2017). 2017 Alzheimer's disease facts and figures. *Alzheimer's & Dementia, 13*, 325–373.

Asai, H., Ikezu, S., Tsunoda, S., Medalla, M., Luebke, J., Haydar, T., et al. (2015). Depletion of microglia and inhibition of exosome synthesis halt tau propagation. *Nature Neuroscience, 18*, 1584–1593.

Babapour Mofrad, R., Tijms, B. M., Scheltens, P., Barkhof, F., van der Flier, W. M., Sikkes, S. A. M., et al. (2020). Sex differences in CSF biomarkers vary by Alzheimer disease stage and APOE epsilon4 genotype. *Neurology, 95*, e2378–e2388.

Barnes, L. L., Wilson, R. S., Bienias, J. L., Schneider, J. A., Evans, D. A., & Bennett, D. A. (2005). Sex differences in the clinical manifestations of Alzheimer disease pathology. *Archives of General Psychiatry, 62*, 685–691.

Barthelemy, N. R., Li, Y., Joseph-Mathurin, N., Gordon, B. A., Hassenstab, J., Benzinger, T. L. S., et al. (2020). A soluble phosphorylated tau signature links tau, amyloid and the evolution of stages of dominantly inherited Alzheimer's disease. *Nature Medicine, 26*, 398–407.

Blennow, K., Fredman, P., Wallin, A., Gottfries, C. G., Karlsson, I., Langstrom, G., et al. (1993). Protein analysis in cerebrospinal fluid. II. Reference values derived from healthy individuals 18–88 years of age. *European Neurology, 33*, 129–133.

Block, M. L., Zecca, L., & Hong, J. S. (2007). Microglia-mediated neurotoxicity: Uncovering the molecular mechanisms. *Nature Reviews Neuroscience, 8*, 57–69.

Bouter, C., Vogelgsang, J., & Wiltfang, J. (2019). Comparison between amyloid-PET and CSF amyloid-beta biomarkers in a clinical cohort with memory deficits. *Clinica Chimica Acta, 492*, 62–68.

Bridel, C., van Wieringen, W. N., Zetterberg, H., Tijms, B. M., Teunissen, C. E., the N. F. L. Group, et al. (2019). Diagnostic value of cerebrospinal fluid neurofilament light protein in neurology: a systematic review and meta-analysis. *JAMA Neurology, 76*, 1035–1048.

Brookmeyer, R., Abdalla, N., Kawas, C. H., & Corrada, M. M. (2018). Forecasting the prevalence of preclinical and clinical Alzheimer's disease in the United States. *Alzheimer's & Dementia, 14*, 121–129.

Brosseron, F., Kolbe, C. C., Santarelli, F., Carvalho, S., Antonell, A., Castro-Gomez, S., et al. (2020). Multicenter Alzheimer's and Parkinson's disease immune biomarker verification study. *Alzheimer's & Dementia*, *16*, 292–304.

Brosseron, F., Traschutz, A., Widmann, C. N., Kummer, M. P., Tacik, P., Santarelli, F., et al. (2018). Characterization and clinical use of inflammatory cerebrospinal fluid protein markers in Alzheimer's disease. *Alzheimer's Research & Therapy*, *10*, 25.

Buckley, R. F., Mormino, E. C., Chhatwal, J., Schultz, A. P., Rabin, J. S., Rentz, D. M., et al. (2019). Associations between baseline amyloid, sex, and APOE on subsequent tau accumulation in cerebrospinal fluid. *Neurobiology of Aging*, *78*, 178–185.

Calsolaro, V., & Edison, P. (2016). Neuroinflammation in Alzheimer's disease: Current evidence and future directions. *Alzheimer's & Dementia*, *12*, 719–732.

Casaletto, K. B., Elahi, F. M., Bettcher, B. M., Neuhaus, J., Bendlin, B. B., Asthana, S., et al. (2017). Neurogranin, a synaptic protein, is associated with memory independent of Alzheimer biomarkers. *Neurology*, *89*, 1782–1788.

Corder, E. H., Ghebremedhin, E., Taylor, M. G., Thal, D. R., Ohm, T. G., & Braak, H. (2004). The biphasic relationship between regional brain senile plaque and neurofibrillary tangle distributions: Modification by age, sex, and APOE polymorphism. *Annals of the New York Academy of Sciences*, *1019*, 24–28.

Corder, E. H., Saunders, A. M., Strittmatter, W. J., Schmechel, D. E., Gaskell, P. C., Small, G. W., et al. (1993). Gene dose of apolipoprotein E type 4 allele and the risk of Alzheimer's disease in late onset families. *Science*, *261*, 921–923.

Dage, J. L., Wennberg, A. M., Airey, D. C., Hagen, C. E., Knopman, D. S., Machulda, M. M., et al. (2016). Levels of tau protein in plasma are associated with neurodegeneration and cognitive function in a population-based elderly cohort. *Alzheimer's & Dementia*, *12*, 1226–1234.

Damoiseaux, J. S., Seeley, W. W., Zhou, J., Shirer, W. R., Coppola, G., Karydas, A., et al. (2012). Gender modulates the APOE epsilon4 effect in healthy older adults: Convergent evidence from functional brain connectivity and spinal fluid tau levels. *Journal of Neuroscience*, *32*, 8254–8262.

Deming, Y., Dumitrescu, L., Barnes, L. L., Thambisetty, M., Kunkle, B., Gifford, K. A., et al. (2018). Sex-specific genetic predictors of Alzheimer's disease biomarkers. *Acta Neuropathologica*, *136*, 857–872.

Duarte-Guterman, P., Albert, A. Y., Inkster, A. M., Barha, C. K., & Galea, L. A. M. (2020). Alzheimer's disease neuroimaging initiative, inflammation in Alzheimer's disease: Do sex and APOE matter? *Journal of Alzheimer's Disease*, *78*, 627–641.

Dumitrescu, L., Barnes, L. L., Thambisetty, M., Beecham, G., Kunkle, B., Bush, W. S., et al. (2019). Sex differences in the genetic predictors of Alzheimer's pathology. *Brain*, *142*, 2581–2589.

Dumurgier, J., Gabelle, A., Vercruysse, O., Bombois, S., Laplanche, J. L., Peoc'h, K., et al. (2013). Exacerbated CSF abnormalities in younger patients with Alzheimer's disease. *Neurobiology of Disease*, *54*, 486–491.

Ekblad, L. L., Rinne, J. O., Puukka, P. J., Laine, H. K., Ahtiluoto, S. E., Sulkava, R. O., et al. (2015). Insulin resistance is associated with poorer verbal fluency performance in women. *Diabetologia*, *58*, 2545–2553.

Fan, C. C., Banks, S. J., Thompson, W. K., Chen, C. H., McEvoy, L. K., Tan, C. H., et al. (2020). Sex-dependent autosomal effects on clinical progression of Alzheimer's disease. *Brain*, *143*, 2272–2280.

Farrer, L. A., Cupples, L. A., Haines, J. L., Hyman, B., Kukull, W. A., Mayeux, R., et al. (1997). Effects of age, sex, and ethnicity on the association between apolipoprotein E genotype and Alzheimer disease. A meta-analysis. APOE and Alzheimer Disease Meta Analysis Consortium. *JAMA, 278*, 1349–1356.

Fatemi, F., Kantarci, K., Graff-Radford, J., Preboske, G. M., Weigand, S. D., Przybelski, S. A., et al. (2018). Sex differences in cerebrovascular pathologies on FLAIR in cognitively unimpaired elderly. *Neurology, 90*, e466–e473.

Ferretti, M. T., Iulita, M. F., Cavedo, E., Chiesa, P. A., Schumacher Dimech, A., Santuccione Chadha, A., et al. (2018). Sex differences in Alzheimer disease – The gateway to precision medicine. *Nature Reviews Neurology, 14*, 457–469.

Fiest, K. M., Roberts, J. I., Maxwell, C. J., Hogan, D. B., Smith, E. E., Frolkis, A., et al. (2016). The prevalence and incidence of dementia due to Alzheimer's disease: A systematic review and meta-analysis. *Canadian Journal of Neurological Sciences, 43*(Suppl 1), S51–S82.

Filon, J. R., Intorcia, A. J., Sue, L. I., Vazquez Arreola, E., Wilson, J., Davis, K. J., et al. (2016). Gender differences in Alzheimer disease: Brain atrophy, histopathology burden, and cognition. *Journal of Neuropathology and Experimental Neurology, 75*, 748–754.

Gaetani, L., Blennow, K., Calabresi, P., Di Filippo, M., Parnetti, L., & Zetterberg, H. (2019). Neurofilament light chain as a biomarker in neurological disorders. *Journal of Neurology, Neurosurgery, and Psychiatry, 90*, 870–881.

Garrido-Garcia, A., de Andres, R., Jimenez-Pompa, A., Soriano, P., Sanz-Fuentes, D., Martinez-Blanco, E., et al. (2019). Neurogranin expression is regulated by synaptic activity and promotes synaptogenesis in cultured hippocampal neurons. *Molecular Neurobiology, 56*, 7321–7337.

Geijselaers, S. L. C., Aalten, P., Ramakers, I., De Deyn, P. P., Heijboer, A. C., Koek, H. L., et al. (2018). Association of cerebrospinal fluid (CSF) insulin with cognitive performance and CSF biomarkers of Alzheimer's disease. *Journal of Alzheimer's Disease, 61*, 309–320.

Giedd, J. N., Raznahan, A., Mills, K. L., & Lenroot, R. K. (2012). Review: Magnetic resonance imaging of male/female differences in human adolescent brain anatomy. *Biology of Sex Differences, 3*, 19.

Grant, R., Condon, B., Lawrence, A., Hadley, D. M., Patterson, J., Bone, I., et al. (1987). Human cranial CSF volumes measured by MRI: Sex and age influences. *Magnetic Resonance Imaging, 5*, 465–468.

Gur, R. C., Gur, R. E., Obrist, W. D., Hungerbuhler, J. P., Younkin, D., Rosen, A. D., et al. (1982). Sex and handedness differences in cerebral blood flow during rest and cognitive activity. *Science, 217*, 659–661.

Gur, R. C., Mozley, P. D., Resnick, S. M., Gottlieb, G. L., Kohn, M., Zimmerman, R., et al. (1991). Gender differences in age effect on brain atrophy measured by magnetic resonance imaging. *Proceedings of the National Academy of Sciences of the United States of America, 88*, 2845–2849.

Gur, R. C., Turetsky, B. I., Matsui, M., Yan, M., Bilker, W., Hughett, P., et al. (1999). Sex differences in brain gray and white matter in healthy young adults: Correlations with cognitive performance. *Journal of Neuroscience, 19*, 4065–4072.

Hickman, S. E., Allison, E. K., & El Khoury, J. (2008). Microglial dysfunction and defective beta-amyloid clearance pathways in aging Alzheimer's disease mice. *Journal of Neuroscience, 28*, 8354–8360.

Hoffman, P. N., Cleveland, D. W., Griffin, J. W., Landes, P. W., Cowan, N. J., & Price, D. L. (1987). Neurofilament gene expression: A major determinant of axonal caliber. *Proceedings of the National Academy of Sciences of the United States of America, 84*, 3472–3476.

Hohman, T. J., Dumitrescu, L., Barnes, L. L., Thambisetty, M., Beecham, G., Kunkle, B., et al. (2018). Sex-specific association of apolipoprotein E with cerebrospinal fluid levels of tau. *JAMA Neurology, 75*, 989–998.

Institute of Medicine. (2001). *Exploring the biological contributions to human health: Does sex matter?*. Washington, DC: The National Academies Press. https://doi.org/10.17226/10028.

Jack, C. R., Jr., Bennett, D. A., Blennow, K., Carrillo, M. C., Dunn, B., Haeberlein, S. B., et al. (2018). NIA-AA research framework: Toward a biological definition of Alzheimer's disease. *Alzheimer's & Dementia, 14*, 535–562.

Jack, C. R., Jr., Knopman, D. S., Jagust, W. J., Petersen, R. C., Weiner, M. W., Aisen, P. S., et al. (2013). Tracking pathophysiological processes in Alzheimer's disease: An updated hypothetical model of dynamic biomarkers. *Lancet Neurology, 12*, 207–216.

Janelidze, S., Mattsson, N., Palmqvist, S., Smith, R., Beach, T. G., Serrano, G. E., et al. (2020). Plasma P-tau181 in Alzheimer's disease: Relationship to other biomarkers, differential diagnosis, neuropathology and longitudinal progression to Alzheimer's dementia. *Nature Medicine, 26*, 379–386.

Janelidze, S., Mattsson, N., Stomrud, E., Lindberg, O., Palmqvist, S., Zetterberg, H., et al. (2018). CSF biomarkers of neuroinflammation and cerebrovascular dysfunction in early Alzheimer disease. *Neurology, 91*, e867–e877.

Karikari, T. K., Pascoal, T. A., Ashton, N. J., Janelidze, S., Benedet, A. L., Rodriguez, J. L., et al. (2020). Blood phosphorylated tau 181 as a biomarker for Alzheimer's disease: A diagnostic performance and prediction modelling study using data from four prospective cohorts. *Lancet Neurology, 19*, 422–433.

Knopman, D. S., Parisi, J. E., Salviati, A., Floriach-Robert, M., Boeve, B. F., Ivnik, R. J., et al. (2003). Neuropathology of cognitively normal elderly. *Journal of Neuropathology and Experimental Neurology, 62*, 1087–1095.

Kodama, L., & Gan, L. (2019). Do microglial sex differences contribute to sex differences in neurodegenerative diseases? *Trends in Molecular Medicine, 25*, 741–749.

Koran, M. E. I., Wagener, M., Hohman, T. J., & Alzheimer's Neuroimaging Initiative. (2017). Sex differences in the association between AD biomarkers and cognitive decline. *Brain Imaging and Behavior, 11*, 205–213.

Kvartsberg, H., Lashley, T., Murray, C. E., Brinkmalm, G., Cullen, N. C., Hoglund, K., et al. (2019). The intact postsynaptic protein neurogranin is reduced in brain tissue from patients with familial and sporadic Alzheimer's disease. *Acta Neuropathologica, 137*, 89–102.

Li, G., Shofer, J. B., Petrie, E. C., Yu, C. E., Wilkinson, C. W., Figlewicz, D. P., et al. (2017). Cerebrospinal fluid biomarkers for Alzheimer's and vascular disease vary by age, gender, and APOE genotype in cognitively normal adults. *Alzheimer's Research & Therapy, 9*, 48.

Liesinger, A. M., Graff-Radford, N. R., Duara, R., Carter, R. E., Hanna Al-Shaikh, F. S., Koga, S., et al. (2018). Sex and age interact to determine clinicopathologic differences in Alzheimer's disease. *Acta Neuropathologica, 136*, 873–885.

Liu, C. C., Hu, J., Zhao, N., Wang, J., Wang, N., Cirrito, J. R., et al. (2017). Astrocytic LRP1 mediates brain Aβ clearance and impacts amyloid deposition. *Journal of Neuroscience, 37*, 4023–4031.

Liu, Y., Paajanen, T., Westman, E., Wahlund, L. O., Simmons, A., Tunnard, C., et al. (2010). Effect of APOE epsilon4 allele on cortical thicknesses and volumes: The AddNeuroMed study. *Journal of Alzheimer's Disease, 21*, 947–966.

Lotze, M., Domin, M., Gerlach, F. H., Gaser, C., Lueders, E., Schmidt, C. O., et al. (2019). Novel findings from 2,838 adult brains on sex differences in gray matter brain volume. *Scientific Reports, 9*, 1671.

Mahley, R. W., & Huang, Y. (2012). Apolipoprotein e sets the stage: Response to injury triggers neuropathology. *Neuron, 76*, 871–885.

Mattsson, N., Andreasson, U., Zetterberg, H., & Blennow, K. (2017). Association of plasma neurofilament light with neurodegeneration in patients with Alzheimer disease. *JAMA Neurology, 74*, 557–566.

Mattsson, N., Insel, P. S., Palmqvist, S., Portelius, E., Zetterberg, H., Weiner, M., et al. (2016). Cerebrospinal fluid tau, neurogranin, and neurofilament light in Alzheimer's disease. *EMBO Molecular Medicine, 8*, 1184–1196.

Mattsson, N., Lonneborg, A., Boccardi, M., Blennow, K., Hansson, O., & Geneva Task Force for the Roadmap of Alzheimer's Biomarkers. (2017). Clinical validity of cerebrospinal fluid Abeta42, tau, and phospho-tau as biomarkers for Alzheimer's disease in the context of a structured 5-phase development framework. *Neurobiology of Aging, 52*, 196–213.

Mattsson, N., Zetterberg, H., Janelidze, S., Insel, P. S., Andreasson, U., Stomrud, E., et al. (2016). Plasma tau in Alzheimer disease. *Neurology, 87*, 1827–1835.

McGeer, P. L., Itagaki, S., Tago, H., & McGeer, E. G. (1987). Reactive microglia in patients with senile dementia of the Alzheimer type are positive for the histocompatibility glycoprotein HLA-DR. *Neuroscience Letters, 79*, 195–200.

Mielke, M. M., Bandaru, V. V., Han, D., An, Y., Resnick, S. M., Ferrucci, L., et al. (2015a). Factors affecting longitudinal trajectories of plasma sphingomyelins: The Baltimore Longitudinal Study of Aging. *Aging Cell, 14*, 112–121.

Mielke, M. M., Bandaru, V. V., Han, D., An, Y., Resnick, S. M., Ferrucci, L., et al. (2015b). Demographic and clinical variables affecting mid- to late-life trajectories of plasma ceramide and dihydroceramide species. *Aging Cell, 14*, 1014–1023.

Mielke, M. M., Ferretti, M. T., Iulita, M. F., Hayden, K., & Khachaturian, A. S. (2018). Sex and gender in Alzheimer's disease – Does it matter? *Alzheimers Dement, 14*, 1101–1103.

Mielke, M. M., Hagen, C. E., Wennberg, A. M. V., Airey, D. C., Savica, R., Knopman, D. S., et al. (2017). Association of plasma total tau level with cognitive decline and risk of mild cognitive impairment or dementia in the Mayo Clinic Study on Aging. *JAMA Neurology, 74*, 1073–1080.

Mielke, M. M., Hagen, C. E., Xu, J., Chai, X., Vemuri, P., Lowe, V. J., et al. (2018). Plasma phospho-tau181 increases with Alzheimer's disease clinical severity and is associated with tau- and amyloid-positron emission tomography. *Alzheimer's & Dementia, 14*, 989–997.

Mielke, M. M., Haughey, N. J., Han, D., An, Y., Bandaru, V. V. R., Lyketsos, C. G., et al. (2017). The association between plasma ceramides and sphingomyelins and risk of Alzheimer's disease differs by sex and APOE in the Baltimore Longitudinal Study of Aging. *Journal of Alzheimer's Disease, 60*, 819–828.

Mielke, M. M., Syrjanen, J. A., Blennow, K., Zetterberg, H., Skoog, I., Vemuri, P., et al. (2019a). Comparison of variables associated with cerebrospinal fluid neurofilament, total-tau, and neurogranin. *Alzheimer's & Dementia, 15*, 1437–1447.

Mielke, M. M., Syrjanen, J. A., Blennow, K., Zetterberg, H., Vemuri, P., Skoog, I., et al. (2019b). Plasma and CSF neurofilament light: Relation to longitudinal neuroimaging and cognitive measures. *Neurology, 93*, e252–e260.

Mielke, M. M., Vemuri, P., & Rocca, W. A. (2014). Clinical epidemiology of Alzheimer's disease: Assessing sex and gender differences. *Clinical Epidemiology, 6*, 37–48.

Nakamura, A., Kaneko, N., Villemagne, V. L., Kato, T., Doecke, J., Dore, V., et al. (2018). High performance plasma amyloid-beta biomarkers for Alzheimer's disease. *Nature, 554*, 249–254.

Nebel, R. A., Aggarwal, N. T., Barnes, L. L., Gallagher, A., Goldstein, J. M., Kantarci, K., et al. (2018). Understanding the impact of sex and gender in Alzheimer's disease: A call to action. *Alzheimer's & Dementia*, *14*, 1171–1183.

Nelson, P. T., Head, E., Schmitt, F. A., Davis, P. R., Neltner, J. H., Jicha, G. A., et al. (2011). Alzheimer's disease is not "brain aging": Neuropathological, genetic, and epidemiological human studies. *Acta Neuropathologica*, *121*, 571–587.

Neu, S. C., Pa, J., Kukull, W., Beekly, D., Kuzma, A., Gangadharan, P., et al. (2017). Apolipoprotein E genotype and sex risk factors for Alzheimer disease: A meta-analysis. *JAMA Neurology*, *74*, 1178–1189.

Nordengen, K., Kirsebom, B. E., Henjum, K., Selnes, P., Gisladottir, B., Wettergreen, M., et al. (2019). Glial activation and inflammation along the Alzheimer's disease continuum. *Journal of Neuroinflammation*, *16*, 46.

Norgren, N., Rosengren, L., & Stigbrand, T. (2003). Elevated neurofilament levels in neurological diseases. *Brain Research*, *987*, 25–31.

Ovod, V., Ramsey, K. N., Mawuenyega, K. G., Bollinger, J. G., Hicks, T., Schneider, T., et al. (2017). Amyloid beta concentrations and stable isotope labeling kinetics of human plasma specific to central nervous system amyloidosis. *Alzheimer's & Dementia*, *13*, 841–849.

Palmqvist, S., Zetterberg, H., Mattsson, N., Johansson, P., Minthon, L., Blennow, K., et al. (2015). Detailed comparison of amyloid PET and CSF biomarkers for identifying early Alzheimer disease. *Neurology*, *85*, 1240–1249.

Parrado-Fernandez, C., Blennow, K., Hansson, M., Leoni, V., Cedazo-Minguez, A., & Bjorkhem, I. (2018). Evidence for sex difference in the CSF/plasma albumin ratio in ~20 000 patients and 335 healthy volunteers. *Journal of Cellular and Molecular Medicine*, *22*, 5151–5154.

Pase, M. P., Beiser, A. S., Himali, J. J., Satizabal, C. L., Aparicio, H. J., DeCarli, C., et al. (2019). Assessment of plasma total tau level as a predictive biomarker for dementia and related endophenotypes. *JAMA Neurology*, *76*, 598–606.

Payami, H., Zareparsi, S., Montee, K. R., Sexton, G. J., Kaye, J. A., Bird, T. D., et al. (1996). Gender difference in apolipoprotein E-associated risk for familial Alzheimer disease: A possible clue to the higher incidence of Alzheimer disease in women. *American Journal of Human Genetics*, *58*, 803–811.

Plassman, B. L., Langa, K. M., Fisher, G. G., Heeringa, S. G., Weir, D. R., Ofstedal, M. B., et al. (2007). Prevalence of dementia in the United States: The aging, demographics, and memory study. *Neuroepidemiology*, *29*, 125–132.

Reiber, H. (1994). Flow rate of cerebrospinal fluid (CSF)—A concept common to normal blood-CSF barrier function and to dysfunction in neurological diseases. *Journal of the Neurological Sciences*, *122*, 189–203.

Roberts, R. O., Aakre, J. A., Kremers, W. K., Vassilaki, M., Knopman, D. S., Mielke, M. M., et al. (2018). Prevalence and outcomes of amyloid positivity among persons without dementia in a longitudinal, population-based setting. *JAMA Neurology*, *75*, 970–979.

Rocca, W. A. (2017). Time, sex, gender, history, and dementia. *Alzheimer Disease and Associated Disorders*, *31*, 76–79.

Rogers, J., Luber-Narod, J., Styren, S. D., & Civin, W. H. (1988). Expression of immune system-associated antigens by cells of the human central nervous system: Relationship to the pathology of Alzheimer's disease. *Neurobiology of Aging*, *9*, 339–349.

Rowe, C. C., Ellis, K. A., Rimajova, M., Bourgeat, P., Pike, K. E., Jones, G., et al. (2010). Amyloid imaging results from the Australian Imaging, Biomarkers and Lifestyle (AIBL) study of aging. *Neurobiology of Aging*, *31*, 1275–1283.

Salloway, S., Sperling, R., Fox, N. C., Blennow, K., Klunk, W., Raskind, M., et al. (2014). Two phase 3 trials of bapineuzumab in mild-to-moderate Alzheimer's disease. *New England Journal of Medicine, 370*, 322–333.

Schoonenboom, N. S., Pijnenburg, Y. A., Mulder, C., Rosso, S. M., Van Elk, E. J., Van Kamp, G. J., et al. (2004). Amyloid beta(1–42) and phosphorylated tau in CSF as markers for early-onset Alzheimer disease. *Neurology, 62*, 1580–1584.

Seshadri, S., Wolf, P. A., Beiser, A., Au, R., McNulty, K., White, R., et al. (1997). Lifetime risk of dementia and Alzheimer's disease. The impact of mortality on risk estimates in the Framingham study. *Neurology, 49*, 1498–1504.

Seyfert, S., Kunzmann, V., Schwertfeger, N., Koch, H. C., & Faulstich, A. (2002). Determinants of lumbar CSF protein concentration. *Journal of Neurology, 249*, 1021–1026.

Strittmatter, W. J., Saunders, A. M., Schmechel, D., Pericak-Vance, M., Enghild, J., Salvesen, G. S., et al. (1993). Apolipoprotein E: High-avidity binding to beta-amyloid and increased frequency of type 4 allele in late-onset familial Alzheimer disease. *Proceedings of the National Academy of Sciences of the United States of America, 90*, 1977–1981.

Tarawneh, R., D'Angelo, G., Crimmins, D., Herries, E., Griest, T., Fagan, A. M., et al. (2016). Diagnostic and prognostic utility of the synaptic marker neurogranin in Alzheimer disease. *JAMA Neurology, 73*, 561–571.

Tibbling, G., Link, H., & Ohman, S. (1977). Principles of albumin and IgG analyses in neurological disorders. I. Establishment of reference values. *Scandinavian Journal of Clinical and Laboratory Investigation, 37*, 385–390.

van Amelsvoort, T., Compton, J., & Murphy, D. (2001). In vivo assessment of the effects of estrogen on human brain. *Trends in Endocrinology and Metabolism, 12*, 273–276.

van Maurik, I. S., Slot, R. E. R., Verfaillie, S. C. J., Zwan, M. D., Bouwman, F. H., Prins, N. D., et al. (2019). Personalized risk for clinical progression in cognitively normal subjects-the ABIDE project. *Alzheimer's Research & Therapy, 11*, 33.

Vergallo, A., Megret, L., Lista, S., Cavedo, E., Zetterberg, H., Blennow, K., et al. (2019). Plasma amyloid beta 40/42 ratio predicts cerebral amyloidosis in cognitively normal individuals at risk for Alzheimer's disease. *Alzheimer's & Dementia, 15*, 764–775.

Verghese, P. B., Castellano, J. M., Garai, K., Wang, Y., Jiang, H., Shah, A., et al. (2013). ApoE influences amyloid-beta (Abeta) clearance despite minimal apoE/Abeta association in physiological conditions. *Proceedings of the National Academy of Sciences of the United States of America, 110*, E1807–E1816.

Wang, M. J., Yi, S., Han, J. Y., Park, S. Y., Jang, J. W., Chun, I. K., et al. (2016). Analysis of cerebrospinal fluid and [11C]PIB PET biomarkers for Alzheimer's disease with updated protocols. *Journal of Alzheimer's Disease, 52*, 1403–1413.

Wellington, H., Paterson, R. W., Portelius, E., Tornqvist, U., Magdalinou, N., Fox, N. C., et al. (2016). Increased CSF neurogranin concentration is specific to Alzheimer disease. *Neurology, 86*, 829–835.

Witte, A. V., Savli, M., Holik, A., Kasper, S., & Lanzenberger, R. (2010). Regional sex differences in grey matter volume are associated with sex hormones in the young adult human brain. *NeuroImage, 49*, 1205–1212.

Wolfsgruber, S., Molinuevo, J. L., Wagner, M., Teunissen, C. E., Rami, L., Coll-Padros, N., et al. (2019). Prevalence of abnormal Alzheimer's disease biomarkers in patients with subjective cognitive decline: Cross-sectional comparison of three European memory clinic samples. *Alzheimer's Research & Therapy, 11*, 8.

Zlokovic, B. V. (2011). Neurovascular pathways to neurodegeneration in Alzheimer's disease and other disorders. *Nature Reviews Neuroscience, 12*, 723–738.

CHAPTER 5

Sex differences in neuroimaging biomarkers in healthy subjects and dementia

Federico Massa[a], Dario Arnaldi[a,b], Michele Balma[c], Matteo Bauckneht[c,d], Andrea Chincarini[e], Pilar M. Ferraro[f], Matteo Grazzini[a], Caterina Lapucci[a,g], Riccardo Meli[a], Silvia Morbelli[c,f], Matteo Pardini[a,b], Enrico Peira[a,e], Stefano Raffa[c], Luca Roccatagliata[c,f], and Flavio Nobili[a,b]

[a]*Department of Neuroscience (DINOGMI), University of Genoa, Genoa, Italy*
[b]*Department of Neurology, IRCCS Polyclinic Hospital San Martino, Genoa, Italy*
[c]*Department of Health Sciences (DISSAL), University of Genoa, Genoa, Italy*
[d]*Nuclear Medicine Unit, IRCCS Polyclinic Hospital San Martino, Genoa, Italy*
[e]*National Institute for Nuclear Physics (INFN), Genoa Section, Genoa, Italy*
[f]*Department of Neuroradiology, IRCCS Polyclinic Hospital San Martino, Genoa, Italy*
[g]*Laboratory of Experimental Neurosciences, HNSR, IRCCS Polyclinic Hospital San Martino, Genoa, Italy*

Abbreviations

AD	**Alzheimer's** disease
ADD	Alzheimer's disease dementia
ADNI	Alzheimer's disease neuroimaging initiative
aMCI	amnestic mild cognitive impairment
APOE	apolipoprotein E
BOLD	blood oxygen level-dependent
CAN	central autonomic network
CBF	cerebral blood flow+
CEN	central executive network
CSF	cerebrospinal fluid
DAN	dorsal attention network
DAT	dopamine transporter
DLB	dementia with Lewy bodies
DMN	default mode network
DTI	diffusion tensor imaging
FA	fractional anisotropy
FC	functional connectivity

FDG-PET	^{18}F-fluorodeoxyglucose positron emission tomography
fMRI	functional magnetic resonance imaging
FPN	frontoparietal network
GM	gray matter
HE	Hurst exponent
HPF	hippocampal parenchymal fraction
^{123}I-β-CIT	^{123}I 2β-carbomethoxy-3β-(4-iodophenyl) tropane
^{123}I-FP-CIT	^{123}I-ioflupane
^{123}I-IMP	N-isopropyl p-I-123-iodoamphetamine
MCI	mild cognitive impairment
MRI	magnetic resonance imaging
NC	normal controls
PD	Parkinson's disease
PET	positron emission tomography
PiB	Pittsburgh compound B
pMRI	perfusion magnetic resonance imaging
QSM	quantitative susceptibility mapping
rCBF	regional cerebral blood flow
ROI	region of interest
RS	resting state
RS-fMRI	resting state-functional magnetic resonance imaging
SBR	specific to nondisplaceable binding ratio
SN	salience network
SPECT	single photon emission computed tomography
SUVR	standardized uptake value ratio
^{99m}Tc-ECD	^{99m}Tc ethylcysteinate dimer
^{99m}Tc-HMPAO	^{99m}Tc-hexamethylpropylene amine oxime
TSPO	translocator protein
VHMC	voxel-mirrored homotopic connectivity
WM	white matter

Introduction

Sex and gender-related differences in terms of human behavior and cognition have been widely reported over the years and are influenced by an interplay of both biological and environmental factors (Ferretti et al., 2018). Furthermore, several neurological conditions, such as dementias, are sex-predisposed, thus suggesting the importance of sexual dimorphism. However, most studies actually consider sex as a nuisance variable, rather than a major factor accounting for the different vulnerabilities and trajectories of normal or pathological brain aging in men and women.

Preclinical animal models as well as postmortem studies in humans have provided useful information on the differences in terms of brain structure and neuropathology between females and males (Cosgrove, Mazure, & Staley, 2007). Within this context, the role of neuroimaging techniques has grown in recent years as they provide in vivo information on brain morphology and functioning, but also on the underpinning neuropathological changes, by using specific radiopharmaceuticals to

Table 1 List of imaging techniques discussed in the text.

	Techniques	Tracers
Structural MRI (sMRI)	Volumetric T1-weighted images Quantitative susceptibility mapping (QSM) Diffusion tensor imaging (DTI)	
Functional MRI (fMRI)	Task-related fMRI Resting state (RS)-fMRI Perfusion MRI (pMRI)	
Perfusion SPECT		^{99m}Tc-HMPAO ^{99m}Tc-ECD ^{133}Xenon ^{123}I-IMP
DAT-SPECT	DAT binding	^{123}I-FP-CIT ^{99m}Tc-TRODAT-1 ^{123}β-CIT
PET	Nigro-striatal assessment Brain metabolism Amyloid binding Tau binding 5-HT(1A) receptor binding TSPO binding	^{18}F-Fluoro-DOPA ^{18}F-FDG ^{11}C-PiB ^{18}F-AV45 (florbetapir) ^{18}F AV-1451 ^{11}C-WAY-1006 ^{11}C-PBR28

image the brain through SPECT and PET technologies. Nevertheless, results from different studies are often conflicting due to technical issues and the lack of a systematic approach, and this limits the consideration of sex as a leading factor in experimental and clinical studies.

Below, we describe the different imaging techniques (Table 1) used to assess sex-related brain differences, both in the healthy and in pathological aging. In addition, we highlight the implications of the findings coming from different studies, and their limitations, which need to be overcome in future neuroimaging studies.

Structural MRI

Prior to the 1990s, few studies examined sex differences in the clinical presentation, disease progression, or treatment of psychiatric and neurological disorders and their correlation with brain macro- and microstructure (Cosgrove et al., 2007). Sex-related differences in brain structure have been largely studied in preclinical animal models, and postmortem studies in humans have initially provided useful information, but methodological factors, i.e., agonal state and postmortem interval, may have affected the results. In this scenario, neuroimaging techniques play an important role in evaluating sex-related differences in brain structure in vivo.

Structural MRI sex differences in healthy subjects

Sex differences in regional brain areas of healthy subjects during adulthood and normal aging have been reported in several studies. The different methodologies applied (i.e., image registration and segmentation algorithms) might explain some conflicting findings. The characterization of the spatial-temporal pattern of GM and WM volume changes in normal aging may also allow better understanding of the mechanisms leading to the pathologic changes in neurodegenerative disorders, the risk of which increases with age (Peng et al., 2016).

Age-related brain volume loss differs between men and women. The volume loss progresses with age in the whole brain, particularly affecting frontal and temporal lobes in men and parietal lobes in women. Moreover, a high degree of heterogeneity was described as for age-related GM volume changes; indeed, some brain regions, including the temporal lobe, hippocampus, and parahippocampal gyrus, are more susceptible to the effect of aging in males (Witelson, Beresh, & Kigar, 2006). In a paper by Peng et al. (2016), a cross-sectional study was conducted of age- and sex-related changes in the GM volume of several brain regions in a population of 124 cognitively normal Chinese adults. In young and middle-aged subjects, female and male subjects showed significant differences in the right middle temporal gyrus, right superior temporal gyrus, left angular gyrus, right middle occipital lobe, left middle cingulate gyrus, and the pars triangularis of the right inferior frontal gyrus, suggesting an interaction between age and sex.

Király et al. (2016) analyzed T1-weighted images from 53 healthy males and 50 age-matched healthy females by using a surface model-based segmentation approach, and demonstrated a significant age-related decrease in males as compared to females.

From a pathophysiological point of view, half a century ago, a postmortem study by Hallgren and Sourander (1958) showed that iron accumulates with varying degrees across brain structures, showing a rapid increase until young adulthood, followed by a smaller rise, and then reaching a plateau after midlife. MRI studies focused on brain iron content in healthy adults yielded conflicting results, showing both linear and nonlinear age trends of iron distribution. Nevertheless, in most of these studies, the iron concentration was higher in the subcortical nuclei as compared to the WM and cortex (Bilgic et al., 2012). In addition to age, sex should also be considered a determinant of brain iron levels variability. QSM, an advanced MRI technique, has been used to provide information about tissue magnetic susceptibility. Using this approach, lower susceptibility values in women than men were found in the thalamus and red nucleus by Gong et al. (2015) and in the substantia nigra, after accounting for age, in a study by Persson et al. (2015), in which, in addition, a linear increase with age of pulvinar susceptibility in men was demonstrated. This latter study represents the first in vivo evidence of lower GM subcortical iron levels selectively in women from the postmenopausal stage, suggesting a role of the hormonal axis in neurodegenerative changes.

As for the WM, aging is a main cause of WM degradation, mostly due to myelin breakdown (Bartzokis et al., 2010). In this context, DTI is a noninvasive in vivo method used to provide a quantitative estimation of the microstructural organization of WM by means of the FA, a DTI parameter ranging from 0, when there is an isotropic movement of water molecules (e.g., CSF) to 1, when the movement of water molecules is anisotropic (e.g., fiber bundles). In particular, across the lifespan, the FA progressively increases during the first two decades of life, which relates to myelin maturation, and then decreases, with a faster rate after 60 years, likely reflecting axonal and myelin changes. It is worthy of note that, in the same way as WM microstructure maturation has been demonstrated to be heterogeneous across brain regions, age-related WM changes seem to follow an anteroposterior gradient, with the most evident changes in the anterior part of the corpus callosum with respect to the splenium (Fan et al., 2019).

Some investigations have reported a lack of significant interactions between sex and age as regarding WM microstructure (Kanaan et al., 2012). However, it may be argued that WM trajectories also present sex specificity, as age-related myelination changes have been described as being more prominent in males than females in animal models (Yang et al., 2008). One of the possible explanations of the lack of sex-specific DTI findings in aging is the use of conventional DTI-derived measures, which are characterized by low sensitivity to axonal microstructural integrity abnormalities. Advanced multishell diffusion-weighted imaging methods may overcome these issues, due to their capability of separating intra- and extra-axonal diffusion compartments. In this context, a recent paper by Toschi et al. (2020) reported that the so called "restricted signal fraction"—a marker of the combined effect of axonal and myelin integrity—has a greater sensitivity relative to traditional DTI measures in detecting the age at which WM microstructural components start to change. In this study, microstructural changes detected with more advanced techniques were found at a greater extent in women than in men. Indeed, in female subjects, the age-related WM decline was found to begin approximately 14 years later than in males and seemed to preferentially affect the frontal regions.

In conclusion, according to sMRI findings, sex should be considered as a major determinant in cross-sectional MRI studies focused on the aging brain. This aspect may be of paramount importance when evaluating the changes of GM structures that are consistently related to several neurodegenerative disorders (e.g., AD).

Structural MRI sex differences in dementia

Sex-related brain structural differences have been investigated in patients with MCI and ADD, and in cognitively normal subjects carrying AD risk factors (i.e., APOE ε4 allele). A higher risk of developing AD (Gao et al., 1998), greater cognitive impairment (Bai et al., 2009), and functional disability (Dodge et al., 2003) were reported in women, but MRI evidence of a "sexual dimorphism" in AD remains controversial.

In females with ADD, either smaller hippocampal volumes (Apostolova et al., 2006) or less atrophy (evaluated through CSF volume) in frontal, temporal, and parietal regions (Kidron et al., 1997) were found as compared to males. In a large cohort of nearly 400 ADD patients, the whole brain volume was unrelated to sex, and two other studies concluded that the frontal and the medial temporal lobes should be included among the brain regions not differentially associated with sex in ADD. Conversely, temporal lobe degeneration over time has been shown to proceed faster in women with ADD than in men (Skup et al., 2011).

Taking into account that sex differences have been suggested among patients with AD and those with aMCI across a variety of domains, including cognition and behavior, Skup et al. (2011) obtained longitudinal sMRI data of 197 individuals with probable ADD and 266 with aMCI compared to 224 healthy controls from the ADNI database to assess sex differences in GM atrophy patterns over 2–3 years. In the study, males showed lower volumes over time, compared to females, in bilateral thalamus and right middle temporal gyrus, in both the ADD and aMCI groups, as well as in the left insula in ADD and in the bilateral caudate nucleus in aMCI groups, respectively.

Conversely, in a 1-year longitudinal MRI study, the 3D profile of progressive atrophy in subjects with probable AD, with amnestic MCI, and healthy controls was mapped, revealing significant age and sex differences in atrophic rates. In particular, brain atrophy rates were about 1%–1.5%/year faster in women than in men (Hua et al., 2010).

As for the hippocampus, which is one of the regions first affected by AD pathology, no significant volume difference between sexes was disclosed in older adults with subjective memory complaints (Cavedo et al., 2018). These results are in line with a metaanalysis conducted by Tan et al. (2016) on 4000 brains, in which no sex differences in the hippocampal volume were detected. In this setting, Ardekani et al. (2019) measured the HPF on 775 MRI volumetric scans of 198 volunteers from a public database (OASIS1, http://oasis-brains.org/), divided into cognitively unimpaired, MCI, or mild/moderate ADD. HPF asymmetry was significantly higher in men after controlling for all the other variables, but there was no sex effect on HPF size. Similar findings were obtained in a recent paper, where no interactive effect of sex on hippocampal volume was detected (Caldwell, Cummings, et al., 2019).

The APOE e4 genotype has been considered as the strongest genetic risk factor for sporadic AD, and higher risk in females than in males. In addition, female APOE ε4 carriers also showed reduced hippocampal volume with respect to their male counterparts in the MCI and ADD conditions, but results are controversial. One longitudinal study in MCI patients reported no significant association between APOE ε4, sex, and hippocampal atrophy over a 2-year period (Spampinato et al., 2016), whereas female sex and APOE ε4 were associated with a longitudinal reduction of hippocampal volumes in the NC and MCI but not in the ADD groups drawn by the ADNI dataset (Shen et al., 2019). Nevertheless, in a previous study by Holland et al. (2013), women in all cohorts (cognitively preserved, MCI, and ADD) demonstrated higher rates of decline than men. Interestingly, in this study, the magnitude of the sex effect on the decline rates was as large as those of ApoE ε4. The different and relatively short follow-up time in the MCI and ADD cohorts cannot be ruled out as a possible explanation of these conflicting findings.

Lastly, as for sex-related effects on AD progression, Lee et al. (2018) no differences were found in cortical thickness between males and females in either AD or normal control groups at baseline, after controlling for age, education, disease duration, age at onset (early onset versus late onset), APOE ε4 allele, and intracranial volume. However, women with ADD showed more accelerated cortical thinning than men over a 5-year follow-up.

Notably, most of the MRI studies tackling sex differences in AD have been longitudinal rather than cross-sectional in nature. Thus, findings likely reflect a faster progression of AD-specific pathology in females in which more severe neurofibrillary degeneration and greater loss of brain parenchyma have been reported and associated with higher cognitive deficit (Filon et al., 2016).

In addition, some technical issues should be considered. Most of the studies are probably underpowered, and the sample size is not large enough to detect a subtle sex effect on atrophy rates. Furthermore, the different technical approaches used to process MR images over the years may be an important contributor to explain the conflicting results in the literature. For instance, whole brain volume estimation may give different results, depending on whether the correction for the intracranial volume (ICV) has been applied or not. Obviously, this bias becomes increasingly important in MRI studies focused on the effect of sex on brain atrophy. Similarly, several approaches for brain segmentation have been applied in the different investigations, partly due to the advance in technical knowledge of MRI analysis over the years. This is the case, for instance, in the choice to use an intensity-based procedure rather than a model-based approach to segment brain structures. This approach has a particular utility in those regions with low tissue contrast and should be preferred for the segmentation of subcortical GM (Király et al., 2016).

Conclusion

An asymmetry of brain volumes and microstructural architecture seems to be present between males and females throughout the lifespan, from adulthood to older age. Furthermore, male and female patients with ADD show different patterns and rate of atrophy progression in crucial sites, although with conflicting results, to which technical issues in MRI analysis and heterogeneity of patients across studies in terms of age, educational level, disease duration, and severity may have contributed.

Fig. 1 summarizes the main morphological and functional MRI potentialities to apply to sex differences research.

Functional MRI

FMRI techniques provide a unique opportunity to elucidate the interplay between sex, brain functions, and behavior. We review evidences of sex-related brain functional differences emerging from distinct fMRI approaches, including task-related fMRI, RS-fMRI, and pMRI.

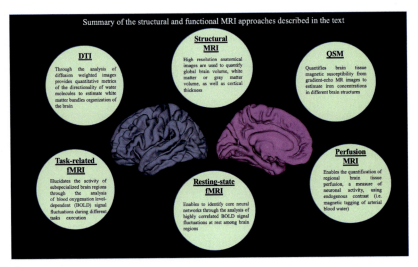

FIG. 1
Summary of the main morphological and functional MRI potentialities to apply to sex differences research, as described in the text.

fMRI sex differences in healthy subjects

Neuronal activation is supported by a higher oxygen supply provided by an increase in rCBF. This process results in a change in the relative levels of oxyhemoglobin and deoxyhemoglobin detectable by MRI using their differential magnetic susceptibilities. This approach is known as BOLD contrast imaging and is traditionally applied to generate maps reflecting the activity of subspecialized brain regions involved in the execution of different tasks (Lv et al., 2018). Overall, converging evidence suggests that, while some cognitive functions and their cortical substrates are differentially modulated by sex-aging interactions, others are not. Hesselmann et al. (2001) have evaluated signal intensity variations related to aging during a motor stimulation paradigm and found a selective significant decrease of signal intensities with age in males.

One study investigated the link between age, sex, handedness, and language lateralization index in a large group of healthy participants using both a semantic decision and a verb generation task (Nenert et al., 2017). Notably, the lateralization indices were found to significantly decrease with age only in right-handed men and in temporoparietal cortical areas, suggesting that the evolution of language lateralization in the human brain may follow different trajectories in men and women. Conversely, for other functions, sex-related differences may not be significantly influenced by aging. Ritchey et al. (2011) found enhanced emotion-related activity of the right amygdala and striatum in females relative to males, independently from age, providing evidence that sex effects on the involvement of these structures may be stable across the lifespan. Intriguingly, for some higher order cognitive functions, neither sex nor aging seem to play a significant role.

Another study has investigated the lateralization of brain hemodynamic activity related to attention processes using an event-related fMRI auditory oddball task (Stevens, Calhoun, & Kiehl, 2005). The authors found greater right hemisphere activity for target detection and novelty processing, but the asymmetry effects did not differ with respect to the age or sex of the participants.

Unlike task-related fMRI, RS-fMRI is acquired in the absence of a stimulus or a task, and the analysis is therefore focused on spontaneous BOLD signal alterations (Lv et al., 2018). With this approach, some studies were able to identify core brain networks sustaining distinct cognitive functions, including: (a) the DMN, which comprises the precuneus/posterior cingulate, lateral parietal, and mesial prefrontal cortex—this network is primarily activated under resting conditions, but it also facilitates or monitors active tasks (working memory, in particular); (b) the DAN, which comprises middle temporal visual areas, superior parietal lobule, the cortical regions near the intraparietal sulcus and ventral premotor cortex, and is mainly engaged during externally directed attentional tasks; (c) the SN, which is primarily composed of the anterior insula and dorsal anterior cingulate cortex and is primarily involved in detecting and filtering salient stimuli, as well as in recruiting CEN and DMN structures; and (d) the FPN, primarily composed of the dorsolateral prefrontal cortex and posterior parietal cortex, particularly engaged during attention and cognitive control process.

Notably, RS fMRI also enables the investigation of connectivity alterations within and between these networks, and evaluation of how different factors, including sex, may differentially mediate these associations. Jamadar et al. (2018) showed greater connectivity in the SN for males compared to females, while the opposite pattern was observed in the DMN.

Other studies focused on the asymmetry of spontaneous cerebral activity in relation to sex. A previous study investigated the relationship between multiple intelligence measures and the degree of coherent functional activity between corresponding cortical areas using VHMC (Santarnecchi et al., 2015), finding a trend towards increased correlation between mirrored connectivity and intelligence quotient scores in the prefrontal cortex and precuneus/cuneus regions in females. Another study has evaluated the lateralization of RS networks (Agcaoglu et al., 2015) finding a higher right lateralization of the lingual gyrus within the visual network and more left lateralization of the inferior frontal gyrus within the frontal network in males. However, it is noteworthy that sex-related connectivity changes are not fixed, as they interact with aging.

Sie et al. (2019) investigated sex-related differences between multiple networks and the CAN, a network primarily involved in the control of visceromotor, neuroendocrine, pain, and behavioral responses. With aging, females demonstrated reduced negative connectivity in the posterior midcingulate gyrus with dorsal precuneus/posterior cingulate cortex and left angular gyrus, possibly suggesting a decay in the suppression of the sympathoexcitation associated with decrease in estrogen levels. Conversely, males showed an increased positive connectivity in posterior midcingulate gyrus with right supramarginal gyrus, and in ventromedial prefrontal cortex with ventral precuneus, suggesting greater parasympathetic regulation with advancing age. Scheinost et al. (2015) showed common and divergent trajectories of age-related connectivity changes across the main RS networks in males and females. In the DMN, males and females both showed age-related decreases in connectivity, while in the FPN, males and females manifested opposing aging trajectories, with an overall negative correlation with age remaining significant only in females. Furthermore, the networks responsible for the basic senses showed differential aging patterns for males and females, with an inverse correlation between connectivity and aging in the visual network selectively observed in females. Overall, these sex differences in aging trajectories may play a role in age-related changes in normal cognition, as well as in the susceptibility to neurological and psychiatric diseases. A subsequent study looking at sex-related effects of aging on DMN, DAN, and SN connectivity, however, found significant global reductions in older males compared to younger males, while for females, age did not modulate intra-network connectivity (Goldstone et al., 2016).

Sex-related differences in VMHC have also been evaluated in relation to aging. A pivotal study from Zuo et al. (2010) demonstrated age-related increases in VMHC of the dorsolateral prefrontal cortex and decreases in VMHC of the amygdala in males, while the opposite pattern was observed in females. Another study, exploring fractal complexity of the RS-fMRI signal across the adult lifespan using HE analysis (Dong et al., 2018), showed that, overall, global mean HE increases with age, indicating a progressive reduction of BOLD activity complexity. However, females exhibited higher HE values in the parietal lobe independently of age, while the interaction between age and sex showed a significant effect in the right parahippocampal gyrus, suggesting that the aging effect on BOLD complexity is different between sexes in this region.

PMRI is an innovative MRI approach that enables the noninvasive quantification of regional brain tissue perfusion using labeled inflowing arterial protons as an endogenous tracer. One study combining pMRI and transcranial Doppler explored sex-related differences in cerebral hemodynamics and their relation to central hemodynamics (Tarumi et al., 2014). Global CBF and wave reflection were higher, while diastolic CBF velocity was lower, in women compared to men, suggesting that female sex may increase central pulse pressure, which in turn may reduce diastolic but raise pulsatile CBF. Another study looked at the effects of physical activity and sex on CBF in older adults, finding greater cortical perfusion in women compared to men, and particularly in women who engaged in strength training compared to women who did not. This effect was absent in men, suggesting that cerebrovascular function may be moderated not only by sex, but also by strength training (Xu et al., 2014). PMRI research is now also focusing on the interaction between sex and aging. A first study comparing CBF between healthy elderly and young subjects showed larger age-related CBF decline in men compared to females (Asllani et al., 2009). However, divergent findings come from a study showing higher CBF in young premenopausal women compared to both young men and older postmenopausal women (Liu, Lou, & Ma, 2016). As outlined by the authors, these findings (replicating older studies with molecular imaging techniques, Krejza, 2001; Ohkura, 1994; Rodriguez, 1988) might be explained by sex hormones differences between women and men. Another study examined the influence of cardiac function on CBF in aged subjects (Henriksen et al., 2014), finding that CBF was higher in females compared to males, and that CBF decrease related to aging tended to be restricted to females.

fMRI sex differences in dementia

Sex-related fMRI differences have also been investigated in patients with ADD, with MCI, and cognitively normal subjects carrying AD risk factors (i.e., APOE ε4 allele). A previous study investigated FC alterations and their behavioral correlates in older females with and without MCI relative to their male counterparts (Huang et al., 2015). The authors found that brain function of subcortical-cortical loops was disrupted in older females with MCI, and that regional RS function of the left precuneus was significantly associated with altered episodic memory in these cases, suggesting a link between network dysregulation and susceptibility to cognitive dysfunction. Converging evidence for a significant involvement of the precuneus in females at risk of AD comes from studies evaluating the interaction between sex, brain functional alterations, and AD risk factors. A pivotal study by Damoiseaux et al. (2012) demonstrated that female APOE ε4 carriers showed significantly reduced DMN connectivity, which was most pronounced in the precuneus, compared with either female APOE ε3 homozygotes or male APOE ε4 carriers, whereas male ε4 carriers differed minimally from male APOE ε3 homozygotes. Furthermore, subsequent studies have suggested that not only the precuneus, but also its functional connections with the hippocampus might be altered in cognitively normal female APOE ε4 carriers and prone to significant age-related decrease (Heise et al., 2014). Taken together, these preliminary observations suggest that greater vulnerability of these connections might be one reason contributing to the increased AD risk in female APOE ε4 carriers.

However, divergent findings come from other studies. Caldwell, Zhuang, et al. (2019) found greater anterior DMN/posterior DMN connectivity related to better verbal learning in cognitively normal women with an APOE ε4 allele and amyloid PET positivity compared to their ε4 negative counterparts, while no similar significant results were observed in men. Another study, looking at the effects of sex on RS FC in cognitively normal individuals with subjective memory complaints has shown a significant reduction of the DMN FC in men compared to women, but the authors did not find any significant effects when looking at the interaction between sex, APOE, and amyloid status in specific hubs (Cavedo et al., 2018).

Conclusion

In healthy aged populations, task-related fMRI studies suggest a complex interaction between sex and neural correlates of common brain processes. For some functions, the involvement of specific brain regions seems to be influenced by both aging and sex, for other functions only by sex, and for other functions by neither of these factors. RS-fMRI studies have evidenced a differential vulnerability of core brain networks in males and females, and an overall trend towards greater lateralization in males and greater homotopic connectivity in females. Notably, both sexes seem to manifest age-related decreases in RS FC, but females have been shown to be more vulnerable to network-specific decline. On the other hand, pMRI studies have been more consistent in reporting higher CBF, as well as more pronounced CBF decline, in females compared to men.

Less evidence is available for sex-related fMRI differences in dementia. The available studies have mainly focused on RS FC alterations in prodromal and symptomatic stages of AD, mainly reporting DMN hubs FC reductions and altered connectivity of these regions with other brain structures in female APOE ε4 carriers, partially explaining the increased vulnerability to AD in these subjects.

In conclusion, while the emerging evidence suggests sex to be a key factor modulating brain functioning, some limitations of the current lines of research need to be highlighted. Overall, there is a considerable paucity of fMRI studies looking at sexual dimorphisms in the human brain compared to sMRI studies. Moreover, while few fMRI studies have specifically investigated sex-related changes in aged populations, exploring this aspect would be pivotal to better understanding how age-related diseases, such as AD, differentially impact on the main correlates of brain functions in males and females. Finally, it is noteworthy that fMRI studies looking at sex differences in dementia have mainly looked at RS FC alterations, while in task-related and pMRI studies sex is often considered as a variable to correct for instead of a modulatory element to investigate on its own. Future studies are therefore warranted to broaden our knowledge on the complex interactions between brain functions, sex, aging, and pathology. See Fig. 1 for a summary of the main fMRI potentialities.

Perfusion SPECT

SPECT aims to measure the nonquantitative brain distribution of lipophilic radio-pharmaceuticals, such as ^{99m}Tc-HMPAO, ^{99m}Tc-ECD, and ^{123}I-IMP. The distribution of these tracers to brain tissue is a function of rCBF and differs one for each as a consequence of the retention mechanism within the brain. Hence, they do not allow quantitative measures and are only roughly correlated with rCBF as measured by quantitative tools, such as $H_2^{15}O$ PET or ^{133}Xenon SPECT, which is an abandoned SPECT (or planar) technique because of the poor spatial resolution. The most appropriate term for SPECT findings is, therefore, "brain perfusion (distribution)," while the term "rCBF," often used to report SPECT findings, should be discouraged.

Perfusion SPECT sex differences in healthy subjects

Early studies with quantitative tools repeatedly showed that females have higher CBF than males in all regions and at all ages, with differences declining in the postmenopausal period (Rodriguez et al., 1988). An effect of estrogens and of a lower oxygen carrying capacity (i.e., a lower hemoglobin concentration) are some among the suggested mechanisms. As for the relative regional distribution of perfusion values, available studies obtained controversial results: the lack of sex differences found by Callen et al. (2004) was inconsistent with the ^{99m}Tc-ECD SPECT study by Van Laere et al. (2001), who found a higher perfusion in men in the bilateral cerebellum and in the left anterior temporal and orbitofrontal cortices, and a significantly higher perfusion in women's right inferior parietal cortex. This was in line with other ^{133}Xenon SPECT studies in which females disclosed either increased absolute global CBF (Devous et al., 1986) or rCBF values in temporoparietal areas in comparison to males (Slosman et al., 2001).

Sex differences in brain perfusion have been reported in older healthy volunteers by means of ^{99m}Tc-ECD SPECT, and also after partial-volume effect correction (Li et al., 2004). Women showed higher regional perfusion in the left inferior frontal gyrus, bilateral middle temporal, and left superior temporal gyri. Such sex differences were consistent with the better performance in women in verbal tasks, which are related to the activity of the left inferior frontal gyrus; whereas, men had higher regional perfusion in the left superior frontal gyrus and in several areas of the right hemisphere, i.e., the cerebellum, middle frontal, fusiform and postcentral gyri, parietal lobule, and precuneus. This is in keeping with the greater ability of men in visuospatial tasks, which involve the right parietal and occipitotemporal regions.

By far the largest study was performed by means of ^{99m}Tc-HMPAO-SPECT in 119 young healthy subjects and in a psychiatric population of 26,683 patients (Amen et al., 2017). Women displayed relatively higher perfusion in prefrontal regions, in the limbic lobe, and in the areas involved in the DMN, namely the posterior cingulate cortex/precuneus, temporo-parietal regions, and medial temporal lobes.

The increased perfusion in limbic areas has been associated with the highest rate of mood disorders in women, as amygdala and limbic lobe are involved in emotional processing. On the other hand, the relative hyperperfusion in the DMN structures, which was described in young females by some authors (Amen et al., 2017; Jones et al., 1998; Slosman et al., 2001), is difficult to interpret. DMN is a pivotal network in memory functioning, especially in episodic memory retrieval, and is typically affected in AD. Indeed, DMN typically displays hypoperfusion even at MCI stage of AD, in keeping with the FDG PET hypometabolic pattern (Morbelli et al., 2015; Fig. 2). In this setting, it was speculated that the increased estrogen-related perfusion (Krejza et al., 2001) might exert a protective role on DMN in young females.

Perfusion SPECT sex differences in dementia

Perfusion SPECT is a useful surrogate marker of neuronal activity and thus it is regarded as a neurodegeneration biomarker. Indeed, patterns of perfusion and brain metabolism closely overlap in conditions of normal brain autoregulation, with more similarities with FDG-PET for ^{99m}Tc-ECD than ^{99m}Tc-HMPAO. However, PET technology allows higher spatial resolution and has thus replaced SPECT, at least in high-income countries.

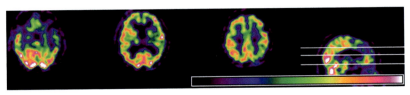

FIG. 2

Perfusion SPECT (^{99m}Tc-HMPAO) shown in three transaxial sections in a 79-year-old woman (5 years of education) with aMCI (mini mental state examination score 23/30, no impairment in autonomy in everyday life activities). The scan shows reduced tracer uptake in the right medial temporal lobe (on *left*), left lateral temporal cortex *(middle)*, and left parietal and posterior cingulate cortex *(right)*.

Studies specifically focusing on sex-related differences of brain perfusion in AD patients are lacking. In a study of 300 ADD patients, females exhibited greater perfusion heterogeneity and asymmetry, as the left hemisphere was more affected (Ott et al., 2000). On the other hand, a greater hypoperfusion in males with AD was described in the parietal and posterior cingulate (Hanyu et al., 2004; Nitrini et al., 2000) and in anterior and middle cingulate cortices (Callen et al., 2004). In the study by Callen et al. (2004), both ^{99m}Tc-HMPAO SPECT and co-registered MRI were used to map the limbic system in 20 men and 20 women with probable ADD compared to 40 age-, sex-, and education-matched normal controls. In the ADD group, men displayed more regions of hypoperfusion, paralleling brain atrophy, in anterior and middle cingulate regions, whereas in women, hypoperfusion was only evident in the anterior thalamus.

In a study with (^{123}I-IMP) SPECT in 30 men and 30 women with AD, Hanyu et al. (2004) reported the typical posterior pattern of hypoperfusion in both sexes. Male patients, however, had a more severe hypoperfusion in the parietal lobe and posterior cingulate, consistent with Nitrini et al. (2000); whereas, females displayed reduced perfusion in additional areas, including the medial frontal lobe and medial temporal regions (Fig. 3).

Men have a more severe decrease of rCBF in the parietooccipital and medial parietal lobes, whereas women have a more severe decrease of rCBF in the lateral, medial, and orbital frontal lobes, and medial and inferior temporal regions. The color of the outer contour corresponds to a Z score of 7.

Notably, the sex differences in brain perfusion found in healthy adults show similarities with those in AD patients, mostly regarding the lower perfusion in parietal and limbic lobes in men (Amen et al., 2017; Jones et al., 1998; Van Laere et al., 2001). The more severe and widespread relative perfusion changes found in men compared to women, despite the similar cognitive status, might suggest that deeper AD-related brain changes are needed for clinical signs to become apparent in men, a concept reminiscent of the cognitive reserve theory. Moreover, it may indicate that the sensitivity of SPECT for the diagnosis of AD may be somehow flattened in female patients in the earliest stages. Such results also support the hypothesis that AD pathology may express differently in men and women, although the underlying biological mechanisms remain mostly unexplained.

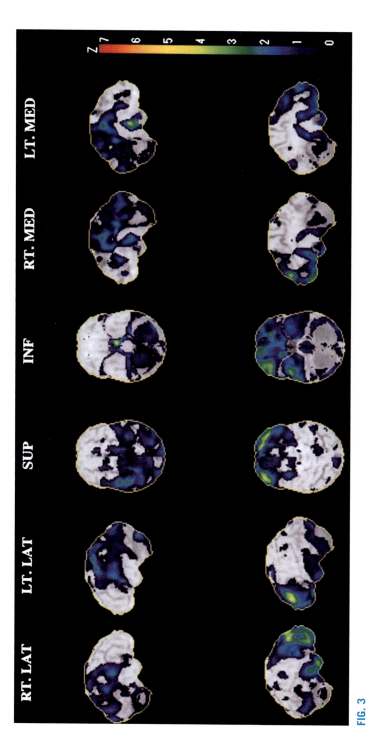

FIG. 3

Statistical maps showing the relative decrease of rCBF in men with AD compared with that in women with AD (top) and in women with AD compared with that in men with AD (bottom).

Reproduced with permission from Hanyu, H., et al. (2004). Differences in regional cerebral blood flow patterns in male versus female patients with Alzheimer disease. American Journal of Neuroradiology, 25(7), 1199–1204.

Estrogens may exert a protective role by reducing the cerebrovascular resistance with the consequent increase in brain perfusion (Krejza et al., 2001; Ohkura et al., 1994) and by promoting the synaptogenesis in the entorhinal cortex via an apolipoprotein E-dependent mechanism (Stone et al., 1998; Chapter 2). Hence, the postmenopausal drop of estrogen might explain the higher vulnerability for AD in females (Mosconi, Berti, Guyara-Quinn, et al., 2017; see also Chapter 9).

Some evidence has suggested a sex effect on brain perfusion due to the APOE ε4 genotype (Lehtovirta et al., 1998). However, according to other authors, neither a correlation between APOE genotype and perfusion patterns (Swartz, Black, & St George-Hyslop, 1999) nor an overall higher female risk of developing AD due to APOE ε4 (Neu et al., 2017) were found. Thus, the genetic role in the sex differences of brain perfusion in AD needs to be further investigated.

Finally, low education has a similarly harmful effect in both sexes, but has been historically more common in women (see Chapter 12). Hence, the studies that evaluated sex differences in brain perfusion could have been biased by cultural effects, as older women might show significant cognitive deficits even with less severe AD pathology.

Conclusion

Sex-related differences in either global or regional brain perfusion have been described in healthy subjects and in AD patients. While higher absolute CBF in women is well established, results are more controversial and heterogeneous regarding regional perfusion distribution. Methodological differences may account for discrepancies, for example, in terms of data analysis (visual versus statistical analysis), as well as others technical issues, such as the considered regions of interest or the tracers, i.e., ^{99m}Tc-HMPAO and ^{99m}Tc-ECD (Nitrini et al., 2000) or ^{123}I-IMP (Hanyu et al., 2004), or whether partial volume-correction was performed (Li et al., 2004).

Several authors have tried to explain such sex differences, but the underlying biological mechanisms are only partially understood. Hormonal balance, education, and genetics have been proposed as factors influencing brain perfusion and might exert either a protective or an enhancing role in neurodegenerative diseases as well. Investigations concerning sex disparities in terms of brain perfusion are meaningful in understanding the different AD vulnerability and the trajectories of normal or pathological brain aging in men and women. In addition, setting up normal databases for statistical image analysis and interpreting the pathological findings according to sex differences might be paramount in clinical practice and in pharmacological trial design.

DAT SPECT

DAT SPECT imaging is a tool for the study of the nigrostriatal dopaminergic system, and is used to confirm nigrostriatal impairment in patients with suspected neurodegenerative parkinsonism and, in the dementia field, for differential diagnosis between AD and DLB. In the current DLB diagnostic criteria, low DAT SBR in basal ganglia is as an indicative biomarker, allowing a diagnosis of probable DLB in the presence of one on more core clinical features (McKeith et al., 2017). ^{123}I-FP-CIT SPECT is currently the most studied and available presynaptic radiopharmaceutical for DAT SPECT imaging.

DAT SPECT sex differences in healthy subjects

In animal models, DAT mRNA measured by in situ hybridization was found to be higher in female compared to male rats. Moreover, early neuroendocrinology studies found a significant positive correlation between estradiol levels and DAT expression, suggesting that sex differences may also be found in humans (Morissette, Biron, & Di Paolo, 1990). Several studies have focused on sex differences in DAT imaging in healthy subjects. A study by Kuikka et al. (1997) investigating 39 healthy subjects with ^{123}I-β-CIT SPECT described higher heterogeneity in women in both the left and right striatum, but no significant differences in average levels between males and females.

Further studies failed to find significant sex differences in overall striatal DAT availability using ^{123}I-β-CIT-SPECT (Best et al., 2005; Ryding et al., 2004; van Dyck et al., 1995). Moreover, in a small sample of 10 women, no significant ^{123}I-β-CIT-SPECT differences were disclosed between the follicular and the luteal phases of the menstrual cycle (Best et al., 2005). However, other studies showed significant sex differences in basal ganglia DAT SBR using ^{123}I-FP-CIT SPECT or ^{99m}Tc-TRODAT-1 SPECT. In detail, women showed from 2.8% to 16.3% higher striatal DAT binding compared with men (Chen et al., 2013; Eusebio et al., 2012; Lavalaye et al., 2000; Mozley et al., 2001; Staley et al., 2001). One possible explanation of such conflicting results is that these studies were all based on ROI analysis, which could have led to an underestimation of a "sex effect." Indeed, MRI studies have shown that basal ganglia in women have a smaller volume than in men (Gunning-Dixon et al., 1998), thus, possibly leading to an relative increase of DAT density in women compared with men. Therefore, Eusebio et al. (2012) conducted a whole-brain, voxel-based analysis of ^{123}I-FP-CIT-SPECT images (thus without predefined ROI) of 51 healthy subjects, and showed a significantly higher tracer SBR in bilateral caudate, putamen, and opercular cortices in women compared with men. This was the first investigation that also focused on the extra-striatal regions and was followed by another study that again described a higher mean ^{123}I-FP-CIT SBR in the thalamus of healthy women compared with men. Furthermore, mean tracer SBR in the pons were slightly higher in men than in women, but this difference did not reach statistical significance (Koch et al., 2014). However, it should be noted that the ^{123}I-FP-CIT is not selective for DAT, but it has an affinity to the serotonin transporter (Arnaldi et al., 2015), thus the extra-striatal regions uptake likely reflects the serotonergic system activity rather than the dopaminergic one in specific regions.

In 2013, a study promoted by the European Association of Nuclear Medicine investigated SBR in the basal ganglia using the software BasGan v2 in 122 healthy controls (67 men) from 13 centers across Europe (ENC-DAT). The mean striatal SBR value was higher in women than in men. Moreover, this difference seems to be more evident for those of younger age (Nobili et al., 2013; Fig. 4). Based on the data of this study, the following formulas can be used to estimate SBR in a single subject, as functions of age and sex:

$$\text{Caudate SBR (Men)} = 6.800 - 0.273 * \text{age} \pm 1.88$$
$$\text{Putamen SBR (Men)} = 6.702 - 0.339 * \text{age} \pm 1.77$$
$$\text{Caudate SBR (Women)} = 7.232 - 0.273 * \text{age} \pm 1.88$$
$$\text{Putamen SBR (Women)} = 7.116 - 0.339 * \text{age} \pm 1.77$$

The result of the ENC-DAT study has been confirmed in the Japanese population, which is known to have a higher prevalence of a significant polymorphism involving a variable number of tandem repeats in the 3′ untranslated region of SLC6A3 gene coding for the DAT. These carriers have a reduced expression of DAT mRNA and protein. Specifically, in a study conducted in 30 healthy controls, the average SBR in males was lower compared with females in each decade (Yamamoto et al., 2017). The importance of a "sex and age correction" in the evaluation of DAT diagnostic exams was also underlined by Nichols et al. (2018) in 132 patients. In the study, DAT-SPECT data, when adjusted by sex and age, could better distinguish patients with PD and DLB from those with essential tremor compared with unadjusted data.

^{18}F-Fluoro-DOPA PET imaging is not a marker of DAT availability, but it is able to investigate presynaptic dopaminergic function by studying the amino acid decarboxylase activity. Studies with ^{18}F-Fluoro-DOPA PET confirmed the results of DAT SPECT studies, by showing that women had significantly higher striatal ^{18}F-Fluoro-DOPA uptake (Ki values) than men, with a more marked difference at caudate level (Laakso et al., 2002).

Overall, despite some conflicting results, it seems that there is a significant effect of sex on brain DAT availability, with women having higher striatal DAT levels compared with men. However, the physiological basis of this finding remains unknown. As this difference usually mitigates in postmenopausal decades, an effect of estrogen levels on DAT production/availability might be suggested, as demonstrated in animal models, but this hypothesis requires confirmation.

DAT SPECT sex differences in dementia

The role of sex in the nigrostriatal dopaminergic system in dementia patients remains poorly understood, and the few studies that investigated sex differences in DAT SPECT in neurodegenerative disorders mainly focus on Parkinson's disease (PD).

In PD patients a 16% higher ^{123}I-FP-CIT SBR was found in women compared with men at motor symptoms onset, without any differences between the rate of decline of the tracer binding over time (Haaxma et al., 2007). Such difference in striatal DAT SBR seems physiological rather than specifically PD-related and also could explain the known delay of PD motor symptoms onset in women compared to men (Twelves, Perkins, & Counsell, 2003). This is consistent with another ^{123}I-FP-CIT SPECT study in a large PD cohort, which showed no significant sex-diagnosis interaction, thus confirming that the sex difference is not strictly related to PD (Kaasinen et al., 2015).

Table 2 summarizes the main papers and results of presynaptic dopaminergic imaging dealing with sex differences.

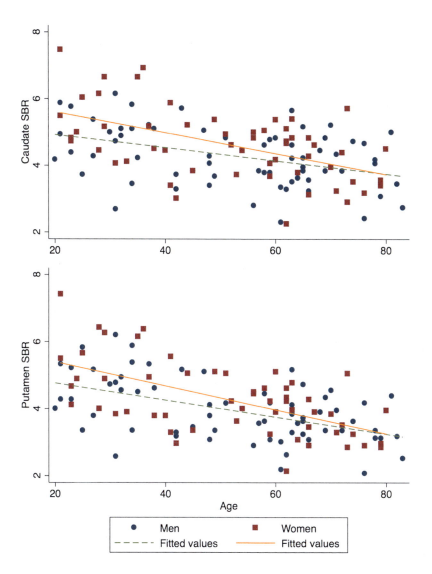

FIG. 4

Bilateral average of Caudate and Putamen SBR in men and women, as a function of age. *Blue circles* represent men and *red squares* represent women. *Green dotted lines* represent fitted values for men and *orange solid lines* represent fitted values for women.

Data from ENC-DAT study Nobili, F., et al. (2013). Automatic semi-quantification of [123I]FP-CIT SPECT scans in healthy volunteers using BasGan version 2: Results from the ENC-DAT database. European Journal of Nuclear Medicine and Molecular Imaging, 40(4), 565–573. doi: 10.1007/s00259-012-2304-8.

Table 2 PET and SPECT studies in healthy subjects reporting sex effect on striatal DAT binding.

Difference	n	Tracer	Notes	No-difference	n	Tracer	Notes
Lavalaye et al. (2000)	45	[123I]FP-CIT		Van Dyck et al. (1995)	28	[123I]β-CIT	
Mozley et al. (2001)	66	[99mTc]TRODAT-1		Kuikka et al. (1997)	39	[123I]β-CIT	Higher heterogeneity in women
Staley et al. (2001)	42	[123I]β-CIT		Ryding et al. (2004)	23	[123I]β-CIT	
Laakso et al. (2002)	35	[18F]FDOPA	Population of premenopausal women	Weng et al. (2004)	40	[99mTc]TRODAT-1	No differences also in 78 PD
Wong, Müller, Kuwabara, Studenski, and Bohnen (2012)	85	[123I]β-CIT	Differences only before 60 years	Best et al. (2005)	122	[123I]β-CIT	
Eusebio et al. (2012)	51	[123I]FP-CIT		van Dyck et al. (2005)	96	[123I]β-CIT	But decline age-related only in women
Nobili et al. (2013)	122	[123I]FP-CIT		Jakobson Mo et al. (2013)	51	[123I]FP-CIT	
Chen et al. (2013)	112	[99mTc]TRODAT-1					
Koch et al. (2014)	103	[123I]FP-CIT	Extra-striatal regions				
Kaasinen et al. (2015)	230	[123I]FP-CIT	Confirmed on 231 PD				
Yamamoto et al. (2017)	30	[123I]FP-CIT	Japanese population				

FDG-PET

Several FDG-PET studies have focused on the effect of sex on brain metabolism to highlight possible metabolic differences and corresponding behavioral discrepancies between men and women. The higher brain volume reported in men, together with the greater percentage of white matter (Cosgrove et al., 2007), or the higher resting rCBF values observed in women (Ragland et al., 2000), may theoretically induce inter-sex differences in FDG distribution. Furthermore, hormones such as estrogen are another potential source of variation in the cerebral metabolism of females (Reiman et al., 1996).

FDG-PET sex differences in healthy subjects

The impact of sex on brain FDG uptake and its distribution in healthy subjects is highly controversial. Some studies reported no differences in global and regional resting cerebral FDG uptake between males and females in the healthy human brain metabolism (Kim, Kim, & Kim, 2009; Miura et al., 1990). However, they also found that the equivalence in brain FDG consumption between sexes was partially contradicted by the analysis of specific age-related metabolic changes. Indeed, higher degrees of insula hypometabolism was observed in aged men, while a sex-specific, age-related hypometabolism involving the caudate nucleus was reported in females. Therefore, the authors indicated the occurrence of sex-specific cerebral metabolic changes associated with aging documented by FDG uptake distribution.

On the other hand, several studies have highlighted the occurrence of sex-specific differences in normal brain FDG distribution in resting conditions regardless of aging. In a pivotal study conducted on a cohort of young adults (mean age of 28 years), men showed higher glucose metabolism in temporal-limbic regions and the cerebellum compared to women (Gur et al., 1995). Some years later, Yoshizawa et al. (2014) analyzed 123 FDG-PET scans from healthy adults by means of a statistical parametric mapping (SPM) approach, showing that the overall cerebral glucose metabolism in females was higher than in males. At regional level, glucose metabolism in the medial frontal lobe, inferior parietal lobule, and posterior cingulate was higher in females, while males had a relatively higher tracer uptake in the cerebellum and in the bilateral inferior temporal lobes. As observed by the authors, this difference in tracer uptake was consistent with sexual differentiation in the neuropsychological profile of enrolled patients. Indeed, females outperformed males on verbal learning tests, while males performed better on visuospatial memory tests. These data are also consistent with older neuropsychological studies showing that healthy females are superior to males in language and verbal learning tasks, while males outperform in spatial and motor assignments (Maccoby & Jacklin, 1974). The results of Yoshizawa and colleagues were only partially confirmed by Hu et al. (2013), who also observed higher levels of brain metabolism restricted to the posterior cortex (including posterior-parietal lobes, occipital lobes, bilateral thalami, and hypothalamus) in females compared to males. The authors also noted significant sex differences within and between brain glucose metabolic networks. Finally, the existence of a regional heterogeneity in brain glucose consumption was confirmed in a large cohort of 963 healthy subjects (Kakimoto et al., 2016). In particular, the study demonstrated sex-specific hypometabolism in the parietal cortex in males and in the ventrolateral frontal cortex in females. As observed by the authors, this sex-related divergence seems to match the well-known popular saying: "men don't listen, and women can't read maps." Interestingly, these differences decline with advancing age, thus restricting the inter-sex differences to young adulthood.

Several factors might account for these conflicting results: on the one hand, the difficulty in recruiting a homogenous sample of patients by age, education, and neuropsychological profile; on the other hand, the technical inconsistencies across studies in terms of image analysis and correction (or no correction) procedures, or the difference in brain size and skull thickness between gender groups. These issues might be confounding factors, ultimately affecting the validity of the results (Miura et al., 1990). Finally, some of the inconsistencies might result from neglecting the possible interaction between different covariates, e.g., the sex-by-APOE interaction. Indeed, while several studies have included sex as a covariate in the analyses, they often did not explicitly test either the presence of APOE genotype in recruited patients or the occurrence of a specific APOE-sex interaction. The finding that the APOE effect on AD risk is stronger in women than in men was extensively reported (Farrer et al., 1997; Payami et al., 1996; Poirier et al., 1993). However, only a few studies have assessed the APOE-by-sex interaction on AD biomarkers. For instance, Sampedro et al. (2015) enrolled a cohort of healthy subjects from the ADNI database with available CSF and/or 3T-MRI and/or FDG-PET. As expected, APOE ε4 carriers had lower CSF Aβ1–42 and higher CSF p-tau181p values than noncarriers, but the APOE-by-sex interaction was significant only for brain metabolism. Sex stratification showed that female APOE ε4 carriers presented widespread brain hypometabolism (and cortical thinning) compared to female noncarriers, whereas, male APOE ε4 carriers showed only a small cluster of hypometabolism and regions of cortical thinning compared to male noncarriers (Fig. 5). In other words, women were metabolically more susceptible to the APOE ε4 genotype. Altogether, these findings suggest that sex can markedly modify the interplay between APOE ε4 genotype and brain metabolism.

FDG-PET sex differences in dementia

If conflicting data are available in the healthy control group, the relationship between sex and brain metabolism is even more complicated in neurodegenerative diseases. Indeed, different protective effects on the brain between males and females might occur, further complicating the interconnection between sex and brain metabolism in pathological conditions. A few available studies have assessed this issue, mainly focusing on the cognitive reserve. Perneczky et al. (2007) suggested a different protective effect of education between men and women. Malpetti et al. (2017) investigated gender differences in brain metabolic activity and resting-state network connectivity

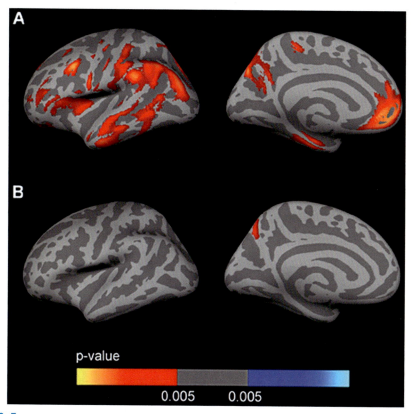

FIG. 5

Sex-stratified FDG analyses in APOE4 carriers and APOE4 noncarriers. Comparison between apolipoprotein E ε4 allele (APOE4) carriers and APOE4 noncarriers ($P<.005$ uncorrected) in females (Panel A) and males (Panel B), co-varied for age and years of education across the lateral and medial views of the cerebral cortex. As shown, women were metabolically more susceptible to APOE4 genotype.

Reproduced from Sampedro, F., et al. (2015). APOE-by-sex interactions on brain structure and metabolism in healthy elderly controls. Oncotarget 6(29), 26663–26674. doi:10.18632/oncotarget.5185.

measured by FDG-PET by also considering the effects of education and occupation in a large dataset of healthy controls and AD patients. Of note, in AD patients the impact of education and occupation on brain metabolism was different according to sex. The correlation between reserve proxies and brain metabolism was observed in the posterior temporoparietal cortex in males and the frontal and limbic cortex in females. Similarly, metabolic connectivity showed greater efficiency in the posterior DMN in males, and in the anterior frontal executive network in females. Based on these data, the authors hypothesized that sex differences in the correlation of education and occupation with brain metabolism in AD might reflect a difference strategy in coping with neurodegeneration, which recruits frontal executive neural resources in females. To interpret this divergence between sexes, it is crucial to take into account the socioeconomic factors that characterized the past century, where women had fewer opportunities for higher education and occupational attainment and, instead, were more engaged in familial and social activities. These historical aspects with socially determined gender roles, behaviors, businesses, and attributes are somehow mirrored in the AD samples of these studies. The sex differences might, therefore, be explained by gender-related aspects, including different levels and types of education and occupation and by other sociodemographic factors that might contribute to cognitive strategies and, consequentially, to brain function and networks.

Amyloid PET

Sex differences in Aβ burden findings are controversial, and too few imaging studies are available to allow a comprehensive overview of the relationship between sex and amyloid load (Ferretti et al., 2018). Sex-related differences are often found in literature as marginal analyses and only a few studies using in vivo PET analyses in AD subjects have focused on the sex-dependent relationship with amyloid burden as a specific factor.

Amyloid PET sex differences in healthy subjects

The similar prevalence of amyloid positivity in male and female normal elderly individuals is a converging piece of evidence from most of the studies (Jack et al., 2015, 2017). Minimal, if any, sex differences have been found in cross-sectional study of the global Aβ burden in clinically normal older adults (Altmann et al., 2014; Buckley et al., 2018; Mielke et al., 2012; Mosconi, Berti, Quinn, et al., 2017). Other results are controversial; for instance, the slightly higher uptake of PiB found in men compared to women in the temporal and occipital lobes by Scheinin et al. (2014) was not confirmed by other reports, which have indicated higher PiB uptake in women than men (Mosconi et al., 2018; Rahman et al., 2020; Vemuri et al., 2017).

Amyloid PET sex differences in dementia

A metaanalysis of PET studies revealed no sex differences in amyloid positivity among individuals with subjective cognitive impairment, aMCI, or nonamnestic MCI (Jansen et al., 2015). A similar metaanalysis focused on patients with AD is currently lacking. However, postmortem studies of AD subjects suggest that there is no sex difference in the occurrence or distribution of Aβ plaques (Barnes et al., 2005). Similarly, sex seems to have no impact on CSF Aβ value in patients with AD dementia and prodromal AD or in cognitively normal individuals (Holland et al., 2013; Mattsson et al., 2017). Some authors suggested that sex differences are more likely to follow the onset of Aβ accumulation (Hohman et al., 2018; Vest & Pike,

2013). This hypothesis has found some traction in a study comparing age, sex, and APOE ε4 effects on memory, brain structure, and amyloid PET (PiB) in cognitively normal individuals aged 30 to 95 years old (Jack et al., 2015).

One of the few studies directly tackling the sex differences in AD using in vivo imaging biomarkers found a significantly higher load of brain amyloid in the anterior cingulate cortex in men than in women (Cavedo et al., 2018). In this study, despite equal levels of global cognition and after controlling for age, education, and clinical comorbidities, men showed higher amyloid load and neurodegeneration and lower FC in the DMN compared with women. These findings suggest that men may have higher brain resilience to the pathophysiological AD processes. On the same line, Pike et al. (2011) observed that women have more evident cognitive impairment than men even with a smaller amyloid burden, suggesting that they might be more susceptible to AD pathology. This also implies that factors other than the brain amyloid load could contribute to clinical outcome at the individual level, such as the menopausal stage (Mosconi et al., 2018; Mosconi, Berti, Quinn, et al., 2017; Rahman et al., 2020), and family history (Villeneuve et al., 2018). Conversely, in one of the few studies focused on the relative contribution and interaction of several factors in the accumulation of cortical amyloid, the effect of sex was marginally significant ($P=.03$) since women showed higher standardized uptake value ratios (SUVRs) than men (Murphy et al., 2013). On the same line, other findings suggested that, although the sex differences in amyloid PET were not significant, elderly women with AD tended towards a greater β-amyloid load (Buckley et al., 2019; Jack et al., 2015; Oveisgharan et al., 2018).

Despite the lack of clear significant sex differences in PET at any age—both for amyloid-negative and amyloid-positive subjects—one study found a trend for a sex × amyloid burden interaction ($P=.062$) with episodic memory, and a significant sex × amyloid burden interaction with visuospatial functions (Pike et al., 2011). Interestingly, no association was evident between sex and APOE genotype, as confirmed by different studies (Cavedo et al., 2018; Jack et al., 2015; Jansen et al., 2015). Another study observed amyloid-moderated sex differences in tau signal was largely restricted to the temporal lobe, suggesting AD-specific female vulnerability to temporal lobe tauopathy in the presence of β-amyloid (Buckley et al., 2020) (for a discussion on sex and gender-differences in CSF measures of amyloid pathology, see Chapter 4).

Conclusion

Strong evidence of sex difference in concentrations of Aβ is still lacking, and this might be due to a low number of studies specifically investigating this topic. Indeed, in most studies about biomarkers the results are adjusted for age and sex, thereby hindering examination of sex differences. Moreover, methodological issues, namely differences in study design, sample size, and the age of recruited subjects, might account for the discrepancies between studies. Even if controversial, overall, such results might suggest that sex does not mediate the effect of amyloid on the volumetric, metabolic, and functional imaging markers of AD, and thus that the effect of sex seems independent from the amyloid status.

Emerging PET modalities

The ductility of PET technology allows investigation in vivo not only of neurodegeneration, but also of brain chemistry, neuroinflammation, and protein deposition. Hence, in recent years efforts have been dedicated to developing specific tracers able to assess the deposition of pathological proteins other than amyloid (Cosgrove et al., 2007; Schain & Kreisl, 2017).

Tau PET sex differences in healthy subjects and dementia

Specific tracers to track tau pathology, such as THK5317, THK5351, AV-1451, and PBB3, have been used in the research setting, both in healthy subjects and in patients with different tauopathies, including AD (Saint-Aubert et al., 2017). Pathological tau is a hallmark of several neurodegenerative diseases. However, various tau isoforms are observed in different neurodegenerative diseases (Spillantini & Goedert, 1998). Normal tau promotes the stability of microtubules in the nervous system, but its pathological hyperphosphorylation leads to the formation of neurofibrillary tangles, which are among the earliest pathophysiological changes in AD, spreading from the entorhinal cortex and hippocampus to the neocortex during the course of the disease (Ziontz et al., 2019). Mounting evidence suggests that women are at higher risk of exhibiting AD pathophysiology, mostly due to differences in the production and the structure of neurofibrillary tangles between sexes (Buckley et al., 2019; Cáceres & González, 2020; Hohman et al., 2018). However, the sex-specific risk of the clinical progression in early AD remains to be fully elucidated.

Sex differences in Aβ deposition alone have not been reported in older adults, supporting the notion that sex differences are more likely to appear downstream, after the onset of Aβ accumulation. Hence, it is meaningful to investigate the influence of gender on the interplay between amyloid and tau deposition in vivo. Elevated CSF tau levels have been reported in women compared with men as a function of APOE ϵ4 status and Aβ, and recently, the availability of TAU PET tracers has allowed us to deepen this finding in terms of quantity, timing, and regional deposition of tau with respect to amyloid (Buckley et al., 2019; see also Chapter 4). In the Mayo Clinic Study of Aging, Jack et al. (2017) aimed to evaluate the clinical characteristics and prevalence of each ATN (i.e., amyloidosis/tauopathy/neurodegeneration) profile in cognitively unimpaired individuals. Participants were thus classified according to normal (A−) or abnormal (A+) amyloid by means of amyloid PET, normal (T−), or abnormal (T+) tau using tau PET, and normal (N−), or abnormal (N+) neurodegeneration, or neuronal injury according to cortical thickness by MR imaging. In both men and women, A−T−N− was the most prevalent until age late 70s, but the prevalence of A+T+N+ and A−T+N+ progressively increased from the age of 50 years and was the most prevalent after 80 years. Of note, by the age of 85 years, more than 90% of men and women had at least one abnormal biomarker. As for the sex differences, only a slight prevalence of A−T−N+ was found in men from age 65 to 75 years. Hence, the prevalence of each ATN group and biomarker abnormality is mostly influenced by age even in individuals who remain cognitively unimpaired over time (Jack et al., 2017).

Similarly, a study with 18F-AV-1451 TAU PET assessed the association between the patterns of brain tau accumulation and other well-established AD factors in a cohort composed of both healthy elderly subjects and early AD patients (Tosun et al., 2017). Highly associated patterns of greater 18F-AV-1451 binding and increased annualized change in cortical amyloid β plaques measured with PET were also explored. In the study, TAU PET tracer retention was associated with age and cross-sectional amyloid PET tracer retention, but not with education, sex, or APOE genotype. However, in the analysis uncorrected for confounding effects, females disclosed greater 18F-AV-1451 binding in diffuse cortical regions, namely lateral temporal, parietal, and frontal regions. Conversely, in 54 cognitively normal subjects, higher 18F-AV-1451 retention, and thus tau pathology, was related to older age, male sex, black race, and amyloid positivity, especially in the frontal and parietal white matter and thalamus (Ziontz et al., 2019).

Finally, the study by Buckley et al. (2019) assessed the association between sex and regional Aβ and tau deposition as measured with 11C-PIB and 18F-AV-1451 PET, respectively, in a large dataset of clinically normal individuals (193 belonging to the Harvard Aging Brain Study and 103 from the ADNI database). In both cohorts, no clear association of sex with regional tau was found, but among those individuals with higher Aβ burden, the females disclosed higher entorhinal cortical tau than the males. In other words, clinically normal older women with higher levels of global Aβ exhibit higher levels of tau burden than men, specifically involving the entorhinal cortex. More recently, the same group examined sex differences in tau-PET signal across the brain, both as a main effect and interaction with global Aβ and APOEε4 carriage in a cohort of 343 clinically normal individuals and 55 MCI individuals (Buckley et al., 2020). The authors observed that women showed higher SUVRs than men, not only in the temporal but also in many extratemporal regions, such as the parietal, middle frontal, lateral occipital, fusiform, supramarginal, cuneus, banks of the superior temporal sulcus, and frontal/temporal pole regions. Of note, many of these regions remained significantly different between the sexes even after adjusting for Aβ status. Higher tau-PET signals in these regions translated to accelerated cognitive decline in women as compared to men.

Taken together, these findings support a biological substrate underpinning sex-related differences in tau deposition in AD, but further studies in large samples are needed.

Neurotransmission PET sex differences in healthy subjects and dementia

The ductility of PET technology and the development of tracers targeting different neurotransmission pathways has allowed us to investigate sex-specific differences in dopaminergic, serotonergic, and GABAergic systems in healthy subjects (Cosgrove et al., 2007). Even though sex differences in AD patients have been poorly investigated, some authors have focused on the serotoninergic system, as serotonin (5-HT) is involved in cognition and plays an important role in AD. In particular the study by Parsey et al. (2002) aimed to determine the effects of age, sex, and severity of lifetime aggressive behavior on 5-HT(1A) receptor binding potential in vivo by means of PET with [carbonyl-C-11]WAY-100635, which is a high affinity 5-HT(1A) antagonist. Significantly higher binding potential was evident in females compared with males in the dorsal raphe, amygdala, anterior cingulate, cingulate body, and medial and orbital prefrontal cortex. This is consistent with previous pharmacological studies, in which lower 5-HT(1A) binding was found in males and in more aggressive individuals. As 5-HT receptors, namely 5-HT(2A), were found to play a role in AD, such evidence might have implications for both the etiological basis and therapeutic management of AD patients. For instance, gender-oriented studies in AD patients might suggest the opportunity to selectively manipulate the hormonal system to influence the clinical and neurocognitive course of symptoms related to the serotoninergic system (Versijpt et al., 2003).

Neuroinflammation PET sex differences in healthy subjects and dementia

In the last 20 years, PET imaging has also focused on different targets to investigate in vivo neuroinflammation (Schain & Kreisl, 2017). In particular, most radioligands are specific for the 18 kDa TSPO, which is considered a useful marker of neuroinflammation as is it highly expressed in activated microglia and reactive astrocytes in the events of brain injury and inflammation. However, it remains unknown whether age and sex have an effect on neuroinflammation, mostly due to the small sample size of the few studies and the high technical challenges associated with production and analysis of PET TSPO radioligands.

In a study on 48 healthy subjects by means of TSPO-specific ^{11}C-PBR28 PET, the total tracer distribution volume was found to increase significantly with age in nearly all regions but it was not affected by sex or body mass index (Paul et al., 2019). In a larger database of 140 healthy subjects studied with the same PET tracer, a significant sex difference was revealed in all brain regions, as females showed a higher volume of distribution of the tracer. Moreover, a subgroup analysis revealed a positive correlation between volume distribution and age in all regions in male subjects, whereas age had no effect on TSPO levels in female subjects (Tuisku et al., 2019). Accordingly, although gender-related data obtained with tracers for neuroinflammation in AD patients are still not available, available studies suggest that age and sex can be confounding factors and should be taken into account in future studies (sex differences in the immune system and microglial function are described in Chapter 3).

Conclusion

Investigations concerning sex disparities are pivotal to understanding the different vulnerability and the trajectories of normal or pathological brain aging in men and women, and neuroimaging techniques play an important role in evaluating in vivo those sex-related differences in brain structure and function. A physiological asymmetry of brain volumes and microstructural architecture throughout the lifespan between sexes, but also differences in the patterns and rate of atrophy progression, have been described. Indeed, a higher susceptibility to AD pathology seems to be present in women, mostly due to divergences in the production and the structure of neurofibrillary tangles, as has emerged from tau-specific PET studies. On the other hand, conflicting results have emerged from functional studies in which a complex interaction between sex and neural correlates of brain processes, regional blood flow, and metabolism seem to be underpinned by factors such as hormonal balance, education, and genetics. However, the weight of methodological differences and technical issues is still not negligible. Indeed, differences in the choice of cohorts, study design, equipment, tracers, data analysis, considered region of interest, brain segmentation, and partial volume correction might explain most of the conflicting results.

In conclusion, there is an urgent need for a more systematic appraisal of sex differences in neuroimaging studies. To set up normal databases for image analysis and to interpret the pathological findings according to the sex differences, rather than considering sex as nuisance factor in biomarker studies, might be of paramount importance in clinical practice and in pharmacological trial design.

Chapter highlights

- Conflicting evidence of sex-related differences in brain structure and functioning have been presented, both in normal and pathological brain aging from neuroimaging studies.
- Methodological and technical issues, as well as differences in biology and environment are crucial factors to be considered.
- A more systematic approach to sex differences in neuroimaging studies may have a substantial impact on clinical practice and in drug trial design.

References

Agcaoglu, O., et al. (2015). Lateralization of resting state networks and relationship to age and gender. *NeuroImage, 104*, 310–325. https://doi.org/10.1016/j.neuroimage.2014.09.001.

Altmann, A., et al. (2014). Sex modifies the APOE-related risk of developing Alzheimer disease. *Annals of Neurology, 75*(4), 563–573. https://doi.org/10.1002/ana.24135.

Amen, D. G., et al. (2017). Gender-based cerebral perfusion differences in 46,034 functional neuroimaging scans. *Journal of Alzheimer's Disease, 60*(2), 605–614. https://doi.org/10.3233/JAD-170432.

Apostolova, L. G., et al. (2006). 3D comparison of hippocampal atrophy in amnestic mild cognitive impairment and Alzheimer's disease. *Brain, 129*(Pt 11), 2867–2873. https://doi.org/10.1093/brain/awl274.

Ardekani, B. A., et al. (2019). Sexual dimorphism and hemispheric asymmetry of hippocampal volumetric integrity in normal aging and Alzheimer disease. *American Journal of Neuroradiology*, *40*(2), 276–282. https://doi.org/10.3174/ajnr.A5943.

Arnaldi, D., et al. (2015). The role of the serotonergic system in REM sleep behavior disorder. *Sleep*, *38*(9), 1505–1509. https://doi.org/10.5665/sleep.5000.

Asllani, I., et al. (2009). Separating function from structure in perfusion imaging of the aging brain. *Human Brain Mapping*, *30*(9), 2927–2935. https://doi.org/10.1002/hbm.20719.

Bai, F., et al. (2009). Abnormal functional connectivity of Hippocampus during episodic memory retrieval processing network in amnestic mild cognitive impairment. *Biological Psychiatry*, *65*(11), 951–958. https://doi.org/10.1016/j.biopsych.2008.10.017.

Barnes, L. L., et al. (2005). Sex differences in the clinical manifestations of Alzheimer disease pathology. *Archives of General Psychiatry*, *62*(6), 685–691. https://doi.org/10.1001/archpsyc.62.6.685.

Bartzokis, G., et al. (2010). Lifespan trajectory of myelin integrity and maximum motor speed. *Neurobiology of Aging*, *31*(9), 1554–1562. https://doi.org/10.1016/j.neurobiolaging.2008.08.015.

Best, S. E., et al. (2005). Striatal dopamine transporter availability with [123I]β-CIT SPECT is unrelated to gender or menstrual cycle. *Psychopharmacology*, *183*(2), 181–189. https://doi.org/10.1007/s00213-005-0158-5.

Bilgic, B., et al. (2012). MRI estimates of brain iron concentration in normal aging using quantitative susceptibility mapping. *NeuroImage*, *59*(3), 2625–2635. https://doi.org/10.1016/j.neuroimage.2011.08.077.

Buckley, R. F., et al. (2018). Sex, amyloid, and APOE ε4 and risk of cognitive decline in preclinical Alzheimer's disease: Findings from three well-characterized cohorts. *Alzheimer's & Dementia*, *14*(9), 1193–1203. https://doi.org/10.1016/j.jalz.2018.04.010.

Buckley, R. F., et al. (2019). Sex differences in the association of global amyloid and regional tau deposition measured by positron emission tomography in clinically normal older adults. *JAMA Neurology*, *76*(5), 542–551. https://doi.org/10.1001/jamaneurol.2018.4693.

Buckley, R. F., et al. (2020). Sex mediates relationships between regional tau pathology and cognitive decline. *Annals of Neurology*, *88*(5), 921–932. https://doi.org/10.1002/ana.25878.

Cáceres, A., & González, J. R. (2020). Female-specific risk of Alzheimer's disease is associated with tau phosphorylation processes: A transcriptome-wide interaction analysis. *Neurobiology of Aging*, *96*, 104–108. https://doi.org/10.1016/j.neurobiolaging.2020.08.020.

Caldwell, J. Z. K., Cummings, J. L., et al. (2019). Cognitively normal women with Alzheimer's disease proteinopathy show relative preservation of memory but not of hippocampal volume. *Alzheimer's Research & Therapy*, *11*(1), 109. https://doi.org/10.1186/s13195-019-0565-1.

Caldwell, J. Z. K., Zhuang, X., et al. (2019). Sex moderates amyloid and apolipoprotein ε4 effects on default mode network connectivity at rest. *Frontiers in Neurology*, *10*(August), 900. https://doi.org/10.3389/fneur.2019.00900.

Callen, D. J. A., et al. (2004). The influence of sex on limbic volume and perfusion in AD. *Neurobiology of Aging*, *25*(6), 761–770. https://doi.org/10.1016/j.neurobiolaging.2003.08.011.

Cavedo, E., et al. (2018). Sex differences in functional and molecular neuroimaging biomarkers of Alzheimer's disease in cognitively normal older adults with subjective memory complaints. *Alzheimer's & Dementia*, 1204–1215. https://doi.org/10.1016/j.jalz.2018.05.014.

Chen, K. C., Yang, Y. K., Howes, O., Lee, I. H., Landau, S., Yeh, T. L., … Bramon, E. (2013). Striatal dopamine transporter availability in drug-naive patients with schizophrenia: A case-control SPECT study with [99mTc]-TRODAT-1 and a meta-analysis. *Schizophrenia Bulletin, 39*(2), 378–386. https://doi.org/10.1093/schbul/sbr163.

Cosgrove, K. P., Mazure, C. M., & Staley, J. K. (2007). Evolving knowledge of sex differences in brain structure, function, and chemistry. *Biological Psychiatry*, 847–855. https://doi.org/10.1016/j.biopsych.2007.03.001.

Damoiseaux, J. S., et al. (2012). Gender modulates the APOE ε4 effect in healthy older adults: Convergent evidence from functional brain connectivity and spinal fluid tau levels. *The Journal of Neuroscience, 32*(24), 8254–8262. https://doi.org/10.1523/JNEUROSCI.0305-12.2012.

Devous, M. D., et al. (1986). Normal distribution of regional cerebral blood flow measured by dynamic single-photon emission tomography. *Journal of Cerebral Blood Flow and Metabolism, 6*(1), 95–104. https://doi.org/10.1038/jcbfm.1986.12.

Dodge, H. H., et al. (2003). Functional transitions and active life expectancy associated with Alzheimer disease. *Archives of Neurology, 60*(2), 253–259. https://doi.org/10.1001/archneur.60.2.253.

Dong, J., et al. (2018). Hurst exponent analysis of resting-state fMRI signal complexity across the adult lifespan. *Frontiers in Neuroscience*, 34. Available at: https://www.frontiersin.org/article/10.3389/fnins.2018.00034.

Eusebio, A., et al. (2012). Voxel-based analysis of whole-brain effects of age and gender on dopamine transporter SPECT imaging in healthy subjects. *European Journal of Nuclear Medicine and Molecular Imaging, 39*(11), 1778–1783. https://doi.org/10.1007/s00259-012-2207-8.

Fan, Q., et al. (2019). Age-related alterations in axonal microstructure in the corpus callosum measured by high-gradient diffusion MRI. *NeuroImage, 191*, 325–336. https://doi.org/10.1016/j.neuroimage.2019.02.036.

Farrer, L. A., et al. (1997). Effects of age, sex, and ethnicity on the association between apolipoprotein E genotype and Alzheimer disease: A meta-analysis. *Journal of the American Medical Association*, 1349–1356. https://doi.org/10.1001/jama.1997.03550160069041.

Ferretti, M. T., et al. (2018). Sex differences in Alzheimer disease—The gateway to precision medicine. *Nature Reviews Neurology*, 457–469. https://doi.org/10.1038/s41582-018-0032-9.

Filon, J. R., et al. (2016). Gender differences in Alzheimer disease: Brain atrophy, histopathology burden, and cognition. *Journal of Neuropathology and Experimental Neurology, 75*(8), 748–754. https://doi.org/10.1093/jnen/nlw047.

Gao, S., et al. (1998). The relationships between age, sex, and the incidence of dementia and Alzheimer disease: A meta-analysis. *Archives of General Psychiatry, 55*(9), 809–815. https://doi.org/10.1001/archpsyc.55.9.809.

Goldstone, A., et al. (2016). Gender specific re-organization of resting-state networks in older age. *Frontiers in Aging Neuroscience, 8*(November). https://doi.org/10.3389/fnagi.2016.00285.

Gong, N. J., et al. (2015). Hemisphere, gender and age-related effects on iron deposition in deep gray matter revealed by quantitative susceptibility mapping. *NMR in Biomedicine, 28*(10), 1267–1274. https://doi.org/10.1002/nbm.3366.

Gunning-Dixon, F. M., et al. (1998). Differential aging of the human striatum: A prospective MR imaging study. *American Journal of Neuroradiology, 19*(8), 1501–1507.

Gur, R. C., et al. (1995). Sex differences in regional cerebral glucose metabolism during a resting state. *Science, 267*(5197), 528–531. https://doi.org/10.1126/science.7824953.

Haaxma, C. A., et al. (2007). Gender differences in Parkinson's disease. *Journal of Neurology, Neurosurgery and Psychiatry, 78*(8), 819–824. https://doi.org/10.1136/jnnp.2006.103788.

Hallgren, B., & Sourander, P. (1958). The effect of age on the non-haemin iron in the human brain. *Journal of Neurochemistry*, *3*(1), 41–51. https://doi.org/10.1111/j.1471-4159.1958.tb12607.x.

Hanyu, H., et al. (2004). Differences in regional cerebral blood flow patterns in male versus female patients with Alzheimer disease. *American Journal of Neuroradiology*, *25*(7), 1199–1204.

Heise, V., et al. (2014). Apolipoprotein E genotype, gender and age modulate connectivity of the hippocampus in healthy adults. *NeuroImage*, *98*, 23–30. https://doi.org/10.1016/j.neuroimage.2014.04.081.

Henriksen, O. M., et al. (2014). Relationship between cardiac function and resting cerebral blood flow: MRI measurements in healthy elderly subjects. *Clinical Physiology and Functional Imaging*, *34*(6), 471–477. https://doi.org/10.1111/cpf.12119.

Hesselmann, V., et al. (2001). Age related signal decrease in functional magnetic resonance imaging during motor stimulation in humans. *Neuroscience Letters*, *308*(3), 141–144. https://doi.org/10.1016/s0304-3940(01)01920-6.

Hohman, T. J., et al. (2018). Sex-specific association of apolipoprotein E with cerebrospinal fluid levels of tau. *JAMA Neurology*, *75*(8), 989–998. https://doi.org/10.1001/jamaneurol.2018.0821.

Holland, D., et al. (2013). Higher rates of decline for women and apolipoprotein e ε4 carriers. *American Journal of Neuroradiology*, *34*(12), 2287–2293. https://doi.org/10.3174/ajnr.A3601.

Hu, Y., et al. (2013). Gender differences of brain glucose metabolic networks revealed by FDG-PET: Evidence from a large cohort of 400 young adults. *PLoS One*, *8*(12), e83821. https://doi.org/10.1371/journal.pone.0083821.

Hua, X., et al. (2010). Sex and age differences in atrophic rates: An ADNI study with n=1368 MRI scans. *Neurobiology of Aging*, *31*(8), 1463–1480. https://doi.org/10.1016/j.neurobiolaging.2010.04.033.

Huang, J., et al. (2015). Identifying brain functional alterations in postmenopausal women with cognitive impairment. *Maturitas*, *81*(3), 371–376. https://doi.org/10.1016/j.maturitas.2015.04.006.

Jack, C. R., et al. (2015). Age, sex, and APOE ε4 effects on memory, brain structure, and β-amyloid across the adult life span. *JAMA Neurology*, *72*(5), 511–519. https://doi.org/10.1001/jamaneurol.2014.4821.

Jack, C. R., et al. (2017). Age-specific and sex-specific prevalence of cerebral β-amyloidosis, tauopathy, and neurodegeneration in cognitively unimpaired individuals aged 50–95 years: A cross-sectional study. *The Lancet. Neurology*, *16*(6), 435–444. https://doi.org/10.1016/S1474-4422(17)30077-7.

Jamadar, S. D., et al. (2018). Sexual dimorphism of resting-state network connectivity in healthy ageing. *The Journals of Gerontology: Series B*, *74*(7), 1121–1131. https://doi.org/10.1093/geronb/gby004.

Jansen, W. J., et al. (2015). Prevalence of cerebral amyloid pathology in persons without dementia: A meta-analysis. *JAMA*, *313*(19), 1924. https://doi.org/10.1001/JAMA.2015.4668.

Jones, K., et al. (1998). Use of singular value decomposition to characterize age and gender differences in SPECT cerebral perfusion. *Journal of Nuclear Medicine*, *39*(6), 965–973. Available at: http://www.ncbi.nlm.nih.gov/pubmed/9627327. (Accessed 21 February 2020).

Kaasinen, V., et al. (2015). Effects of aging and gender on striatal and extrastriatal [123I]FP-CIT binding in Parkinson's disease. *Neurobiology of Aging*, *36*(4), 1757–1763. https://doi.org/10.1016/j.neurobiolaging.2015.01.016.

Kakimoto, A., et al. (2016). Age-related sex-specific changes in brain metabolism and morphology. *Journal of Nuclear Medicine*, *57*(2), 221–225. https://doi.org/10.2967/jnumed.115.166439.

Kanaan, R. A., et al. (2012). Gender differences in white matter microstructure. *PLoS One*, *7*(6), e38272. https://doi.org/10.1371/journal.pone.0038272.

Kidron, D., et al. (1997). Quantitative MR volumetry in Alzheimer's disease: Topographic markers and the effects of sex and education. *Neurology*, *49*(6), 1504–1512. https://doi.org/10.1212/WNL.49.6.1504.

Kim, I. J., Kim, S. J., & Kim, Y. K. (2009). Age- and sex-associated changes in cerebral glucose metabolism in normal healthy subjects: Statistical parametric mapping analysis of F-18 fluorodeoxyglucose brain positron emission tomography. *Acta Radiologica*, *50*(10), 1169–1174. https://doi.org/10.3109/02841850903258058.

Király, A., et al. (2016). Male brain ages faster: The age and gender dependence of subcortical volumes. *Brain Imaging and Behavior*, *10*(3), 901–910. https://doi.org/10.1007/s11682-015-9468-3.

Koch, W., et al. (2014). Extrastriatal binding of [123I]FP-CIT in the thalamus and pons: Gender and age dependencies assessed in a European multicentre database of healthy controls. *European Journal of Nuclear Medicine and Molecular Imaging*, *41*(10), 1938–1946. https://doi.org/10.1007/s00259-014-2785-8.

Krejza, J., et al. (2001). Effect of endogenous estrogen on blood flow through carotid arteries. *Stroke*, *32*(1), 30–36. https://doi.org/10.1161/01.str.32.1.30.

Kuikka, J. T., et al. (1997). Fractal analysis of striatal dopamine re-uptake sites. *European Journal of Nuclear Medicine*, *24*(9), 1085–1090. https://doi.org/10.1007/bf01254238.

Laakso, A., et al. (2002). Sex differences in striatal presynaptic dopamine synthesis capacity in healthy subjects. *Biological Psychiatry*, *52*(7), 759–763. https://doi.org/10.1016/S0006-3223(02)01369-0.

Lavalaye, J., et al. (2000). Effect of age and gender on dopamine transporter imaging with [123I]FP-CIT SPET in healthy volunteers. *European Journal of Nuclear Medicine*, *27*(7), 867–869. https://doi.org/10.1007/s002590000279.

Lee, J., et al. (2018). Sex-related reserve hypothesis in Alzheimer's disease: Changes in cortical thickness with a five-year longitudinal follow-up. *Journal of Alzheimer's Disease*, *65*(2), 641–649. https://doi.org/10.3233/JAD-180049.

Lehtovirta, M., et al. (1998). Longitudinal SPECT study in Alzheimer's disease: Relation to apolipoprotein E polymorphism. *Journal of Neurology, Neurosurgery, and Psychiatry*, *64*(6), 742–746. https://doi.org/10.1136/jnnp.64.6.742.

Li, Z.-J., et al. (2004). Gender difference in brain perfusion 99mTc-ECD SPECT in aged healthy volunteers after correction for partial volume effects. *Nuclear Medicine Communications*, *25*(10), 999–1005. https://doi.org/10.1097/00006231-200410000-00003.

Liu, W., Lou, X., & Ma, L. (2016). Use of 3D pseudo-continuous arterial spin labeling to characterize sex and age differences in cerebral blood flow. *Neuroradiology*, *58*(9), 943–948. https://doi.org/10.1007/s00234-016-1713-y.

Lv, H., et al. (2018). Resting-state functional MRI: Everything that nonexperts have always wanted to know. *American Journal of Neuroradiology*, 1390–1399. https://doi.org/10.3174/ajnr.A5527.

Maccoby, E. E., & Jacklin, C. N. (1974). *The psychology of sex differences*. Stanford University Press.

Malpetti, M., et al. (2017). Gender differences in healthy aging and Alzheimer's dementia: A 18F-FDG-PET study of brain and cognitive reserve. *Human Brain Mapping*, *38*(8), 4212–4227. https://doi.org/10.1002/hbm.23659.

Mattsson, N., et al. (2017). Clinical validity of cerebrospinal fluid Aβ42, tau, and phospho-tau as biomarkers for Alzheimer's disease in the context of a structured 5-phase development framework. *Neurobiology of Aging*, 196–213. https://doi.org/10.1016/j.neurobiolaging.2016.02.034.

McKeith, I. G., et al. (2017). Diagnosis and management of dementia with Lewy bodies. *Neurology*, *89*(1), 88–100. https://doi.org/10.1212/WNL.0000000000004058.

Mielke, M. M., et al. (2012). Indicators of amyloid burden in a population-based study of cognitively normal elderly. *Neurology*, *79*(15), 1570–1577. https://doi.org/10.1212/WNL.0b013e31826e2696.

Miura, S. A., et al. (1990). Effect of gender on glucose utilization rates in healthy humans: A positron emission tomography study. *Journal of Neuroscience Research*, *27*(4), 500–504. https://doi.org/10.1002/jnr.490270410.

Morbelli, S., et al. (2015). Visual versus semi-quantitative analysis of 18F-FDG-PET in amnestic MCI: An European Alzheimer's Disease Consortium (EADC) project. *Journal of Alzheimer's Disease*, *44*(3), 815–826. https://doi.org/10.3233/JAD-142229.

Morissette, M., Biron, D., & Di Paolo, T. (1990). Effect of estradiol and progesterone on rat striatal dopamine uptake sites. *Brain Research Bulletin*, *25*(3), 419–422. https://doi.org/10.1016/0361-9230(90)90231-N.

Mosconi, L., Berti, V., Guyara-Quinn, C., et al. (2017). Perimenopause and emergence of an Alzheimer's bioenergetic phenotype in brain and periphery. *PLoS One*, *12*(10), e0185926. https://doi.org/10.1371/journal.pone.0185926.

Mosconi, L., Berti, V., Quinn, C., et al. (2017). Sex differences in Alzheimer risk. *Neurology*, *89*(13), 1382–1390. https://doi.org/10.1212/WNL.0000000000004425.

Mosconi, L., et al. (2018). Increased Alzheimer's risk during the menopause transition: A 3-year longitudinal brain imaging study. *PLoS One*, *13*(12), e0207885. https://doi.org/10.1371/journal.pone.0207885.

Mozley, L. H., et al. (2001). Striatal dopamine transporters and cognitive functioning in healthy men and women. *American Journal of Psychiatry*, *158*(9), 1492–1499. https://doi.org/10.1176/appi.ajp.158.9.1492.

Murphy, K. R., et al. (2013). Mapping the effects of ApoE4, age and cognitive status on 18F-florbetapir PET measured regional cortical patterns of beta-amyloid density and growth. *NeuroImage*, *78*, 474–480. https://doi.org/10.1016/j.neuroimage.2013.04.048.

Nenert, R., et al. (2017). Age-related language lateralization assessed by fMRI: The effects of sex and handedness. *Brain Research*, *1674*, 20–35. https://doi.org/10.1016/j.brainres.2017.08.021.

Neu, S. C., et al. (2017). Apolipoprotein E genotype and sex risk factors for Alzheimer disease: A meta-analysis. *JAMA Neurology*, *74*(10), 1178–1189. https://doi.org/10.1001/jamaneurol.2017.2188.

Nichols, K. J., et al. (2018). Interpreting 123I–ioflupane dopamine transporter scans using hybrid scores. *European Journal of Hybrid Imaging*, *2*(1). https://doi.org/10.1186/s41824-018-0028-0.

Nitrini, R., et al. (2000). SPECT in Alzheimer's disease: Features associated with bilateral parietotemporal hypoperfusion. *Acta Neurologica Scandinavica*, *101*(3), 172–176. https://doi.org/10.1034/j.1600-0404.2000.101003172.x.

Nobili, F., et al. (2013). Automatic semi-quantification of [123I]FP-CIT SPECT scans in healthy volunteers using BasGan version 2: Results from the ENC-DAT database. *European Journal of Nuclear Medicine and Molecular Imaging*, *40*(4), 565–573. https://doi.org/10.1007/s00259-012-2304-8.

Ohkura, T., et al. (1994). Evaluation of estrogen treatment in female patients with dementia of the Alzheimer type. *Endocrine Journal, 41*(4), 361–371. https://doi.org/10.1507/endocrj.41.361.

Ott, B. R., et al. (2000). Lateralized cortical perfusion in women with Alzheimer's disease. *The Journal of Gender-Specific Medicine, 3*(6), 29–35.

Oveisgharan, S., et al. (2018). Sex differences in Alzheimer's disease and common neuropathologies of aging. *Acta Neuropathologica, 136*(6), 887–900. https://doi.org/10.1007/s00401-018-1920-1.

Parsey, R. V., et al. (2002). Effects of sex, age, and aggressive traits in man on brain serotonin 5-HT1A receptor binding potential measured by PET using [C-11]WAY-100635. *Brain Research, 954*(2), 173–182. https://doi.org/10.1016/S0006-8993(02)03243-2.

Paul, S., et al. (2019). Building a database for brain 18 kDa translocator protein imaged using [11C]PBR28 in healthy subjects. *Journal of Cerebral Blood Flow and Metabolism, 39*(6), 1138–1147. https://doi.org/10.1177/0271678X18771250.

Payami, H., et al. (1996). Gender difference in apolipoprotein E—Associated risk for familial Alzheimer disease: A possible clue to the higher incidence of Alzheimer disease in women. *American Journal of Human Genetics, 58*(4), 803–811.

Peng, F., et al. (2016). A cross-sectional voxel-based morphometric study of age-and sex-related changes in gray matter volume in the Normal aging brain. *Journal of Computer Assisted Tomography, 40*(2), 307–315. https://doi.org/10.1097/RCT.0000000000000351.

Perneczky, R., et al. (2007). Gender differences in brain reserve: An (18)F-FDG PET study in Alzheimer's disease. *Journal of Neurology, 254*(10), 1395–1400. https://doi.org/10.1007/s00415-007-0558-z.

Persson, N., et al. (2015). Age and sex related differences in subcortical brain iron concentrations among healthy adults. *NeuroImage, 122*, 385–398. https://doi.org/10.1016/j.neuroimage.2015.07.050.

Pike, K. E., et al. (2011). Cognition and beta-amyloid in preclinical Alzheimer's disease: Data from the AIBL study. *Neuropsychologia, 49*(9), 2384–2390. https://doi.org/10.1016/j.neuropsychologia.2011.04.012.

Poirier, J., et al. (1993). Apolipoprotein E polymorphism and Alzheimer's disease. *The Lancet, 342*(8873), 697–699. https://doi.org/10.1016/0140-6736(93)91705-Q.

Ragland, J. D., et al. (2000). Sex differences in brain-behavior relationships between verbal episodic memory and resting regional cerebral blood flow. *Neuropsychologia, 38*(4), 451–461. https://doi.org/10.1016/S0028-3932(99)00086-X.

Rahman, A., et al. (2020). Sex-driven modifiers of Alzheimer risk: A multimodality brain imaging study. *Neurology, 95*(2), E166–E178. https://doi.org/10.1212/WNL.0000000000009781.

Reiman, E. M., et al. (1996). The application of positron emission tomography to the study of the normal menstrual cycle. *Human Reproduction, 11*(12), 2799–2805. https://doi.org/10.1093/oxfordjournals.humrep.a019214.

Ritchey, M., et al. (2011). Emotion processing in the aging brain is modulated by semantic elaboration. *Neuropsychologia, 49*(4), 640–650. https://doi.org/10.1016/j.neuropsychologia.2010.09.009.

Rodriguez, G., et al. (1988). Sex differences in regional cerebral blood flow. *Journal of Cerebral Blood Flow and Metabolism, 8*(6), 783–789. https://doi.org/10.1038/jcbfm.1988.133.

Ryding, E., et al. (2004). A new model for separation between brain dopamine and serotonin transporters in 123I-β-CIT SPECT measurements: Normal values and sex and age dependence. *European Journal of Nuclear Medicine and Molecular Imaging, 31*(8), 1114–1118. https://doi.org/10.1007/s00259-004-1489-x.

Saint-Aubert, L., et al. (2017). Tau PET imaging: Present and future directions. *Molecular Neurodegeneration*. https://doi.org/10.1186/s13024-017-0162-3.

Sampedro, F., et al. (2015). APOE-by-sex interactions on brain structure and metabolism in healthy elderly controls. *Oncotarget*, *6*(29), 26663–26674. https://doi.org/10.18632/oncotarget.5185.

Santarnecchi, E., et al. (2015). Intelligence-related differences in the asymmetry of spontaneous cerebral activity. *Human Brain Mapping*, *36*(9), 3586–3602. https://doi.org/10.1002/hbm.22864.

Schain, M., & Kreisl, W. C. (2017). Neuroinflammation in neurodegenerative disorders—A review. *Current Neurology and Neuroscience Reports*, *1*. https://doi.org/10.1007/s11910-017-0733-2.

Scheinin, N. M., et al. (2014). Cortical 11C-PIB uptake is associated with age, APOE genotype, and gender in "healthy aging". *Journal of Alzheimer's Disease*, *41*(1), 193–202. https://doi.org/10.3233/JAD-132783.

Scheinost, D., et al. (2015). Sex differences in normal age trajectories of functional brain networks. *Human Brain Mapping*, *36*(4), 1524–1535. https://doi.org/10.1002/hbm.22720.

Shen, S., et al. (2019). Sex differences in the association of APOE ε4 genotype with longitudinal hippocampal atrophy in cognitively normal older people. *European Journal of Neurology*, *26*(11), 1362–1369. https://doi.org/10.1111/ene.13987.

Sie, J.-H., et al. (2019). Gender- and age-specific differences in resting-state functional connectivity of the central autonomic network in adulthood. *Frontiers in Human Neuroscience*, *13*, 369. https://doi.org/10.3389/fnhum.2019.00369.

Skup, M., et al. (2011). Sex differences in grey matter atrophy patterns among AD and aMCI patients: Results from ADNI. *NeuroImage*, *56*(3), 890–906. https://doi.org/10.1016/j.neuroimage.2011.02.060.

Slosman, D. O., et al. (2001). (133)Xe SPECT cerebral blood flow study in a healthy population: Determination of T-scores. *Journal of Nuclear Medicine*, *42*(6), 864–870. Available at: http://www.ncbi.nlm.nih.gov/pubmed/11390549. (Accessed 21 February 2020).

Spampinato, M. V., et al. (2016). Gender, apolipoprotein E genotype, and mesial temporal atrophy: 2-year follow-up in patients with stable mild cognitive impairment and with progression from mild cognitive impairment to Alzheimer's disease. *Neuroradiology*, *58*(11), 1143–1151. https://doi.org/10.1007/s00234-016-1740-8.

Spillantini, M. G., & Goedert, M. (1998). Tau protein pathology in neurodegenerative diseases. *Trends in Neurosciences*, 428–433. https://doi.org/10.1016/S0166-2236(98)01337-X.

Staley, J. K., et al. (2001). Sex differences in [123I]β-CIT SPECT measures of dopamine and serotonin transporter availability in healthy smokers and nonsmokers. *Synapse*, *41*(4), 275–284. https://doi.org/10.1002/syn.1084.

Stevens, M. C., Calhoun, V. D., & Kiehl, K. A. (2005). Hemispheric differences in hemodynamics elicited by auditory oddball stimuli. *NeuroImage*, *26*(3), 782–792. https://doi.org/10.1016/j.neuroimage.2005.02.044.

Stone, D. J., et al. (1998). Increased synaptic sprouting in response to estrogen via an apolipoprotein E-dependent mechanism: Implications for Alzheimer's disease. *Journal of Neuroscience*, *18*(9), 3180–3185. https://doi.org/10.1523/jneurosci.18-09-03180.1998.

Swartz, R. H., Black, S. E., & St George-Hyslop, P. (1999). Apolipoprotein E and Alzheimer's disease: A genetic, molecular and neuroimaging review. *The Canadian Journal of Neurological Sciences*, *26*(2), 77–88. Available at: http://www.ncbi.nlm.nih.gov/pubmed/10352866. (Accessed 22 February 2020).

Tan, A., et al. (2016). The human hippocampus is not sexually-dimorphic: Meta-analysis of structural MRI volumes. *NeuroImage, 124*(Pt A), 350–366. https://doi.org/10.1016/j.neuroimage.2015.08.050.

Tarumi, T., et al. (2014). Cerebral hemodynamics in normal aging: Central artery stiffness, wave reflection, and pressure pulsatility. *Journal of Cerebral Blood Flow and Metabolism, 34*(6), 971–978. https://doi.org/10.1038/jcbfm.2014.44.

Toschi, N., et al. (2020). Multishell diffusion imaging reveals sex-specific trajectories of early white matter degeneration in normal aging. *Neurobiology of Aging, 86*, 191–200. https://doi.org/10.1016/j.neurobiolaging.2019.11.014.

Tosun, D., et al. (2017). Association between tau deposition and antecedent amyloid-β accumulation rates in normal and early symptomatic individuals. *Brain, 140*(5), 1499–1512. https://doi.org/10.1093/brain/awx046.

Tuisku, J., et al. (2019). Effects of age, BMI and sex on the glial cell marker TSPO—A multicentre [11C]PBR28 HRRT PET study. *European Journal of Nuclear Medicine and Molecular Imaging, 46*(11), 2329–2338. https://doi.org/10.1007/s00259-019-04403-7.

Twelves, D., Perkins, K. S. M., & Counsell, C. (2003). Systematic review of incidence studies of Parkinson's disease. *Movement Disorders*, 19–31. https://doi.org/10.1002/mds.10305.

van Dyck, C. H., et al. (1995). Age-related decline in striatal dopamine transporter binding with iodine-123-beta-CITSPECT. *Journal of Nuclear Medicine, 36*(7), 1175–1181. Available at: http://europepmc.org/abstract/MED/7790941.

Van Laere, K., et al. (2001). 99mTc-ECD brain perfusion SPET: Variability, asymmetry and effects of age and gender in healthy adults. *European Journal of Nuclear Medicine, 28*(7), 873–887. https://doi.org/10.1007/s002590100549.

Vemuri, P., et al. (2017). Evaluation of amyloid protective factors and Alzheimer disease neurodegeneration protective factors in elderly individuals. *JAMA Neurology, 74*(6), 718–726. https://doi.org/10.1001/jamaneurol.2017.0244.

Versijpt, J., et al. (2003). Imaging of the 5-HT2A system: Age-, gender-, and Alzheimer's disease-related findings. *Neurobiology of Aging, 24*, 553–561. https://doi.org/10.1016/S0197-4580(02)00137-9.

Vest, R. S., & Pike, C. J. (2013). Gender, sex steroid hormones, and Alzheimer's disease. *Hormones and Behavior*, 301–307. https://doi.org/10.1016/j.yhbeh.2012.04.006.

Villeneuve, S., et al. (2018). Proximity to parental symptom onset and amyloid-β burden in sporadic Alzheimer disease. *JAMA Neurology, 75*(5), 608–619. https://doi.org/10.1001/jamaneurol.2017.5135.

Witelson, S., Beresh, H., & Kigar, D. (2006). Intelligence and brain size in 100 postmortem brains: Sex, lateralization and age factors. *Brain, 129*, 386–398. https://doi.org/10.1093/brain/awh696.

Xu, X., et al. (2014). Cerebrovascular perfusion among older adults is moderated by strength training and gender. *Neuroscience Letters, 560*, 26–30. https://doi.org/10.1016/j.neulet.2013.12.011.

Yamamoto, H., et al. (2017). Age-related effects and gender differences in Japanese healthy controls for [123I] FP-CIT SPECT. *Annals of Nuclear Medicine, 31*(5), 407–412. https://doi.org/10.1007/s12149-017-1168-1.

Yang, S., et al. (2008). Sex differences in the white matter and myelinated nerve fibers of Long-Evans rats. *Brain Research, 1216*, 16–23. https://doi.org/10.1016/j.brainres.2008.03.052.

Yoshizawa, H., et al. (2014). Characterizing the normative profile of 18F-FDG PET brain imaging: Sex difference, aging effect, and cognitive reserve. *Psychiatry Research: Neuroimaging, 221*(1), 78–85. https://doi.org/10.1016/j.pscychresns.2013.10.009.

Ziontz, J., et al. (2019). Tau pathology in cognitively normal older adults. *Alzheimer's & Dementia: Diagnosis, Assessment & Disease Monitoring*, *11*, 637–645. https://doi.org/10.1016/j.dadm.2019.07.007.

Zuo, X. N., et al. (2010). Growing together and growing apart: Regional and sex differences in the lifespan developmental trajectories of functional homotopy. *Journal of Neuroscience*, *30*(45), 15034–15043. https://doi.org/10.1523/JNEUROSCI.2612-10.2010.

Jakobson Mo, S., Larsson, A., Linder, J., Birgander, R., Edenbrandt, L., Stenlund, H., … Riklund, K. (2013). 123I-FP-Cit and 123I-IBZM SPECT uptake in a prospective normal material analysed with two different semiquantitative image evaluation tools. *Nuclear Medicine Communications*, *34*(10), 978–989. https://doi.org/10.1097/MNM.0b013e328364aa2e.

van Dyck, C. H., Malison, R. T., Jacobsen, L. K., Seibyl, J. P., Staley, J. K., Laruelle, M., … Gelernter, J. (2005). Increased dopamine transporter availability associated with the 9-repeat allele of the SLC6A3 gene. *The Journal of Nuclear Medicine*, *46*(5), 745–751.

Wong, K. K., Müller, M. L., Kuwabara, H., Studenski, S. A., & Bohnen, N. I. (2012). Gender differences in nigrostriatal dopaminergic innervation are present at young-to-middle but not at older age in normal adults. *Journal of Clinical Neuroscience*, *19*(1), 183–184. https://doi.org/10.1016/j.jocn.2011.05.013.

Weng, Y. H., Yen, T. C., Chen, M. C., Kao, P. F., Tzen, K. Y., Chen, R. S., … Lu, C. S. (2004). Sensitivity and specificity of 99mTc-TRODAT-1 SPECT imaging in differentiating patients with idiopathic Parkinson's disease from healthy subjects. *The Journal of Nuclear Medicine*, *45*(3), 393–401.

CHAPTER 6

Sex and gender differences in neuropsychological symptoms for clinical diagnosis of Alzheimer's disease

Emnet Z. Gammada[a], Rhoda Au[b,c], and Nancy S. Foldi[d,e]

[a]*Department of Psychiatry and Biobehavioral Sciences and Semel Institute for Neuroscience and Human Behavior, David Geffen School of Medicine at UCLA, Los Angeles, CA, United States*
[b]*Departments of Anatomy & Neurobiology, Neurology and Framingham Heart Study, Boston University School of Medicine, Boston, MA, United States*
[c]*Department of Epidemiology, Boston University School of Public Health, Boston, MA, United States*
[d]*Department of Psychology, Queens College and The Graduate Center, City University of New York, New York, NY, United States*
[e]*Department of Psychiatry, NYU Langone Hospital—Long Island, NYU Langone Health, Mineola, NY, United States*

Introduction

Neuropsychological domains of cognition are associated with complex underlying neural networks that characterize brain-behavior relationships throughout the life span. The detection and progression of Alzheimer's disease (AD) is evident in altered cognitive (Banks et al., 2019; Honarpisheh & McCullough, 2019) and biological markers (Jack et al., 2018; Liesinger et al., 2018). Multiple neuropsychological domains are susceptible to the disease, although memory, language, and executive function play prominent roles. As women have a significantly greater lifetime risk of developing AD (Alzheimer's Association, 2019), sex/gender-specific cognitive differences (Sundermann, Biegon, et al., 2016; Sundermann, Maki, et al., 2016) are critical and must be characterized both prior to disease onset and across the continuum of disease progression (Banks et al., 2019; Honarpisheh & McCullough, 2019; Nebel et al., 2018).

Interestingly, while neuropsychological assessments have been developed for disease detection over many decades, they have not traditionally applied sex/gender-specific norms of standardized tests for adults. Aging is part of the continuous developmental process, and it is striking that, while psychological test development for early childhood and adolescence have standardly provided age-group based sex/gender-specific cognitive norms, adult and late-life sex/gender-specific cognitive norms are only now being established (Banks et al., 2019; Miller et al., 2015; Sundermann et al., 2019). The first aim of this chapter is to help characterize sex/gender-specific neuropsychological differences in memory, language, and executive functions in late life, in the service of early disease detection. The second aim is to illustrate why these particular cognitive domains provide critical information and can capture disease profiles and progression in women and men.

The terminology of "sex" versus "gender" warrants clarification. Sex refers to the biological construct of chromosomal, gonadal, and hormonal features (e.g., male, female, intersex). Gender refers to the cultural and psychosocial factors that shape masculine and feminine identities via social and work-related stressors, education, and occupation (e.g., masculine, feminine, androgynous). These two expressions interact to form what is called "men" and "women" in humans. Both sex and gender play important roles in the development and expression of disease, including AD (Carter, Resnick, Mallampalli, & Kalbarczyk, 2012; Mielke, Vemuri, & Rocca, 2014). While often congruent, sex and gender may act independently or synergistically in determining disease risk. The current chapter uses "sex/gender" to reinforce that any observed differences in AD could be due to biological mechanisms, social mechanisms, or synergistic effects of both.

The focus of this chapter emphasizes how sex/gender changes the course of healthy aging and of disease development, emphasizing three cognitive domains, namely memory, language, and executive function. Each domain reviewed includes representative tasks and studies that have yielded sex/gender differences. Cognitive function changes can stand alone, or they can be behavioral manifestation of neurodegeneration as evidenced by relevant disease-related fluid- and imaging-based biomarkers, e.g., regional volumetrics, white matter connectivity, disease load, neurochemical, or genetic contribution (Braak & Braak, 1991; Seeley, Crawford, Zhou, Miller, & Greicius, 2009; Weintraub, Wicklund, & Salmon, 2012). It is important to note that multiple interpretations of data are possible, and that sex/gender-specific interactions of cognition can vary as a function of underlying neurobiology, demographics, and experiential events. For instance, a verbal memory recall task where women perform higher than men could be explained by multiple possible accounts: (a) older women, on average, have higher baseline recall performance than older men, and that disparity remains evident at disease onset and subsequent progression; (b) both groups start at a similar point, but the rate of decline in women is slower than in men; (c) there is a sex-specific vulnerability of hippocampal volume during early disease development (Hua et al., 2010) such that men may be more susceptible and perform more poorly on verbal recall at initial disease states; and (d) both men and women have similar focal hippocampal disease load, yet women—but not men—can draw on cognitive reserve (Stern, 2002) or neural compensation to recruit alternate brain networks and show higher task performance.

Thus, sex/gender differences may be easy to detect, but not always easy to explain. The ultimate long-term goal of the field will be to tease apart the source of and reasons for sex-specific cognitive performance differences. The characterization of sex/gender differences in memory, language, and executive functions will highlight differences of underlying theory or mechanisms across these three prominent domains. Furthermore, spearheaded by the reformative research of Sundermann et al. (2019, 2020), the relationship between sex/gender-specific cognitive markers of disease detection, measurement, progression, and treatment efficacy in women and men will be explored. Distinctive sex/gender representations of cognitive function follow divergent developmental trajectories. Failure to appreciate these trajectories may continue to delay detection and/or misdiagnosis of AD and related disorders.

Memory
Introduction

Memory pertains to the ability to learn, retain, recall, or recognize information in any primary modality of visual, auditory, tactile, or olfactory modalities. The focus of this discussion is primarily on AD disease-related deficits of episodic and semantic memory functions. Development of AD pathology in medial temporal lobe structures (e.g., hippocampus, entorhinal, and perirhinal cortex) (Braak & Braak, 1991, 1995) disrupts neural networks underlying both episodic and semantic memory functions. The profile of memory decline, along with an inability to learn and retain new information (i.e., anterograde amnesia), has long been a clinical hallmark of AD pathology (Salmon, 2000). Patients with AD are impaired on episodic memory tasks found in a variety of cognitive procedures (e.g., free recall, recognition, paired-associate learning) across multiple modalities (e.g., auditory, visual, or olfaction) (Buckley et al., 2019; Weintraub et al., 2012). It is widely accepted that the episodic memory deficits in AD are due to ineffective consolidation and storage of new information (Delis, Kaplan, Kramer, & Ober, 2000). However, the literature has only begun to capture sex/gender-specific differences using verbal measures from standard list learning tasks [e.g., Rey Auditory Verbal Learning Test (RAVLT; Schmidt, 1996), California Verbal Learning Test (CVLT; Delis et al., 2000), or the Consortium to Establish a Registry for Alzheimer's disease (CERAD; Welsh et al., 1994)]. Qualitative metrics of impaired processing of information (Egli et al., 2014; Millar et al., 2017; Thomas et al., 2018; Milberg & Hebben, 2013) detail why the consolidation is susceptible; sex/gender differences will be instructive in these processes as well. Verbal memory, in particular, has key qualitative, long-standing sex/gender differences, as described below.

Sex/gender differences in verbal memory in healthy adults

Particular verbal memory list-learning tasks have captured sex/gender differences. The California Verbal Learning Test (CVLT: Delis et al., 2000) requires the participant to learn a wordlist over several trials. The list is purposely constructed with embedded semantic categories, which could elicit an organization strategy. When

(Kramer, Delis, and Daniel (1988) examined performance of healthy older men and women, women scored significantly higher than men across the five learning trials, and for both immediate and delayed free recall conditions. Importantly, women demonstrated higher instances of semantic clustering in their responses, suggesting they had self-initiated semantic categorization during learning and recall. In contrast, men were more likely to use passive organization, recalling items following the original serial presentation or serial clustering. Examination (McCarrey, An, Kitner-Triolo, Ferrucci, & Resnick, 2016) of cognitive trajectories from clinically healthy older adults replicated these sex/gender differences, wherein women outperformed men in immediate and delayed recalls of the CVLT. On a verbal paired-associates list learning task, sex/gender differences were examined in young adulthood and adolescence (Waters & Schreiber, 1991), and again, women out-performed men on a task that did not explicitly indicate or require elaboration. Yet, when researchers encouraged strategy use and elaboration to both men and women, sex/gender differences disappeared; this study suggests self-generated initiation of in-depth semantic processing may be a more intuitive strategy to promote better encoding and retrieval.

Sex/gender differences in verbal memory in mild cognitive impairment

It is important to determine whether these sex/gender differences persist in the early stages of disease development. In a seminal series of studies (Sundermann, Biegon, et al., 2016; Sundermann, Maki, et al., 2016), Sundermann and colleagues examined sex differences in memory of verbal list-learning material in women and men diagnosed with mild cognitive impairment (MCI) using the Rey Auditory Verbal Learning Test (RAVLT) (Schmidt, 1996), which lacks explicit semantic categories. They found that women outperformed men on total word recall at learning and at delay recall, despite equal levels of brain pathology; yet, both groups presented with comparable hippocampal volume atrophy and with hypometabolism quantified by decreased temporal lobe glucose metabolic rates. A posited alternate access to semantic associations could aid in processing and retrieving verbal information; but, in turn, this could obscure the degree of actual underlying pathological load. Supportive performance was also seen in an even older sample (Golchert et al., 2019), where women appear to use verbal skills to maintain performance. Sundermann, Maki, et al. (2016) proposed that women may have greater availability of a sex-specific cognitive reserve (Stern, 2012), which may underlie and support performance in verbal memory domains, or may. However, if women are circumventing the effects of actual disease pathology, it may be masking what otherwise would be a diagnosis of MCI. These important findings suggest that those women who subsequently transition from MCI to AD had superior cognitive reserve; however, it delayed their clinical diagnosis.

The role of cognitive reserve and resilience is complicated as it is linked to years of education (Wilson et al., 2019) or rate of change (Lavrencic et al., 2018) and may be not fully explain conversion to disease (see also Chapter 12). Sundermann,

Biegon, et al. (2016) and Sundermann, Maki, et al. (2016) have underscored that the magnitude of the female advantage in verbal memory may vary on severity of atrophy. That is, women's advantage in verbal memory was evident despite minimal to moderate temporal hypometabolism and minimal to moderate hippocampal atrophy; however, this advantage was attenuated when hypometabolism or atrophy levels were more severe. The proposed argument is that women show better verbal memory performance than men, despite comparable levels of brain pathophysiology as measured by structural and functional neuroimaging, particularly in the early stages of disease.

These findings suggest that MCI may only be clinically detected at a more advanced disease stage in women compared to men, because women are better able to compensate for greater underlying neuropathology during the early stages of the disease process. It is also possible that compensatory strategies are masked by insensitivity of standard neuropsychological tests to detect them. In either case, the consequence is that women receive a diagnosis of MCI later in the disease course, and when they transition to AD, they may have greater underlying pathology than men. These findings help to explain the paradoxical sex differences in MCI and AD prevalence (Alzheimer's Association, 2019; Brookmeyer et al., 2011; Petersen et al., 2010; Roberts et al., 2012).

Sex/gender differences in verbal memory in AD

When meeting criteria for an AD diagnoses, findings suggest that women perform worse than men on verbal recall memory tasks. Henderson and Buckwalter (1994) found that women diagnosed with AD showed lower recall than men using the Consortium to Establish a Registry for Alzheimer's Disease (CERAD) word list, after controlling for age, education, and duration of illness. Similarly, Pusswald et al. (2015) also examined CERAD list-learning performance, revealing that women in the early stage of AD recalled fewer items on average than did men. These data corroborate Sundermann et al.'s findings (Sundermann, Biegon, et al., 2016; Sundermann, Maki, et al., 2016), showing that, in contrast to performance of healthy older adults and individuals diagnosed with MCI, once the clinical manifestation of AD ensues, women lose their verbal memory advantage and perform worse than men (i.e., a threshold effect).

Sex/gender differences and rates of verbal memory decline

Word list learning, recall, and recognition are commonly used to assess memory change. Throughout life, healthy women generally outperform healthy men on these typical memory measures in healthy aging and early disease stages (Sundermann et al., 2017). Studies suggest that women are less likely to receive a diagnosis of MCI than men because of attenuated test performance decline (e.g., cognitive resilience; Caldwell, Cummings, Banks, Palmqvist, & Hansson, 2019; Roberts et al., 2012; Sachdev et al., 2012). However, once diagnosed with MCI, women progress faster than men from MCI to AD (Koran, Wagener and Hohman, 2017; Roberts et al., 2014; Tschanz et al., 2011), and once diagnosed with AD, women exhibit a more rapid cognitive decline (Alzheimer Association, 2019; Mielke et al., 2014; Nebel et al., 2018), suggesting that the underlying pathological burden is much greater relative to men at the clinical threshold of diagnosis.

Summary

Advances in our understanding of verbal memory tasks reveal increased awareness of sex/gender differences at all stages, including healthy premorbid status to early diagnosis to progression. It is increasingly clear that sex/gender-specific profiles need to be reevaluated and integrated into diagnostics. This has motivated development of sex/gender-specific verbal memory norms, such as those introduced by Sundermann et al. (2019). When these sex/gender-specific list-learning norms and cut scores are incorporated into the MCI diagnostic criteria, a subset of 10% of women—previously classified as healthy according to previous "standard" diagnostic criteria—was reclassified as MCI (false negatives). Concordantly, sex/gender-specific diagnostic criteria reclassified a subset of 10% of men—previously classified as having MCI—to normal healthy aging (false positives). Thus, it is increasingly important to account for a verbal memory advantage in women; redistribution of the membership in MCI and healthy control samples should improve diagnostic accuracy.

Language
Introduction

Language is a cognitive system that is uniquely human and its neural representation involves multiple neural systems that overlap with networks of AD pathology. Language is composed of the three domains of phonology, syntax, and semantics. Phonology refers to the finite number of language-specific, meaningful sound units, each of which is defined as a phoneme (Blumstein, Baker, & Goodglass, 1977). Syntax refers to the finite, language-specific rules of grammar: the rules that dictate how to generate word sequences to form meaningful organized sentence structures (Chomsky, 1957; Matchin & Hickok, 2020). Semantics refers to the meaning assigned to each unit, or word, that is agreed upon by the language community; every human language has an infinite number of semantic units. The three language domains of phonology, syntax, and semantics are mediated by interlocking central neural networks (Fridriksson et al., 2018). Each of the three language domains is represented in all six mechanisms of language use, namely: production, repetition, comprehension, naming, reading, and writing.

The neural representation of language (Friederici, Opitz, & von Cramon, 2000; Hickok & Poeppel, 2007; Poeppel, Emmorey, Hickok, & Pylkkanen, 2012) provides a hierarchical and integrated system underlying each of these three domains of the language system. The semantic network (Devereux, Clarke, Marouchos, & Tyler,

2013) is the key source of linguistic deficit in AD. To appreciate how a sex/gender-specific architecture supporting the language system could be particularly affected by AD, it is important to first consider several complimentary and overlapping variables including laterality, handedness, and white matter interconnectivity.

Laterality, handedness, and connectivity of the language system

Language representation in the brain needs to be considered within the context of neural representation of handedness, the lateralization of brain regions subserving language (e.g., left language dominance), as well as sex/gender-specific profiles of neural location and interconnectivity that become affected during the course of disease development.

First, language representation is asymmetrical and related to handedness. The language network is heavily lateralized (Sommer, Aleman, Bouma, & Kahn, 2004), such that right-handers have greater left hemisphere representation of language compared to left-handers. Nenert et al. (2017) report that language functions in right-handers are predominantly left lateralized; only 5%–7% do not show that profile. In contrast, left-handers show more atypical lateralization of language functions (22%–25%) where language is either right lateralized or represented bilaterally (Wallentin, 2009).

Second, semantic functions are affected in AD, whereas phonological or syntactic functions are not; in fact, the presence of phonological or syntactic impairment should signal non-AD etiology. Hickok and Poeppel (Hickok & Poeppel, 2004) demonstrate that the wide lexical-semantic network has some bilateral distribution, compared to either syntactic or phonological representation, which are predominantly represented unilaterally. The semantic network (Forseth et al., 2018) is reliant on the access integrity of the middle fusiform, superior temporal gyri, and ventral stream. There are mixed findings of the structural lateralization underlying language in men and women. For instance, Sommer et al. (2004) suggest that women do not have greater bilateral language distribution, as had been believed. However, finer grade analyses of white matter (Jung et al., 2019) measuring fractional anisotropy and radial diffusivity do show that distinct language-related pathways can differ in men and women. The network approach of language functions and representation need to engage in both volumetric regional areas and white matter interconnecting pathways. Nonetheless, it is even more striking that AD related sex differences predominantly affect the semantic network.

Third, the interconnectivity associated with language networks represent interlocking dorsal and ventral neural networks (Binder & Desai, 2011) underlying each of the phonological, syntactic, and semantic systems (Hickok & Poeppel, 2004, 2015; Poeppel & Hickok, 2004). The combinatorial semantic network (Binder & Desai, 2011) involves regional parcellation and binding of the anterior superior temporal gyrus, planum temporale, and anterior temporal lobe, and convergence into higher integrated representations involving ventral, fusiform regions, lateral temporal regions, and the inferior parietal angular gyrus (Forseth et al., 2018; Hickok et al., 2018; Poeppel et al., 2012). It is of interest that in early life, syntactic development is dependent on completed arcuate fasciculus interconnectivity (Perani et al., 2011). This is followed by subsequent dissociation of the arcuate fasciculus from superior temporal streams, which are initially interconnected (Skeide, Brauer, & Friederici, 2014). The integration of the dorsal streams with ventral anterior temporal pole and regions of medial temporal cortex in the dominant hemispheres (Humphries, Willard, Buchsbaum, & Hickok, 2001) remains critical for a functioning semantic network. It is worth noting that in AD, local volumetric depletion and cortical thinning as well as white matter integrity are at risk; therefore sex/gender-specific differences of the semantic system could emerge from changes not only in gray matter regions within the semantic network, but also in access and interconnectivity of these underlying networks (see also Chapter 5).

Semantic dysfunction in neural disorders other than AD

As mentioned, language deficits in AD emerge in the semantic domain, with phonologic or syntactic deficits conspicuously absent. Importantly, semantic deficits are not exclusive to AD, and occur in focal vascular aphasias (e.g., left angular gyrus lesions), semantic and logopenic variants of primary progressive aphasias (PPA; Gorno-Tempini et al., 2011; Grossman, 2018; Powers et al., 2013; Staffaroni et al., 2020), and semantic dementia (Irish, Addis, Hodges, & Piguet, 2012). Unlike AD, the PPAs are distinguished by preserved episodic memory skills well into the progression of the disease. The focus of this chapter is on AD and posits that the semantic system—that is, knowledge, representation, and access to agreed-upon meaningful semantic labels—is highly sensitive to early AD pathology, and critically interlinked with amnestic deficits in episodic and semantic memory we will examine this in the next section.

Critical semantic disruption in AD

The semantic network is posited as one of the most sensitive markers of AD development (Egli et al., 2014; Foldi, 2011). The vulnerability of semantic encoding can be captured by qualitative measures of list-learning tasks such as California Verbal Learning Test (Delis et al., 2000) or the Rey Auditory Verbal Learning Test (Rey, 1958). Accurate list-learning recall follows the principle of serial position (e.g., list word order). Primacy list items are defined as those positioned at the beginning of serially presented words and recall is dependent on engaging deep semantic encoding processes (Gainotti, Marra, Villa, Parlato, & Chiarotti, 1998). Poor semantic encoding results in lower levels of learning, and subsequent poor recall of primacy items is a harbinger of disease risk in healthy controls (Bruno et al., 2015; Egli et al., 2014; Howieson et al., 2011; Kasper et al., 2016). Semantic vulnerability prior to disease diagnosis is similarly seen in word generation (verbal fluency) with lower performance on semantic category cues compared to letter cues (Vonk et al., 2020). Poor semantic memory compared to episodic memory (Hirni, Kivisaari, Monsch, & Taylor, 2013) also captures semantic deficits, reflecting deficient function of the anterior middle temporal lobe regions. The role of semantic network, organization, and retrieval remains a critical and unique determiner of prognosis.

Much like the research in the memory domain, why sex/gender performance differs and why the semantic ability is so sensitive to disease development needs to be considered. Gainotti, Spinelli, Scaricamazza, and Marra (2013) refute the idea that differences result from experiences and familiarity of distinct categories (e.g., tools for men or kitchen items for women); rather, documented gender differences more likely reflect generational experiences. A second explanation is that the neural networks and representation of language functions differ in healthy men and women, where women have greater cortical distribution representing the same semantic skill and knowledge. Thus, when women experience AD-related focal hippocampal pathology, other remaining cortical resources are still available to compensate. This supposition is supported by Banks et al. (2019), who suggest that composite scores showing change in language and executive skills better capture initial decline. A third explanation may be sex/gender differences in the white matter networks: as language relies on intact white matter interconnectivity (Jung et al., 2019), sex/gender differences may reflect the progression of disconnection between critical regions. Finally, an alternate possibility is that different sex/gender profiles of language just represent an epiphenomenon. It may be that AD pathology "happens" to overlap with the neurological regions and interconnectivity of the semantic network and, because of different distribution and representation of the language network in men and women, its intersection with AD pathology yields different sex/gender longitudinal profiles.

Executive function
Introduction

Executive function refers to the broad category of cognitive, behavioral, motor, and emotional tasks allowing an individual to generate or respond to events in the environment (Bonelli & Cummings, 2007; Grissom & Reyes, 2019; Stuss & Alexander, 2000). Higher order top-down control of executive skills (Miller & D'Esposito, 2005; Stuss & Knight, 2013), which regulate or override lower level skills, are broad and involve cognitive tasks of switching set, flexibility, planning, generativity, inhibition, sequencing, problem solving, and components of working memory. Executive skills (Diamond, 2013) extend to higher order judgment, moderating emotional and behavioral responses to social situations (Burgess, Veitch, de Lacy Costello, & Shallice, 2000; Damasio, 1995; Funahashi, 2017; Grafman & Litvan, 1999; Guarino et al., 2019; Stuss & Alexander, 2000; Stuss, Shallice, Alexander, & Picton, 1995). Higher order complex executive functions reflect involvement of the underlying neurological interconnectivity between secondary and tertiary frontal regions and cortico-cortical networks (e.g., frontal local and distal regions with cortical temporal, visual, and parietal regions) as well as frontal cortical-subcortical networks (Bonelli & Cummings, 2007). Executive function interconnectivity mechanisms rely on the default-mode

(Cacciaglia et al., 2018), the dorsal-attentional, and the fronto-parietal networks, which are all susceptible to aging (Grady, Sarraf, Saverino, & Campbell, 2016).

The effects of AD on these executive functions appear to be broad. It is important to appreciate that disease-related mechanisms (e.g., amyloid or plaque accumulation, cortical thinning, white matter hyperintensities) can disrupt executive performance due not only by local regional but also distal network dysfunction. Thus, focal frontal involvement (e.g., Dickerson et al., 2009; Salat, Kaye, & Janowsky, 2001) as well as distal disruption due to diaschisis—secondary to temporal or parietal gray matter volume depletion or to severed white matter connectivity—can severely impact executive function integrity. Both focal and distal dysfunctions profoundly affect cognitive tasks attributed to frontal control or executive performance (Bondi et al., 2002; Levy et al., 2002; Rabinovici, Stephens, & Possin, 2015). It is not surprising that diverse executive functions are highly susceptible, as they may present as some of the earliest and most sensitive cognitive symptoms of AD disease process. Speed or efficiency used to retrieve previously learned information may be more representative of executive than memory performance (Salat et al., 2001) and AD affects the interpretation of cognitive and behavioral tasks.

Sex/gender differences in executive function

Sex/gender comparisons of executive functions emerge from several sources. Early developmental connectivity demonstrates clear sex/gender differences (Li et al., 2014). Executive functions, like other domains of cognition, have sex-specific norms for childhood, but not for adult men and women. Yet, sex/gender differences impact age-related or disease-related decline in multiple ways (Grissom & Reyes, 2019). For example, sex/gender performance may appear similarly on a cognitive measure, but not take into account differing rate of decline; or, performance can appear equivalent, but not take into account that the same task is mediated by alternate networks, again supporting the concept of different underlying sex/gender-specific strategies. Speed or efficiency used to retrieve previously learned information may influence executive more than memory performance (Salat et al., 2001) and AD affects the interpretation of cognitive and behavioral tasks.

A sex/gender difference in AD may be explained by showing how task performance appears similar, but results from different underlying neurobiological mechanisms used to perform the task (Cross, Copping, & Campbell, 2011; Grissom & Reyes, 2019; Reber & Tranel, 2017). The same cognitive problem can be solved using different strategies, activating and recruiting alternate neural circuits. In attentional tasks, Phillips, Rogers, Haworth, Bayer, and Tales (2013) showed that, while healthy men and women showed no difference, women with MCI show decreased accuracy and increased intra-individual RT variability compared to men in simple decisions tasks.

In young adults, women demonstrate better spatial working memory (i.e., ability to temporarily store and hold information "on-line") compared to verbal working memory tasks (Duff & Hampson, 2001; Lejbak, Vrbancic, & Crossley, 2009). These studies of attentional working memory suggest a possibility that healthy young women may be more efficient at maintaining and updating information in a readily accessible form to perform ongoing tasks. However, this skill may not hold into late life (D'Antuono, Maini, Marin, Boccia, & Piccardi, 2020) even without disease. Several studies from focal lesion literature support this notion (Cross et al., 2011; Grissom & Reyes, 2019; Reber & Tranel, 2017). Tranel, Damasio, Denburg, and Bechara (2005) investigated a decision-making task in men and women and found sex-related functional asymmetry of the prefrontal cortices, especially the ventromedial prefrontal cortices, which are critical for social conduct, emotional processing, and decision-making. Specifically, they found that the right-sided ventromedial prefrontal cortex is important in men for decision-making, while the left-sided ventromedial prefrontal cortex is important in women but not men. Thus, men and women may be accessing different circuits and drawing on different strategies to solve the same problem. For example, men may use a more holistic, gestalt-type strategy, and women may use a more analytic, verbally mediated strategy. These differences could reflect asymmetric, gender-related differences in the neurobiology of left and right ventromedial prefrontal cortices sectors. These findings illustrate how the experiences of sex/gender may shape neuroarchitecture for men and women, and result in differential recruitment of brain regions.

Sutterer, Koscik, and Tranel (2015) replicated and extended the findings of sex-related asymmetry of the ventromedial prefrontal cortex. They found that men with right-sided and women with left-sided damage show similar deficits in decision-making under conditions of risk and ambiguity. Hence, while the ultimate behavioral performance may be indistinguishable across men and women, there is a sex-related asymmetry in the brain structures underlying those challenging skills.

Tranel and Bechara (2009) also found the same sex-related functional asymmetry in another brain area associated with social conduct, emotional processing, personality, and complex decision making: the amygdala. In men, patients with right-sided amygdala damage were impaired in this function, and patients with left-sided amygdala damage were not; the opposite pattern was obtained in women. These findings provide support for the notion that sex-related functional asymmetry of the amygdala may reflect (as either a cause or effect) differences in the manner in which men and women apprehend, process, and execute emotion-related information. These sex-specific signaling patterns may be driving the cognitive performance observed as sex/gender differences at a molecular level driving the same cognitive performance.

Relatedly, Malpetti et al. (2017) examined sex/gender differences in brain metabolic activity and resting state network connectivity in healthy older adults and patients with Alzheimer's disease, and found greater efficiency in the posterior default mode network for men, and in the anterior frontal executive network in women. Other neuroimaging studies (Christakou et al., 2009; Hill, Laird, & Robinson, 2014) also report different brain activation patterns in men and women during cognitive control and working memory tasks, suggesting a higher involvement of the prefrontal cortex in adult women and parietal cortex in men. Thus, although men and women may present with similar-appearing cognitive ability, their strategies may reflect different neurobiological mechanisms and networks. It is still unclear whether disease risk is predicated on the vulnerability of one or another network being disrupted during disease development.

Sex/gender differences in cognitive reserve mechanisms

Cognitive compensation (Cabeza et al., 2018; Stern, 2002) may mask underlying cognitive decline through greater activation or broader recruitment of brain regions. The hemispheric asymmetry reduction in older adults (HAROLD) model (Cabeza, 2002; Cabeza et al., 2018) differentiates reserve, maintenance, and compensation as neurological functions change in old age, which shift to mechanisms that maintain optimal aging. The prefrontal region and its interconnectivity may allow for alternate strategies to complete executive tasks. Cabeza and colleagues suggest that this model may result from a global reorganization of neurocognitive networks as well as from regional neural changes. Furthermore, bilateral activity in older adults may reflect compensatory processes as well as dedifferentiation processes. Berlingeri, Danelli, Bottini, Sberna, and Paulesu (2013) revisited this model and found that the HAROLD model captured only some of the age-related changes of brain pattern observed in aging. These researchers expand the HAROLD-like pattern to regions outside the prefrontal cortex, including temporal regions and parieto-occipital regions. Moreover, in a study examining participants with MCI, Lenzi et al. (2011) found that, in addition to the selective memory deficit, these patients also showed changes of brain activity within networks associated with language and attention, suggesting the presence of compensation mechanisms in patients at the earliest clinical stages of AD. These findings suggest that the compensation mechanisms may become progressively reduced with the evolution of the disease, until a critical "clinical threshold" is overcome.

Whether these age-related compensatory processes differ by sex/gender is a new question. To address this, Berger, Demin, Holtkamp, and Bengner (2018) examined men and women with temporal lobe epilepsy and frontal lobe epilepsy to investigate women's verbal memory advantage. These researchers surprisingly found verbal memory advantage in women with temporal lobe epilepsy, but not in women with frontal lobe epilepsy. This finding is consistent with other investigations (Berenbaum, Baxter, Seidenberg, & Hermann, 1997; Berger, Oltmanns, Holtkamp, & Bengner, 2017) that have also demonstrated that women's verbal memory advantage remains unaltered even after temporal lobe epilepsy surgery, suggesting that temporal lobe structures may not be as necessary for women's memory advantage. Rather, frontal lobe structures may be supporting memory encoding and retrieval through organizational and control processes (Fletcher & Henson, 2001; Ojemann & Kelley, 2002). This hypothesis is further supported by functional neuroimaging studies, showing increased activation of frontal regions in women compared to men during working memory tasks (Goldstein et al., 2005; Hill et al., 2014). These finding are also in line with observations of sex/gender differences in verbal memory. As highlighted above, Sundermann, Biegon, et al. (2016) demonstrated sex-specific verbal memory advantage for women with MCI despite mild-to-moderate levels of hippocampal atrophy. Thus, the women's verbal memory advantage may be mediated by the frontal system.

Conclusion

Sex/gender differences in AD reflect a complex interplay of developmental, neuroendocrine, and psychosocial factors, which result in lifelong neural mechanisms that underlie cognitive processes. While measurement of some cognitive abilities differ in men and women, other tasks may appear "similar" yet be supported by alternate underlying cognitive strategies or neurological networks. Detecting which biological networks are vulnerable is important for disease detection; however, the recent surge to capture sex/gender differences of neurobiological mechanisms must simultaneously incorporate precision cognitive tasks to appreciate how sex-specific mechanisms function. We refer to these as "cognitive biomarkers" of disease. For example, Sundermann, Biegon, et al. (2016) demonstrated that the consequence of women having a sex-specific verbal memory advantage over men can potentially be a missed diagnosis. Women's "better" verbal skill masks underlying disease-related impairment in the early stage of disease, such that women then require more neurodegeneration than men before clinical impairment is detectable. Consequently, women are not assigned the MCI diagnosis, only to later meet criteria of AD with greater underlying pathology. To avoid this cascade and move into the era of precision medicine, it will be important to contextualize both cognitive and disease metrics with known sex/gender differences and sex-specific norms to improve diagnostic accuracy.

While this chapter highlights important sex/gender cognitive differences in language, memory, and executive function, some limitations need to be acknowledged. First, continued comparison of both cross-sectional and additional longitudinal studies will shed light on the effect of each cognitive domain and their interactions. Even knowledge of early life as well as sex/gender-specific processes, will illuminate development of those differences in late life. Second, we acknowledge that an intersectional analysis is warranted when examining health disparities. Given marked racial and ethnic disparities in the prevalence of AD, it will be important for future projects to examine the intersection of sex/gender with race/ethnicity in AD (Barnes et al., 2005; Manly et al., 2008; Vila-Castelar et al., 2020). Many of the studies discussed assume equivalence of sex and gender. Without measures of self-report, we do not adequately capture these biological and sociocultural implications. Lastly, many of the studies analyzed selected convenience samples, which may not hold true in communities representing the general population.

In summary, early cognitive changes in AD of memory, language, and executive functioning increasingly highlight the need to examine sex-specific differences (see Table 1). It is critical for future research to appreciate the complex interplay of neurological, neuroendocrine, developmental, and psychosocial factors that can affect cognitive trajectories in men and women. Attention to strategy differences as well

Table 1 Highlighted areas of sex/gender difference in verbal memory, language, and executive function.

Verbal memory *Ability to learn, retain, recall, or recognize verbal information*	Language *Production, repetition, comprehension, naming, reading, and writing*	Executive function *Broad abilities associated with complex, higher-level cognitive functions*
Healthy controls • Women outperform men across learning, immediate and delayed free verbal recall • Women's advantage in semantic clustering suggests better self-initiating categorization during learning and retrieval	**Laterality** • Language representation is lateralized asymmetrically; degree of left lateralization is a function of hand dominance • The semantic system has components of bilateral neural representation • The semantic network is reliant on within-hemisphere and cross-hemisphere interconnectivity	**Source of executive disruption in AD** • Executive functions are susceptible, earliest and sensitive cognitive symptoms of AD • Dysfunction may reflect executive dysfunction direct from frontal regions, or regions with cortico-cortical networks as well as frontal cortical-subcortical networks
Mild cognitive impairment (MCI) • Women outperform men on total verbal scores at learning and at delay recall • With their verbal memory advantage, women's diagnosis of MCI may be clinically detected only with more advanced disease load • Verbal memory advantage in women may also reflect availability of alternate neural substrates to compensate for disease	**Semantic dysfunction in AD** • In AD, the semantic network is affected, but syntactic and phonological systems remain intact • The semantic network in AD is the most sensitive marker of disease development	**Sex/gender differences in AD** • Sex/gender performance on executive function tasks can appear "equivalent," however the strategies employed may be mediated by alternate networks resulting in sex/gender-specific advantage • Disease risk may be predicated on the vulnerability of the network disrupted during the disease course
Alzheimer's disease (AD) • Men outperform women on verbal memory recall • With clear clinical manifestation of AD, women lose their verbal memory advantage and perform worse than the men	**Sex/gender differences in language in AD** • Sex-specific language networks differ in men and women in AD • Women's ability to retain linguistic and verbal memory may rely on alternate spared semantic mechanisms • Women's semantic skills may be preserved, because of their compensatory strategy or networks	**Cognitive compensation** • Sex differences may depend on ability to reorganize to mask underlying cognitive decline • Compensatory upregulation of skill, but it may mask underlying cognitive decline • Compensatory reorganization by recruiting skills to manage novel tasks • Women's sex-specific verbal memory advantage may be associated with recruitment of frontal regions

as accuracy will provide more meaningful measurement, detection, and treatment of a cognitive course. Together, the sex/gender influences of language, memory, and executive profiles provide critical and sensitive measures of disease risk.

Chapter highlights

- Sex differences in memory, language, and executive functioning have been described in cognitive healthy aging as well as in the AD continuum.
- The contribution of neurological, neurodevelopmental, and neuroendocrine, as well as psychological and psychosocial factors to the different cognitive trajectories in men and women need to be elucidated.
- Differences in performance, as well as strategy and accuracy, in neuropsychological tests of men and women might be exploited for more meaningful diagnostic tests.

Support

Support for Dr. Au was provided, in part, by National Institute on Aging grants AG054156; AG062109; AG049810; AG068753. Support for Dr. Foldi was provided by grants from NIH-National Institute of General Medicine—SC3GM122662 and by Professional Staff Congress—City University of New York, A49-211; A48-133.

References

Alzheimer's Association. (2019). Alzheimer facts and figures report. *Alzheimer's & Dementia: The Journal of the Alzheimer's Association*, *15*(3), 321–387. https://doi.org/10.1016/j.jalz.2019.01.010.

Banks, S. J., Shifflett, B., Berg, J. L., Sundermann, E., Peavy, G., Bondi, M. W., & Edland, S. D. (2019). Sex-specific composite scales for longitudinal studies of incipient Alzheimer's disease. *Alzheimers Dement (N Y)*, *5*, 508–514. https://doi.org/10.1016/j.trci.2019.07.003.

Barnes, L., Wilson, R. S., Li, Y., Aggarwal, N. T., Gilley, D. W., McCann, J. J., & Evans, D. A. (2005). Racial differences in the progression of cognitive decline in Alzheimer disease. *The American Journal of Geriatric Psychiatry*, *13*(11), 959–967.

Berenbaum, S., Baxter, L., Seidenberg, M., & Hermann, B. (1997). Role of the hippocampus in sex differences in verbal memory: Memory outcome following left anterior temporal lobectomy. *Neuropsychology*, *11*(4), 585–591.

Berger, J., Demin, K., Holtkamp, M., & Bengner, T. (2018). Female verbal memory advantage in temporal, but not frontal lobe epilepsy. *Epilepsy Research*, *139*, 129–134. https://doi.org/10.1016/j.eplepsyres.2017.11.018.

Berger, J., Oltmanns, F., Holtkamp, M., & Bengner, T. (2017). Sex differences in verbal and nonverbal learning before and after temporal lobe epilepsy surgery. *Epilepsy & Behavior*, *66*, 57–63. https://doi.org/10.1016/j.yebeh.2016.11.037.

Berlingeri, M., Danelli, L., Bottini, G., Sberna, M., & Paulesu, E. (2013). Reassessing the HAROLD model: Is the hemispheric asymmetry reduction in older adults a special case of compensatory-related utilisation of neural circuits? *Experimental Brain Research*, *224*(3), 393–410. https://doi.org/10.1007/s00221-012-3319-x.

Binder, J. R., & Desai, R. H. (2011). The neurobiology of semantic memory. *Trends in Cognitive Sciences*, *15*(11), 527–536. https://doi.org/10.1016/j.tics.2011.10.001.

Blumstein, S. E., Baker, E., & Goodglass, H. (1977). Phonological factors in auditory comprehension in aphasia. *Neuropsychologia*, *15*(1), 19–30. https://doi.org/10.1016/0028-3932(77)90111-7.

Bondi, M. W., Serody, A. B., Chan, A. S., Eberson-Shumate, S. C., Delis, D. C., Hansen, L. A., & Salmon, D. P. (2002). Cognitive and neuropathologic correlates of Stroop Color-Word Test performance in Alzheimer's disease. *Neuropsychology*, *16*(3), 335.

Bonelli, R. M., & Cummings, J. L. (2007). Frontal-subcortical circuitry and behavior. *Dialogues in Clinical Neuroscience*, *9*(2), 141–151.

Braak, H., & Braak, E. (1991). Neuropathological stageing of Alzheimer-related changes. *Acta Neuropathologica*, *82*(4), 239–259.

Braak, H., & Braak, E. (1995). Staging of Alzheimer's disease-related neurofibrillary changes. *Neurobiology of Aging*, *16*(3), 271–278.

Brookmeyer, R., Evans, D. A., Hebert, L., Langa, K. M., Heeringa, S. G., Plassman, B. L., & Kukull, W. A. (2011). National estimates of the prevalence of Alzheimer's disease in the United States. *Alzheimers Dement*, *7*(1), 61–73. https://doi.org/10.1016/j.jalz.2010.11.007.

Bruno, D., Grothe, M. J., Nierenberg, J., Teipel, S. J., Zetterberg, H., Blennow, K., & Pomara, N. (2015). The relationship between CSF tau markers, hippocampal volume and delayed primacy performance in cognitively intact elderly individuals. *Alzheimers Dement (Amst)*, *1*(1), 81–86. https://doi.org/10.1016/j.dadm.2014.11.002.

Buckley, R. F., Mormino, E. C., Rabin, J. S., Hohman, T. J., Landau, S., Hanseeuw, B. J., … Sperling, R. A. (2019). Sex differences in the Association of Global Amyloid and Regional tau Deposition Measured by positron emission tomography in clinically normal older adults. *JAMA Neurology*, *76*(5), 542–551. https://doi.org/10.1001/jamaneurol.2018.4693.

Burgess, P. W., Veitch, E., de Lacy Costello, A., & Shallice, T. (2000). The cognitive and neuroanatomical correlates of multitasking. *Neuropsychologia*, *38*(6), 848–863.

Cabeza, R. (2002). Hemispheric asymmetry reduction in older adults: The HAROLD model. *Psychology and Aging*, *17*(1), 85–100.

Cabeza, R., Albert, M., Belleville, S., Craik, F. I. M., Duarte, A., Grady, C. L., … Rajah, M. N. (2018). Maintenance, reserve and compensation: The cognitive neuroscience of healthy ageing. *Nature Reviews. Neuroscience*, *19*(11), 701–710. https://doi.org/10.1038/s41583-018-0068-2.

Cacciaglia, R., Molinuevo, J. L., Sánchez-Benavides, G., Falcón, C., Gramunt, N., Brugulat-Serrat, A., … ALFA Study. (2018). Episodic memory and executive functions in cognitively healthy individuals display distinct neuroanatomical correlates which are differentially modulated by aging. *Human Brain Mapping*, *39*(11), 4565–4579. https://doi.org/10.1002/hbm.24306.

Caldwell, J., Cummings, J. L., Banks, S. J., Palmqvist, S., & Hansson, O. (2019). Cognitively normal women with Alzheimer's disease proteinopathy show relative preservation of memory but not of hippocampal volume. *Alzheimer's Research & Therapy*, *11*(1), 109. https://doi.org/10.1186/s13195-019-0565-1.

Carter, C. L., Resnick, E. M., Mallampalli, M., & Kalbarczyk, A. (2012). Sex and gender differences in Alzheimer's disease: Recommendations for future research. *Journal of Women's Health (2002)*, *21*(10), 1018–1023. https://doi.org/10.1089/jwh.2012.3789.

Chomsky, N. (1957). *Syntactic structures*. The Hague: Mouton & Co.

Christakou, A., Halari, R., Smith, A. B., Ifkovits, E., Brammer, M., & Rubia, K. (2009). Sex-dependent age modulation of frontostriatal and temporo-parietal activation during cognitive control. *NeuroImage*, *48*(1), 223–236. https://doi.org/10.1016/j.neuroimage.2009.06.070.

Cross, C. P., Copping, L. T., & Campbell, A. (2011). Sex differences in impulsivity: A meta-analysis. *Psychological Bulletin*, *137*(1), 97.

Damasio, A. R. (1995). Toward a neurobiology of emotion and feeling: Operational concepts and hypotheses. *The Neuroscientist*, *1*(1), 19–25.

D'Antuono, G., Maini, M., Marin, D., Boccia, M., & Piccardi, L. (2020). Effect of ageing on verbal and visuo-spatial working memory: Evidence from 880 individuals. *Applied Neuropsychology. Adult*. https://doi.org/10.1080/23279095.2020.1732979.

Delis, D. C., Kaplan, E., Kramer, J. H., & Ober, B. A. (2000). *California Verbal Learning Test—II* (2nd ed.). San Antonio, TX: The Psychological Corporation.

Devereux, B. J., Clarke, A., Marouchos, A., & Tyler, L. K. (2013). Representational similarity analysis reveals commonalities and differences in the semantic processing of words and objects. *The Journal of Neuroscience: The Official Journal of the Society for Neuroscience*, *33*(48), 18906–18916. https://doi.org/10.1523/JNEUROSCI.3809-13.2013.

Diamond, A. (2013). Executive functions. *Annual Review of Psychology*, *64*, 135–168. https://doi.org/10.1146/annurev-psych-113011-143750.

Dickerson, B. C., Bakkour, A., Salat, D. H., Feczko, E., Pacheco, J., Greve, D. N., … Rosas, H. D. (2009). The cortical signature of Alzheimer's disease: Regionally specific cortical thinning relates to symptom severity in very mild to mild AD dementia and is detectable in asymptomatic amyloid-positive individuals. *Cerebral Cortex*, *19*(3), 497–510.

Duff, S. J., & Hampson, E. (2001). A sex difference on a novel spatial working memory task in humans. *Brain and Cognition*, *47*(3), 470–493.

Egli, S. C., Beck, I. R., Berres, M., Foldi, N. S., Monsch, A. U., & Sollberger, M. (2014). Serial position effects are sensitive predictors of conversion from MCI to Alzheimer's disease dementia. *Alzheimer's & Dementia*, *10*(5 Suppl), S420–S424. https://doi.org/10.1016/j.jalz.2013.09.012.

Fletcher, P., & Henson, R. (2001). Frontal lobes and human memory: Insights from functional neuroimaging. *Brain*, *124*(Pt 5), 849–881.

Foldi, N. S. (2011). Getting the hang of it: Preferential gist over verbatim story recall and the roles of attentional capacity and the episodic buffer in Alzheimer disease. *Journal of the International Neuropsychological Society*, *17*(1), 69–79. https://doi.org/10.1017/S1355617710001165.

Forseth, K. J., Kadipasaoglu, C. M., Conner, C. R., Hickok, G., Knight, R. T., & Tandon, N. (2018). A lexical semantic hub for heteromodal naming in middle fusiform gyrus. *Brain*, *141*(7), 2112–2126. https://doi.org/10.1093/brain/awy120.

Fridriksson, J., den Ouden, D. B., Hillis, A. E., Hickok, G., Rorden, C., Basilakos, A., … Bonilha, L. (2018). Anatomy of aphasia revisited. *Brain: A Journal of Neurology*, *141*(3), 848–862. https://doi.org/10.1093/brain/awx363.

Friederici, A. D., Opitz, B., & von Cramon, D. Y. (2000). Segregating semantic and syntactic aspects of processing in the human brain: An fMRI investigation of different word types. *Cerebral Cortex*, *10*(7), 698–705. https://doi.org/10.1093/cercor/10.7.698.

Funahashi, S. (2017). Working memory in the prefrontal cortex. *Brain Sciences*, *7*(5), 49.

Gainotti, G., Marra, C., Villa, G., Parlato, V., & Chiarotti, F. (1998). Sensitivity and specificity of some neuropsychological markers of Alzheimer's dementia. *Alzheimer Disease and Associated Disorders*, *12*, 152–162.

Gainotti, G., Spinelli, P., Scaricamazza, E., & Marra, C. (2013). Asymmetries in gender-related familiarity with different semantic categories. Data from normal adults. *Behavioural Neurology, 27*(2), 175–181. https://doi.org/10.3233/BEN-120277.

Golchert, J., Roehr, S., Luck, T., Wagner, M., Fuchs, A., Wiese, B., … Riedel-Heller, S. G. (2019). Women outperform men in verbal episodic memory even in oldest-old age: 13-year longitudinal results of the AgeCoDe/AgeQualiDe study. *Journal of Alzheimer's Disease, 69*(3), 857–869. https://doi.org/10.3233/JAD-180949.

Goldstein, J., Jerram, M., Poldrack, R., Anagnoson, R., Breiter, H., Makris, N., … Seidman, L. (2005). Sex differences in prefrontal cortical brain activity during fMRI of auditory verbal working memory. *Neuropsychology, 19*(4), 509–519. https://doi.org/10.1037/0894-4105.19.4.509.

Gorno-Tempini, M. L., Hillis, A. E., Weintraub, S., Kertesz, A., Mendez, M., Cappa, S. F., … Grossman, M. (2011). Classification of primary progressive aphasia and its variants. *Neurology, 76*(11), 1006–1014. https://doi.org/10.1212/WNL.0b013e31821103e6.

Grady, C., Sarraf, S., Saverino, C., & Campbell, K. (2016). Age differences in the functional interactions among the default, frontoparietal control, and dorsal attention networks. *Neurobiology of Aging, 41*, 159–172.

Grafman, J., & Litvan, I. (1999). Importance of deficits in executive functions. *The Lancet, 354*(9194), 1921–1923.

Grissom, N., & Reyes, T. (2019). Let's call the whole thing off: Evaluating gender and sex differences in executive function. *Neuropsychopharmacology, 44*(1), 86–96.

Grossman, M. (2018). Linguistic aspects of primary progressive aphasia. *Annual Review of Linguistics, 4*, 377–403. https://doi.org/10.1146/annurev-linguistics-011516-034253.

Guarino, A., Favieri, F., Boncompagni, I., Agostini, F., Cantone, M., & Casagrande, M. (2019). Executive functions in Alzheimer disease: A systematic review. *Frontiers in Aging Neuroscience, 10*, 437.

Henderson, V., & Buckwalter, J. (1994). Cognitive deficits of men and women with Alzheimer's disease. *Neurology, 44*(1), 90–96.

Hickok, G., & Poeppel, D. (2004). Dorsal and ventral streams: A framework for understanding aspects of the functional anatomy of language. *Cognition, 92*(1–2), 67–99. https://doi.org/10.1016/j.cognition.2003.10.011.

Hickok, G., & Poeppel, D. (2007). The cortical organization of speech processing. *Nature Reviews. Neuroscience, 8*(5), 393–402. https://doi.org/10.1038/nrn2113.

Hickok, G., & Poeppel, D. (2015). Neural basis of speech perception. *Handbook of Clinical Neurology, 129*, 149–160. https://doi.org/10.1016/B978-0-444-62630-1.00008-1.

Hickok, G., Rogalsky, C., Matchin, W., Basilakos, A., Cai, J., Pillay, S., … Fridriksson, J. (2018). Neural networks supporting audiovisual integration for speech: A large-scale lesion study. *Cortex, 103*, 360–371. https://doi.org/10.1016/j.cortex.2018.03.030.

Hill, A., Laird, A., & Robinson, J. (2014). Gender differences in working memory networks: A BrainMap meta-analysis. *Biological Psychology, 102*, 18–29. https://doi.org/10.1016/j.biopsycho.2014.06.008.

Hirni, D. I., Kivisaari, S. L., Monsch, A. U., & Taylor, K. I. (2013). Distinct neuroanatomical bases of episodic and semantic memory performance in Alzheimer's disease. *Neuropsychologia, 51*(5), 930–937. https://doi.org/10.1016/j.neuropsychologia.2013.01.013.

Honarpisheh, P., & McCullough, L. D. (2019). Sex as a biological variable in the pathology and pharmacology of neurodegenerative and neurovascular diseases. *British Journal of Pharmacology, 176*(21), 4173–4192. https://doi.org/10.1111/bph.14675.

Howieson, D. B., Mattek, N., Seeyle, A. M., Dodge, H. H., Wasserman, D., Zitzelberger, T., & Jeffrey, K. (2011). Serial position effects in mild cognitive impairment. *Journal of Clinical* and *Experimental Neuropsychology, 33*(3), 292–299. https://doi.org/10.1080/13803395.20 10.516742.

Hua, X., Hibar, D. P., Lee, S., Toga, A. W., Jack, C. R., Jr., Weiner, M. W., et al. (2010). Sex and age differences in atrophic rates: An ADNI study with n=1368 MRI scans. *Neurobiology of Aging, 31*, 1463–1480.

Humphries, C., Willard, K., Buchsbaum, B., & Hickok, G. (2001). Role of anterior temporal cortex in auditory sentence comprehension: An fMRI study. *Neuroreport, 12*(8), 1749–1752. https://doi.org/10.1097/00001756-200106130-00046.

Irish, M., Addis, D. R., Hodges, J. R., & Piguet, O. (2012). Considering the role of semantic memory in episodic future thinking: Evidence from semantic dementia. *Brain, 135*(7), 2178–2191. https://doi.org/10.1093/brain/aws119.

Jack, C. R., Jr., Bennett, D. A., Blennow, K., Carrillo, M. C., Dunn, B., Haeberlein, S. B., … Contributors. (2018). NIA-AA research framework: Toward a biological definition of Alzheimer's disease. *Alzheimers Dement, 14*(4), 535–562. https://doi.org/10.1016/j.jalz.2018.02.018.

Jung, M., Mody, M., Fujioka, T., Kimura, Y., Okazawa, H., & Kosaka, H. (2019). Sex differences in white matter pathways related to language ability. *Frontiers in Neuroscience, 13*, 898. https://doi.org/10.3389/fnins.2019.00898.

Kasper, E., Brueggen, K., Grothe, M. J., Bruno, D., Pomara, N., Unterauer, E., … Buerger, K. (2016). Neuronal correlates of serial position performance in amnestic mild cognitive impairment. *Neuropsychology, 30*(8), 906–914. pii: 2016-24163-001.

Koran, M., Wagener, M., Hohman, T. J., & The Alzheimer's Neuroimaging Initiative. (2017). Sex differences in the association between AD biomarkers and cognitive decline. *Brain Imaging and Behavior, 11*(1), 205–213. https://doi.org/10.1007/s11682-016-9523-8.

Kramer, J., Delis, D., & Daniel, M. (1988). Sex differences in verbal learning. *Journal of Clinical Psychology, 44*(6), 907–915. https://doi.org/10.1002/1097-4679(198811)44:6<907::AID-JCLP2270440610>3.0.CO;2-8.

Lavrencic, L. M., Richardson, C., Harrison, S. L., Muniz-Terrera, G., Keage, H. A. D., Brittain, K., … Stephan, B. C. M. (2018). Is there a link between cognitive reserve and cognitive function in the oldest-old? *The Journals of Gerontology. Series A, Biological Sciences and Medical Sciences, 73*(4), 499–505. https://doi.org/10.1093/gerona/glx140.

Lejbak, L., Vrbancic, M., & Crossley, M. (2009). The female advantage in object location memory is robust to verbalizability and mode of presentation of test stimuli. *Brain and Cognition, 69*(1), 148–153.

Lenzi, D., Serra, L., Perri, R., Pantano, P., Lenzi, G. L., Paulesu, E., … Macaluso, E. (2011). Single domain amnestic MCI: A multiple cognitive domains fMRI investigation. *Neurobiology of Aging, 32*(9), 1542–1557. https://doi.org/10.1016/j.neurobiolaging.2009.09.006.

Levy, G., Jacobs, D. M., Tang, M. X., Côté, L. J., Louis, E. D., Alfaro, B., … Marder, K. (2002). Memory and executive function impairment predict dementia in Parkinson's disease. *Movement Disorders: Official Journal of the Movement Disorder Society, 17*(6), 1221–1226.

Li, G., Nie, J., Wang, L., Shi, F., Lyall, A. E., Lin, W., … Shen, D. (2014). Mapping long hemispheric asymmetries of the human cerebral cortex from birth to 2 years of age. *Cerebral Cortex, 24*(5), 1289–1300. https://doi.org/10.1093/cercor/bhs413.

Liesinger, A. M., Graff-Radford, N. R., Duara, R., Carter, R. E., Hanna Al-Shaikh, F. S., Koga, S., … Murray, M. E. (2018). Sex and age interact to determine clinicopathologic differences in Alzheimer's disease. *Acta Neuropathologica, 136*(6), 873–885. https://doi.org/10.1007/s00401-018-1908-x.

Malpetti, M., Ballarini, T., Presotto, L., Garibotto, V., Tettamanti, M., & Perani, D. (2017). Gender differences in healthy aging and Alzheimer's Dementia: A 18 F-FDG-PET study of brain and cognitive reserve. *Human Brain Mapping.* https://doi.org/10.1002/hbm.23659.

Manly, J., Tang, M., Schupf, N., Stern, Y., Vonsattel, J., & Mayeux, R. (2008). Frequency and course of mild cognitive impairment in a multiethnic community. *Annals of Neurology: Official Journal of the American Neurological Association and the Child Neurology Society, 63*(4), 494–506.

Matchin, W., & Hickok, G. (2020). The cortical organization of syntax. *Cerebral Cortex, 30*(3), 1481–1498. https://doi.org/10.1093/cercor/bhz180.

McCarrey, A., An, Y., Kitner-Triolo, M., Ferrucci, L., & Resnick, S. (2016). Sex differences in cognitive trajectories in clinically normal older adults. *Psychology and Aging, 31*(2), 166–175. https://doi.org/10.1037/pag0000070.

Mielke, M., Vemuri, P., & Rocca, W. (2014). Clinical epidemiology of Alzheimer's disease: Assessing sex and gender differences. *Clinical Epidemiology, 6*, 37–48. https://doi.org/10.2147/CLEP.S37929.

Milberg, W., & Hebben, N. (2013). In L. Ashendorf, R. Swenson, & D. Libon (Eds.), *Historical foundations of the process approach and modern neuropsychology at the Boston VA Medical Center* (pp. 31–45). Oxford University Press.

Millar, P. R., Balota, D. A., Maddox, G. B., Duchek, J. M., Aschenbrenner, A. J., Fagan, A. M., … Morris, J. C. (2017). Process dissociation analyses of memory changes in healthy aging, preclinical, and very mild Alzheimer disease: Evidence for isolated recollection deficits. *Neuropsychology, 31*(7), 708–723. https://doi.org/10.1037/neu0000352.

Miller, B. T., & D'Esposito, M. (2005). Searching for "the top" in top-down control. *Neuron, 48*(4), 535–538.

Miller, I. N., Himali, J. J., Beiser, A. S., Murabito, J. M., Seshadri, S., Wolf, P. A., & Au, R. (2015). Normative data for the cognitively intact oldest-old: The Framingham Heart Study. *Experimental Aging Research, 41*(4), 386–409. https://doi.org/10.1080/0361073X.2015.1053755.

Nebel, R. A., Aggarwal, N. T., Barnes, L. L., Gallagher, A., Goldstein, J. M., Kantarci, K., & Maki, P. M. (2018). Understanding the impact of sex and gender in Alzheimer's disease: A call to action. *Alzheimer's & Dementia, 14*(9), 1171–1183. https://doi.org/10.1016/j.jalz.2018.04.008.

Nenert, R., Allendorfer, J. B., Martin, A. M., Banks, C., Vannest, J., Holland, S. K., & Szaflarski, J. P. (2017). Age-related language lateralization assessed by fMRI: The effects of sex and handedness. *Brain Research, 1674*, 20–35. https://doi.org/10.1016/j.brainres.2017.08.021.

Ojemann, J., & Kelley, W. (2002). The frontal lobe role in memory: A review of convergent evidence and implications for the Wada memory test. *Epilepsy & Behavior, 3*(4), 309–315.

Perani, D., Saccuman, M. C., Scifo, P., Anwander, A., Spada, D., Baldoli, C., … Friederici, A. (2011). The neural language networks at birth. *Proceedings of the National Academy of Sciences of the United States of America, 108*(38), 16056–16061.

Petersen, R., Roberts, R., Knopman, D., Geda, Y., Cha, R., Pankratz, V., … Rocca, W. (2010). Prevalence of mild cognitive impairment is higher in men. The Mayo Clinic study of aging. *Neurology, 75*(10), 889–897. https://doi.org/10.1212/WNL.0b013e3181f11d85.

Phillips, M., Rogers, P., Haworth, J., Bayer, A., & Tales, A. (2013). Intra-individual reaction time variability in mild cognitive impairment and Alzheimer's disease: Gender, processing load and speed factors. *PLoS One, 8*(6), e65712. https://doi.org/10.1371/journal.pone.0065712. PMID: 23762413; PMCID: PMC3677873.

Poeppel, D., Emmorey, K., Hickok, G., & Pylkkanen, L. (2012). Towards a new neurobiology of language. *Journal of Neuroscience, 32*(41), 14125–14131. https://doi.org/10.1523/JNEUROSCI.3244-12.2012.

Poeppel, D., & Hickok, G. (2004). Towards a new functional anatomy of language. *Cognition, 92*(1–2), 1–12. https://doi.org/10.1016/j.cognition.2003.11.001.

Powers, J. P., McMillan, C. T., Brun, C. C., Yushkevich, P. A., Zhang, H., Gee, J. C., & Grossman, M. (2013). White matter disease correlates with lexical retrieval deficits in primary progressive aphasia. *Frontiers in Neurology*, 4, 212. https://doi.org/10.3389/fneur.2013.00212.

Pusswald, G., Lehrner, J., Hagmann, M., Dal-Bianco, P., Benke, T., Marksteiner, J., ... Schmidt, R. (2015). Gender-specific differences in cognitive profiles of patients with Alzheimer's Disease: Results of the prospective dementia registry Austria (PRODEM-Austria). *Journal of Alzheimer's Disease*, 46(3), 631–637. https://doi.org/10.3233/JAD-150188.

Rabinovici, G. D., Stephens, M. L., & Possin, K. L. (2015). Executive dysfunction. *Continuum (Minneapolis, Minn.)*, 21(3 behavioral neurology and neuropsychiatry), 646–659. https://doi.org/10.1212/01.CON.0000466658.05156.54.

Reber, J., & Tranel, D. (2017). Sex differences in the functional lateralization of emotion and decision making in the human brain. *Journal of Neuroscience Research*, 95(1–2), 270–278.

Rey, A. (1958). Memorisation d'une serie de 15 mots en 5 répétitions. In *L'examen clinique en psychologie* (pp. 26–42). Paris: Press Universitaires de France.

Roberts, R., Geda, Y., Knopman, D., Cha, R., Pankratz, V., Boeve, B., ... Petersen, R. (2012). The incidence of MCI differs by subtype and is higher in men: The Mayo Clinic Study of Aging. *Neurology*, 78(5), 342–351. pii:WNL203376.

Roberts, R. O., Knopman, D. S., Mielke, M. M., Cha, R. H., Pankratz, V. S., Christianson, T. J., ... Rocca, W. A. (2014). Higher risk of progression to dementia in mild cognitive impairment cases who revert to normal. *Neurology*, 82(4), 317–325.

Sachdev, P. S., Lipnicki, D. M., Crawford, J., Reppermund, S., Kochan, N. A., Trollor, J. N., ... Mather, K. A. (2012). Risk profiles for mild cognitive impairment vary by age and sex: The Sydney Memory and Ageing Study. *The American Journal of Geriatric Psychiatry*, 20(10), 854–865.

Salat, D. H., Kaye, J. A., & Janowsky, J. S. (2001). Selective preservation and degeneration within the prefrontal cortex in aging and Alzheimer disease. *Archives of Neurology*, 58(9), 1403–1408.

Salmon, D. P. (2000). Disorders of memory in Alzheimer's disease. In *Vol. 2. Handbook of neuropsychology: Memory and its disorders* (2nd ed., pp. 155–195). Amsterdam: Elsevier.

Schmidt, M. (1996). *Rey auditory verbal learning test: A handbook*. Los Angeles: Western Psychological Services.

Seeley, W., Crawford, R., Zhou, J., Miller, B., & Greicius, M. (2009). Neurodegenerative diseases target large-scale human brain networks. *Neuron*, 62(1), 42–52. https://doi.org/10.1016/j.neuron.2009.03.024.

Skeide, M. A., Brauer, J., & Friederici, A. D. (2014). Syntax gradually segregates from semantics in the developing brain. *NeuroImage*, 100, 106–111. https://doi.org/10.1016/j.neuroimage.2014.05.080.

Sommer, I. E., Aleman, A., Bouma, A., & Kahn, R. S. (2004). Do women really have more bilateral language representation than men? A meta-analysis of functional imaging studies. *Brain*, 127(Pt 8), 1845–1852. https://doi.org/10.1093/brain/awh207.

Staffaroni, A. M., Bajorek, L., Casaletto, K. B., Cobigo, Y., Goh, S. M., Wolf, A., ... ARTFL/LEFFTDS Consortium. (2020). Assessment of executive function declines in presymptomatic and mildly symptomatic familial frontotemporal dementia: NIH-EXAMINER as a potential clinical trial endpoint. *Alzheimers Dement*, 16(1), 11–21. https://doi.org/10.1016/j.jalz.2019.01.012.

Stern, Y. (2002). What is cognitive reserve? Theory and research application of the reserve concept. *Journal of the International Neuropsychological Society*, 8(3), 448–460.

Stern, Y. (2012). Cognitive reserve in ageing and Alzheimer's disease. *The Lancet. Neurology*, *11*(11), 1006–1012. https://doi.org/10.1016/S1474-4422(12)70191-6.

Stuss, D., & Alexander, M. (2000). Executive functions and the frontal lobes: A conceptual view. *Psychological Research*, *63*(3–4), 289–298.

Stuss, D. T., & Knight, R. T. (2013). *Principles of frontal lobe function*. New York: Oxford University Press.

Stuss, D. T., Shallice, T., Alexander, M. P., & Picton, T. W. (1995). A multidisciplinary approach to anterior attentional functions. *Annals of the New York Academy of Sciences*, *769*(1), 191–212.

Sundermann, E. E., Biegon, A., Rubin, L. H., Lipton, R. B., Landau, S., & Maki, P. M. (2017). Does the female advantage in verbal memory contribute to underestimating Alzheimer's disease pathology in women versus men? *Journal of Alzheimers Disease*, *56*(3), 947–957. https://doi.org/10.3233/JAD-160716.

Sundermann, E. E., Biegon, A., Rubin, L. H., Lipton, R. B., Mowrey, W., Landau, S., … Alzheimer's Disease Neuroimaging Initiative. (2016). Better verbal memory in women than men in MCI despite similar levels of hippocampal atrophy. *Neurology*, *86*(15), 1368–1376. https://doi.org/10.1212/WNL.0000000000002570.

Sundermann, E. E., Maki, P., Biegon, A., Lipton, R., Mielke, M., Machulda, M., … Alzheimer's Disease Neuroimaging Initiative. (2019). Sex-specific norms for verbal memory tests may improve diagnostic accuracy of amnestic MCI. *Neurology*, *93*(20), e1881–e1889. https://doi.org/10.1212/WNL.0000000000008467.

Sundermann, E. E., Maki, P. M., Reddy, S., Bondi, M. W., Biegon, A., & Alzheimer's Disease Neuroimaging Initiative. (2020). Women's higher brain metabolic rate compensates for early Alzheimer's pathology. *Alzheimer's & Dementia (Amsterdam, Netherlands)*, *12*(1), e12121. https://doi.org/10.1002/dad2.12121.

Sundermann, E. E., Maki, P., Rubin, L., Lipton, R., Landau, S., Biegon, A., & Alzheimer's Disease Neuroimaging Initiative. (2016). Female advantage in verbal memory: Evidence of sex-specific cognitive reserve. *Neurology*, *87*(18), 1916–1924. pii:WNL.0000000000003288.

Sutterer, M. J., Koscik, T. R., & Tranel, D. (2015). Sex-related functional asymmetry of the ventromedial prefrontal cortex in regard to decision-making under risk and ambiguity. *Neuropsychologia*, *75*, 265–273.

Thomas, K. R., Edmonds, E. C., Eppig, J., Salmon, D. P., Bondi, M. W., & Initi, A. s. D. N. (2018). Using neuropsychological process scores to identify subtle cognitive decline and predict progression to mild cognitive impairment. *Journal of Alzheimers Disease*, *64*(1), 195–204. https://doi.org/10.3233/Jad-180229.

Tranel, D., & Bechara, A. (2009). Sex-related functional asymmetry of the amygdala: Preliminary evidence using a case-matched lesion approach. *Neurocase*, *15*(3), 217–234.

Tranel, D., Damasio, H., Denburg, N. L., & Bechara, A. (2005). Does gender play a role in functional asymmetry of ventromedial prefrontal cortex? *Brain*, *128*(12), 2872–2881.

Tschanz, J. T., Corcoran, C. D., Schwartz, S., Treiber, K., Green, R. C., Norton, M. C., … Lyketsos, C. G. (2011). Progression of cognitive, functional, and neuropsychiatric symptom domains in a population cohort with Alzheimer dementia: The Cache County dementia progression study. *The American Journal of Geriatric Psychiatry: Official Journal of the American Association for Geriatric Psychiatry*, *19*(6), 532–542. https://doi.org/10.1097/JGP.0b013e3181faec23.

Vila-Castelar, C., Guzmán-Vélez, E., Pardilla-Delgado, E., Buckley, R. F., Bocanegra, Y., Baena, A., … Quiroz, Y. T. (2020). Examining sex differences in markers of cognition and neurodegeneration in autosomal dominant Alzheimer's disease: Preliminary findings from the Colombian Alzheimer's Prevention Initiative Biomarker Study. *Journal of Alzheimer's Disease: JAD*, *77*(4), 1743–1753. https://doi.org/10.3233/JAD-200723.

Vonk, J. M. J., Bouteloup, V., Mangin, J. F., Dubois, B., Blanc, F., Gabelle, A., … MEMENTO Cohort Study Group. (2020). Semantic loss marks early Alzheimer's disease-related neurodegeneration in older adults without dementia. *Alzheimers Dement (Amst)*, *12*(1), e12066. https://doi.org/10.1002/dad2.12066.

Wallentin, M. (2009). Putative sex differences in verbal abilities and language cortex: A critical review. *Brain and Language*, *108*(3), 175–183. https://doi.org/10.1016/j.bandl.2008.07.001.

Waters, H., & Schreiber, L. (1991). Sex differences in elaborative strategies: A developmental analysis. *Journal of Experimental Child Psychology*, *52*(3), 319–335.

Weintraub, S., Wicklund, A., & Salmon, D. (2012). The neuropsychological profile of Alzheimer disease. *Cold Spring Harbor Perspectives in Medicine*, *2*(4), a006171. https://doi.org/10.1101/cshperspect.a006171.

Welsh, K., Butters, N., Mohs, R., Beekly, D., Edland, S., Fillenbaum, G., & Heyman, A. (1994). The consortium to establish a registry for Alzheimer's Disease (CERAD). Part V. A normative study of the neuropsychological battery. *Neurology*, *44*(4), 609.

Wilson, R. S., Yu, L., Lamar, M., Schneider, J. A., Boyle, P. A., & Bennett, D. A. (2019). Education and cognitive reserve in old age. *Neurology*, *92*(10), e1041–e1050. https://doi.org/10.1212/wnl.0000000000007036.

CHAPTER 7

Sex differences in psychiatric disorders and their implication for dementia

Ewelina Biskup[a,b,c], Valeria Jordan[a], Beatrice Nasta[a,d], and Katrin Rauen[a,d,e]

[a]*Women's Brain Project, Guntershausen, Switzerland*
[b]*Department of Advanced Biomedical Sciences, Federico II University of Naples, Naples, Italy*
[c]*College of Clinical Medicine, Shanghai University of Medicine and Health Sciences, Shanghai, China*
[d]*Department of Geriatric Psychiatry, Psychiatric Hospital Zurich, University of Zurich, Zurich, Switzerland*
[e]*Institute for Stroke and Dementia Research, University Hospital, LMU Munich, Munich, Germany*

Abbreviations

BPSD	Behavioral and Psychological Symptoms of Dementia
ICD-10	International Classification of Diseases, 10th revision
MMSE	Mini-Mental State Examination
NPI-Q	Neuropsychiatric Inventory Questionnaire
OECD	Organisation for Economic Co-operation and Development
OR	Odds Ratio
SSRI	Selective Serotonin Reuptake Inhibitor
WHO	World Health Organization

Psychiatric disorders matter as modifiable risk factors for dementia over the entire life span

Psychiatric disorders are a major global health burden and play a key role in most of the potentially modifiable risk factors for dementia over the entire life span. According to the 2020 *Lancet* Commission report, 12 modifiable risk factors occur during early, mid, and later life accounting for up to 40% of dementia risk worldwide (see also Chapter 10 on lifestyle risk factors and Chapter 12 on socioeconomic risk factors) (Livingston, Huntley, Sommerlad, et al., 2020). This proposed model, covering the 12 life-course risk factors that may theoretically help to prevent or delay dementia, needs our attention from a psychiatric perspective. Psychiatric disorders play a major role in at least 7 out of these 12 modifiable risk factors from early childhood to later life, and thus impact at least 24% out of 40% of dementia risk worldwide (Fig. 1). Low education and of a lower standard during early life accounts for 7% of dementia risk and is well-known to affect mental health due to socioeconomic inequalities (Reiss, 2013). Excessive alcohol consumption during midlife, defined as a weekly alcohol intake beyond 21 units (168 g), is associated with brain atrophy and cognitive and physical impairment, and its prevention might reduce the risk of developing early onset dementia, i.e., age at onset below 65 years, by 1%. Although alcohol disorders affect more males than females, namely 16.5% of males versus only 4% of females, they increase the risk of developing dementia about threefold in both sexes (Schwarzinger, Pollock, Hasan, Dufouil, & Rehm, 2018). Thus, treating patients' alcohol dependency is important for the prevention of early onset dementia regardless of sex.

Obesity accounts for 1% of dementia risk during midlife and is at least partially associated with psychiatric conditions such as depression, anxiety, or eating disorders in both sexes (Brumpton, Langhammer, Romundstad, Chen, & Mai, 2013; Tronieri, Wurst, Pearl, & Allison, 2017; Udo, McKee, White, et al., 2013). In contrast to common assumptions, males and females report similar histories and symptoms of binge eating, with males experiencing worse metabolic health compared to females (Udo et al., 2013). Smoking impacts 5% of dementia risk worldwide, and is thus another important and potentially modifiable risk factor for dementia during later life (Livingston et al., 2020). According to the 10th revision of the International Classification of Diseases (ICD-10), tobacco consumption, like alcohol consumption, is a behavioral disorder through psychotropic substances and has most likely a bidirectional relation to psychiatric disorders such as depression and anxiety (Fluharty, Taylor, Grabski, & Munafò, 2017). Smoking seems to affect males and females differently; the evidence is sparse and controversial in terms of the bidirectional relation between smoking and depression, and to date inconclusive.

Furthermore, depression is undoubtedly a potentially modifiable risk factor for dementia and accounts for 4% of the population-attributable fraction (Livingston et al., 2020). Depressive symptoms in mid to later life are associated with risk of developing dementia, and it is important to differentiate depressive symptoms as either a pure psychiatric disease or as a prodrome of Alzheimer's disease. It is worthy of note that recurrent depression during mid and later life is particularly associated with vascular dementia, with an adjusted hazard ratio of 3.5 compared to 1.9 for Alzheimer's disease (Barnes, Yaffe, Byers, et al., 2012). These results have been adjusted for sex, race and education for mid and later life periods, but they have not been separately reported for both sexes so far, thus, potential sex- and gender-related differences in dementia risks remain underreported and unclear. Likewise, social isolation accounts for 4% of the population-attributable fraction of potentially modifiable risk factors for dementia and most probably both sexes are equally affected (Livingston et al., 2020). However, social isolation is a key feature in psychiatric disorders such as depression, anxiety, social phobia, psychosis, and at least in some cases of psychotropic drugs addiction. Finally, physical inactivity is relevant in most psychiatric diseases due to the lack of motivation, power, willingness, and eagerness, and is relevant as a potentially modifiable risk factor in 2% of dementia risk.

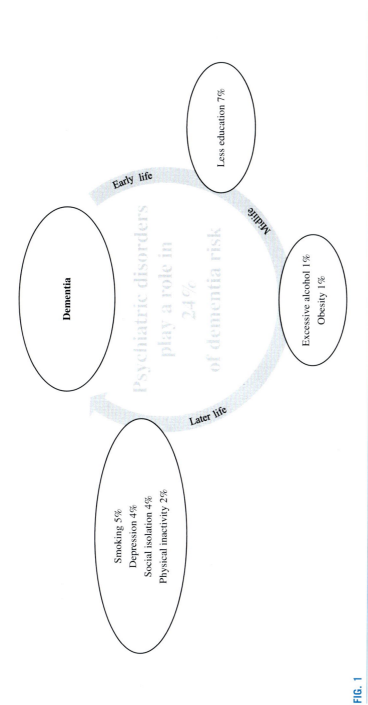

FIG. 1

According to the Lancet Commission report 2020 (Livingston et al., 2020), a 12 risk factor life-course model of dementia prevention has been suggested, helping to theoretically prevent or delay dementia. Analyzing this population-attributable fraction of modifiable risk factors from a psychiatric perspective uncovers that most, namely 7 out of 12, risk factors for dementia are related to psychiatric disorders and account for 24% out of 40% of dementia risk worldwide. Thus, identifying psychiatric disorders early and providing efficient treatment—besides the tremendous stigma of mental health diseases—is a major challenge with utmost relevance in dementia prevention.

Taken together, at least 24 out of 40% modifiable dementia risk is related to psychiatric disorders. This population attributable fraction is related to 7 out of 12 potentially modifiable risk factors for dementia. Thus, firstly, good mental health is a key player in preventing dementia and, secondly, reducing stigma of mental illness is most relevant to increase prevention, early diagnosis, and treatment of psychiatric disorders as risk factors or prodrome of dementia.

Major depression: A relevant modifiable risk factor for dementia with sex- and gender-related implications

Major depression is a huge global burden that is still stigmatized worldwide, despite it being curable; the diagnostic criteria of depression according to the ICD-10 are given in Table 1 (Dilling et al., 2016). The World Health Organization (WHO) has ranked major depression as the third largest contributor to the current global burden of disease, with females being affected twice as often as males. The WHO estimates that, by 2030, major depression will be the leading cause of the global burden of disease (Malhi & Mann, 2018; Rauen, Vetter, Eisele, et al., 2020; World Health Organization, 2008). The lifetime risk of major depression is estimated to be 15–18% (Bromet, Andrade, Hwang, et al., 2011; Kessler & Bromet, 2013), and it is of note that the global burden of disease study ranked major depression for all ages and both sexes within the highest disability class along with active psychosis, severe migraine, quadriplegia, and terminal stage cancer (World Health Organization, 2008).

Previous assumptions that affective disorders are equally distributed between the sexes prior to puberty, and that their distribution changes thereafter to a male to female ratio of 1:2 throughout the entire adult life span (Bale, 2019; Kaczkurkin, Raznahan, & Satterthwaite, 2019; Rauen et al., 2020), have been challenged. Currently, there is increasing evidence that sex- and gender-related differences have already emerged at age 12, with an odds ratio of 2.4, peaking during adolescence (age 13–16 years) to a threefold higher risk of depression in females compared to males. Thereafter, females maintain a stable twofold increased risk of depression compared to males over the adult life span (Salk, Hyde, & Abramson, 2017). A recent meta-analysis on the relationship between income inequality and magnitude of the gender difference in depression found little to no evidence of a relationship (Salk et al., 2017), a counterintuitive finding that calls for our attention and suggests that gender equity might have both beneficial and detrimental effects on females' mental health. Currently, the multifactorial pathogenesis of sex- and gender-related disparity in depression is not fully clear. To date, genetic factors, sex hormones, and/or gender-related educational issues have been discussed (Bale, 2019; Kaczkurkin et al., 2019).

More than two decades ago, the neuroprotective effect of estrogen with respect to neuronal degeneration had been suggested and the increased risk to females of developing Alzheimer's disease and/or depression after postmenopausal estrogen withdrawal emphasized (see also Chapters 2 and 9) (Seeman, 1997). In addition to the beneficial effect of estrogens, this latter review pinpoints the detrimental cyclic

Table 1 Diagnostic criteria of depression according to the International Classification of Diseases (ICD-10: F32).

General criteria	
G1	Duration of depressive symptoms for at least 2 weeks
G2	No history of manic or hypomanic episodes (ICD-10: F30)
G3	Depressive symptoms are not caused by psychotropic drugs (ICD-10: F1) or by organic brain diseases (ICD-10: F0)
Specific criteria	
A	General criteria G1–G3 are present
B	At least two out of three core features of depression are present: (1) depressive symptoms independent from circumstances (2) Lack of interest or joy with respect to usually pleasant activities (3) Reduced motivation or increased fatigue
C	One or more symptoms of: (1) Lack of confidence or self-worth (2) Unfounded feelings of guilt (3) Repetitive thoughts of death or suicidal ideations or suicidal behavior (4) Complaints or evidence of reduced ability to think or concentrate or indecision (5) Psychomotor agitation or inhibition (6) Sleep disorder (7) Lack of appetite or increased appetite with weight changes
Severity	
Mild depression	General criteria G1–G3, two criteria of B and a total of 3–4 symptoms out of B and C are present
Moderate depression	General criteria G1–G3, two criteria of B and a total of 5–6 symptoms out of B and C are present
Severe depression = Major depression	General criteria G1–G3, three criteria of B and a total of ≥7 symptoms out of B and C are present, no hallucinations

Major depression is a synonym for severe depression, as indicated (table was translated and modified) (Dilling, Mombour, Schmidt, & Schulte-Markwort, 2016).

fluctuations of estrogens and progesterone that enhance the female stress response as well as personality factors that might further enhance the female susceptibility to depression. In detail, females invest their emotions more frequently in relationships compared to males and thus suffer not only from their own detrimental life events but from those of their close network. Moreover, females tend to internalize their feelings more often, blaming themselves for incompetence or failure and have a ruminative passive behavior compared to males (Seeman, 1997). Furthermore, the psychopathology in depression differs between females and males, with females suffering more often from atypical signs such as weight gain, bulimia, anxiety, hypersomnia, and somatoform disorders, while males are more prone to impulsiveness and substance dependencies (Blanco, Vesga-López, Stewart, et al., 2012; Marcus, Kerber, Rush, et al., 2008; Vetter, Spiller, Cathomas, et al., 2020). These sex- and gender-related differences in the prevalence and psychopathology of depression bear the risk of over-diagnosing females and overlooking major depression in males (Salk et al., 2017).

The HUNT study, having analyzed 28,916 participants (50.2% women) aged 30–60 years, suggests that psychological distress, characterized by general symptoms of depression and anxiety, predicts dementia 25 years later with a hazard ratio of 1.3, which can be reduced by physical activity during midlife—albeit adjusted for age, sex, education, marital status, smoking, alcohol, longstanding illnesses—results are not given for both sexes separately, and thus need our focus in the future (Zotcheva, Bergh, Selbæk, et al., 2018). It is well-known that depression prevalence does not differ between high-, middle-, and low-income countries, underlining that its causes go far beyond modern lifestyle and poverty (Global Burden of Disease Study 2013 Collaborators, 2015; Malhi & Mann, 2018; Rauen et al., 2020; Vos, Flaxman, Naghavi, et al., 2012). A large body of patients still remain undiagnosed (Briggs, Tobin, Kenny, & Kennelly, 2018; Georgakakou-Koutsonikou & Williams, 2017; Stein & Fazel, 2015), and almost half untreated (Kohn, Saxena, Levav, & Saraceno, 2004; Ludtke, Pult, Schroder, Moritz, & Bucker, 2018). Lack of awareness, failure in recognizing depressive symptoms, the limited therapy capacities, and the stigma of mental disorders are the main reasons for untreated depression (Georgakakou-Koutsonikou & Williams, 2017; Kohn et al., 2004; Ludtke et al., 2018; Mohr, Ho, Duffecy, et al., 2010), which is particularly relevant in the young (Andrade, Alonso, Mneimneh, et al., 2014; Davey & McGorry, 2019; Georgakakou-Koutsonikou & Williams, 2017; Johnson, Dupuis, Piche, Clayborne, & Colman, 2018).

Aiming to improve dementia prevention, it is most important to reduce the stigma of depression and start both pharmacological and nonpharmacological treatment early to improve the patient's wellbeing. Early treatment is of utmost relevance, as selective serotonin reuptake inhibitors (SSRIs), e.g., citalopram, are the first-line recommendation for pharmacological treatment of depression and also have the potential to delay conversion from mild cognitive impairment to Alzheimer's dementia (Cirrito, Disabato, Restivo, et al., 2011; Fisher, Wallace, Tripoli, Sheline, & Cirrito, 2016; Shen, Smith, Chang, et al., 2011). In detail, progression to Alzheimer's disease was delayed by approximately 3 years in patients suffering from mild cognitive impairment with a history of depression and long-term SSRI treatment of 4 years compared to short-term treatment, other antidepressants, or no treatment. In contrast to the observed beneficial effect in cognition, SSRI treatment did not change neurodegenerative biomarkers in the cerebrospinal fluid (CSF) (Bartels, Wagner, Wolfsgruber, Ehrenreich, & Schneider, 2018). Again, this study reported sex distribution of study groups, but did not report results under sex- and gender-related aspects. Thus, avoiding psychological distress, being physically active during midlife and SSRI long-term treatment of depression have implications in reducing the risk of dementia in patients suffering from major depression. Current evidence of these beneficial aspects has not been sex- and gender-stratified, thus further research is necessary to unravel sex- and gender-related treatment of major depression and its implication for Alzheimer's disease.

Social signal transduction theory of depression: A hypothesis to explain the female's increased vulnerability during childhood and puberty

The biological multilevel theory, namely the *social signal transduction theory of depression*, was proposed, which suggests a link between neural, physiological, molecular, and genomic mechanisms and adverse social-environmental experiences that drive depression pathogenesis, maintenance, and its recurrence (Slavich & Irwin, 2014; Slavich & Sacher, 2019). The authors focus on stressors with respect to social threats such as social conflicts, rejection, isolation, and exclusion that trigger inflammation resulting in hampered mood, anhedonia, fatigue, psychomotor retardation, and social-behavioral withdrawal, and have recently extended their hypothesis with respect to sex-related differences in prevalence of major depression (Slavich & Sacher, 2019). While progesterone and testosterone are considered to be antiinflammatory, estrogen in low concentration is proinflammatory and in high concentration antiinflammatory (see also Chapter 3) (Klein, 2000).

Low estrogen levels explain females' vulnerability to the new onset of inflammation-related major depression without history during hormonal transition periods such as postpartum and during menopause (Freeman, Sammel, Lin, & Nelson, 2006; Frokjaer, Pinborg, Holst, et al., 2015; Slavich & Sacher, 2019), and need our attention to develop screening and treatment to protect females' brains from this major burden, which not only increases their own risk of hampered mental health, but also affects their children's. This latter transition of disadvantages in mental health for the next generation is based on a 20% higher risk of unsecure bonding (Barnes & Theule, 2019), which in turn increases the risk of experiencing depression and/or anxiety. It is well-known that children's early social-emotional development is shaped by their environment, which underlines the need to diagnose and treat the mother's depression early, thereby protecting infants from detrimental social-emotional conditions that, in principle, can be compensated for by fathers (Behrendt, Scharke, Herpertz-Dahlmann, Konrad, & Firk, 2019). Whether mother's, or parent's, depression affects girls and boys differently is not clear yet, but it can be assumed that mother's/parent's depression during female puberty, with increasing inflammation-related vulnerability through ovarian cycles, might trigger the disparity in the prevalence of depression between sexes. In addition, the abovementioned socioeconomic inequality that underlies less education for females, with a 7% risk of dementia, depression during childhood most probably negatively affects education, and thus needs our research and clinical attention, not only to avoid educational deficits but also to prevent dementia.

Late life versus earlier life depression and risk of developing dementia

Major depression is common over the entire life span and shares pathological hallmarks with dementia, such as vascular diseases, alterations in glucocorticoid levels, hippocampal atrophy, increased amyloid-ß plaques deposition, proinflammation, and deficits of nerve growth factors (Byers & Yaffe, 2011; Harrington, Lim, Gould, & Maruff, 2015). The arising and still controversial question concerns the timing of depression and its association with dementia, namely whether early- or late-lifetime depression is associated with a higher risk of developing dementia. Currently, early-lifetime depression is suggested to entail a twofold higher risk of dementia, while the association of late-lifetime depression with dementia is more controversial, with reports on a two- to fivefold increased risk of dementia (Byers & Yaffe, 2011). To tackle this question in future studies, it is important to acknowledge that clinical diagnosis of depression is a more reliable clinical outcome compared to self-rating by patients, which might have confounded study results during late life, as discussed later.

Within the Framingham study, 949 participants (63.6% females) with a mean age of 79 years were followed up over 17 years to uncover the association between depression and Alzheimer's disease. Depressed participants had more than a 50% increase in risk of developing Alzheimer's disease. Factors that were more common in depressed than nondepressed subjects were being older, being female, and being less educated beyond high school (Saczynski, Beiser, Seshadri, et al., 2010). Further reports on the association between depression and Alzheimer's disease did not consider sex and gender differences in their analysis beyond reporting on sex distribution of participants (Andersen, Lolk, Kragh-Sørensen, Petersen, & Green, 2005; Gatz, Tyas, St John, & Montgomery, 2005). In contrast to Alzheimer's disease, the probably of developing vascular dementia was estimated with an incidence rate of 3.79 within the Canadian population. A variety of significant risks were analyzed with depression playing a major role. In detail, risk factors were age (OR=1.05), residing in a rural area (OR=2.03), living in an institution (OR=2.33), suffering from diabetes (OR=2.15), suffering from depression (OR=2.41), having an apolipoprotein E ε4 status (OR=2.34), having hypertension for females (OR=2.05), having heart problems for males (OR=2.52), taking aspirin (OR=2.33), and having been occupational exposed to pesticides or fertilizers (OR=2.05); on the other hand, eating shellfish (OR=0.46), and exercise for females (OR=0.46) were protective. No effects were reported for sex distribution, education, or alcohol intake (Hébert, Lindsay, Verreault, et al., 2000). One large retrospective study of 13,535 Americans (57.9% females) pinpoints an adjusted hazard of all-cause dementia by approximately 20% for midlife depression, 70% for later life, and 80% for participants having experienced midlife and later life depression. Differentiating dementia revealed that participants with midlife and later life depression had a twofold increased risk for Alzheimer's disease and even a threefold increased risk for vascular dementia without reporting sex- and gender-stratified results (Barnes et al., 2012).

This latter study emphasizes the pronounced association between midlife and later life depression that particularly lead to vascular dementia, which can be explained by the "vascular-depression-dementia hypothesis." This hypothesis claims that the damaged frontostriatal brain regions contribute to cognitive deficits, hampered executive functioning, psychomotor slowing, and resistance to treatment in later life depression, as previously reviewed (Byers & Yaffe, 2011). Thus, treatment for refractory depression in later life particularly needs our clinical and research attention with respect to developing new treatment strategies and to sex- and gender-related dementia prevention.

Depression or dementia? A key diagnostic challenge in the elderly

Depression and dementia are often concurrent and differential diagnosis is often difficult due to overlapping symptoms (Table 2) (Leyhe, Reynolds 3rd, Melcher, et al., 2017). Major depression increases mortality up to two and a half times in patients with mild dementia compared to no depressive or only mild depressive symptoms within 3 years of follow-up (Petersen, Waldorff, Siersma, et al., 2017), underlining the relevance of a precise diagnosis. Although results were adjusted for age, sex, smoking, alcohol consumption, education, body mass index, household status, cognitive status measured by the Mini-Mental State Examination (MMSE), the Charlson Comorbidity Index (CCI), Quality of Life Scale for Alzheimer's Disease (QoL-AD), Neuropsychiatric Inventory Questionnaire (NPI-Q), Alzheimer's Disease Cooperative Study Activity of Daily Living Scale (ADCS-ADL), medication, and randomization (with or without psychological interventions according to the Danish Alzheimer's Intervention Study (DAISY)), sex-related results themselves have not been reported so far, and need our focus. Nevertheless, differentiating major depression from dementia and diagnosing major depression in demented patients is a key challenge due to overlapping symptoms (Leyhe et al., 2017). In contrast to younger adults, major depression in the elderly frequently comes with pronounced cognitive disturbances, and careful neuropsychological diagnostics can help to differentiate major depression from cognitive decline evolving to dementia (Table 3).

In addition to the neuropsychological patterns that differ in patients suffering from major depression from those in Alzheimer's disease, the following clinical features require clinical expertise for decision-making and the correct diagnosis. The elderly frequently suffer from delusions of poverty, poisoning, influence by neighbors or family members that might overlap with dementia making differential diagnosis challenging. Furthermore, they may suffer from social isolation as a risk factor for dementia, from pronounced negative thinking due to a variety of negative life experiences, and somatic complaints. Differentiating major depression from dementia might be even more difficult as recent evidence pinpoints sex- and gender-related differences in patients' psychopathological features, as mentioned earlier, with females being more prone to depressive mood, atypical features, anxiety, somatoform

Table 2 Overlapping symptoms in major depression and Alzheimer's disease.

Loss of interest in previously enjoyable activities and hobbies
Depressed mood and/or apathy
Social withdrawal
Distinct cognitive disorders
Sleeping disorders including lack of sleep or hypersomnia or disturbed circadian rhythm

Table 3 Differentiating neuropsychological patterns in major depression and Alzheimer's disease (table translated and modified) (Hatzinger & Savaskan, 2019; Leyhe et al., 2017).

	Major depression	Alzheimer's disease
General cognitive profile	• No clear deficits	• Memory deficits independent of time and failure
New memory	• Slow with deficits by time limits • Deficits by failure • Relatively good recognition • No genuine storage deficit, but attentional deficits that impair encoding • Improvement with repeated exposure, normal recall, retrieval cues	• Disturbed recognition • Guesswork • Flat learning curve despite repeated exposure • Rapid forgetting • Inefficacy of cueing for recall
Drawing	• Inaccurate drawing	• Constructive practical errors
Orientation	• Good orientation	• Disturbed orientation
Speech	• Slow and hypophonia	• Aphasia, confabulation
Spatial-constructive abilities	• Inaccurate	• Apraxia

complaints, and feelings of guilt than males (Seeman, 1997; Blanco et al., 2012; Marcus et al., 2008; Vetter et al., 2020). In contrast, males with major depression suffer more frequently from impulsivity and substance abuse than females. These male-like hallmarks of depression are often overlooked, and diagnosing depression in males with dementia can be increasingly difficult, as impulsivity in particular overlaps with behavioral and psychological symptoms of dementia (BPSD).

Despite these different sex- and gender-related psychopathological features in major depression, analysis of brain network structures does not differ between sexes (Vetter et al., 2020), and needs our further focus in depression research and clinical practice. Importantly, self-rating of somatic and depressive symptoms might be sex- and gender-biased, as males and females differ with respect to symptom reporting, symptom recognition, and treatment. Males are less likely to be diagnosed and treated for major depression due to their tendency of not admitting their symptoms. While somatic complaints are the most robust sign of prodromal Alzheimer's disease in males and females, the depressive affect was only relevant in females as a prodrome of Alzheimer's (Norton, Carrière, Pérès, et al., 2019). To differentiate depression in the elderly from dementia remains difficult and needs distinct neuropsychiatric and neuropsychological expertise. Magnetic resonance imaging can support differential diagnosis by distinguishing neurodegenerative atrophy patterns of Alzheimer's disease, vascular dementia, or other causes of an organic affective disorder. In doubtable cases, the absence of fluid neurodegenerative biomarkers in the cerebrospinal fluid, reduces the likelihood of Alzheimer's disease. Thus, differentiating cognitive disturbances in major depression from prodrome or the full picture of dementia remains a multidisciplinary challenge and the development of blood biomarkers would be helpful.

Pharmacotherapy in the elderly: A major challenge with the risk of detrimental polypharmacy

Pharmacotherapy in the elderly is particularly challenging due to a variety of comorbidities and is a key component in dementia treatment. Here, we pinpoint sex-related detrimental effects of antidepressants, detrimental polypharmacy in dementia, and the sex-related disparity in prescribing antipsychotics (please see section "Behavioral and psychological symptoms of dementia").

Antidepressants in dementia

First-line therapy to treat major depression in dementia is a nonpharmacological approach including psychological and behavioral interventions as well as supportive clinical management, as the efficacy of pharmacotherapy is doubtable (Leyhe et al., 2017). If the nonpharmacological approach is not sufficient, we strive for an antidepressant monotherapy according to the current guidelines. Antidepressants that are suitable are escitalopram, citalopram, mirtazapine, and duloxetine, as they do not have anticholinergic side effects, thereby avoiding drug-induced harm to cognition.

To date, the question of whether antidepressants mitigate dementia progression in patients suffering from major depression is still not answered (Livingston et al., 2020). Only a few randomized clinical trials are available on the efficacy of antidepressants in patients suffering from Alzheimer's dementia, and no robust conclusions—particularly as no sex- and gender-stratified results are available—can be drawn so far (Orgeta, Tabet, Nilforooshan, & Howard, 2017). A recent Cochrane review—that did not stratify results with respect to sex and gender—on the efficacy of antidepressants for treating depression in patients with dementia did not provide strong support for antidepressants, particularly beyond 12 weeks. These clinical results in patients with depression and dementia showed either low or no effects of antidepressants, while remission rates of depression slightly favored the use of antidepressants (Dudas, Malouf, McCleery, & Dening, 2018).

In contrast experimental data suggest that SSRI intake reduces amyloid-ß in the brain interstitial fluid, amyloid-ß plaques in the brain, and cognitive burden in

Alzheimer's disease animal models (Cirrito et al., 2011; Fisher et al., 2016; Shen et al., 2011). Two of the three studies incorporated mice, of which one analyzed female littermates and the other did not report on the animals' sex. The third study incorporated male rats. Therefore, further experimental and clinical research is necessary to unravel the pathophysiology and efficacy of antidepressants in terms of slowing down conversion or disease progression in Alzheimer's disease. However, the Australian longitudinal Alzheimer's Disease Neuroimaging Initiative found, in 137 (68 males, 69 females) patients with mild cognitive impairment and a history of depression that the use of SSRIs, e.g., citalopram, was associated with a delayed onset of Alzheimer's by more than 4 years (Bartels et al., 2018). Again, results have not been reported in a sex-stratified manner, and thus, further sex- and gender-stratified research on the benefits and harms of antidepressants is needed.

Polypharmacy

Polypharmacy, with detrimental drug-disease or drug-drug interactions, in psychiatric disorders including dementia is well-known and particularly relevant in the elderly due to a variety of comorbidities, with polypharmacy often outweighing the benefits (Hukins, Macleod, & Boland, 2019). To date, sex- and gender-related differences of drug pharmacokinetics and dynamics have been identified, but their clinical significance in dementia is not yet clear (Trenaman, Rideout, & Andrew, 2019). However, there is some evidence that community-dwelling females receive more potentially inappropriate medications, including psychotropic medications such as antipsychotics, benzodiazepines, and antidepressants, compared to males (Trenaman et al., 2019). A variety of population-based studies uncovered that inappropriate polypharmacy is particularly relevant in patients with dementia, compared to those without. In detail, potentially inappropriate medication ranged from 13 to 74% and from 11 to 39% in patients with and without dementia, respectively, indicating that dementia patients are more prone to inappropriate prescribing; however, results have not been sex stratified as yet (Hukins et al., 2019).

A large Danish nationwide, register-based study on 1,032,120 subjects with ($N=35,476$) and without ($N=994,231$) dementia revealed that potentially inappropriate medication was more frequent among older people with dementia than without, after stratifying for age, sex, and comorbidities (Kristensen, Nørgaard, Jensen-Dahm, et al., 2018). In a large English mental health data-based study on 4668 patients with dementia, 1128 (24.2%) were prescribed four to six medications, and 739 (15.8%) seven or more medications, with polypharmacy increasing the risk of hospitalization by 3% and mortality within 2 years by 5% for each additional drug compared to baseline; again results have not been stratified for sex-differences as yet (Mueller, Molokhia, Perera, et al., 2018). Another population-based study in the United Kingdom on comorbidities and polypharmacy in dementia pinpoints the relevance of the detrimental impact of comorbidity and polypharmacy in patients with dementia compared to nondementia subjects, suggesting the need of multidisciplinary care and careful prescribing in dementia (Clague, Mercer, McLean, Reynish,

& Guthrie, 2017). Taken together, it is important to avoid inappropriate polypharmacy that might causes adverse side effects such as falls, dizziness, confusion, cognitive dysfunction, or delirium. The OECD report emphasizes that adverse side effects cause not only personal harm, but 8.6 million unplanned hospitalizations in Europe annually, making polypharmacy one of the three key action areas of the WHO Global Patient Safety Challenge (OECD, 2019).

Behavioral and psychological symptoms of dementia

BPSD such as agitation, aggression, psychosis, depression, or apathy contribute to patients' and caregivers' burden, increases early institutionalization, and more than double health costs in comparison to dementia patients without BPSD (Herrmann, Lanctôt, Sambrook, et al., 2006). More severe cognitive impairment, measured by lower scores on the MMSE, older age, female sex, and dementia other than Alzheimer's disease, particularly raise indirect costs of care. Thus, diagnosing and treating BPSD early is relevant to improve patients' and caregivers' well-being and help to reduce health care costs. Greater symptom severity is a predictor for disease progression with cognitive decline, loss of independence, and higher mortality (Li, Hu, Tan, Yu, & Tan, 2014). BPSD differs between males and females, according to a limited number of studies, as reviewed by Ferretti, Iulita, Cavedo, et al. (2018). Males have been reported to be more apathetic, agitated, aggressive, abusive, suffer from diurnal rhythm disturbances, and develop more socially inappropriate behavior than females (Kitamura, Kitamura, Hino, Tanaka, & Kurata, 2012; Ott, Lapane, & Gambassi, 2000; Ott, Tate, Gordon, & Heindel, 1996). In contrast, females seem to be more prone to depressive symptoms, affect lability, reclusiveness, and delusions (Ferretti et al., 2018; Kitamura et al., 2012; Ott et al., 1996).

Whether BPSD shares the pathology responsible for cognitive decline or has a different pathway is still unclear. Analyzing postmortem brains has revealed that neuropsychiatric symptoms—measured by the NPI-Q—primarily correlate with subcortical neurofibrillary tangles when adjusted for sex, and thus link to the tau pathology in Alzheimer's disease in both sexes (Ehrenberg, Suemoto, França Resende, et al., 2018). The most frequent neuropsychiatric symptoms in Alzheimer's disease during Braak stages I and II are agitation, anxiety, appetite dysfunction, depression, and sleep disturbances, of which agitation continues and is accompanied by delusions and progression of cognitive decline during Braak stages III and IV (Ehrenberg et al., 2018). These findings underline that neuropsychiatric symptoms occur early during prodromal phases of Alzheimer's disease (Ehrenberg et al., 2018; Lyketsos, Carrillo, Ryan, et al., 2011). In clinical practice these early neuropsychiatric symptoms during prodromal Alzheimer's disease are often overlooked or misdiagnosed. In contrast to these research findings suggesting predominately neuropsychiatric symptoms during early Braak stages, we clinically experience agitation, aggression, circadian rhythm sleep-wake disorders, and hallucinations, thus BPSD, during moderate and severe Alzheimer's disease concomitant with Braak stages III and beyond. This discrepancy between clinical experience and postmortem findings needs our careful analysis with respect to other reasons for BPDS in Alzheimer's disease such as polypharmacy-relevant adverse side effects or delirium.

Treatment of BPSD: A key challenge in dementia care

First-line recommendation is a nonpharmacological approach including psychosocial interventions that should be patient- and caregiver-centered for successful treatment of BPSD (Dyer, Harrison, Laver, Whitehead, & Crotty, 2018; Tible, Riese, Savaskan, & von Gunten, 2017). However, a patient's agitation, aggression, disturbed sleep-wake-cycles, and psychotic symptoms often demand psychopharmacological treatment. Comorbidities and pain should be sufficiently treated as these factors might aggravate BPSD. The effect of antidementia drugs on BPSD is still controversial, with some beneficial effect of cholinesterase inhibitors on negative symptoms such as apathy and depression (Birks & Harvey, 2006; Loy & Schneider, 2006; Tible et al., 2017), while memantine has a beneficial effect on positive symptoms such as agitation, hallucinations, and delusions in moderate to severe Alzheimer's disease (McShane, Areosa Sastre, & Minakaran, 2006; Tible et al., 2017).

Although adverse effects of benzodiazepines and antipsychotics are well known, particularly in the elderly, including falls, decreased alertness, anticholinergic, and extrapyramidal side effects, decreased mobility, and increased mortality, these drugs are commonly prescribed (de Jong, Van der Elst, & Hartholt, 2013). In patients with Alzheimer's disease, use of antipsychotics to control BPSD is widespread, albeit a second-line recommendation. Particularly, atypical antipsychotics such as risperidone and aripiprazole (off-label) are effective to control BSPD but should be avoided whenever possible due to adverse side effects and increased mortality. The OECD particularly emphasizes in their report *Health at a glance 2019*, the detrimental effects of antipsychotics due to falls, confusion, or even delirium, as well as increased mortality, with females 23% more likely to be prescribed antipsychotics than males in the elderly (65+) (OECD, 2019). Thus, females are at higher risk of detrimental adverse side effects by antipsychotics than males, which needs our careful attention in clinical research and practice aiming to reduce this harmful sex- and gender-related disparity in the future. We particularly stress the increased risk of recurrent falls, particularly in females taking antidepressants, benzodiazepines, or antipsychotics (de Jong et al., 2013), and the heterogeneity of study groups in clinical trials that have accounted for the multiple failures in developing more effective treatments so far (see also Chapter 11) (Ferretti, Martinkova, Biskup, et al., 2020).

Benzodiazepines in the elderly

Benzodiazepines are still commonly prescribed in the elderly, primarily for treatment of anxiety and sleep disorders (see also Chapter 8). However, it is well-known that these hypnotics increase the risk of falls, dementia, mortality, and sleep disorders due to disturbed sleep architecture, and lead to tolerance and dependency and might result in paradoxical effects with increasing anxiety and awakening (Savaskan, 2016). It is worthy of note that the FDA has reduced dosages for zolpidem due to slowed hepatic metabolization in the elderly. In addition, females metabolize Z-substances, namely zolpidem, zopiclone, and zaleplon, 50% slower than males. Thus, females are at a particularly higher risk of adverse side effects through benzodiazepines and Z-substances (Cubała, Wiglusz, Burkiewicz, & Gałuszko-Wegielnik, 2010), which should only be used for short term interventions during hospitalization.

Conclusion

We have outlined that psychiatric disorders account for at least 24% out of 40% of dementia risk, with 7 out of 12 of the population-attributable fractions of potentially modifiable risk factors for dementia. Major depression is of utmost relevance, with females being affected twice as often as males over the adult life span. Depression during midlife and later life doubles the risk for Alzheimer's disease and almost quadruples the risk for vascular dementia. Major depression and Alzheimer's disease often occur concomitantly and differential diagnosis is a key challenge due to a variety of overlapping symptoms, including cognitive deficits. However, distinct neuropsychological patterns in disturbed cognition can help in paving the way to precise diagnosis and treatment. Although SSRIs might delay conversion to Alzheimer's disease, the current evidence for their beneficial effect in dementia is doubtable and results have not been sex- and gender-stratified as yet. A second major challenge in Alzheimer's dementia is BPSD, with sex differences in clinical symptoms. First-line recommendation for treating major depression in dementia as well as BPSD is a nonpharmacological approach. Despite this current knowledge, harmful benzodiazepines and antipsychotics are particularly prescribed in females, resulting in a harmful sex- and gender-related disparity that needs our attention in clinical research and practice.

Chapter highlights

- Psychiatric disorders account for at least 24% out of 40% of dementia risk with 7 out of 12 population-attributable fractions of potentially modifiable risk factors for dementia.
- Depression is a relevant risk factor for dementia, with females being affected twice as often as males. Depression during midlife and later life double the risk for Alzheimer's disease and almost quadruples the risk for vascular dementia.
- Antidepressants, benzodiazepines, and antipsychotics have well-known adverse side effects and are prescribed more frequently in females than males. Thus, females are at greater risk of pharmaceutical harm, which needs our attention in personalized medicine.

References

Andersen, K., Lolk, A., Kragh-Sørensen, P., Petersen, N. E., & Green, A. (2005). Depression and the risk of Alzheimer disease. *Epidemiology, 16*, 233–238.

Andrade, L. H., Alonso, J., Mneimneh, Z., et al. (2014). Barriers to mental health treatment: Results from the WHO World Mental Health surveys. *Psychological Medicine, 44*, 1303–1317.

Bale, T. L. (2019). Sex matters. *Neuropsychopharmacology, 44*, 1–3.

Barnes, J., & Theule, J. (2019). Maternal depression and infant attachment security: A meta-analysis. *Infant Mental Health Journal, 40*, 817–834.

Barnes, D. E., Yaffe, K., Byers, A. L., et al. (2012). Midlife vs late-life depressive symptoms and risk of dementia: Differential effects for Alzheimer disease and vascular dementia. *Archives of General Psychiatry, 69*, 493–498.

Bartels, C., Wagner, M., Wolfsgruber, S., Ehrenreich, H., & Schneider, A. (2018). Impact of SSRI therapy on risk of conversion from mild cognitive impairment to Alzheimer's dementia in individuals with previous depression. *American Journal of Psychiatry, 175*, 232–241.

Behrendt, H. F., Scharke, W., Herpertz-Dahlmann, B., Konrad, K., & Firk, C. (2019). Like mother, like child? Maternal determinants of children's early social-emotional development. *Infant Mental Health Journal, 40*, 234–247.

Birks, J., & Harvey, R. J. (2006). Donepezil for dementia due to Alzheimer's disease. *Cochrane Database of Systematic Reviews*. Cd001190.

Blanco, C., Vesga-López, O., Stewart, J. W., et al. (2012). Epidemiology of major depression with atypical features: Results from the National Epidemiologic Survey on Alcohol and Related Conditions (NESARC). *Journal of Clinical Psychiatry, 73*, 224–232.

Briggs, R., Tobin, K., Kenny, R. A., & Kennelly, S. P. (2018). What is the prevalence of untreated depression and death ideation in older people? Data from the Irish Longitudinal Study on Aging. *International Psychogeriatrics, 30*, 1393–1401.

Bromet, E., Andrade, L. H., Hwang, I., et al. (2011). Cross-national epidemiology of DSM-IV major depressive episode. *BMC Medicine, 9*, 90.

Brumpton, B., Langhammer, A., Romundstad, P., Chen, Y., & Mai, X. M. (2013). The associations of anxiety and depression symptoms with weight change and incident obesity: The HUNT Study. *International Journal of Obesity, 37*, 1268–1274.

Byers, A. L., & Yaffe, K. (2011). Depression and risk of developing dementia. *Nature Reviews Neurology, 7*, 323–331.

Cirrito, J. R., Disabato, B. M., Restivo, J. L., et al. (2011). Serotonin signaling is associated with lower amyloid-β levels and plaques in transgenic mice and humans. *Proceedings of the National Academy of Sciences, 108*, 14968–14973.

Clague, F., Mercer, S. W., McLean, G., Reynish, E., & Guthrie, B. (2017). Comorbidity and polypharmacy in people with dementia: Insights from a large, population-based cross-sectional analysis of primary care data. *Age and Ageing, 46*, 33–39.

Cubała, W. J., Wiglusz, M., Burkiewicz, A., & Gałuszko-Węgielnik, M. (2010). Zolpidem pharmacokinetics and pharmacodynamics in metabolic interactions involving CYP3A: Sex as a differentiating factor. *European Journal of Clinical Pharmacology, 66*, 955. author reply 957–958.

Davey, C. G., & McGorry, P. D. (2019). Early intervention for depression in young people: A blind spot in mental health care. *Lancet Psychiatry, 6*, 267–272.

de Jong, M. R., Van der Elst, M., & Hartholt, K. A. (2013). Drug-related falls in older patients: Implicated drugs, consequences, and possible prevention strategies. *Therapeutic Advances in Drug Safety, 4*, 147–154.

Dilling, H., Mombour, W., Schmidt, M. H., & Schulte-Markwort, E. (2016). *ICD-10 Internationale Klassifikation psychischer Störungen, Diagnostische Kriterien für Forschung und Praxis. 6. überarbeitete Auflage unter Berücksichtigung der Änderungen gemäß*. ICD-10-GM ed Bern: Hogrefe. 260 p.

Dudas, R., Malouf, R., McCleery, J., & Dening, T. (2018). Antidepressants for treating depression in dementia. *Cochrane Database of Systematic Reviews, 8*. Cd003944.

Dyer, S. M., Harrison, S. L., Laver, K., Whitehead, C., & Crotty, M. (2018). An overview of systematic reviews of pharmacological and non-pharmacological interventions for the treatment of behavioral and psychological symptoms of dementia. *International Psychogeriatrics, 30*, 295–309.

Ehrenberg, A. J., Suemoto, C. K., França Resende, E. P., et al. (2018). Neuropathologic correlates of psychiatric symptoms in Alzheimer's disease. *Journal of Alzheimer's Disease, 66*, 115–126.

Ferretti, M. T., Iulita, M. F., Cavedo, E., et al. (2018). Sex differences in Alzheimer disease—The gateway to precision medicine. *Nature Reviews Neurology, 14*, 457–469.

Ferretti, M. T., Martinkova, J., Biskup, E., et al. (2020). Sex and gender differences in Alzheimer's disease: Current challenges and implications for clinical practice: Position paper of the Dementia and Cognitive Disorders Panel of the European Academy of Neurology. *European Journal of Neurology, 27*, 928–943.

Fisher, J. R., Wallace, C. E., Tripoli, D. L., Sheline, Y. I., & Cirrito, J. R. (2016). Redundant Gs-coupled serotonin receptors regulate amyloid-β metabolism in vivo. *Molecular Neurodegeneration, 11*, 45.

Fluharty, M., Taylor, A. E., Grabski, M., & Munafò, M. R. (2017). The association of cigarette smoking with depression and anxiety: a systematic review. *Nicotine & Tobacco Research, 19*, 3–13.

Freeman, E. W., Sammel, M. D., Lin, H., & Nelson, D. B. (2006). Associations of hormones and menopausal status with depressed mood in women with no history of depression. *Archives of General Psychiatry, 63*, 375–382.

Frokjaer, V. G., Pinborg, A., Holst, K. K., et al. (2015). Role of serotonin transporter changes in depressive responses to sex-steroid hormone manipulation: A positron emission tomography study. *Biological Psychiatry, 78*, 534–543.

Gatz, J. L., Tyas, S. L., St John, P., & Montgomery, P. (2005). Do depressive symptoms predict Alzheimer's disease and dementia? *Journals of Gerontology. Series A, Biological Sciences and Medical Sciences, 60*, 744–747.

Georgakakou-Koutsonikou, N., & Williams, J. M. (2017). Children and young people's conceptualizations of depression: A systematic review and narrative meta-synthesis. *Child: Care, Health and Development, 43*, 161–181.

Global Burden of Disease Study 2013 Collaborators. (2015). Global, regional, and national incidence, prevalence, and years lived with disability for 301 acute and chronic diseases and injuries in 188 countries, 1990–2013: A systematic analysis for the Global Burden of Disease Study 2013. *Lancet, 386*, 743–800.

Harrington, K. D., Lim, Y. Y., Gould, E., & Maruff, P. (2015). Amyloid-beta and depression in healthy older adults: A systematic review. *The Australian and New Zealand Journal of Psychiatry, 49*, 36–46.

Hatzinger, M., & Savaskan, E. (2019). *Empfehlungen für die Diagnostik und Therapie der Depression im Alter*. Bern: Hogrefe.

Hébert, R., Lindsay, J., Verreault, R., et al. (2000). Vascular dementia: Incidence and risk factors in the Canadian study of health and aging. *Stroke, 31*, 1487–1493.

Herrmann, N., Lanctôt, K. L., Sambrook, R., et al. (2006). The contribution of neuropsychiatric symptoms to the cost of dementia care. *International Journal of Geriatric Psychiatry, 21*, 972–976.

Hukins, D., Macleod, U., & Boland, J. W. (2019). Identifying potentially inappropriate prescribing in older people with dementia: A systematic review. *European Journal of Clinical Pharmacology, 75*, 467–481.

Johnson, D., Dupuis, G., Piche, J., Clayborne, Z., & Colman, I. (2018). Adult mental health outcomes of adolescent depression: A systematic review. *Depression and Anxiety, 35*, 700–716.

Kaczkurkin, A. N., Raznahan, A., & Satterthwaite, T. D. (2019). Sex differences in the developing brain: Insights from multimodal neuroimaging. *Neuropsychopharmacology, 44*, 71–85.

Kessler, R. C., & Bromet, E. J. (2013). The epidemiology of depression across cultures. *Annual Review of Public Health, 34*, 119–138.

Kitamura, T., Kitamura, M., Hino, S., Tanaka, N., & Kurata, K. (2012). Gender differences in clinical manifestations and outcomes among hospitalized patients with behavioral and psychological symptoms of dementia. *Journal of Clinical Psychiatry, 73*, 1548–1554.

Klein, S. L. (2000). The effects of hormones on sex differences in infection: From genes to behavior. *Neuroscience and Biobehavioral Reviews, 24*, 627–638.

Kohn, R., Saxena, S., Levav, I., & Saraceno, B. (2004). The treatment gap in mental health care. *Bulletin of the World Health Organization, 82*, 858–866.

Kristensen, R. U., Nørgaard, A., Jensen-Dahm, C., et al. (2018). Polypharmacy and potentially inappropriate medication in people with dementia: A nationwide study. *Journal of Alzheimer's Disease, 63*, 383–394.

Leyhe, T., Reynolds, C. F., 3rd, Melcher, T., et al. (2017). A common challenge in older adults: Classification, overlap, and therapy of depression and dementia. *Alzheimer's & Dementia, 13*, 59–71.

Li, X. L., Hu, N., Tan, M. S., Yu, J. T., & Tan, L. (2014). Behavioral and psychological symptoms in Alzheimer's disease. *BioMed Research International, 2014*, 927804.

Livingston, G., Huntley, J., Sommerlad, A., et al. (2020). Dementia prevention, intervention, and care: 2020 report of the lancet commission. *Lancet, 396*, 413–446.

Loy, C., & Schneider, L. (2006). Galantamine for Alzheimer's disease and mild cognitive impairment. *Cochrane Database of Systematic Reviews*. Cd001747.

Ludtke, T., Pult, L. K., Schroder, J., Moritz, S., & Bucker, L. (2018). A randomized controlled trial on a smartphone self-help application (Be Good to Yourself) to reduce depressive symptoms. *Psychiatry Research, 269*, 753–762.

Lyketsos, C. G., Carrillo, M. C., Ryan, J. M., et al. (2011). Neuropsychiatric symptoms in Alzheimer's disease. *Alzheimer's & Dementia, 7*, 532–539.

Malhi, G. S., & Mann, J. J. (2018). Depression. *Lancet, 392*, 2299–2312.

Marcus, S. M., Kerber, K. B., Rush, A. J., et al. (2008). Sex differences in depression symptoms in treatment-seeking adults: Confirmatory analyses from the Sequenced Treatment Alternatives to Relieve Depression study. *Comprehensive Psychiatry, 49*, 238–246.

McShane, R., Areosa Sastre, A., & Minakaran, N. (2006). Memantine for dementia. *Cochrane Database of Systematic Reviews*. Cd003154.

Mohr, D. C., Ho, J., Duffecy, J., et al. (2010). Perceived barriers to psychological treatments and their relationship to depression. *Journal of Clinical Psychology, 66*, 394–409.

Mueller, C., Molokhia, M., Perera, G., et al. (2018). Polypharmacy in people with dementia: Associations with adverse health outcomes. *Experimental Gerontology, 106*, 240–245.

Norton, J., Carrière, I., Pérès, K., et al. (2019). Sex-specific depressive symptoms as markers of pre-Alzheimer dementia: Findings from the Three-City cohort study. *Translational Psychiatry, 9*, 291.

OECD. (2019). *Health at a glance 2019: OECD indicators.* Paris: OECD Publishing.

Orgeta, V., Tabet, N., Nilforooshan, R., & Howard, R. (2017). Efficacy of antidepressants for depression in Alzheimer's disease: Systematic review and meta-analysis. *Journal of Alzheimer's Disease, 58*, 725–733.

Ott, B. R., Lapane, K. L., & Gambassi, G. (2000). Gender differences in the treatment of behavior problems in Alzheimer's disease. SAGE Study Group. Systemic Assessment of Geriatric drug use via Epidemiology. *Neurology, 54*, 427–432.

Ott, B. R., Tate, C. A., Gordon, N. M., & Heindel, W. C. (1996). Gender differences in the behavioral manifestations of Alzheimer's disease. *Journal of the American Geriatrics Society, 44*, 583–587.

Petersen, J. D., Waldorff, F. B., Siersma, V. D., et al. (2017). Major depressive symptoms increase 3-year mortality rate in patients with mild dementia. *International Journal of Alzheimer's Disease, 2017*, 7482094.

Rauen, K., Vetter, S., Eisele, A., et al. (2020). Internet cognitive behavioral therapy with or without face-to-face psychotherapy: A 12-weeks clinical trial of patients with depression. *Frontiers in Digital Health, 2*, 1–10. https://doi.org/10.3389/fdgth.2020.00004.

Reiss, F. (2013). Socioeconomic inequalities and mental health problems in children and adolescents: A systematic review. *Social Science & Medicine, 90*, 24–31.

Saczynski, J. S., Beiser, A., Seshadri, S., et al. (2010). Depressive symptoms and risk of dementia: The Framingham Heart Study. *Neurology, 75*, 35–41.

Salk, R. H., Hyde, J. S., & Abramson, L. Y. (2017). Gender differences in depression in representative national samples: Meta-analyses of diagnoses and symptoms. *Psychological Bulletin, 143*, 783–822.

Savaskan, E. (2016). Benzodiazepin-Abhängigkeit im Alter: Wie geht man damit um? *Praxis, 105*, 637–641.

Schwarzinger, M., Pollock, B. G., Hasan, O. S. M., Dufouil, C., & Rehm, J. (2018). Contribution of alcohol use disorders to the burden of dementia in France 2008–13: A nationwide retrospective cohort study. *The Lancet Public Health, 3*, e124–e132.

Seeman, M. V. (1997). Psychopathology in women and men: Focus on female hormones. *American Journal of Psychiatry, 154*, 1641–1647.

Shen, F., Smith, J. A., Chang, R., et al. (2011). 5-HT(4) receptor agonist mediated enhancement of cognitive function in vivo and amyloid precursor protein processing in vitro: A pharmacodynamic and pharmacokinetic assessment. *Neuropharmacology, 61*, 69–79.

Slavich, G. M., & Irwin, M. R. (2014). From stress to inflammation and major depressive disorder: A social signal transduction theory of depression. *Psychological Bulletin, 140*, 774–815.

Slavich, G. M., & Sacher, J. (2019). Stress, sex hormones, inflammation, and major depressive disorder: Extending Social Signal Transduction Theory of Depression to account for sex differences in mood disorders. *Psychopharmacology, 236*, 3063–3079.

Stein, K., & Fazel, M. (2015). Depression in young people often goes undetected. *Practitioner, 259*, 17–22. 12–13.

Tible, O. P., Riese, F., Savaskan, E., & von Gunten, A. (2017). Best practice in the management of behavioural and psychological symptoms of dementia. *Therapeutic Advances in Neurological Disorders*, *10*, 297–309.

Trenaman, S. C., Rideout, M., & Andrew, M. K. (2019). Sex and gender differences in polypharmacy in persons with dementia: A scoping review. *SAGE Open Medicine*, *7*. 2050312119845715.

Tronieri, J. S., Wurst, C. M., Pearl, R. L., & Allison, K. C. (2017). Sex differences in obesity and mental health. *Current Psychiatry Reports*, *19*, 29.

Udo, T., McKee, S. A., White, M. A., et al. (2013). Sex differences in biopsychosocial correlates of binge eating disorder: A study of treatment-seeking obese adults in primary care setting. *General Hospital Psychiatry*, *35*, 587–591.

Vetter, J. S., Spiller, T. R., Cathomas, F., et al. (2020). Sex differences in depressive symptoms and their networks in a treatment-seeking population – A cross-sectional study. *Journal of Affective Disorders*, *278*, 357–364.

Vos, T., Flaxman, A. D., Naghavi, M., et al. (2012). Years lived with disability (YLDs) for 1160 sequelae of 289 diseases and injuries 1990–2010: A systematic analysis for the Global Burden of Disease Study 2010. *Lancet*, *380*, 2163–2196.

World Health Organization. (2008). *The global burden of disease: 2004 update*. Available from https://www.who.int/healthinfo/global_burden_disease/2004_report_update/en/.

Zotcheva, E., Bergh, S., Selbæk, G., et al. (2018). Midlife physical activity, psychological distress, and dementia risk: The HUNT study. *Journal of Alzheimer's Disease*, *66*, 825–833.

CHAPTER 8

Sleep disorders and dementia

Beatrice Nasta[a,b], MaryJane Hill-Strathy[b], Ewelina Biskup[a,c,d], and Katrin Rauen[a,b,e,*]

[a]*Women's Brain Project, Guntershausen, Switzerland*
[b]*Department of Geriatric Psychiatry, Psychiatric Hospital Zurich, University of Zurich, Zurich, Switzerland*
[c]*Department of Advanced Biomedical Sciences, Federico II University of Naples, Naples, Italy*
[d]*College of Clinical Medicine, Shanghai University of Medicine and Health Sciences, Shanghai, China*
[e]*Institute for Stroke and Dementia Research, University Hospital, LMU Munich, Munich, Germany*

Abbreviations

BMI	Body Mass Index
CPAP	Continuous Positive Airway Pressure
CSF	Cerebrospinal Fluid
EEG	Electroencephalography
ICSD	International Classification of Sleep Disorders
MCI	Mild Cognitive Impairment
MMSE	Mini Mental State Examination
NREM	Non-Rapid Eye Movement
OSAS	Obstructive Sleep Apnea Syndrome
RBD	REM Sleep Behavior Disorder
REM	Rapid Eye Movement
SNRI	Selective Norepinephrine Reuptake Inhibitor
SSRI	Selective Serotonin Reuptake Inhibitor

Why do we spend a third of life sleeping? An introduction to sleep and its main characteristics

Sleep is a vital biological process with important recuperative functions that follows a circadian rhythm (~24 h), which is regulated by the suprachiasmatic nucleus of the hypothalamus, our endogenous clock. Moreover, external factors, so-called "zeitgeber," such as alterations of daylight and darkness, working or activity patterns,

---
[*] Senior contributor

and meals, all influence our sleep-wake rhythm and the sleep pressure increases the longer the period since the last sleep (Schupp & Hanning, 2003). Increasing sleep pressure by preventing patients from napping during daytime and establishing recurrent "zeitgeber" are important tools for the non-pharmacological treatment of sleep disorders.

Sleep research is relatively young and first started in the 1920s with electroencephalographic findings during sleep and was significantly influenced through the discovery of rapid eye movement (REM) sleep by Aserinsky and Kleitman (1953) (Dement, 2003). Further development of sleep science and sleep medicine has been intertwined with polysomnography since the late 1950s (Deak & Epstein, 2009), which is a multiparametric recording of biophysiological changes that occur during sleep and monitors a variety of body functions. Based on polysomnographic data, non-rapid eye movement (NREM) sleep stages account for 75% to 85% of the total sleep time, and REM sleep can be determined by the following techniques: electroencephalography (EEG) for assessing brain activity, electrocardiography (ECG) and pulse oximetry to record heart rate and oxygenation, electrooculogram (EOG) to observe eye movements, electromyography (EMG) for deriving muscle activity, and video monitoring to watch sleep behaviors.

Sleep has its physiologically defined architecture and consists of four sleep cycles that each last for about 90–120 min. Let's shine a light on one sleep cycle with its four sleep stages, namely three NREM sleep stages (N1, N2, and N3) and one REM sleep stage. In detail, sleep physiologically starts with NREM sleep stage N1 (drowsiness); followed by NREM sleep stage N2 (subdued sleep), when brain activity slows down, and heart rate and body temperature drop; then NREM sleep stage N3 (deep sleep) follows with further decline of brain activity and body relaxation indicated by slow waves in the EEG but with persistent muscle activity. NREM stages N1 and N2 account for light sleep. After NREM sleep stage N3 (deep sleep), REM sleep ensues and is defined by its rapid eye movements, muscle atony, and sympathetic and awake-like brain activity with patients having lively dreams that are not acted out due to the loss of muscle activity in healthy humans. The recurrent sleep cycles physiologically change during the night and shift from more deep sleep (NREM stage N3) to a longer proportion of NREM stage N2 and REM sleep in the second half of the night (Anderson & Bradley, 2013; Institute of Medicine Committee on Sleep Medicine and Research, 2006; Patel, Steinberg, & Patel, 2018; Schupp & Hanning, 2003). The REM sleep stage is particularly relevant in this chapter as REM sleep behavior disorders (RBD) are a hallmark in neurodegenerative diseases such as Parkinson's disease, dementia with Lewy bodies, and multisystem atrophy (Boeve, Silber, Ferman, et al., 2003).

During aging, physiological sleep changes occur with respect to sleep duration and sleep architecture. Sleep duration decreases over the human life span, with children sleeping 10 to 14h out of 24h, and young adults 6.5 to 8.5h per night. Thereafter, sleep duration decreases to 5 to 7h per night during midlife, remaining physiologically stable beyond the age of 60. Starting from midlife, healthy adults spend less time in deep sleep (NREM stage 3) and REM sleep (Patel et al., 2018).

These physiological factors during aging—reduced duration of sleep, less deep (NREM stage 3) and REM sleep—often account for subjective sleep complaints and need to be targeted during non-pharmacological sleep therapy.

The introductory question on why we spend a third of our lives sleeping, leads us to the multiple functions of sleep that encompass, among other factors, memory consolidation, improving emotional regulation and decision making, regeneration of the immune and metabolic systems, neuronal plasticity, and the waste clearance of the brain by the glymphatic system (Walker, 2017). Thus, sleep improves learning, memorization, decision making, and also recalibrates our brain circuits dedicated to emotions—allowing us to cope with the social and psychological challenges of the next day. Moreover, sleep rebalances the immune system, the cardiovascular system by lowering heart rate and blood pressure, and improves the metabolic state by adjusting insulin, blood glucose, appetite, and body weight, and thus keeps us healthy.

To date, the exact function of sleep with respect to cognition and memory reconsolidation is still not fully clear. However, there is evidence that sleep improves memory recall and increases resistance of memories to subsequent interference, and that the hippocampus is relevant with respect to memory and behavior. Currently, sleep-dependent, neurobiological processes that directly lead to the consolidation of declarative memories can be assumed (Ellenbogen, Payne, & Stickgold, 2006). Furthermore, hampered sleep in turn results in neurobehavioral changes with decreased executive functioning, decreased attention, increased reaction time as well as increased errors in judgment and decision making (Institute of Medicine Committee on Sleep Medicine and Research, 2006).

Sleep disorders and physiological sleep changes during aging

Sleep disorders are defined as any disturbance of the patient's normal sleep pattern and are grouped according to the 3rd edition of the international classification of sleep disorders (ICSD) into: (i) insomnia, (ii) sleep-related breathing disorders, (iii) central disorders of hypersomnolence, (iv) circadian rhythm sleep-wake disorders, (v) parasomnias, and (vi) sleep-related movement disorders (International classification of sleep disorders—Third edition (ICSD-3), 2019). Here, we focus on insomnia, obstructive sleep apnea syndrome (OSAS) as a serious sleep related breathing disorder, and REM sleep behavior disorder (RBD) as REM sleep is relevant for patients' cognition and RBD often occurs in neurodegenerative disorders (Bubu, Brannick, & Mortimer, 2017; de Almondes, Costa, Malloy-Diniz, & Diniz, 2016; Haba-Rubio, Marti-Soler, Tobback, et al., 2017; Shi, Chen, Ma, et al., 2018).

Physiological aging is often accompanied by quantitative and qualitative sleep changes that affect the four sleep stages of NREM and REM sleep. As mentioned above, NREM sleep is divided into three stages, namely NREM stage N1 (drowsiness, light sleep), subdued sleep with slowed brain activity, temperature drop, muscle relaxation, slowed breathing and reduced heart rate (NREM stage N2, light sleep), and deep sleep with slow waves and further body relaxation (NREM stage N3, deep sleep). During aging, a variety of alterations, e.g., increased sleep onset latency, decreased sleep duration, more fragile sleep, and pronounced light sleep stages (NREM stages N1 and N2), might arise. Diminished REM sleep might occur during aging or in patients suffering from neurodegenerative diseases (Mander, Winer, & Walker, 2017). However, it is not necessarily associated with sleep changes or sleep disorders (Vitiello, 2009).

Almost two decades ago, a meta-analysis uncovered sex- and gender-related differences of sleep patterns during normal aging, with females having a longer sleep onset latency, more deep sleep (NREM stage N3), and longer REM sleep compared to males. In contrast, males experienced more subdued sleep (NREM stage N2) and were more likely to wake up after sleep onset than females. Sleep efficiency and light sleep (NREM stage N1) did not differ between sexes (Ohayon, Carskadon, Guilleminault, & Vitiello, 2004). The decrement of slow wave sleep (NREM stage N3) has been described in males from early adulthood to older age and is associated with hormonal changes of growth hormone and cortisol release—findings that are not seen in females (Van Cauter, Leproult, & Plat, 2000). Although there is a large body of literature on sleep changes during healthy aging, the debate is still controversial, with questions arising as to why the elderly might be less able to generate sufficient sleep or simply need less sleep (Mander et al., 2017). Poor sleep efficiency is often underdiagnosed and has been suggested to worsen cognitive function in older males; interestingly this was found to be independent of comorbid depression (Biddle, Naismith, Griffiths, et al., 2017); nevertheless, this study did not include females, and thus we proceed to the current knowledge on sex- and gender-related differences in sleep disorders.

Sex- and gender-related differences in sleep and sleep disorders

The US National Sleep Foundation dedicated a major symposium on the topic of females' sleep in 2007 and the Society for Women's Health Research further specified sex- and gender-related differences in sleep in 2013 (Mallampalli & Carter, 2014). Since then, a variety of differences between male and female sleep have been discovered regarding: (i) the epidemiology of sleep in the healthy population, (ii) the characteristics of normal sleep patterns in animal models, (iii) the epidemiology of sleep disorders, (iv) obstructive sleep apnea syndrome (OSAS), and (v) the treatment of sleep disorders that are summarized in the research report of the Society for Women's Health (Mallampalli & Carter, 2014).

Here, we particularly pinpoint that females have a 40% increased risk of insomnia in comparison to males (Mallampalli & Carter, 2014; Zhang & Wing, 2006), and highlight sex- and gender-related differences in OSAS, namely differences in clinical symptoms, anthropometric measures, age of onset, self-reported sleepiness using the Epworth Sleepiness Scale, continuous positive airway pressure (CPAP) treatment, and comorbid depression (Anttalainen, Saaresranta, Kalleinen, et al., 2007; Baldwin, Kapur, Holberg, Rosen, & Nieto, 2004; Gabbay & Lavie, 2012; Jordan & McEvoy, 2003; Macey, Kumar, Yan-Go, Woo, & Harper, 2012; Mallampalli & Carter, 2014; Ralls & Grigg-Damberger, 2012; Subramanian, Jayaraman, Majid, Aguilar, & Surani, 2012; Wheaton, Perry, Chapman, & Croft, 2012). Moreover, assessing self-rated sleep quality using the Pittsburgh Sleep Quality Index—at least in male patients—might help identifying patients with a 17% higher likelihood of developing cognitive impairment during the following year when reporting worse sleep quality by 1 point (Potvin, Lorrain, Forget, et al., 2012). This latter finding was not seen in women in a sex- and gender-stratified analysis, after adjusting for age, education, baseline scores in the Mini Mental Status Examination (MMSE), psychotropic drug use, anxiety, depressive episodes, cardiovascular conditions, and chronic diseases.

Current knowledge on sex- and gender-related differences in sleep disorders and their implications for cognitive impairment evolving to dementia is sparse, and the underlying mechanisms with increased β-amyloid deposition in the brain, reduced glymphatic clearance during disturbed sleep, hypoxia, and cardiovascular diseases due to OSAS are still unclear (Livingston, Huntley, Sommerlad, et al., 2020). Thus, we further focus on sex- and gender-related differences that might help to unravel this gap of knowledge and pave the way for personalized medicine in the future.

Sleep disorders in Alzheimer's disease

Alzheimer's disease frequently comes along with sleep disturbances; up to 45% of Alzheimer's patients have a sleep disorder with a major impact on patient's and caregiver's well-being, and is a main reason for early institutionalization (Peter-Derex, Yammine, Bastuji, & Croisile, 2015). Sleep alterations occur during early stages and increase in moderate to severe Alzheimer's disease. Disrupted sleep architecture with sleep fragmentation, decreased sleep length, involuntary daytime napping, the sundown syndrome, and/or inversion of the sleep-wake cycle are common in Alzheimer's disease (Peter-Derex et al., 2015; Savaskan, 2015). Alterations in the sleep-wake cycle are linked to pathological changes in the suprachiasmatic nucleus and melatonin secretion (Weldemichael & Grossberg, 2010). In healthy middle-aged males, it has been shown that one night of total sleep deprivation is enough to decrease amyloid Aβ42 protein in the cerebrospinal fluid (CSF) and results in detrimental mood changes. Thus, chronic sleep deprivation might elevate the risk of developing Alzheimer's disease (Ooms, Overeem, Besse, et al., 2014). Recently, this observation was further supported by increased amyloid-β in the right hippocampus and thalamus after one night of sleep deprivation compared to baseline in 10 males and 10 females using ^{18}F-positron emission tomography (PET) with the tracer Florbetaben, thereby suggesting preliminary evidence for the effect of sleep deprivation on increased β-amyloid pathology in male and female brains (Shokri-Kojori, Wang, Wiers, et al., 2018). In contrast, a study analyzing 13 healthy subjects (69.2% males) after 5 to 8 consecutive nights of partial sleep deprivation showed preserved slow-wave sleep

(NREM stage N3) and increased orexin—a neurotransmitter that regulates wakefulness—in the CSF, with no changes of amyloid and associated biomarkers (Olsson, Ärlig, Hedner, Blennow, & Zetterberg, 2018). Thus, partial sleep deprivation does not seem to increase protein turnover in healthy brains and does not cause acute neuronal damage that can be detected in the CSF—findings that are potentially associated with the preserved slow-wave sleep (deep sleep NREM stage N3).

Successful compensation for partial sleep deprivation physiologically occurs through increased sleep pressure that leads to deep sleep (NREM stage N3), which in turn keeps the protein turnover stable and protects the brain from neuronal damage. In contrast, deep sleep (NREM stage N3) is often hampered in Alzheimer's disease. These results need to be replicated in larger samples including sex-stratification as the latter has yet to be done. To date, a bidirectional relationship between sleep disorders and Alzheimer's disease is likely, as disrupted sleep-wake cycles increase cerebral amyloid-β deposit and its accumulation aggravates the detrimental cascade with increased wakefulness and altered sleep patterns (Ju, Lucey, & Holtzman, 2014). Experimental models show that sleep deprivation increases soluble amyloid-β in the brain, which in turn increases amyloid-β plaques, while sleep extension does the opposite. These findings underline the bidirectional relation and pinpoint the importance of treating sleep disturbances early.

Sleep architecture in Alzheimer's disease

Sleep architecture in patients with Alzheimer's disease changes compared to aged-matched controls (Musiek, Xiong, & Holtzman, 2015). In detail, sleep deprivation and circadian dysfunction increase neuronal activity and decrease the glymphatic protein clearance during sleep, thereby leading to increased accumulation of amyloid-β aggregates and synaptic damage in the brain, which in turn increases circadian dysfunction and detrimentally disturbs the patient's sleep further (Fig. 1).

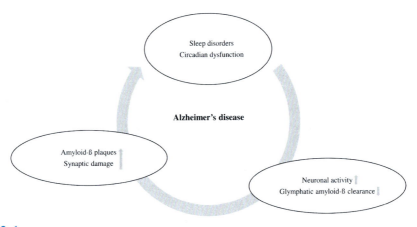

FIG. 1

Bidirectional relationship between sleep disorders and Alzheimer's disease.

Patients with Alzheimer's disease experience less REM sleep and less deep slow-wave sleep (NREM stage N3). These sleep stages, namely REM and deep NREM slow-wave sleep (NREM stage N3), are the most important for memory consolidation, with slow-wave sleep contributing to the consolidation of recently encoded neuronal memory into long-term memory and REM sleep ensuring the stabilization of transformed memories (Rasch & Born, 2013). These mechanisms are most probably relevant for both hippocampus- and non-hippocampus-dependent memories. Thus, deprivation of REM and NREM slow-wave sleep in patients with Alzheimer's disease aggravates memory consolidation and its long-term stabilization; whether these findings are equally relevant in male and female patients is still not clear.

Treating sleep disorders in Alzheimer's disease

The treatment of sleep disorders in Alzheimer's disease necessitates meticulous diagnostics, including the general recommendations of excluding common organic reasons for the sleep failure. Thereafter, it is recommended to integrate self-assessment, not solely from patients but also from their caregivers, in addition to objective medical assessments. Sleep assessment should move from subjective measures such as the Pittsburgh Sleep Quality Index (PSQI) or the Epworth Sleepiness Scale (ESS)—neither instrument has been validated in dementia, but both are generally suitable for longitudinally measuring self-rated sleep disturbances—to objective measures, e.g., sleep logs accompanied with actigraphy and polysomnography (McCurry, Gibbons, Logsdon, Vitiello, & Teri, 2003; Ooms & Ju, 2016). Moreover, dementia-specific scales such as the Sleep Disturbance Inventory (SDI) for assessing the caregiver's burden due to sleep disturbance in patients with Alzheimer's disease, or the Behavior Pathology in Alzheimer's Disease Rating Scale (BEHAVE-AD) should be applied (Ooms & Ju, 2016; Tractenberg, Singer, Cummings, & Thal, 2003).

In addition to identifying and treating causal factors, e.g., cardiovascular, endocrine, or psychiatric comorbidities as a result of a proper diagnostic, a non-pharmacological approach focusing on sufficient daytime activities, adapting lifestyle habits, and striving for a rhythmic bedtime are the basis to help improving the patient's sleep. Light therapy early in the morning, for example with 3000 lux for 30 to 90 min, has been shown to improve insomnia in neurodegenerative diseases (Amara, Chahine, & Videnovic, 2017). Moreover, in community-dwelling subjects with Alzheimer's disease, walking, bright light exposure, or both interventions improved sleep compared to controls when applied for at least 30 min at 4 days per week (McCurry, Pike, Vitiello, et al., 2011; Ooms & Ju, 2016). Thus, bright light exposure and walking for 30 min at least 4 days per week on a regular basis can improve the sleep-wake cycle in patients suffering from Alzheimer's disease and is recommended within the new guidelines for insomnia by the German Society of Neurology (Mayer, 2020).

Pharmacological treatment should be carefully adapted to the patient's comorbidities, the drug's side effects, and the patient's specific sleep burden such as insomnia, disturbed sleep-wake cycle, behavioral disorders, or RBD (Weldemichael & Grossberg, 2010). Furthermore, sleep-related breathing disorders should be sufficiently treated to avoid oxygen desaturation, as hypoxia disrupts myelin, which is notably vulnerable in females during menopause (Klosinski, Yao, Yin, et al., 2015; Mosconi, Berti, Quinn, et al., 2017). In particular, neuropsychiatric and behavioral symptoms, including the sundown syndrome, need pharmacological treatment, according to current dementia guidelines. Decision-making should always include the increased risk of extrapyramidal side effects and increased mortality through antipsychotics (see also Chapter 7). Risperidone and aripiprazole (off-label) decrease agitation and aggression in dementia, and haloperidol below 3 mg can also decrease aggression, however, all of them are having an increased risk of detrimental extrapyramidal side effects and higher mortality. Agitation can be treated with pipamperone, which has a sedative effect. Melatonin and clonazepam are well tolerated and effective to treat RBD, however the efficacy of melatonin in dementia is controversial (Jansen, Forbes, Duncan, Morgan, & Malouf, 2006; McCleery, Cohen, & Sharpley, 2016).

Sleep disorders and Alzheimer's disease: The caregiver's burden

Sleep disorders in Alzheimer's disease do not only have a detrimental effect on disease progression, but significantly increase the caregiver's burden. Nocturnal awakenings, nocturnal wandering, and snoring were associated with an increased caregiver's burden, as was analyzed in a cohort of 50% female patients with Alzheimer's disease and 61% female caregivers (Gehrman, Gooneratne, Brewster, Richards, & Karlawish, 2018). Thus, sufficient treatment of sleep disorders and caregiver's burden are core components in the treatment of patients with Alzheimer's disease. A recent analysis of 496 Japanese caregivers (males: 49.8%; females 50.2%) of patients with Alzheimer's disease (males: 27.8%; females: 72.2%) pinpoints the equal sex distribution of caregivers, while disease distribution favors females. This study emphasizes that approximately half of patients did not take their sleep medication and sleep disorders significantly hampered the caregiver's health and quality of life (Okuda, Tetsuka, Takahashi, et al., 2019). In contrast to this latter study, numerous studies report an even larger proportion, with up to 70% of females within the caregiver group (Mahoney, Regan, Katona, & Livingston, 2005; Ory, Hoffman 3rd, Yee, Tennstedt, & Schulz, 1999). This is particularly relevant as there are more female patients suffering from Alzheimer's disease and more female caregiver's suffering from the caregiving burden, thus clearly indicating a gender imbalance (see also Chapter 14).

Without a doubt, the caregiving burden differs between dementia versus non-dementia patients. Caregivers of patients suffering from dementia spend more hours per week on caregiving, have more employment complications, more mental and physical health problems, less time for leisure and other family members, and more family conflicts, compared to caregivers of non-dementia patients (Ory et al., 1999). These findings, together with the larger portion of female caregivers, need careful consideration in research and clinical practice to provide better support and to diminish the caregiver's burden in the future. Psychiatric disorders such as anxiety (23.5%) and depression (10.5%) are common in caregivers of patients with

Alzheimer's disease, and clinicians should be particularly aware of these burdens (Mahoney et al., 2005; Pinquart & Sörensen, 2006). Moreover, a poor-quality relationship between the caregiver and care recipient predicts both, the caregiver's depression and anxiety (Mahoney et al., 2005). Focusing on the physical and mental health of the patient's caregiver is important, not only for the caregiver's quality of life and health, but also to support the patient's care by specifically trained caregivers, as this can result in improved sleep-wake rhythms, increased day time activities, and better patient compliance to sleep educational interventions by the caregivers (McCurry et al., 2003). Consequently, diagnosing and treating sleep disorders in Alzheimer's disease are highly relevant to improving the patient's and caregiver's bidirectional burden.

Key points

- Sleep disorders affect up to 45% of patients with Alzheimer's disease, occur early, and increase during moderate to severe disease stages.
- Sleep disorders in Alzheimer's disease hamper the patient's and caregiver's wellbeing and are a relevant factor for early institutionalization.
- Disrupted sleep architecture with sleep fragmentation, decreased sleep length, involuntary day time napping, and inversion of the sleep-wake cycle, including the sundown syndrome, are common signs in patients with Alzheimer's disease that decrease the glymphatic clearance and increase amyloid-β pathology.
- Sex- and gender-stratified research focusing on sleep disorders and their role for neuronal damage and neurodegenerative biomarkers in Alzheimer's disease is necessary.
- Diagnosing and treating sleep disorders in Alzheimer's disease is a major challenge and includes non-pharmacological and pharmacological approaches that need our careful attention in clinical practice.

Insomnia: An independent risk factor for cognitive impairment

Insomnia is defined as the difficulty falling asleep and/or staying asleep. Falling asleep normally takes 5–10 min, and is considered pathologic when exceeding 30 min on at least 3 occasions per week, persisting throughout at least 1 month (International classification of sleep disorders—Third edition (ICSD-3), 2019). Patients suffering from insomnia often complain about subjective cognitive impairment, and objective assessments uncover mild to moderate cognitive dysfunctions. Insomnia particularly hampers the cognitive domains of attention, episodic memory, working memory, and executive functioning in comparison to healthy subjects (Fortier-Brochu, Beaulieu-Bonneau, Ivers, & Morin, 2012). Patients with insomnia usually underestimate total sleep time and overestimate sleep onset latency. However, subjective complaints often overestimate objective findings, and this discrepancy comes with increased affective and anxiety disorders (Pang, Guo, Wu, et al., 2018; Taylor, Lichstein, Durrence, Reidel, & Bush, 2005).

Females have a 40% increased risk of insomnia in comparison to males, which might be at least partially explained by females' greater awareness, sensitive body vigilance, and the tendency of overreporting (Mallampalli & Carter, 2014; Zhang & Wing, 2006). Insomnia is a frequent symptom in affective and anxiety disorders that often outlasts remission of the psychiatric disease (Rauen & Weidt, 2017), and therefore, these psychiatric burdens, namely the higher females' prevalence of depression and anxiety disorders, most probably contribute to this sex- and gender-related imbalance of insomnia. More than half of the elderly population complain about their sleep (Vitiello, 2009; Yaremchuk, 2018), and approximately one third suffer from sleep disorders as a barrier to successful aging, and again, females are more affected (Tardy, Gonthier, Barthelemy, Roche, & Crawford-Achour, 2015). This is of importance as current evidence suggests insomnia as an independent risk factor for cognitive impairment (Pang et al., 2018; Wardle-Pinkston, Slavish, & Taylor, 2019). However, studies on insomnia and cognitive performance have a broad heterogeneity, so far; thus, consistent use of operationalized diagnosis of insomnia and comprehensive test batteries for assessing cognitive performance are required. In addition, confounding factors such as comorbidities, medication, and previous nights' sleep should also be considered in future studies (Wardle-Pinkston et al., 2019).

Looking closer into the brains of patients with insomnia uncovers that the neural networks of the awakening, affective control, and cognitive systems are involved. In particular, pathological changes in the hippocampus and medial prefrontal cortex support the clinical picture of impaired memory integration in patients with insomnia and mild cognitive impairment (MCI) (Pang et al., 2018). This latter study reported that brain activity during functional neuroimaging positively correlated with subjective sleep quality assessed by the Pittsburgh Sleep Quality Index (PSQI) as well as with cognitive function assessed by the Montreal Cognitive Assessment (MoCA) (Pang et al., 2018), thereby supporting subjective and objective sleep disturbances in patients with MCI.

The large Swiss HypnoLaus study revealed that patients aged above 65 years with mild dementia (Clinical Dementia Rating > 0) experience a disrupted sleep architecture (Haba-Rubio et al., 2017). In detail, these patients had more light sleep (NREM stage N1), less deep sleep (NREM stage N3), less REM sleep, a lower sleep efficiency, higher intra-sleep wake, and higher sleepiness scores. Moreover, sleep-related breathing disorder, particularly a higher apnea/hypopnea index and a higher oxygen desaturation index, were independently associated with the patients' cognitive impairment, indicating the detrimental relevance of sleep fragmentation and hypoxia in dementia.

Thus, we will highlight obstructive sleep apnea as a modifiable risk for cognitive impairment evolving to dementia, after discussing treatment options for insomnia in the elderly with respect to cognitive dysfunction.

Treating sleep disorders in the elderly

How to treat insomnia in the elderly? The first line treatment is a non-pharmacological approach using cognitive behavioral therapy to improve and stabilize the patient's sleep-wake rhythm (Zdanys & Steffens, 2015). Important aspects are sleep education focusing, for example, on sleep hygiene, sufficient and rhythmic activities during the day, as well as relaxation techniques particularly before bedtime, and/or specific light therapy in the morning. Although still rare, psychological and educative group therapy is efficient to improve insomnia and sleep quality in the elderly (Lovato, Lack, Wright, & Kennaway, 2014; Sadler, McLaren, Klein, Harvey, & Jenkins, 2018).

Secondly, additional pharmacotherapy is necessary, but needs careful attention due to comorbidities, polypharmacy, the higher risk of adverse side effects, and decreased metabolism in the elderly. Trazodone—a dual serotonergic antidepressant without anticholinergic side effects—is recommended for the pharmacological treatment of insomnia, particularly because trazodone has been shown to reduce cognitive decline 2.6-fold compared to non-trazodone users in a small, controlled study sample of 9 females and 16 males with an average age of 75.4 ± 7.5 years and an initial score of 28 out of 30 in the MMSE over 4 years. These patients suffered from sleep disturbances including insomnia and were diagnosed with either MCI, predicted Alzheimer's pathology, or were cognitively healthy. A decrease in cognitive decline was associated with subjectively improved sleep. Impressively, the beneficial trazodone effect in terms of better cognitive performance in the MMSE was also seen in patients with predicted Alzheimer's pathology (La, Walsh, Neylan, et al., 2019). This study needs replication with respect to larger sex- and gender-stratified sample sizes.

Despite this promising evidence on trazodone, and the broad knowledge of the detrimental adverse side effects of benzodiazepines and the so-called z-drugs (zolpidem, zopiclone, and zaleplon), benzodiazepines and z-drugs are still commonly prescribed and frequently used. In terms of drug metabolism, it is notable that the elderly metabolize zolpidem twice as slowly as younger patients, and females metabolize zolpidem twice as slowly as males; thus, these drugs particularly harm the elderly and notably female patients (Cubała, Wiglusz, Burkiewicz, & Gałuszko-Węgielnik, 2010). Why are benzodiazepines and z-drugs particularly harmful in the elderly? Harmful side effects are the tolerance, dependency, rebound insomnia, paradoxical effects with increased agitation and anxiety, hampered sleep architecture, sedation with postural instability accompanied by an increased risk of falls, and cognitive impairment (Atkin, Comai, & Gobbi, 2018; Savaskan, 2016). Thus, benzodiazepines and z-drugs should only be prescribed for short periods of time (below 3–4 weeks) during inpatient treatment and in particular, should not be prescribed in the elderly (see also Chapter 7). Further recommended options for the treatment of insomnia in the elderly might be melatonin, mirtazapine, or quetiapine, and off-label prescription can be considered.

Key points

- Insomnia is an independent risk factor for cognitive impairment and females have a 40% increased risk of insomnia compared to males.
- First-line treatment of insomnia in the elderly is the non-pharmacological approach, including cognitive behavioral therapy and group therapy.
- In the elderly, pharmacotherapy needs particular attention due to comorbidities, polypharmacy, slower metabolism, and adverse side effects.
- Trazodone improves sleep and delays cognitive decline, while benzodiazepines and z-drugs should be avoided due to the detrimental side effects with increased risk of falls, tolerance, dependency, paradoxical effect, and cognitive impairment.
- Sex- and gender-stratified outcome reporting with respect to non-pharmacological and pharmacological treatment of insomnia is necessary.

Obstructive sleep apnea syndrome: A risk factor for cognitive impairment and Alzheimer's disease

OSAS is one of the most common sleep-related breathing disorders and is associated with an increased risk of cardiovascular diseases such as high blood pressure, heart disease, and stroke, which in turn increases the risk of cognitive impairment (Livingston et al., 2020; MFMER, 2020a). OSAS is associated with a partial or complete airway obstruction, with typical symptoms being loud snoring, nocturnal awakening, night time sweating, morning headaches, excessive daytime sleepiness or drowsiness, mood changes, decreased libido, difficulties concentrating, and hampered cognitive functioning (Maspero, Giannini, Galbiati, Rosso, & Farronato, 2015; Patel, 2019). To date, male sex, increased age, a higher body mass index (BMI), hypertension, and a history of snoring with witnessed apneas are currently recognized to be the most important predictors of moderate to severe OSAS (Jung, Junna, Mandrekar, & Morgenthaler, 2017). Sleep-related breathing disorders are associated with a 26% higher likelihood of cognitive impairment, with executive functioning particularly hampered. Applying sufficient overnight oxygen showed improved cognition, suggesting hypoxia to be the relevant trigger for cognitive impairment—albeit the mechanisms are still yet to be fully understood and have only been studied in males (Blackwell, Yaffe, Laffan, et al., 2015; Leng, McEvoy, Allen, & Yaffe, 2017). Nevertheless, there is evidence that females have almost a two-fold increased risk of developing MCI or even dementia when experiencing a sleep-related breathing disorder, and again, hypoxia seems to be the relevant trigger, while sleep fragmentation or length of sleep is not (Yaffe, Laffan, Harrison, et al., 2011).

Obstructive sleep apnea syndrome and the different clinical pictures in male and female patients

Current evidence suggests that OSAS in general affects males twice as often as females (Heinzer, Vat, Marques-Vidal, et al., 2015; Maspero et al., 2015; Valipour,

2012), while in turn females compared to males are twice as likely to develop a cognitive impairment due to a sleep-related breathing disorder. Reasons for OSAS being more frequent in males might be related to differences in pharyngeal collapsibility and central respiratory drive. Interestingly, female patients experience OSAS later in life, particularly during menopause, and those suffering from OSAS have a higher BMI compared to males (Valipour, 2012). Almost two decades ago, a large study on 830 male and female patients with OSAS uncovered similar severity of OSAS in male and female patients during REM sleep but milder OSAS in females during NREM sleep—a relevant finding that has not yet been fully understood (O'Connor, Thornley, & Hanly, 2000). Although women seem to experience milder OSAS with a lower apnea-hypopnea index and shorter apneas and hypopneas than males, they remain more often undiagnosed with relevant consequences in terms of morbidity and mortality (Wimms, Woehrle, Ketheeswaran, Ramanan, & Armitstead, 2016).

One important factor for overseeing OSAS in females might be their atypical symptoms, with insomnia, depression, and/or restless legs syndrome—clinical features that do not routinely require a polysomnography, which in turn would be necessary and the current gold standard to diagnose OSAS (Valipour, 2012). Thus, the current estimates with a male to female ratio of 2:1 might be misleading, as twice as many male than female patients (13.3% versus 6.9%) received medical examination including polysomnography due to abnormal sleep habits that were recognized by their bed partners—suggesting a possible bias of the current OSAS prevalence due to the lower awareness of diagnosing OSAS in females (Auer, Frauscher, Hochleitner, & Högl, 2018). To date, it is well-known that treating OSAS reduces cardiovascular risks, depression, anxiety, and cognitive impairment, and thus extending efforts in diagnosing OSAS in females will help to improve precision medicine in the future (Tamanna and Geraci, 2013).

Obstructive sleep apnea syndrome in relation to cognitive impairment and Alzheimer's disease

Age and sex matters in terms of OSAS and the risk of developing cognitive dysfunction over the entire life span. Snoring in infants and children is associated with lower intelligence, and middle-aged adults have an increased risk of cognitive impairment compared to older adults suffering from similar apnea severity. Moreover, elderly females with OSAS might experience MCI or even dementia 5 years after onset of the sleep-related breathing disorders (Grigg-Damberger & Ralls, 2012). Interestingly, newly diagnosed, and so far untreated patients with OSAS showed a reduced myelin and axonal integrity in multiple and particularly left-sided brain areas including the medulla oblongata, the basal ganglia, and the limbic system—areas that are also relevant for cardiovascular, respiratory, and mood regulations. In particular, myelin was more vulnerable to hypoxemia (Kumar, Pham, Macey, et al., 2014) a potential finding that might explain the increased risk of females suffering OSAS during menopause—a time frame in which female myelin is per se more vulnerable (Klosinski et al., 2015; Mosconi et al., 2017). Moreover, substantial loss of white matter integrity in females compared to males was found and was related to the higher portion of anxiety and depression in females suffering from OSAS in comparison to their male counterparts (Macey et al., 2012).

In contrast, a recent study on 1084 middle-aged male and female patients with OSAS did not find sex-related differences with respect to subjective cognitive impairment, while female sex/gender was an independent predictor for tiredness, delayed sleep onset, and morning headaches, whereas males more frequently reported loud snoring and experienced apnea (Nigro, Dibur, Borsini, et al., 2018). These findings suggest that females are potentially more affected and restricted in their work performance and quality of life due to sleepiness and headaches, compared to males. When it comes to cognitive dysfunctions, it is well-known that patients with OSAS suffer from impaired concentration, memory, and executive functioning (Vaessen, Overeem, & Sitskoorn, 2015), and it is highly relevant to distinguish between subjective and objective findings, as both restrict the patient's quality of life. However, research on subjective cognitive complaints in patients suffering from OSAS is sparse. Treating OSAS using CPAP is beneficial in terms of subjective and objective cognitive impairments but available data needs to be sex- and gender-stratified in the future (Bubu, Andrade, Umasabor-Bubu, et al., 2020; Crawford-Achour, Dauphinot, Martin, et al., 2015; Kanbay, Demir, Tutar, et al., 2017; Mulgrew, Ryan, Fleetham, et al., 2007; Perez-Cabezas, Ruiz-Molinero, & Jimenez-Rejano, 2020; Turner, Zambrelli, Lavolpe, et al., 2019). Finally, applying CPAP demands knowledge of sex-related differences in terms of applying less pressure in females compared to males (Mallampalli & Carter, 2014; Ralls & Grigg-Damberger, 2012).

Biomarkers in OSAS and Alzheimer's disease

Studying OSAS and cognitive impairment advances to proteomic analysis with recently identified biomarkers, namely insulin, angiopoietin-1, and IL-1B, in cognitive-impaired females suffering from OSAS. These biomarkers are also relevant in Alzheimer's disease, suggesting a link between both diseases that might have a potential for diagnosing patients' sequels early (Lal, Hardiman, Kumbhare, & Strange, 2019). To date, it is unclear if these biomarkers are only valid for a subgroup of postmenopausal females, and thus, further research is needed. Additionally, OSAS and Alzheimer's disease seem to share amyloid and tau pathology, inflammation, oxidative stress, and metabolic disturbances that can be detected by fluid cerebrospinal and blood biomarkers, e.g., amyloid-β, tau proteins, inflammatory cytokines, acute-phase proteins, antioxidants and oxidized products, homocysteine and clusterin protein (apolipoprotein J) (Baril, Carrier, Lafrenière, et al., 2018; Livingston et al., 2020). Thus, these biomarkers might have the ability to detect patients with OSAS that are at risk of developing Alzheimer's disease early.

Despite knowing the importance of sex-related differences in both OSAS and Alzheimer's disease, research primarily reports on sex distribution in terms of included subjects as well as on socioeconomic factors, but still struggles to consequently report on sex- and gender-stratified results. A recently published systematic review on OSAS and Alzheimer's disease included 68 out of 2717 studies and pinpoints that: (i) OSAS is often associated with cognitive impairment in young and middle-aged adults; (ii) older adults with OSAS and MCI or Alzheimer's disease are more likely to seek medical treatment due to sleep disturbance; (iii) OSAS and Alzheimer's are linked with respect to neurodegenerative biomarkers, e.g., amyloid-β40, amyloid-β42, total amyloid-β, and p-tau 181, in cognitive-normal subjects of all age groups; (iv) OSAS particularly worsens metabolic injury in middle-aged patients by deteriorating neuronal injury with pronounced memory and cognitive impairment in older adults; (v) OSAS might induce neurodegeneration by intermittent hypoxia, sleep fragmentation, reduced slow wave sleep (NREM stages N3), and intrathoracic pressure swings; and (vi) CPAP treatment might improve cognition in patients suffering from OSAS and Alzheimer's disease (Bubu et al., 2020). There is currently no doubt about the link between OSAS and Alzheimer's disease as well as the effective reduction of cognitive complaints and restrictions by sufficient CPAP treatment. Nevertheless, to date, sex- and gender-stratified results are sparse and need our focus to improve personalized medicine in the future.

Key points

- OSAS is as modifiable risk factor of Alzheimer's disease with a male to female ratio of 2:1; differences in clinical presentation in female and male patients might lead to underdiagnosis of females.
- CPAP treatment is effective in stabilizing or even improving cognitive function in patients suffering from OSAS and Alzheimer's disease.
- Neurodegenerative, inflammatory, and metabolic fluid biomarkers pinpoint the link between OSAS and Alzheimer's disease.
- Sex- and gender-stratified outcome analyses in OSAS are necessary. Better diagnosing of the atypical presentation of OSAS in females might contribute to helping to reduce Alzheimer's disease and females' burden of dementia.

REM sleep behavior disorder: A relevant parasomnia and an early clinical biomarker for neurodegenerative diseases

RBD is a relevant parasomnia that can be either idiopathic or secondary, with a mean onset age between 50 and 65 years (ranging from childhood to 80 years of age) (Boeve et al., 2003). Secondary RBD is associated with the intake of antidepressants—selective serotonin reuptake inhibitors (SSRIs), selective norepinephrine reuptake inhibitors (SNRIs), or tricyclic antidepressants—and other neurological diseases, e.g., narcolepsy type 1 (Barone & Henchcliffe, 2018; Dauvilliers, Schenck, Postuma, et al., 2018; St Louis & Boeve, 2017). To date, it is insufficiently understood whether antidepressant-related RBD in particular is a harmless drug side effect or an early marker of prodromal neurodegeneration (Barone & Henchcliffe, 2018).

However, there is evidence that both forms of RBD are strongly associated with α-synucleinopathies such as Parkinson's disease, dementia with Lewy bodies, or multisystem atrophy (Dauvilliers et al., 2018; Shenker & Singh, 2017; St Louis & Boeve, 2017). As RBD occurs decades before the clinical manifestation of neurodegeneration (Claassen, Josephs, Ahlskog, et al., 2010), it might be a suitable clinical biomarker that helps detecting subthreshold neurodegeneration early and its sufficient treatment might delay conversion to the clinically evident neurodegenerative disease.

According to the 3rd edition of the ICSD, RBD is defined through (1) repeated episodes of behavior or vocalization during REM sleep that are either supported by polysomnography or are presumed according to reports on dream enactment, and (2) evidence of REM sleep without atonia assessed by polysomnography. If REM sleep without atonia is not observed during polysomnography, a probable RBD diagnosis can be given on the basis of strong and suggestive clinical signs (International classification of sleep disorders—Third edition (ICSD-3), 2019). Diagnosing RBD includes a physical and neurological exam, taking a sleep history from the patient's bed partner, and polysomnography as an objective measurement (MFMER, 2020b; St Louis & Boeve, 2017). Specific findings are repeated arousals during sleep where the patient talks, makes noise, or performs complex motor behaviors, e.g., punching, kicking, or running movements, which are often related to the patient's dreams. Furthermore, the patient recalls the dreams and is alert when awaking during these episodes, not being confused or disoriented. These clinical findings are supported by increased muscle activity during REM sleep, which can be recorded by electromyography during polysomnography and is not caused by any other sleep or mental health disorder, medication, or substance abuse (MFMER, 2020b).

Why is it important to detect RBD early? Firstly, RBD is treatable by melatonin 3 to 12 mg or clonazepam 0.25 to 2 mg at bedtime (St Louis & Boeve, 2017). While melatonin is well-tolerated and has few adverse side effects, clonazepam might lead to daytime sleepiness, disturbed balance, and increased sleep apnea, which needs consideration in decision-making (St Louis & Boeve, 2017). Moreover, clonazepam might increase the risk of dementia (Postuma, Iranzo, Hogl, et al., 2015). To date, there is no knowledge whether melatonin or clonazepam has a sex-specific drug efficacy. However, zolpidem—a benzodiazepine-like drug, and thus related to clonazepam—is metabolized 50% slower in females compared to males (Cubała et al., 2010). Thus, sex-stratified research on the drug efficacy of melatonin, and particularly of clonazepam is suggested. Secondly, one major aspect is protecting both, the patient and bed partner, from injury by the involuntary movements of the patient acting out dreams (Boeve, Silber, Saper, et al., 2007). Both recommended drugs, i.e., melatonin and clonazepam, reduce dream enactment; however non-pharmacological bed safety recommendations—such as removal of potentially harmful furniture close to the patient's bedside, enough distance between the patient and the bed partner, or even placing the mattress directly on the floor to avoid falling out of the bed—should be applied as well. Thirdly, RBD hampers not only the patient's but also the bed partner's quality of life and daily performance, and thereby potentially the couple relationship (Lam, Wong, Li, et al., 2016). Thus, diagnosing and treating RBD early is important to diminish the caring burden. Fourthly and finally, RBD is an early clinical biomarker for neurodegenerative diseases as the pathological hallmark of α-synucleinopathies such as Parkinson's disease, dementia with Lewy bodies, multisystem atrophy, but also occurs in Alzheimer's disease, and thus diagnosing and treating RBD early might be suitable to delay conversion to an overt neurodegenerative disease (MFMER, 2020b).

REM sleep behavior disorder and sex- and gender-related differences

The overall prevalence of RBD is uncertain and estimated as 0.4%–0.5% in the general population. The prevalence increases with age up to 2% in the 6th and up to 6% in the 7th decade of life, with males being predominantly affected and with estimates of up to 80% (Barone & Henchcliffe, 2018; Boeve et al., 2003). However, females might be underdiagnosed due to a different clinical picture with less violent and less acting-out movements (Barone & Henchcliffe, 2018). Moreover, females on average have a higher life expectancy, and thus acting-out of dreams might be less recognized due to absent bed partners. As RBD is strongly associated with α-synucleinopathies, such as Parkinson's disease, multisystem atrophy, and dementia with Lewy bodies, the higher male prevalence of RBD might be linked to the higher male proportion of Parkinson's disease. Interestingly, a clinical trial on a relatively large sample size in current RBD research included 63 males and 27 females with RBD and revealed that females were younger at RBD onset and diagnosis, took more antidepressants, and had less dream-related behaviors compared to males. Polysomnography revealed that females with RBD had more deep sleep, indicated by slow wave sleep (NREM stage N3), and less light sleep (NREM stage N1) compared to males, while electromyographic findings—thus, muscle activity—did not differ between sexes (Zhou, Zhang, Li, et al., 2015).

REM sleep behavior disorder and the risk of clinical manifestation of a neurodegenerative disease

A recent clinical trial of 305 RBD patients pinpoints that 33% of patients convert to a clinically manifested neurodegenerative disease with an increasing risk over time, namely 25% at 3 years, and 41% at 5 years (Postuma et al., 2015). Age, but not sex, was relevant for conversion to clinically apparent neurodegeneration. Moreover, a positive family history of dementia doubled the likelihood of this conversion. Importantly, and accordingly to our abovementioned point on pharmacological treatment, clonazepam increased the risk of converting to dementia almost three-fold. Thus, we suggest melatonin in RBD treatment whenever sufficient. A large cross-sectional analysis on 263 patients with Parkinson's disease and 158 patients with Parkinson's disease and probable RBD uncovered differences in clinical and fluid biomarkers (Pagano, De Micco, Yousaf, et al., 2018). In detail, patients with Parkinson's disease and probable RBD suffered from a higher burden of non-motor symptoms, faster motor progression, and cognitive decline over a 60-months follow-up period compared to Parkinson's disease without RBD. In terms of fluid biomarkers, patients with Parkinson's disease and probable RBD had lower β-amyloid 1–42 (Aβ42) levels and a higher total tau to Aβ42 ratio in the CSF compared to Parkinson's disease without RBD. The presence of RBD was a predictor for cognitive decline only in patients with Parkinson's disease who had both low CSF Aβ42 and low CSF α-synuclein levels, while RBD in controls without Parkinson's disease was not associated with cognitive decline. However, these results have not yet been sex- and gender-stratified.

Nevertheless, there is evidence that the risk to convert from probable RBD to MCI or Parkinson's disease is increased 2.2-fold after stratifying for age, sex, education, and comorbidities, but none of the patients deteriorated to dementia within the follow-up period of 4 years (Boot, Boeve, Roberts, et al., 2012), suggesting longer observational periods are needed. Despite stratifying for sex differences, this study did not report on the difference between females and males with respect to clinical manifestation of MCI or Parkinson's disease, which is needed in the future. Recently, a multicenter trial analyzed 1280 patients with RBD from 24 centers and confirmed a high risk of conversion to overt neurodegenerative disease. The sample size included 80% males, and thus represents the current estimates of the male to female ratio; but again, results have not yet been sex- and gender-stratified. The same multicenter study revealed that the only clearly differentiating variable between dementia-first and Parkinsonism-first was cognition itself (Postuma, Iranzo, Hu, et al., 2019). However, the underlying pathology is still unclear, and might be related to either α-synuclein spreading first to the cortex and thereafter to the substantia nigra, or comorbid amyloid cortical pathology that rapidly progresses to dementia-first (Adler & Beach, 2016; Chételat, La Joie, Villain, et al., 2013; Postuma et al., 2019). To conclude, sex- and gender-stratified evidence on RBD and the risk of neurodegeneration including Alzheimer's disease is still sparse.

Sundown syndrome in Alzheimer's disease is associated with RBD

A major concern in Alzheimer's disease is the sundown syndrome—a syndrome characterized by aggravation of neuropsychiatric symptoms such as agitation, anxiety, aggressive behavior, hallucinations, and disorientation that occurs in 28% of patients with Alzheimer's disease during the late afternoon, and facilitates amyloid pathology (Pyun, Kang, Yun, Park, & Kim, 2019). This phenomenon was also seen in altered circadian locomotor activity in transgenic APP23 mice, which developed activity disturbances with aging at 6 and 12 months of age compared to controls (C57BL/6 mice); this was similar to the patient's sundown phenomenon, and is thus suitable for experimental research of behavior and psychological symptoms in dementia (BPSD) (Vloeberghs, Van Dam, Engelborghs, et al., 2004). RBD, APOE ε4 carrier status, and more severe dementia were significantly associated with an increased risk of the sundown syndrome. Females suffered more often from sundown syndrome than males with an odds ratio of 1.5 after univariate analysis and of 2.3 after multivariate analysis. However, both values have not been statistically significant in a small sample of 29 patients (9 males; 20 females) with Alzheimer's disease and sundown syndrome (Pyun et al., 2019). Currently, the underlying mechanisms of the sundown syndrome are not fully understood and it remains questionable whether sex- and/or gender-related factors are relevant. Finally, it remains unclear whether RBD is relevant in Alzheimer's disease. Current evidence from longitudinal studies estimates Alzheimer's disease in 3% to 11% of RBD patients, however this proportion might be overestimated due to solely using clinical criteria for diagnosing Alzheimer's disease and due to mixed dementia of Alzheimer's disease and dementia with Lewy bodies (Galbiati, Carli, Hensley, & Ferini-Strambi, 2018).

In conclusion, RBD is a relevant sleeping disorder that primarily affects males, with an increased risk of conversion to particularly α-synucleinopathies such as Parkinson's disease, dementia with Lewy bodies, and multisystem atrophy. Nevertheless, there is evidence that RBD occurs in Alzheimer's disease as well, and might increase the risk of sundown syndrome with behavioral changes at sunset, which in turn affects females more often than males. RBD can be treated by melatonin at a dosage of 3 to 12 mg or clonazepam at a dosage of 0.25 to 2 mg at bedtime with the latter having more adverse side effects such as daytime sleepiness, disturbed balance, increased sleep apnea, and an increased risk of dementia, which need careful consideration in decision-making.

Key points

- RBD is a relevant parasomnia that primarily affects males and can be either idiopathic or secondary with an average age of onset between 50 and 65 years.
- RBD is strongly associated with α-synucleinopathies such as Parkinson's disease, dementia with Lewy bodies, or multisystem atrophy, but might also occur in Alzheimer's disease.
- Females with RBD are younger at onset, take more antidepressants, have less dream-related behaviors, and have a different sleep architecture compared to males.
- RBD is diagnosed by taking a history including the bed partner and a polysomnography.
- RBD is treatable by melatonin 3 to 12 mg or clonazepam 0.25 to 2 mg at bedtime with clonazepam having more adverse side effects including a higher risk of dementia.
- Sundown syndrome is a common clinical phenomenon with 28% of patients with Alzheimer's disease being affected. Sundown syndrome presents with neuropsychiatric symptoms such as agitation, hallucinations, behavioral changes, or aggression in the late afternoon. It seems to be associated with RBD, APOE ε4 carrier, and more severe Alzheimer's disease with females being affected more than twice as often as males.

Conclusion

Sleep disorders and cognitive impairment evolving to dementia have a bidirectional relationship with a variety of sex- and gender-related aspects that are not fully understood yet. Poor sleep is often underdiagnosed and the clinical picture of OSAS and RBD differs between females and males, which might impede diagnosis in females. Early non-pharmacological and pharmacological treatments can substantially improve the patient's and bed partner's sleep, cognition, and quality of life. Insomnia, OSAS, and RBD are modifiable risk factors for cognitive impairment evolving to dementia. Thus, focusing on sleep disorders might help to slow down the conversion to clinically manifested dementia and need our careful attention in research and clinical practice. Proper understanding of sleep disorders, including the sex and gender differences in their pathophysiology, diagnosis, and management are necessary steps to achieve targeted care to improve lives of both, affected patients and their caregivers.

Chapter highlights

- Knowledge on sex- and gender-related differences in sleep disorders and Alzheimer's disease is sparse.
- Sleep disorders and dementia have a bidirectional relationship:
    - Insomnia is an independent risk factor for cognitive impairment with females having a 40% higher risk than males.
    - OSAS is a modifiable risk factor for cognitive impairment and dementia with a male to female ratio of 2:1, but female patients might be underdiagnosed due to a different clinical presentation.
    - RBD is a prodromal marker for α-synucleinopathies and can be present in Alzheimer's disease.
- Almost half of patients with Alzheimer's disease suffer from sleep disorders with disrupted sleep-wake cycles, behavioral changes including sundown syndrome, which increases amyloid-β plaques in the brain and results in a vicious circle of increasing the sleep disturbances.
- Diagnosing and treating sleep disorders in Alzheimer's disease early improves patient's and caregiver's wellbeing and delay patient's institutionalization.

References

Adler, C. H., & Beach, T. G. (2016). Neuropathological basis of nonmotor manifestations of Parkinson's disease. *Movement Disorders, 31*, 1114–1119.

Amara, A. W., Chahine, L. M., & Videnovic, A. (2017). Treatment of sleep dysfunction in Parkinson's disease. *Current Treatment Options in Neurology, 19*, 26.

Anderson, K. N., & Bradley, A. J. (2013). Sleep disturbance in mental health problems and neurodegenerative disease. *Nature and Science of Sleep, 5*, 61–75.

Anttalainen, U., Saaresranta, T., Kalleinen, N., et al. (2007). CPAP adherence and partial upper airway obstruction during sleep. *Sleep & Breathing, 11*, 171–176.

Aserinsky, E., & Kleitman, N. (1953). Regularly occurring periods of eye motility, and concomitant phenomena, during sleep. *Science*, *118*, 273–274.

Atkin, T., Comai, S., & Gobbi, G. (2018). Drugs for insomnia beyond benzodiazepines: Pharmacology, clinical applications, and discovery. *Pharmacological Reviews*, *70*, 197–245.

Auer, M., Frauscher, B., Hochleitner, M., & Högl, B. (2018). Gender-specific differences in access to polysomnography and prevalence of sleep disorders. *Journal of Women's Health*, *27*, 525–530.

Baldwin, C. M., Kapur, V. K., Holberg, C. J., Rosen, C., & Nieto, F. J. (2004). Associations between gender and measures of daytime somnolence in the Sleep Heart Health Study. *Sleep*, *27*, 305–311.

Baril, A. A., Carrier, J., Lafrenière, A., et al. (2018). Biomarkers of dementia in obstructive sleep apnea. *Sleep Medicine Reviews*, *42*, 139–148.

Barone, D. A., & Henchcliffe, C. (2018). Rapid eye movement sleep behavior disorder and the link to alpha-synucleinopathies. *Clinical Neurophysiology*, *129*, 1551–1564.

Biddle, D. J., Naismith, S. L., Griffiths, K. M., et al. (2017). Associations of objective and subjective sleep disturbance with cognitive function in older men with comorbid depression and insomnia. *Sleep Health*, *3*, 178–183.

Blackwell, T., Yaffe, K., Laffan, A., et al. (2015). Associations of sleep disordered breathing, nocturnal hypoxemia and subsequent cognitive decline in older community-dwelling men: The MrOS sleep study. *Journal of the American Geriatrics Society*, *63*, 453–461.

Boeve, B. F., Silber, M. H., Ferman, T. J., et al. (2003). REM sleep behavior disorder in Parkinson's disease, dementia with lewy bodies, and multiple system atrophy. In M.-A. Bédard, Y. Agid, S. Chouinard, et al. (Eds.), *Mental and behavioral dysfunction in movement disorders* (pp. 383–397). Totowa, NJ: Humana Press.

Boeve, B. F., Silber, M. H., Saper, C. B., et al. (2007). Pathophysiology of REM sleep behaviour disorder and relevance to neurodegenerative disease. *Brain*, *130*, 2770–2788.

Boot, B. P., Boeve, B. F., Roberts, R. O., et al. (2012). Probable REM sleep behavior disorder increases risk for mild cognitive impairment and Parkinson's disease: A population-based study. *Annals of Neurology*, *71*, 49–56.

Bubu, O. M., Brannick, M., Mortimer, J., et al. (2017). Sleep, cognitive impairment, and Alzheimer's disease: A systematic review and meta-analysis. *Sleep*, *40*, 1–18.

Bubu, O. M., Andrade, A. G., Umasabor-Bubu, O. Q., et al. (2020). Obstructive sleep apnea, cognition and Alzheimer's disease: A systematic review integrating three decades of multidisciplinary research. *Sleep Medicine Reviews*, *50*, 101250.

Chételat, G., La Joie, R., Villain, N., et al. (2013). Amyloid imaging in cognitively normal individuals, at-risk populations and preclinical Alzheimer's disease. *NeuroImage: Clinical*, *2*, 356–365.

Claassen, D. O., Josephs, K. A., Ahlskog, J. E., et al. (2010). REM sleep behavior disorder preceding other aspects of synucleinopathies by up to half a century. *Neurology*, *75*, 494–499.

Crawford-Achour, E., Dauphinot, V., Martin, M. S., et al. (2015). Protective effect of long-term CPAP therapy on cognitive performance in elderly patients with severe OSA: The PROOF study. *Journal of Clinical Sleep Medicine*, *11*, 519–524.

Cubała, W. J., Wiglusz, M., Burkiewicz, A., & Gałuszko-Węgielnik, M. (2010). Zolpidem pharmacokinetics and pharmacodynamics in metabolic interactions involving CYP3A: Sex as a differentiating factor. *European Journal of Clinical Pharmacology*, *66*, 955.

Dauvilliers, Y., Schenck, C. H., Postuma, R. B., et al. (2018). REM sleep behaviour disorder. *Nature Reviews. Disease Primers*, *4*, 19.

de Almondes, K. M., Costa, M. V., Malloy-Diniz, L. F., & Diniz, B. S. (2016). Insomnia and risk of dementia in older adults: Systematic review and meta-analysis. *Journal of Psychiatric Research, 77*, 109–115.

Deak, M., & Epstein, L. J. (2009). The history of polysomnography. *Sleep Medicine Clinics, 4*, 313–321.

Dement, W. C. (2003). Knocking on Kleitman's door: The view from 50 years later. *Sleep Medicine Reviews, 7*, 289–292.

Ellenbogen, J. M., Payne, J. D., & Stickgold, R. (2006). The role of sleep in declarative memory consolidation: Passive, permissive, active or none? *Current Opinion in Neurobiology, 16*, 716–722.

Fortier-Brochu, E., Beaulieu-Bonneau, S., Ivers, H., & Morin, C. M. (2012). Insomnia and daytime cognitive performance: A meta-analysis. *Sleep Medicine Reviews, 16*, 83–94.

Gabbay, I. E., & Lavie, P. (2012). Age- and gender-related characteristics of obstructive sleep apnea. *Sleep & Breathing, 16*, 453–460.

Galbiati, A., Carli, G., Hensley, M., & Ferini-Strambi, L. (2018). REM sleep behavior disorder and Alzheimer's disease: Definitely no relationship? *Journal of Alzheimer's Disease, 63*, 1–11.

Gehrman, P., Gooneratne, N. S., Brewster, G. S., Richards, K. C., & Karlawish, J. (2018). Impact of Alzheimer disease patients' sleep disturbances on their caregivers. *Geriatric Nursing, 39*, 60–65.

Grigg-Damberger, M., & Ralls, F. (2012). Cognitive dysfunction and obstructive sleep apnea: From cradle to tomb. *Current Opinion in Pulmonary Medicine, 18*, 580–587.

Haba-Rubio, J., Marti-Soler, H., Tobback, N., et al. (2017). Sleep characteristics and cognitive impairment in the general population the HypnoLaus study. *Neurology, 88*, 463–469.

Heinzer, R., Vat, S., Marques-Vidal, P., et al. (2015). Prevalence of sleep-disordered breathing in the general population: The HypnoLaus study. *The Lancet Respiratory Medicine, 3*, 310–318.

Institute of Medicine Committee on Sleep Medicine and Research. (2006). The National Academies Collection: Reports funded by National Institutes of Health. In H. R. Colten, & B. M. Altevogt (Eds.), *Sleep disorders and sleep deprivation: An unmet public health problem*. Washington, DC: National Academies Press.

International classification of sleep disorders—Third edition (ICSD-3). (2019). Darien, IL: American Academy of Sleep Medicine. Available from: https://learn.aasm.org/Public/Catalog/Details.aspx?id=%2FgqQVDMQIT%2FEDy86PWgqgQ%3D%3D&returnurl=%2fUsers%2fUserOnlineCourse.aspx%3fLearningActivityID%3d%252fgqQVDMQIT%252fEDy86PWgqgQ%253d%253d.

Jansen, S. L., Forbes, D., Duncan, V., Morgan, D. G., & Malouf, R. (2006). Melatonin for the treatment of dementia. *Cochrane Database of Systematic Reviews*, (1), CD003802. https://doi.org/10.1002/14651858.CD003802.pub3.

Jordan, A. S., & McEvoy, R. D. (2003). Gender differences in sleep apnea: Epidemiology, clinical presentation and pathogenic mechanisms. *Sleep Medicine Reviews, 7*, 377–389.

Ju, Y.-E. S., Lucey, B. P., & Holtzman, D. (2014). Sleep and Alzheimer disease pathology—A bidirectional relationship. *Nature Reviews. Neurology, 10*, 115–119.

Jung, Y., Junna, M. R., Mandrekar, J. N., & Morgenthaler, T. I. (2017). The National Healthy Sleep Awareness Project Sleep Health Surveillance Questionnaire as an obstructive sleep apnea surveillance tool. *Journal of Clinical Sleep Medicine, 13*, 1067–1074.

Kanbay, A., Demir, N. C., Tutar, N., et al. (2017). The effect of CPAP therapy on insulin-like growth factor and cognitive functions in obstructive sleep apnea patients. *The Clinical Respiratory Journal, 11*, 506–513.

Klosinski, L. P., Yao, J., Yin, F., et al. (2015). White matter lipids as a ketogenic fuel supply in aging female brain: Implications for Alzheimer's disease. *eBioMedicine, 2,* 1888–1904.

Kumar, R., Pham, T. T., Macey, P. M., et al. (2014). Abnormal myelin and axonal integrity in recently diagnosed patients with obstructive sleep apnea. *Sleep, 37,* 723–732.

La, A. L., Walsh, C. M., Neylan, T. C., et al. (2019). Long-term trazodone use and cognition: A potential therapeutic role for slow-wave sleep enhancers. *Journal of Alzheimer's Disease, 67,* 911–921.

Lal, C., Hardiman, G., Kumbhare, S., & Strange, C. (2019). Proteomic biomarkers of cognitive impairment in obstructive sleep apnea syndrome. *Sleep & Breathing, 23,* 251–257.

Lam, S. P., Wong, C. C., Li, S. X., et al. (2016). Caring burden of REM sleep behavior disorder—Spouses' health and marital relationship. *Sleep Medicine, 24,* 40–43.

Leng, Y., McEvoy, C. T., Allen, I. E., & Yaffe, K. (2017). Association of sleep-disordered breathing with cognitive function and risk of cognitive impairment: A systematic review and meta-analysis. *JAMA Neurology, 74,* 1237–1245.

Livingston, G., Huntley, J., Sommerlad, A., et al. (2020). Dementia prevention, intervention, and care: 2020 report of the Lancet Commission. *Lancet, 396,* 413–446.

Lovato, N., Lack, L., Wright, H., & Kennaway, D. J. (2014). Evaluation of a brief treatment program of cognitive behavior therapy for insomnia in older adults. *Sleep, 37,* 117–126.

Macey, P. M., Kumar, R., Yan-Go, F. L., Woo, M. A., & Harper, R. M. (2012). Sex differences in white matter alterations accompanying obstructive sleep apnea. *Sleep, 35,* 1603–1613.

Mahoney, R., Regan, C., Katona, C., & Livingston, G. (2005). Anxiety and depression in family caregivers of people with Alzheimer disease: The LASER-AD study. *The American Journal of Geriatric Psychiatry, 13,* 795–801.

Mallampalli, M. P., & Carter, C. L. (2014). Exploring sex and gender differences in sleep health: A Society for Women's Health Research Report. *Journal of Women's Health, 23,* 553–562.

Mander, B. A., Winer, J. R., & Walker, M. P. (2017). Sleep and human aging. *Neuron, 94,* 19–36.

Maspero, C., Giannini, L., Galbiati, G., Rosso, G., & Farronato, G. (2015). Obstructive sleep apnea syndrome: A literature review. *Minerva Stomatologica, 64,* 97–109.

Mayer, G. (2020). *S2k-Leitlinie: Insomnie bei neurologischen Erkrankungen: Deutsche Gesellschaft für Neurologie (DGN).* Version 3: 02.03.2020. Available from: https://dgn.org/leitlinien/ll-030-045-insomnie-bei-neurologischen-erkrankungen-2020/.

McCleery, J., Cohen, D. A., & Sharpley, A. L. (2016). Pharmacotherapies for sleep disturbances in dementia. *Cochrane Database of Systematic Reviews, 11,* Cd009178.

McCurry, S. M., Gibbons, L. E., Logsdon, R. G., Vitiello, M., & Teri, L. (2003). Training caregivers to change the sleep hygiene practices of patients with dementia: The NITE-AD project. *Journal of the American Geriatrics Society, 51,* 1455–1460.

McCurry, S. M., Pike, K. C., Vitiello, M. V., et al. (2011). Increasing walking and bright light exposure to improve sleep in community-dwelling persons with Alzheimer's disease: Results of a randomized, controlled trial. *Journal of the American Geriatrics Society, 59,* 1393–1402.

MFMER. (2020a). *Obstructive sleep apnea:* © *1998–2020 Mayo Foundation for Medical Education and Research (MFMER).* Available from: https://www.mayoclinic.org/diseases-conditions/obstructive-sleep-apnea/symptoms-causes/syc-20352090.

MFMER. (2020b). *REM sleep behavior disorder:* © *1998–2020 Mayo Foundation for Medical Education and Research (MFMER).* Available from: https://www.mayoclinic.org/diseases-conditions/rem-sleep-behavior-disorder/diagnosis-treatment/drc-20352925.

Mosconi, L., Berti, V., Quinn, C., et al. (2017). Sex differences in Alzheimer risk: Brain imaging of endocrine vs chronologic aging. *Neurology, 89*, 1382–1390.

Mulgrew, A. T., Ryan, C. F., Fleetham, J. A., et al. (2007). The impact of obstructive sleep apnea and daytime sleepiness on work limitation. *Sleep Medicine, 9*, 42–53.

Musiek, E. S., Xiong, D. D., & Holtzman, D. M. (2015). Sleep, circadian rhythms, and the pathogenesis of Alzheimer disease. *Experimental & Molecular Medicine, 47*, e148.

Nigro, C. A., Dibur, E., Borsini, E., et al. (2018). The influence of gender on symptoms associated with obstructive sleep apnea. *Sleep & Breathing, 22*, 683–693.

O'Connor, C., Thornley, K. S., & Hanly, P. J. (2000). Gender differences in the polysomnographic features of obstructive sleep apnea. *American Journal of Respiratory and Critical Care Medicine, 161*, 1465–1472.

Ohayon, M. M., Carskadon, M. A., Guilleminault, C., & Vitiello, M. V. (2004). Meta-analysis of quantitative sleep parameters from childhood to old age in healthy individuals: Developing normative sleep values across the human lifespan. *Sleep, 27*, 1255–1273.

Okuda, S., Tetsuka, J., Takahashi, K., et al. (2019). Association between sleep disturbance in Alzheimer's disease patients and burden on and health status of their caregivers. *Journal of Neurology, 266*, 1490–1500.

Olsson, M., Ärlig, J., Hedner, J., Blennow, K., & Zetterberg, H. (2018). Sleep deprivation and cerebrospinal fluid biomarkers for Alzheimer's disease. *Sleep, 41*, 1–8.

Ooms, S., & Ju, Y. E. (2016). Treatment of sleep disorders in dementia. *Current Treatment Options in Neurology, 18*, 40.

Ooms, S., Overeem, S., Besse, K., et al. (2014). Effect of 1 night of total sleep deprivation on cerebrospinal fluid β-amyloid 42 in healthy middle-aged men a randomized clinical trial. *JAMA Neurology, 71*, 971–977.

Ory, M. G., Hoffman, R. R., 3rd, Yee, J. L., Tennstedt, S., & Schulz, R. (1999). Prevalence and impact of caregiving: A detailed comparison between dementia and nondementia caregivers. *The Gerontologist, 39*, 177–185.

Pagano, G., De Micco, R., Yousaf, T., et al. (2018). REM behavior disorder predicts motor progression and cognitive decline in Parkinson disease. *Neurology, 91*, e894–e905.

Pang, R., Guo, R., Wu, X., et al. (2018). Altered regional homogeneity in chronic insomnia disorder with or without cognitive impairment. *AJNR. American Journal of Neuroradiology, 39*, 742–747.

Patel, S. R. (2019). Obstructive sleep apnea. *Annals of Internal Medicine, 171*, Itc81–itc96.

Patel, D., Steinberg, J., & Patel, P. (2018). Insomnia in the elderly: A review. *Journal of Clinical Sleep Medicine, 14*, 1017–1024.

Perez-Cabezas, V., Ruiz-Molinero, C., Jimenez-Rejano, J. J., et al. (2020). Continuous positive airway pressure treatment in patients with Alzheimer's disease: A systematic review. *Journal of Clinical Medicine, 9*, 1–9.

Peter-Derex, L., Yammine, P., Bastuji, H., & Croisile, B. (2015). Sleep and Alzheimer's disease. *Sleep Medicine Reviews, 19*, 29–38.

Pinquart, M., & Sörensen, S. (2006). Gender differences in caregiver stressors, social resources, and health: An updated meta-analysis. *The Journals of Gerontology. Series B, Psychological Sciences and Social Sciences, 61*, P33–P45.

Postuma, R. B., Iranzo, A., Hogl, B., et al. (2015). Risk factors for neurodegeneration in idiopathic rapid eye movement sleep behavior disorder: A multicenter study. *Annals of Neurology, 77*, 830–839.

Postuma, R. B., Iranzo, A., Hu, M., et al. (2019). Risk and predictors of dementia and parkinsonism in idiopathic REM sleep behaviour disorder: A multicentre study. *Brain, 142*, 744–759.

Potvin, O., Lorrain, D., Forget, H., et al. (2012). Sleep quality and 1-year incident cognitive impairment in community-dwelling older adults. *Sleep, 35*, 491–499.

Pyun, J. M., Kang, M. J., Yun, Y., Park, Y. H., & Kim, S. (2019). APOE ε4 and REM sleep behavior disorder as risk factors for sundown syndrome in Alzheimer's disease. *Journal of Alzheimer's Disease, 69*, 521–528.

Ralls, F. M., & Grigg-Damberger, M. (2012). Roles of gender, age, race/ethnicity, and residential socioeconomics in obstructive sleep apnea syndromes. *Current Opinion in Pulmonary Medicine, 18*, 568–573.

Rasch, B., & Born, J. (2013). About sleep's role in memory. *Physiological Reviews, 93*, 681–766.

Rauen, K., & Weidt, S. (2017). *Praxis (Bern 1994). 106* (pp. 715–721).

Sadler, P., McLaren, S., Klein, B., Harvey, J., & Jenkins, M. (2018). Cognitive behavior therapy for older adults with insomnia and depression: A randomized controlled trial in community mental health services. *Sleep, 41*.

Savaskan, E. (2015). Sleep disorders in dementia patients. *Zeitschrift für Gerontologie und Geriatrie, 48*, 312–317.

Savaskan, E. (2016). Benzodiazepine dependency in the elderly: How to deal with it. *Praxis (Bern 1994), 105*, 637–641.

Schupp, M., & Hanning, C. D. (2003). Physiology of sleep. *BJA CEPD Reviews, 3*, 69–74.

Shenker, J. I., & Singh, G. (2017). Sleep and Dementia. *Missouri Medicine, 114*, 311–315.

Shi, L., Chen, S. J., Ma, M. Y., et al. (2018). Sleep disturbances increase the risk of dementia: A systematic review and meta-analysis. *Sleep Medicine Reviews, 40*, 4–16.

Shokri-Kojori, E., Wang, G. J., Wiers, C. E., et al. (2018). β-Amyloid accumulation in the human brain after one night of sleep deprivation. *Proceedings of the National Academy of Sciences of the United States of America, 115*, 4483–4488.

St Louis, E. K., & Boeve, B. F. (2017). REM sleep behavior disorder: Diagnosis, clinical implications, and future directions. *Mayo Clinic Proceedings, 92*, 1723–1736.

Subramanian, S., Jayaraman, G., Majid, H., Aguilar, R., & Surani, S. (2012). Influence of gender and anthropometric measures on severity of obstructive sleep apnea. *Sleep & Breathing, 16*, 1091–1095.

Tamanna, S., & Geraci, S. A. (2013). Major sleep disorders among women: (Women's health series). *Southern Medical Journal, 106*, 470–478.

Tardy, M., Gonthier, R., Barthelemy, J. C., Roche, F., & Crawford-Achour, E. (2015). Subjective sleep and cognitive complaints in 65 year old subjects: A significant association. The PROOF cohort. *The Journal of Nutrition, Health & Aging, 19*, 424–430.

Taylor, D. J., Lichstein, K. L., Durrence, H. H., Reidel, B. W., & Bush, A. J. (2005). Epidemiology of insomnia, depression, and anxiety. *Sleep, 28*, 1457–1464.

Tractenberg, R. E., Singer, C. M., Cummings, J. L., & Thal, L. J. (2003). The sleep disorders inventory: An instrument for studies of sleep disturbance in persons with Alzheimer's disease. *Journal of Sleep Research, 12*, 331–337.

Turner, K., Zambrelli, E., Lavolpe, S., et al. (2019). Obstructive sleep apnea: Neurocognitive and behavioral functions before and after treatment. *Functional Neurology, 34*, 71–78.

Vaessen, T. J., Overeem, S., & Sitskoorn, M. M. (2015). Cognitive complaints in obstructive sleep apnea. *Sleep Medicine Reviews, 19*, 51–58.

Valipour, A. (2012). Gender-related differences in the obstructive sleep apnea syndrome. *Pneumologie, 66*, 584–588.

Van Cauter, E., Leproult, R., & Plat, L. (2000). Age-related changes in slow wave sleep and REM sleep and relationship with growth hormone and cortisol levels in healthy men. *Journal of the American Medical Association, 284*, 861–868.

Vitiello, M. V. (2009). Recent advances in understanding sleep and sleep disturbances in older adults: Growing older does not mean sleeping poorly. *Current Directions in Psychological Science*, *18*, 316–320.

Vloeberghs, E., Van Dam, D., Engelborghs, S., et al. (2004). Altered circadian locomotor activity in APP23 mice: A model for BPSD disturbances. *The European Journal of Neuroscience*, *20*, 2757–2766.

Walker, M. (2017). *Why we sleep—Unlocking the power of sleep and dreams.* New York: Scribner.

Wardle-Pinkston, S., Slavish, D. C., & Taylor, D. J. (2019). Insomnia and cognitive performance: A systematic review and meta-analysis. *Sleep Medicine Reviews*, *48*, 101205.

Weldemichael, D. A., & Grossberg, G. T. (2010). Circadian rhythm disturbances in patients with Alzheimer's disease: A review. *International Journal of Alzheimer's Disease*, *2010*, 1–9.

Wheaton, A. G., Perry, G. S., Chapman, D. P., & Croft, J. B. (2012). Sleep disordered breathing and depression among U.S. adults: National Health and Nutrition Examination Survey, 2005–2008. *Sleep*, *35*, 461–467.

Wimms, A., Woehrle, H., Ketheeswaran, S., Ramanan, D., & Armitstead, J. (2016). Obstructive sleep apnea in women: Specific issues and interventions. *BioMed Research International*, *2016*, 1764837.

Yaffe, K., Laffan, A. M., Harrison, S. L., et al. (2011). Sleep-disordered breathing, hypoxia, and risk of mild cognitive impairment and dementia in older women. *Journal of the American Medical Association*, *306*, 613–619.

Yaremchuk, K. (2018). Sleep disorders in the elderly. *Clinics in Geriatric Medicine*, *34*, 205–216.

Zdanys, K. F., & Steffens, D. C. (2015). Sleep disturbances in the elderly. *The Psychiatric Clinics of North America*, *38*, 723–741.

Zhang, B., & Wing, Y. K. (2006). Sex differences in insomnia: A meta-analysis. *Sleep*, *29*, 85–93.

Zhou, J., Zhang, J., Li, Y., et al. (2015). Gender differences in REM sleep behavior disorder: A clinical and polysomnographic study in China. *Sleep Medicine*, *16*, 414–418.

CHAPTER 9

Hormones and dementia

Cassandra Szoeke[a], Sue Downie[b], Susan Phillips[b], and Stephen Campbell[c]

[a]Centre for Medical Research, Royal Melbourne Hospital, University of Melbourne, Melbourne, VIC, Australia
[b]Department of Medicine (RMH), University of Melbourne, Melbourne, VIC, Australia
[c]Australian Healthy Ageing Organisation, Melbourne, VIC, Australia

Sex differences are hormone differences

To better understand dementia etiology and identify risk factors, it is crucial to examine the sexes separately, yet women are underrepresented in the published literature (Snyder et al., 2016). While the sex differences outlined in previous chapters can have both gender and sex components (Sachdev et al., 2012), this chapter will focus on the influence of sex hormones on cognition, cognitive decline, and the risk of dementia, as there are strong indicators that sex hormones have an important role in cognition.

Given that more than 100 years of dementia research has yielded no disease-modifying therapy or cure, it is clear our understanding of this complex neurodegenerative disease is incomplete. In 2015, Calcoen and colleagues (Calcoen, Elias, & Yu, 2015) summarized the position of Alzheimer's research as having almost 10 times the failure rate of the industry standard. A snapshot of dementia research shows a predominance of research on older individuals (well after the onset of early changes in working memory circuitry (Jacobs et al., 2017)), which often excludes those with vascular pathology (Ritchie, Terrera, & Quinn, 2015; Sperling et al., 2011). Importantly, there is also an absence of reporting differences by sex, which removes the opportunity to examine biological sex differences in results (Laws, Irvine, & Gale, 2016). Yet, it is known that two-thirds of all dementia cases are women (Alzheimer Association, 2014), and vascular risk and disease is a fundamental component of disease manifestation (de la Torre, 2010a; Harrison et al., 2014; Wiesmann, Kiliaan, & Claassen, 2013)—itself an area with well documented sex differences (Sobhani et al., 2018)—and it takes three decades for the neuropathological changes characteristic of Alzheimer's dementia to reach levels clinically matched with a diagnosis (Villemagne et al., 2013).

In this chapter we will focus on the following:

(1) hormones have an influence on neural activity, performance, brain structure, function, and inflammation; and the evidence of hormone impact on cognition in women and men;
(2) the menopausal transition occurs in the key age-window identified by dementia researchers as likely responsible for the chronic evolution of neurodegenerative processes from age 45 to manifestation of disease over 70 years of age;
(3) menopause impacts the trajectory of cognitive decline, and those with early menopause (including hysterectomized women) have a higher risk of negative cognitive change;
(4) results of randomized controlled hormone therapy trials; and
(5) the impact of hormones on other known key risk factors for dementia.

Hormones and cognition

Sex hormones are essential for a wide range of functions beyond their role in reproduction. They are not only produced in the gonads, but also the adrenal glands and peripheral tissues. Experimental, epidemiological, and clinical studies suggest that androgens, estrogens, and perhaps even progestogens can reduce the risk for dementia (Pike, Carroll, Rosario, & Barron, 2009). The hormone most commonly examined has been estrogen. However, research has also examined progestogen, testosterone and its primary precursor dehydroepiandrosterone (DHEA), and the sulfate (DHEA-S). Some observational studies have also examined follicle-stimulating hormone (FSH), luteinizing hormone (LH), and prolactin (PRL). Of course, feedback loops and interactive synthesis pathways dictate connections between many of these.

In women, estrogens and progestogens are the main sex hormones. Estrogens are synthesized from androgens by the ovaries and also, albeit in lower quantities, by the liver, adrenal glands, breasts, and fat cells. Progestogen synthesis occurs in the corpus luteum and the adrenals, as well as in the placenta during pregnancy. In women, testosterone is synthesized in small quantities by the adrenal glands, thecal cells of the ovaries, and placenta during pregnancy. In men, testosterone is the main sex hormone synthesized by the Leydig cells in the testes, and estrogens are synthesized in the Leydig cells, Sertoli cells, and mature spermatocytes.

Sex hormone synthesis is controlled by the hypothalamic-pituitary-gonadal (HPG) axis, involving central pulsatile release of gonadotropin-releasing hormone (GnRH), which stimulates the pituitary to release luteinizing hormone (LH) and follicle-stimulating hormone (FSH) into general circulation, which then bind to target cells that coordinate the transfer of cholesterol to the inner mitochondrial membrane to initiate steroidogenesis. The first step is the conversion of cholesterol to pregnenolone, which is then converted to specific sex hormones, such as estrogens, progestogens, and androgens.

In this chapter, we refer to hormone therapy (HT) to encompass various terms utilized in the literature: hormone replacement therapy (HRT), menopausal hormone therapy (MHT), and estrogen therapy (ET), all of which include estrogen alone or combined with a progestin (most often used by women with an intact uterus to reduce the risk of endometrial cancer). HT is routinely prescribed to manage symptoms associated with the menopause and has long been thought to improve cognition. Testosterone administered to men and to women has not been proven to enhance cognitive function. Similarly, androgen deprivation therapy (ADT), which is widely used to reduce testosterone production in men with prostate cancer, has produced varying and inconclusive outcomes on cognition and dementia risk (Lee, Park, Joung, & Kim, 2020).

Estrogen

There is evidence that ongoing estrogen production, when there is a delay of menopause, increases a woman's chance of survival. Each additional year before becoming menopausal is associated with 2% lower (age-adjusted) mortality (Cagnacci & Venier, 2019). This represents a balance of estrogen's net effect due to decreased risk of cardiovascular disease and of atherosclerosis (Jacobsen, Nilssen, Heuch, & Kvale, 1997; van der Schouw, van der Graaf, Steyerberg, Eijkemans, & Banga, 1996; van der Voort, van der Weijer, & Barentsen, 2003), and lower bone fracture risk (van der Voort et al., 2003), which are offset by the increased risk of breast cancer growth and endometrial cancer (Cagnacci & Venier, 2019).

Estrogen is the most well-studied hormone influencing cognition (see also Chapter 2). It has been shown to increase cerebral blood flow and glucose utilization and increase synaptogenesis in the hippocampus (Almeida, 1999). Higher estradiol has been associated with an increased density of neuronal synapses (McEwen & Milner, 2007). In animal models, higher estradiol has also been shown to reduce two key biomarkers of Alzheimer's: tau phosphorylation (Alvarez-de-la-Rosa et al., 2005) and amyloid deposition (Yue et al., 2005), as well as improve learning and memory (Antov & Stockhorst, 2018). Several hundred research publications have demonstrated that estrogen has a favorable effect on brain tissue, physiology, and cognition in later life (Barrett-Connor & Laughlin, 2009), thus establishing its neuroprotective effect.

Progesterone

Interest in progesterone and cognition has accelerated in recent years. Progesterone is produced in the adrenals, ovaries, and Leydig's cells, and is synthesized from cholesterol, although it is predominantly a female reproductive hormone that increases before each ovulation and reaches high levels during pregnancy to promote uterine growth (Barros, Tufik, & Andersen, 2015). It is routinely combined with estrogen in hormone therapy to reduce the risk of endometrial cancer in women with an intact uterus, and this provides an opportunity to observe differences between women receiving progesterone and those not. However, this is complicated by the underlying differences in indication for the different choices of therapy. Reviews in this area have demonstrated that progesterone exhibits neuroprotective properties and a complex interaction with estrogen. Examination of the studies analyzed indicates that effects may depend on dose, time of administration, subject age, and type of hormone used (Barros et al., 2015). Given its role in routine combination with estrogen and the known side effects of both larger progesterone doses and medroxyprogesterone acetate (MPA), the main focus for treatment impact remains estrogen.

Testosterone and DHEA

Testosterone is produced by the testes in men and by the ovaries in women, although in much smaller amounts. In both men and women, testosterone is also synthesized from cholesterol by the adrenal glands. In both sexes, testosterone can be converted to estrogen and also has vital biological effects through estrogenic action. Testosterone may act directly via androgen receptors, or by reduction to the more potent androgen dihydrotestosterone (DHT) and/or aromatization to estradiol. In women, concentrations decline during the reproductive years, then appear to be maintained beyond the age of 65 years (Davis, Baber, et al., 2019). One constraint in analyzing testosterone has been the ability to accurately measure serum testosterone, especially the minute amounts present in female serum (Davis, Bell, et al., 2019; Handelsman, Sikaris, & Ly, 2016). Using more precise measurements, a recent analysis of 55,000 blood samples of females aged 0–99 years showed that testosterone peaked in late adolescence and declined gradually over the next two decades but remained stable across and beyond menopause (Handelsman et al., 2016).

The ovaries release testosterone directly into the blood stream, but testosterone can also be synthesized from other hormones originating from the ovaries and adrenal glands, such as DHEA and androstenedione (IMS, 2019). After secretion from the adrenals, DHEA and DHEA-S are then converted into androgens and/or estrogens in peripheral tissue, and account for about 50% of total androgens in adult men, approximately 75% in women before menopause, and almost 100% in postmenopaual women (Labrie, Bélanger, Cusan, Gomez, & Candas, 1997). In the 1990s, DHEA was popularized as a treatment to alleviate menopausal symptoms and to improve sexual function and wellbeing (Jane & Davis, 2014). In 2003, Labrie et al. suggested that DHEA should be included in hormone therapy compounds (Labrie et al., 2003). However, in 2011, Davis and colleagues reported that their randomized clinical trial of postmenopausal women who were administered DHEA indicated it did not improve low sexual desire, diminished wellbeing, or cognitive function (Davis, Panjari, & Stanczyk, 2011).

Testosterone therapy, on the other hand, showed some promise for improving specific cognitive functions. In 2014, the same research team reported (Davis et al., 2014) that their randomized clinical trial, in which postmenopausal women not on HT were given transdermal testosterone for 26 weeks, showed a statistically significant better performance for verbal learning and memory, compared with placebo, although there were no significant differences for other cognitive domains.

There is also evidence that testosterone, like estrogen, reduces beta-amyloid accumulation (Pike et al., 2009). While most research to date has focused on estrogen, the newer assay techniques along with these early findings have led researchers in the field to comment: "testosterone may be as, or even more, important than estrogens in determining disease risk in elderly women" (Davis, Bell, et al., 2019).

The International Menopause Society's Global Consensus Position Statement on the Use of Testosterone Therapy for Women, published in September 2019 (Davis, Baber, et al., 2019), concluded: "There is insufficient evidence to support the use of testosterone to enhance cognitive performance, or to delay cognitive decline, in postmenopausal women." The statement also called for more adequately powered randomized clinical trials of the effects of testosterone on cognitive performance, in particular with a focus on measuring total testosterone as the main biomarker rather than "free" testosterone, as evidence that "free" testosterone is the biologically active testosterone fraction is lacking.

Menopause and cognition

Today, it is well known that most dementias develop gradually. In the past 5 years we have seen that the hallmark of Alzheimer's disease (AD), amyloid protein, takes three decades to accumulate to the levels evident in those with diagnosable dementia (Villemagne et al., 2013). The International Dominantly Inherited Alzheimer Network (DIAN) study, which closely examined those genetically predisposed to develop AD, corroborated this 30-year timeline (Bateman et al., 2012) of changes including amyloid accrual, brain cell loss, reduced metabolism, and in the later decades, cognitive decline, providing a timescale to the previous "hypothetical model" of AD development (Jack et al., 2013). Of particular interest is that this timeline of three decades of evolution before disease onset (which occurs over age 70) aligns with the mean age of menopause (see Fig. 1). This is further supported by studies examining the neuropathological antecedents of AD (Mosconi & Brinton, 2018). Studies that examined hypometabolism found that atrophy and amyloid beta deposition are significantly present in peri- and postmenopausal women compared to premenopausal women and age-matched men (Mosconi, Berti, Guyara-Quinn, et al., 2017; Mosconi, Berti, Quinn, et al., 2017). Exactly how these differences are mediated will be central to our understanding of such differences (Fig. 1).

Natural menopause

Menopause occurs in all women and represents a dramatic decline in ovarian sex steroid production, specifically estradiol (up to 90% decline) and progesterone. It is important to note that the average age at menopause (defined as 12 months after the final menstrual period) is 52 years (range 45–55) and is preceded by perimenopause or the menopausal transition, which typically lasts several years and involves a period of fluctuating hormone levels accompanied by physical, mental, and emotional changes (Pinkerton & Stovall, 2010).

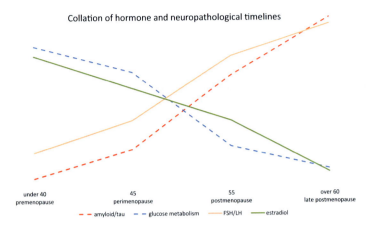

FIG. 1

Collation of hormone and neuropathological timelines. Demonstrates the changes in neuropathology (*dashed lines*) and hormonal profile (*solid lines*) over time across the menopausal transition (age 45–55 years). Timeline of amyloid/tau provided from Villemagne et al. (2013) and Bateman et al., (2012) as 30 years from disease onset. Timeline of glucose metabolism as 30 years from disease onset provided from Bateman et al. (2012). Alzheimer's disease occurs over 70. Timeline of hormones provided by Jameson et al. (2018).

Results from small prospective trials and observational studies nearly three decades ago established that dementia and vascular disease occurred in postmenopausal women at a much higher rate than expected for age alone (Yaffe, Sawaya, Lieberburg, & Grady, 1998). Vascular risk is a known strong risk factor for increasing risk of dementia, and therefore there are clear pathophysiological changes that occur with menopause which can impact the development of dementia.

For many women, from the onset of menopause onwards, diminishing memory and recall of events are often described in general terms as "forgetfulness" (Maki, 2015). Studies show that cognitive changes during perimenopause are prevalent (Ammann et al., 2013; Coker et al., 2010; Shao et al., 2012; Sharma, 2003; van der Voort et al., 2003; Yaffe et al., 1998), with an impact on attention, concentration, and ability to complete memory tasks (Legault et al., 2009). Significantly, these also translate to higher rates of subsequent dementia in later life (Hendrie et al., 2006; Yaffe et al., 1998).

Fluctuations in estrogen levels during the menstrual cycle have been demonstrated to affect both memory and recall (Vranic & Hromatko, 2008) and depression (Lithgow & Moussavi, 2017; Mulligan, Hajcak, Klawohn, Nelson, & Meyer, 2019); which itself is also known to impact cognitive performance (Chapter 7). Interestingly, looking across the different cognitive domains, the strongest associations appear to be between estrogen and verbal memory, rather than a global cognitive effect.

Surgical menopause

Epidemiological evidence suggests that both surgical menopause (under age 45 years) and premature ovarian insufficiency (menopause < 40 years) are associated with 1.5–2-fold increase in vascular risk (Anagnostis et al., 2019), which is a well-known risk factor for dementia. Studies also show that women who have premature menopause from hysterectomy/oophorectomy are more likely to have memory or cognitive decline (Phillips & Sherwin, 1992; Rocca, Grossardt, & Maraganore, 2008; Ryan et al., 2014). Furthermore, women who experienced early menopause (under age 45 years) and did not take hormone therapy were found to have increased risk for dementia (Rivera et al., 2009). Clinical findings have also demonstrated pathological correlations in women who undergo surgically-induced menopause at less than 45 years of age showing both faster cognitive decline and increased AD pathology (Ryan et al., 2014), including higher burdens of neuritic plaques (Bove et al., 2014).

Observational studies of hormone therapy use

HT is prescribed to peri- and postmenopausal women to reduce the frequency and severity of vasomotor symptoms, including hot flashes, bone loss, and osteoporotic fractures, and symptoms of vaginal atrophy (Cagnacci & Venier, 2019).

Since the mid-1970s, HT has been examined sporadically for its effect on memory and what was then referred to as "mental performance." Through the 1990s, small observational studies suggested estrogen benefited memory (Caldwell, 1954; Kampen & Sherwin, 1994; Phillips & Sherwin, 1992; Vanhulle & Demol, 1976), and other work demonstrated its impact on neuropathology, with MRIs showing lower rates of vascular damage along with improved cognition in those who were taking HT (Schmidt et al., 1996). This research indicated that the mechanism of estrogen's impact on cognition may be via its well-known vascular effects.

Hysterectomized/oophorectomized women who take HT have lower rates of dementia and heart disease than their non-HT user counterparts (Mikkola et al., 2017). However, a meta-analysis of 15 epidemiologic studies reporting on HT use did not demonstrate that "any" form of HT reduced the risk of AD compared to no HT (O'Brien, Jackson, Grodstein, Blacker, & Weuve, 2014). A retrospective analysis of those with AD on a national registry did not find a consistent positive benefit on diagnosis of AD (Imtiaz et al., 2017). Similarly, the Finnish case-control study involving a national register analysis of 84,739 postmenopausal women who used HT and an equal number who did not, found that the use of systemic HT between 1999 and 2013 was associated with a 9%–17% increased risk of AD (Savolainen-Peltonen et al., 2019). Accepting the well-known bias and difficulties with registry dementia diagnosis, it is important to note that in the Finnish study the risk did not differ significantly between use of estradiol-only HT and combined estrogen-progestogen HT, nor the age at initiation. A recent meta-analysis examining risk of dementia diagnosis in 28 studies confirmed a relationship between HT and AD (odds ratio − 1.08) and all-cause dementia (odds ratio − 1.16) in menopausal women (Wu et al., 2020).

However, in more detailed studies which examined cognitive change or neuropathology, relationships between these factors and HT were consistently demonstrated. The Cache County study reported that, among older women, longer duration of use of HT was associated with better cognitive scores (Matyi, Rattinger, Schwartz, Buhusi, & Tschanz, 2019). Similar findings were reported in the Kuopio CAIDE study, which examined older women (aged 65–79) taking estradiol-based HT for more than 8 years and showed that these women had superior global cognition, episodic memory, and cognitive speed than those who used HT for less than 5 years or were nonusers (Imtiaz, Tolppanen, Solomon, Soininen, & Kivipelto, 2017). A small meta-analysis that examined brain activation changes in postmenopausal women who had taken HT, using functional MRI (fMRI) of neural responses during working memory tasks, found a positive correlation between activation and task performance, suggesting that HT may benefit working memory (Benson, Kirichek, Beral, & Green, 2015; Li et al., 2015). The most recent meta-analysis of more specific outcomes indicated that HT can improve cognitive function in female patients with AD (Zhou et al., 2020). It appears that the relationship between estrogen and cognition is complex and is impacted by timing, duration, and interaction with other concurrent symptoms and pathologies.

While the above reports are not randomized controlled trials of HT, they are the most recently published data examining HT and significant cognitive decline or disease, and they demonstrate the difficulty of assessing outcomes of chronic disease with long timelines using the current randomized controlled trials of HT in younger women.

Interventional HT use

Although several current randomized controlled trials are examining the impact of maintaining estrogen levels past menopause, these have only commenced in the past 5 years, and therefore will not be able to demonstrate an impact on dementia development, or even cognitive decline (where clinically significant trajectories are now proven to occur only after age 70 (Pietrzak et al., 2015)), with any power for several decades. Therefore, the evidence we have on maintaining estrogen from menopause into aging is still predominantly based on observational research.

We do now have 18-year data on the massive NIH-funded Women's Health Initiative (WHI), a randomized clinical trial that administered HT from 1995 to 2002. This has made clear that once women pass menopause (average age 52), there is no benefit in starting HT (mean age of participants was 63 years) nor for women who do not suffer clinically significant menopause symptoms (given those with significant symptoms were excluded from the study) (Shumaker et al., 1998; The Women's Health Initiative Study Group, 1998). This 18-year follow-up found: no increases in overall mortality; no increased risk of all-cause, cardiovascular, or cancer mortality; but an increased risk of breast cancer among those who had been on combined estrogen-progestogen therapy; although a reduced risk of breast cancer among estrogen-alone users (Manson et al., 2017). It is noteworthy that the increased breast cancer risk demonstrated earlier in the study had persisted at this follow-up despite cessation of therapy many years earlier. In this sense, the follow-up confirmed that HT should not be initiated in women 60 or older, a decade or so past menopause, without significant menopausal symptoms.

It is important to discuss this WHI study as it is highly influential in the HT area, not just due to its findings, but also because its size influenced the many meta-analyses summarizing the evidence in the field since. WHI enrolled 27,000 women in its HT trial to evaluate the effect of 8 years of HT on the most common causes of death and disability in postmenopausal women, specifically cardiovascular disease, cancer, and osteoporosis (Shumaker et al., 1998). Postmenopausal women aged 50–79 were randomized to receive conjugated equine estrogen (CEE) alone (if hysterectomized), or CEE plus medroxyprogesterone acetate (MPA), or placebo. The first results were published in 2002 after a mean 5.2 years of treatment, reporting that among the CEE+MPA participants an increased incidence of coronary heart disease and breast cancer was observed, together with a reduction of osteoporotic fractures and colorectal cancer (Rossouw et al., 2002). These differences appeared after only 5 years of use. The risks of treatment in this group of older women outweighed the benefits, and the trial was prematurely discontinued. Nineteen months later, the CEE-alone part of the trial reported an increased risk of stroke, no benefit for coronary heart disease, and decreased risk of hip fracture, and this too was terminated before completion (Anderson et al., 2004). Although the CEE-alone study showed that the benefits of reduced osteoporotic fracture and colon cancer were maintained and there was no increased risk of breast cancer or cardiac disease, the overall message on HT remained negative.

Following the publication of the WHI findings, the Committee on Safety of Medicines issued guidance in 2003 (Medicines and Healthcare Products Regulatory Agency, 2003), advising that each decision to start HT should be made on a case-by-case basis and treatment should be appraised at least once a year. A further update in 2007 recommended: "For all women, the lowest effective dose should be used for the shortest time" (Medicines and Healthcare Products Regulatory Agency, 2007).

Hormone therapy and cognition

The WHI Memory Study (WHIMS), a substudy of cognitive function, examined women who were even older than those in the larger WHI trial (recruitment over 65 years of age). This study showed decline in memory scores (Rapp et al., 2003) which was persistent over time (Espeland et al., 2010) and a doubling of risk for developing dementia for those on CEE+MPA (Shumaker et al., 2004). This was far from the protective effect indicated by observational trials, although again, this was in women who commenced HT over 65, quite remote from menopause (Espeland et al., 2013; Gleason et al., 2015; Henderson et al., 2016; Maki, Girard, & Manson, 2019).

The WHI Study of Cognitive Ageing (WHISCA) enrolled women 3 years after WHI randomization (Resnick et al., 2004), therefore participants had been taking HT for 3 years before their first WHISCA assessment. At testing, those women (mean age 74) taking CEE+MPA for 4 years (Resnick et al., 2006) had a less favorable verbal memory but better figural memory than the placebo group. Importantly, these differences were not due to mood influence, as there was no difference in positive or negative affect between the groups (Resnick et al., 2006). On the other hand, those on CEE-alone had worse spatial ability compared to placebo but demonstrated no changes in the other domains and no effect on memory (Resnick et al., 2009). The influence of HT on neuropathology was also evaluated with evidence of greater atrophy in those taking HT (Resnick et al., 2009) compared to the placebo group, although this did not persist over time and there was no change in cerebral vascular pathology (Coker et al., 2014). The most recent follow-up showed no significant changes and reported that there may be no long-term detrimental effects on cognition, however there was a reduced power with loss to follow-up (Goveas et al., 2016). Again, it is important to note that these results reflect impact on older women (mean age 74) taking HT well after menopause.

The Heart and Estrogen/Progestin Replacement Study (HERS), a randomized clinical trial, the timing of which overlapped with the WHI HT trial, showed that older postmenopausal women (mean age 71) on 4 years of CEE+MPA did not demonstrate better cognitive function (Grady et al., 2002). However, many of these participants had established coronary disease. On the other hand, the Prospective Epidemiological Risk Factor (PERF) study, a smaller, shorter randomized clinical trial that examined HT commencing in women who were younger (mean age 54), closer to menopause, and free of cardiovascular disease, showed that an average of 10 years after ceasing HT, the risk of cognitive impairment was decreased by 64% (Bagger et al., 2005).

Hormone therapy in younger women

By this stage, the potential for vascular risk benefit among younger women was well described, and therefore, WHI participants aged 50–55 at randomization formed the WHIMS-Young (WHIMS-Y) cohort to assess protective effects on cognition in younger postmenopausal women receiving CEE-alone or combined with MPA (Vaughan et al., 2013). Analyses showed no acute benefit or risk to cognitive function, with only long-term use (i.e., more than 10 years) appearing to convey benefit (Espeland et al., 2013).

It is difficult to extrapolate findings from the post hoc analyses of WHI subgroups. While the required duration of follow-up and detail of hormone use alongside vascular and mood risk factors is available in epidemiological work, without randomization there may be other confounders driving HT use that could explain the observed positive impact on cognition. Certainly, higher education levels and sociodemographic bias in women who were prescribed HT have been reported.

Therefore, there will be much interest in the two studies underway that examine estrogen treatment at the time of menopause. The cognition arm of the Early vs Late Intervention Trial with Estradiol (ELITE-Cog) initially showed that after 5 years there was no negative impact on cognitive function, whether participants took estradiol-based therapy at mean age 55 and within 6 years of menopause, or at mean age 65 and more than 10 years after menopause (Henderson et al., 2016). When a small subcohort of these women were placed under stressful conditions, those with more than 4 years of HT performed better on working memory tasks than those on placebo (Herrera, Hodis, Mack, & Mather, 2017). This is important early work because—as mentioned above—the cognitive decline seen in aging is only detected after age 70; therefore, this study indicates there may be early detectable changes in cognition for those on HT. This could bring our understanding from randomized controlled trials (RCTs) forward by decades.

The Kronos Early Estrogen Prevention Study (KEEPS), which began soon after the WHI HT trial terminated, recruited women aged 42–58 within 3 years of menopause and with no preclinical vascular disease, and randomized them to a lower-dose CEE, or transdermal 17β-estradiol, or placebo (Wharton, Gleason, Miller, & Asthana, 2013). Cognitive assessment after 4 years of treatment showed no significant effects on cognition (Miller et al., 2019). Neuropathological work by KEEPS showed that these recently postmenopausal women taking low-dose CEE had less decline in cerebral volumes (Kantarci et al., 2018) compared to placebo, although there was no change between HT users and placebo for global cognition (Gleason et al., 2015) or in the development of white matter hyperintensities in the brain (Miller et al., 2019). Interestingly, 3 years after discontinuation of HT, there were no differences in cerebral volume detected between groups, suggesting only active therapy has an impact here. We need to start considering the other effects of estrogen therapy, as will be discussed below, given that the most recent follow-up in KEEPS notes a trend for reduced accumulation of coronary artery calcium with CEE, and positive effects on mood, sleep, sexual function, and reduced hot flashes (Miller et al., 2019). The cognitive measures in both ELITE-Cog and KEEPS and imaging for tau deposition among KEEPS participants (Miller et al., 2019) are ongoing and will provide valuable information on cognition as participants move toward the age at which dementia usually occurs.

Encouragingly, all of these trials—WHIMS-Y (Espeland et al., 2013), ELITE-Cog (Henderson et al., 2016), and KEEPS (Gleason et al., 2015)—show no adverse effect of HT on cognition in younger postmenopausal women.

The timing hypothesis

Since the WHI HT findings, there has been a shift toward starting to administer HT in younger women and those closer to menopause. A 2009 meta-analysis of studies in women who initiated HT within 10 years of menopause onset and/or in women aged younger than 60 years (Salpeter, Cheng, Thabane, Buckley, & Salpeter, 2009) showed a mortality benefit. More recently, a 2015 Cochrane Review confirmed

HT initiated in younger women (before age 60, and less than 10 years after menopause) lowered coronary heart disease by 50% and all-cause mortality by 30%, and increased the risk of thrombosis, but not that of stroke (Boardman et al., 2015; NAMS, 2017) (see Fig. 2).

A prominent review was prepared for the US Preventive Services Task Force in which 18 HT trials were included, involving 40,058 women. It is important to note that more than half the participants ($n = 27,347$) originated from the WHI HT trial (Gartlehner et al., 2017). The analysis showed that women randomized to estrogen-only therapy had lower rates of osteoporotic fracture and diabetes, but a higher rate of stroke, thromboembolic disease, gallbladder disease, and urinary incontinence compared with women randomized to placebo. Women randomized to estrogen plus progestin had a lower rate of diabetes, osteoporotic fracture, and colon cancer, but a higher rate of invasive breast carcinoma, stroke, urinary incontinence, thromboembolic disease, and dementia. HT was not associated with a difference in quality of life or all-cause mortality (Gartlehner et al., 2017). This led to well-known detailed recommendations on HT use that advised initiating HT before age 60 or less than 10 years after menopause for symptom relief but not prevention of chronic diseases

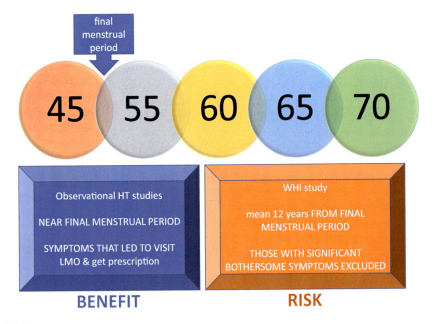

FIG. 2

Summary of the evidence for hormones and cognitive decline by age of cohorts and proximity to final menstrual period when commencing treatment. *LMO*, local medical officer; *WHI*, Women's Health Initiative.

Graphic created by P.S. Campbell.

(Grossman, Curry, Owens, Barry, & Davidson, 2017). However, there has been much discussion on the evidence that led to these recommendations as the vast majority (92%) of the women on HT in the analysis were using high doses of MPA and/or CEE, whereas the current recommendations of the International Menopause Society (IMS) are for different preparations and in lower doses (de Villiers et al., 2016). Furthermore, only three of the 18 trials started HT within 12 years of menopause, with these women representing only 8% of the total participants included in the review (Salpeter et al., 2009). Today, it is recommended that HT be initiated before age 60 or less than 10 years after menopause (de Villiers et al., 2016; Jane & Davis, 2014; NAMS, 2017). It is also important that in the future we collect more information on transdermal therapy, which is known to have a better side-effect profile than other forms of HT (IMS, 2019).

The IMS Consensus Statement on Hormone Therapy (de Villiers et al., 2016) acknowledged that: "[HT] initiated in early menopause has no substantial effect on cognition, but, based on observational studies, it may prevent AD in later life. In RCTs, oral MHT initiated in women aged 65 or older also has no substantial effect on cognition and increases the risk of dementia."

Side-effect profile

An important consideration for HT is its side effect profile. Estrogen promotes the growth of estrogen receptor positive cancers and also has prothrombotic properties. We have good experience with long-term therapy from oral contraceptive pill use; however, postmenopause data are from HT studies in which little long-term follow-up data on the new estrogen preparations are available (see Fig. 3).

The recent publication in *The Lancet* from the Collaborative Group on Hormonal Factors in Breast Cancer's meta-analysis concluded that the risk of breast cancer for HT users was highest among those over age 60 and those using estrogen-progesterone, compared with women using estrogen-only HT (Collaborative Group, 2019). For women of average weight in developed countries, 5 years of HT use starting at age 50 would increase breast cancer incidence at ages 50–69 years by about 1 in every 50 users of estrogen plus *daily* progestogen, one in 70 users of estrogen plus *intermittent* progestogen, and one in every 200 users of estrogen-only preparations. The IMS responded "by," pointing out that much of the data was derived from old studies including the WHI HT trials that had used different preparations (IMS, 2019). The IMS noted that the WHI HT trials "contributed substantially to our understanding of the benefits and risks of HT," for example, most of the WHI regimens involved formulations and doses that are known to have adverse effects and hence, are no longer routinely recommended (IMS, 2019). The IMS confirmed that the use of the progestogens medroxyprogesterone acetate (MPA) and norethisterone (norethindrone) "is now discouraged because of their known adverse effects, but these account for nearly all of the data for combined estrogen-progestogen therapy" that has been reported (IMS, 2019). An important finding of this detailed meta-analysis was

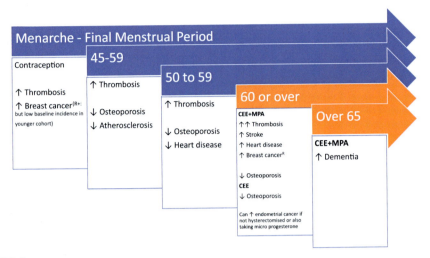

FIG. 3
Data on hormone-based treatment by age at commencement. Breast cancer in WHI, 8 more cases per 10,000 in CEE+MPA group. FDA rules regarding risk: "Rare" means 10 more cases in every 10,000 people. Very rare ≤ 1 more case in every 10,000 people. *CEE*, conjugated equine estrogen; *MPA*, medroxyprogesterone.

Graphic created by P.S. Campbell.

that risk factors for breast cancer include obesity, and from the age of 50 the increase in breast cancer risk among women taking estrogen-only therapy approximates that of obese women not taking hormone therapy (Collaborative Group, 2019). While the issues of HT are debated, it is crucial that we look more closely at the interaction of weight with risk, in the context of hormone therapy.

Hormones and cognition in men

In men, testosterone production decreases with age, as does that of other closely interrelated hormones (e.g., dehydroepiandrosterone, growth hormone, thyroxine, and melatonin). This natural decline of androgens and resultant symptoms is termed symptomatic late-onset hypogonadism (LOH) or symptomatic androgen deficiency of the aging male (ADAM) (Morales, 2004). Andropause refers to a loss of testicular function due to accident, disease, or surgical or medical castration (for example, as part of prostate cancer treatment), although it is sometimes loosely (and inaccurately) interchanged with hypogonadism, and compared (inaccurately) with female menopause (Morales, 2004)—especially given that symptoms of LOH include sexual dysfunction, muscle weakness, obesity, osteoporosis, hot flushes, insomnia, fatigue, poor concentration, and depression (Huhtaniemi, 2014).

Since the early 1980s, studies have shown that testosterone supplementation in men with low levels and/or hypogonadism may improve some cognitive functions including memory, attention, executive function, and visuospatial and visuoperceptual function (Hua, Hildreth, & Pelak, 2016). Observational and clinical trials of endogenous testosterone in men have included its effects on performance in many cognitive domains (Hua et al., 2016). However, a systematic review of testosterone therapy on cognition by Hua et al. found that study results ranged widely, and the variability in outcomes is likely related in part to the lack of consensus on methods for testosterone measurement and supplementation, as well as the disparate measures of cognitive function (Hua et al., 2016). A 2020 review of 27 studies involving 18,599 men also reported inconsistent findings, although their meta-analysis showed an increased risk of all-cause dementia with decreasing total testosterone and concluded that testosterone supplement treatment may improve general cognitive function and motor response in the short term (Zhang, Kang, & Li, 2020).

The most recent important testosterone-cognition study, the Cognitive Function Trial, which was conducted at 12 US academic medical centers (Resnick et al., 2017), showed that 1 year of testosterone therapy did not improve cognitive function in men aged 65 or older with a low serum testosterone level, nor did it improve impaired sexual function, physical function, or vitality. The Journal of the American Medical Association (JAMA) editorial accompanying the study's report declared: "Today, eight decades since the first clinical use of testosterone, the sole unequivocal indication for testosterone treatment is as replacement therapy for men with pathological hypogonadism" (Handelsman, 2017). On the same day, *Alzforum* (the Alzheimer's research network) announced: "Case Closed: Testosterone Does Not Boost Cognition." This bold statement, however, was in line with the FDA's 2015 Drug Safety Communication (US Food & Drug Administration, 2015), which cautioned that prescription testosterone products are approved only for men with hypogonadism, that is, not to improve cognitive function. It is worth noting that both the 2016 systematic review and the 12-center study of testosterone and cognition mentioned above involved older men and showed limited benefit. Some of these issues mirror early studies of estrogen and cognition that were conducted among older women and showed limited benefit, but when the focus switched to women under age 60, outcomes were more positive. That said, it is important that midlife timing be further explored in men, and it will be particularly of interest to examine areas noted below that are current gaps in knowledge.

In the reverse situation, testosterone suppression is used in androgen deprivation therapy (ADT) to treat prostate cancer by blocking the production of testosterone in order to reduce or halt the proliferation of testosterone-dependent prostate cancer cells. Numerous studies have looked at the effect of ADT on cognition and the possible development of dementia, including analyzing metabolic changes in brain function (Cherrier, Rose, & Higano, 2003) and neuronal activation (Cherrier,

Borghesani, Shelton, & Higano, 2010), with some very large retrospective studies currently being carried out (Jayadevappa et al., 2019; Nead et al., 2016; Tully et al., 2021). After almost two decades, however, research to date has failed to produce conclusive evidence that testosterone suppression reduces cognitive function (Lee et al., 2020).

Gaps in knowledge
The impact of hormones on known key risk factors for cognitive decline

Sex hormones impact more than cognition. Over the past half century, laboratory, observational, and randomized clinical trials have quantified the impact of HT on coronary heart disease, cardiovascular diseases, cancers (colorectal, endometrial, and breast), inflammation, vascular disease, thrombosis, osteoporosis, sleep, stress, sexual function, and cognition, noting the positive effect of estrogen (Barrett-Connor & Laughlin, 2009). Changes in hormones (estrogen, progesterone, FSH, LH, testosterone, and DHEA) may affect numerous health outcomes including vasomotor symptoms, cardiovascular disease, osteoporosis, depression, mood disorders, sexual function, vaginal atrophy (Pinkerton & Stovall, 2010), gut inflammation, diabetes, stroke, affective disorders, sleep disturbances, and cognitive changes (Nelson, 2008). While mechanisms are not well elucidated (Neves-e-Castro et al., 2015), many of these factors are known risks for dementia and therefore investigating the influence of HT on these is crucial to our understanding of the impact of estrogen on cognition. In particular, the observations of estrogen's effect on heart disease, dementia, cholesterol, hypertension, BMI, sleep, stress, and vasomotor symptoms warrant examination of the interplay between hormones, vascular risk, and cognition (as detailed in Chapter 10).

Vascular risk and disease (BMI, HT, lipids (APOE4))
The important overlaps in vascular and amyloid pathologies in the development of dementia have been known for some time (Szoeke, Campbell, Chiu, & Ames, 2009). The primary biomarkers associated with AD are amyloid, tau, and the apolipoprotein (APOE) genotype, so their connections with vascular pathologies are important when considering the role of hormones, given that estrogen has both cardiovascular and cerebrovascular effects. It is now known that vascular risk factors and vascular disease augment the development of neurodegeneration, which leads to cell loss, amyloid deposition, and cognitive decline. Therefore, the impact of hormones on dementia is incomplete without considering the impact on vascular risk (de la Torre, 2010b).

Let's not forget that in 1906, Alois Alzheimer noted microvascular changes in his postmortem of Auguste Deter, a younger woman with earlier onset dementia who had pathological evidence of what we now know as plaques and tangles (Toodayan, 2016).

In 2019, more than 100 years later, when launching the World Health Organization (WHO)'s dementia risk reduction guidelines, the WHO Director-General, Dr Tedros Adhanom Ghebreyesus, said: "what is good for our heart, is also good for our brain" (World Health Organization, 2019). These WHO dementia guidelines recommend people exercise regularly, avoid smoking and harmful use of alcohol, control their weight, eat a healthy diet, and maintain healthy blood pressure, cholesterol, and blood sugar levels (World Health Organization, 2019). These overlap with heart risk reduction guidelines (American Heart Association, 2019), underscoring the similarity of risk factors between heart disease and dementia.

The implications of sex differences on cardiovascular risk factors for AD have been poorly studied. Most research on vascular risk has focused on whole populations or populations consisting mostly of men (Teodorescu, Vavra, & Kibbe, 2013), yet (or perhaps due to this) since 1984 the death rate due to vascular disease has been consistently higher among women than men (Wenger, 2013). It has been established that there are underlying pathophysiological differences that underpin these differences. Women experience more microvascular disease than men, while men have higher prevalence of coronary artery disease than premenopausal women, which is believed to be due to the protective effects of estrogen against atherosclerosis, oxidative stress, and inflammation (Miller et al., 2019). Therefore, the evolution of disease in women is distinct.

Clinical studies have shown that HT favorably impacts the risk factors for cardiovascular disease, decreasing cardiovascular disease risk and all-cause mortality when initiated in younger women (under 60 years of age) or within 10 years of menopause (Salpeter, Walsh, Greyber, Ormiston, & Salpeter, 2004; Salpeter et al., 2006). Furthermore, women who discontinue HT before the age of 60 have an increased cardiac mortality risk (Mikkola et al., 2015).

There is an increased risk of cardiovascular disease in women experiencing early menopause (before 45 years of age) who do not take hormones (Rivera et al., 2009). When HT is initiated under age 60 and/or within 10 years of menopause, results demonstrate no significant increased risk of heart disease (Manson et al., 2013), and a reduction in cardiovascular disease (Schierbeck et al., 2012), with half the rate of coronary heart disease (Boardman et al., 2015), less coronary artery bypass grafting/percutaneous coronary interventions, and fewer myocardial infarctions (MI) (Rossouw et al., 2007).

The Danish Osteoporosis Prevention Study (DOPS) in younger women also showed vascular protection after 10 years of treatment with HT (Schierbeck et al., 2012). Both ELITE (Hodis et al., 2016) and KEEPS (Miller et al., 2019) randomized trials reported a protective vascular effect of HT in young women close to menopause. In the KEEPS study, there was a trend for reduced accumulation of coronary artery calcium with CEE. Significantly, the study also noted the impact of HT on reducing hot flashes (Miller et al., 2019). It is important to consider hot flashes and vascular risk markers together. Risk factor profiles developed to predict cardiovascular disease and stroke risk have also been demonstrated to predict risk of cognitive decline, MCI, and dementia (Harrison et al., 2014). Data shows that after a first myocardial infarction, HT users have a lower mortality rate than nonusers (Shlipak et al., 2001; Tackett et al., 2010; Windler, Stute, Ortmann, & Mueck, 2015). While precise mechanisms of this cardiac protection is not entirely defined, we know that HT protects against high cholesterol (Shepardson et al., 2011), hypertension (Verghese et al., 2003), and high body mass index (BMI) (Anstey, Cherbuin, Budge, & Young, 2011). It is important that subsequent research evaluate the impact of HT on all of these factors known to influence the pathophysiology of dementia.

Estrogen has a direct impact on lowering blood levels of low-density lipoprotein and apolipoprotein E (APOE) (Almeida et al., 2006; Gregersen et al., 2019) and increasing levels of the heart-protective high-density lipoprotein, as well as having vasodilator effects that reduce blood pressure (Gartlehner et al., 2017). The impact of estrogen on blood pressure and cardiovascular functions was established many years ago (McEwen, Alves, Bulloch, & Weiland, 1998). The higher than expected rates for age of both myocardial infarction and stroke in postmenopausal women (Yaffe et al., 1998) suggests a clear hormonal component to vascular risk. Newer work has shown that hot flashes, a common menopausal symptom, had a high correlation with subclinical vascular disease (Bechlioulis et al., 2010; Thurston, Kuller, Edmundowicz, & Matthews, 2010; Thurston et al., 2011) (aortic calcification, poor endothelial function, greater intima media thickness) compared to those without symptoms. It is well known that estrogen can reduce hot flashes and that this is a primary indication for therapy. Hot flashes are known to be associated with higher risk of stroke, and heart disease and palpitations and, therefore, the importance of estrogen treatment, symptoms, and disease evolution needs further investigation.

The APOE4 allele is the strongest genetic risk factor for sporadic AD (Altmann, Tian, Henderson, & Greicius, 2014). Altmann and colleagues showed that APOE4 carriers, both men and women, had the highest risk of progressing to MCI or from MCI to Alzheimer's compared with noncarriers. For women, the risk was 1.8-fold compared with noncarriers (Altmann et al., 2014). APOE is a lipoprotein required for transport of cholesterol, and APOE4 is a common genetic risk factor for vascular disease (Eichner et al., 2002). We also know that APOE codes for an apo-lipoprotein integral to the vascular system in the body. The influence of this genotype in the interaction of hormones and cognition is important (Rosenson et al., 2018). Yet most of the studies reported above do not comment on differences in outcome by genotype and there is a paucity of information on the impact of the strongest genetic risk factor for dementia that appears to play a central role in the complex relationship between vascular factors, hormones, and neurodegeneration (Depypere, Vierin, Weyers, & Sieben, 2016).

There is evidence that APOE genotype mediates the HT effect, which may have significant implications for patient selection. A small cross-sectional study has shown that women taking unopposed estrogen for at least 12 months and who were not APOE4 carriers had the highest cognitive performance on tests of memory and learning, whereas APOE4 carriers on HT performed the same as nonusers (Burkhardt et al., 2004). Almost 300 women were studied, comparing current HT users to past

HT users and nonusers. It was shown that cognitive performance among current users declined over 6 years by 1.5 points, compared to never-users declining by 2.7 points, demonstrating a significant interaction with APOE genotypes such that estrogen use was not associated with decline in the APOE4-positive women (Yaffe, Haan, Byers, Tangen, & Kuller, 2000).

Diabetes and impaired glucose tolerance

Large, randomized controlled trials have suggested HT reduces the incidence of diabetes in women (Canonico et al., 2014; Espeland et al., 2004; Kanaya et al., 2003; Reboussin, Greendale, & Espeland, 1998; Salpeter et al., 2006). HT improves β-cell insulin secretion, glucose effectiveness, and insulin sensitivity, lipid and glucose metabolism dysregulation, as well as body fat redistribution, leading to abdominal obesity. A 30% reduction in incidence of diabetes mellitus has been observed among women with preexisting coronary artery disease that are on HT (Kanaya et al., 2003). There have been discussions that estrogen's ability to regulate the source of energy utilized by the brain may have a significant contribution to its role in worsening cognitive decline in those with diabetes (Espeland et al., 2015). The disrupted glucose homeostasis that occurs after menopause (Yan et al., 2019) and it's contribution to vascular health is an area for future research.

Metabolic syndrome and inflammation

The impact of estrogen on vascular risk factors including glucose utilization and its influence on BMI suggest it may be an important factor in the development of metabolic disturbance, which leads to chronic underlying inflammation, now demonstrated to underpin many of the chronic diseases of aging. Inflammatory diseases such as the rheumatological conditions (Stevens-Lapsley & Kohrt, 2010) and inflammatory conditions of the brain, such as multiple sclerosis, are well known to have significant sex differences, with women affected more than men (Disanto & Ramagopalan, 2013). Obesity itself has also been shown to impact cognitive decline (Bove et al., 2013). There is evidence that estrogen has both anti-inflammatory (Sohrabji & Bake, 2006) and antioxidant properties (Almeida, 1999). The role of inflammation in the pathophysiology of dementia has been reviewed elsewhere (Borshchev, Uspensky, & Galagudza, 2019), showing that inflammation has an important role in both disease evolution and progression. There is early data showing a strong relationship between estrogen and the gut microbiome (Baker, Al-Nakkash, & Herbst-Kralovetz, 2017), which is increasingly demonstrating a key role in both inflammation and influence on the development of chronic diseases of aging, including dementia. There is also research on women who have undergone surgical or natural menopause that shows increased levels of proinflammatory markers and systematic inflammation (Abu-Taha et al., 2009; Cioffi et al., 2002), with a demonstrated relationship with declining estrogen levels (Pfeilschifter, Köditz, Pfohl, & Schatz, 2002).

We already know that bone and estrogen are linked, with all studies showing a consistent benefit of estrogen on bone remodeling and strength. The most common menopausal symptom is, in fact, aches and joint pains (Szoeke, Cicuttini, Guthrie,

& Dennerstein, 2008), and the impact of pain on impairing cognitive performance is well-known. Pain and inflammation (as described in Chapter 3) are two areas that need further investigation in the context of cognitive decline in aging and their interaction with hormonal impacts on cognition.

Depression
Women have a higher risk of developing depression in their lifetime compared to men (Eid, Gobinath, & Galea, 2019) (see Chapter 7). There is a twofold increased risk of AD and vascular dementia among women with late-life depression (Barnes et al., 2012). It is worth noting the new evidence from randomized trials that examine outcomes more broadly. For instance, the KEEPS follow-up in 2019 (Miller et al., 2019) reported positive effects of HT on mood and sexual function. Examining the symptoms and sequelae of depression alongside cognitive decline will be important in developing our understanding of the complex evolution of dementia, as well as estrogen's contribution in the incidence and progression of this disease.

While there is some work on depression to date, the importance of stress and anxiety should also be considered in this context, as animal work has demonstrated that the interaction between stress and 17β-estradiol (E2) can change brain structure and function in critical regions such as the hippocampus, amygdala, and prefrontal cortex (McEwen, Nasca, & Gray, 2016).

Sleep
Women are more likely than men to experience periods of chronic sleep disturbance throughout their lives (see Chapter 8). Such chronic disturbance in sleep can change the production and clearance of amyloid beta peptides that are associated with the sleep-wake cycle, leading to increased amyloid beta accumulation (a hallmark of AD). Sleep disturbances have been associated with poorer cognition and increased risk of AD (Nebel et al., 2018). The association of sleep and cognitive impairment may also be working through an inflammatory pathway as we see interactions between inflammation and sleep (Clark & Vissel, 2014). It is important to note, however, that there is only emerging evidence on this subject, as this is a less well explored area of hormone impact, but it is considered in the longer term follow-up from KEEPS researchers (Miller et al., 2019) who noted better sleep metrics in their treatment arm. As cognitive outcomes become apparent in these new studies, it will be crucial to look at the ancillary symptoms known to be influenced by estrogen as interactive in the relationship between estrogen and cognition.

Midlife to late-life longitudinal prospective studies including hormone, cognitive, and neuropathological biomarkers

Many of the studies seeking to examine the menopausal transition were designed to follow-up women from 45 to 60 years of age and lacked meaningful cognitive measures or clinical cognitive outcomes, since cognitive decline would not clinically manifest until much later in life (Sperling et al., 2011). Those that do exist often do not have specialized neuroimaging for the hallmarks of dementia (such as atrophy and amyloid). Clearly, we need to measure both hormones and cognition at midlife, alongside neuropathological biomarkers, with regular follow up to at least age 70, preferably 80, but this is yet to be done. Only once the timing and duration of hormone exposures and their influence on cognition are understood can we tap the potential for carefully timed and dosed therapy to mitigate cognitive decline in women.

This issue is a significant one not just in dementia research but for many chronic diseases of aging. Epidemiological studies that begin in midlife are required to determine the quantity, timing, and duration of modifiable risk exposures in order to create intervention guidelines (Daviglus et al., 2010). The US National Institute of Health (NIH) 2010 State-of-the-Science Conference statement "Preventing Alzheimer Disease and Cognitive Decline" noted that there is insufficient evidence to propose a midlife intervention, since the optimal age to target is unknown, and there is a lack of information on the interactions between the various risk factors (Daviglus et al., 2010). The gaps in knowledge were outlined as it is unknown whether midlife risk exposure is cumulative, or even reversible (Norton, Matthews, Barnes, Yaffe, & Brayne, 2014). Existing studies that examine only midlife or late-life periods, but not both, are limited. The research field has echoed the call for studies starting in midlife, well before disease development, to identify those who are at risk for later life disease and neurodegenerative changes at an earlier point in time (Biessels, 2014). A life-course approach is required to examine the effects of exogenous and endogenous sex steroid exposures, mood, and cognitive decline, together with other confounding morbidities in order to determine the exposures that relate to pathology (Rapp et al., 2003).

Timing and therapeutic windows

The failure of later life interventional strategies indicate that midlife is a crucial period of disease development and is the most likely target for altering risk of disease development (Anstey, Cherbuin, & Herath, 2013). The critical window for initiating HT appears to be before age 60 and/or within a decade of menopause. Favorable outcomes for those on HT are seen for all-cause mortality, myocardial infarction (MI) (Rossouw et al., 2007), and coronary heart disease (CHD) (Boardman et al., 2015). However, most dementia studies have recruited people over 60 years of age without recording measurements of hormone levels or HT use.

The research field now makes it clear that the timing of intervention is relevant to effects on cognition, also on vascular risk, with high cholesterol in those under age 70 associated with later development of dementia, but high cholesterol in those over age 70 protecting against development of dementia (Shepardson et al., 2011). Such U-shaped relationships require longitudinal prospective studies to span the prodrome of disease.

Having established that HT administered a decade or so after menopause demonstrates a greater risk than benefit profile is not to say there may not be potential for improvement in people who have already received the terminal diagnosis of Alzheimer's dementia. In fact, a recent meta-analysis indicates that HT can improve cognitive function in female patients with AD (Zhou et al., 2020).

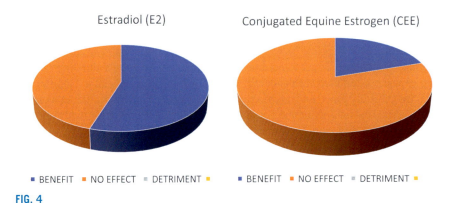

FIG. 4

The type of estrogen has an impact: benefit was seen for women up to 59 years of age in just over half the studies using estradiol (E2) but only 20% of the studies using conjugated equine estrogen.

Information on all types of HT preparation

Not all preparations of estrogen appear to exert the same clinical effects and side-effect profile. In the WHI trial, women administered 0.625 mg of oral CEE with MPA had increased risk of CHD, but those on CEE alone showed no change (Anderson et al., 2004; Rossouw et al., 2002). The incidence of thrombosis has been observed to increase with oral estrogen use, but large observational studies do not identify an increased risk with transdermal estradiol use (Vinogradova, Coupland, & Hippisley-Cox, 2019). Lower doses of oral estrogen therapy demonstrate lower risk of thrombosis than higher doses (Speroff, 2010), however there is an absence of comparative randomized control data. Other studies suggest micronized progesterone may be less thrombogenic than other progestins (Windler et al., 2015); and no excess risk has explicitly been identified with vaginal estrogen, although this could reflect the smaller number of users of this formulation. Limited observational data also suggest less risk with transdermal compared with oral estrogen (Canonico et al., 2014; L'Hermite, Simoncini, Fuller, & Genazzani, 2008), even in women with obesity or an underlying thrombophilia. Mechanisms of the low side-effect profile of the transdermal estrogens is suggested to be due to avoiding hepatic first pass effect, and therefore having no interaction with coagulation factors or hepatic-binding globulins (Sitruk-Ware, 2007). It will be important to consider outcomes by HT type, as well as dose and duration, as results of more recent studies become available (see Fig. 4).

Conclusion

Confirming estrogen as a preventive therapy for cognitive decline remains as elusive today as in 1954 when Caldwell measured the effects of estrogen, progesterone, and testosterone administered to older women and concluded that improvement in "intellectual functioning," specifically memory, would be possible with sex hormones (Caldwell, 1954).

Timing is a key issue in cognitive decline, with clear evidence for therapeutic windows which do not only optimize treatment impact but, in the case of cognitive decline, can range from being protective to doubling the risk of disease depending on timing. This is true for both hormone impact and vascular risk.

This evidence, together with the 30-year disease prodrome, highlight the importance of supporting lifespan research to be able to mitigate chronic disease of aging, and in particular, neurodegeneration.

Without clarification on timing and cumulative and latent effects, it is not possible to properly design an intervention that derives empirical evidence from the target population and the timing and duration to achieve a known outcome (Hendrie et al., 2006).

We are only just beginning to look at the impact of reproductive aging on cognitive aging. A 2019 review showed how few studies have considered this (Taylor, Pritschet, Yu, & Jacobs, 2019), yet it is clearly an important question for at least two-thirds of individuals living with dementia.

Understanding the relationship between HT use and subsequent health is of key importance to women deciding whether and when to take HT (Hickey & Banks, 2016). A current intervention would not show significant cases of dementia for another several decades. Can we wait that long? The WHI study required over $260 million of public investment—referred to by the *New York Times* as the $625 million study for just 5 years of follow-up back in the early 2000s (Roth et al., 2014)—and many papers have discussed its inability to answer these questions and the fact that it will never be replicated. There is, therefore, a call for longitudinal studies as the best means to examine timing (Mercer, Gunn, & Wyke, 2011) and to determine which causes to target to maintain health (Barnett et al., 2012). Furthermore, there is evidence that exogenous sex hormones alter the risk of cognitive decline in men (Verdile et al., 2014), yet this area has been very poorly researched thus far. Despite this, a systematic review found very few longitudinal studies in women that examined morbidity (France et al., 2012), with those that do exist focusing on menopausal transition. In particular, studies on postmenopausal women are lacking.

We now know that modifiable risk factors make a significant contribution to the prevalence of dementia (for an extensive overview and discussion, see Chapters 10 and 12), and it is estimated that up to 3 million diagnoses of AD worldwide could be avoided with just a 10%–25% reduction in recognized modifiable midlife risk factors (Barnes & Yaffe, 2011). However, the optimal age to target is unknown, along with whether midlife risk exposure is cumulative or even reversible, and there is a lack of information on the interactions between the various risk factors, which are known to be highly related (Norton et al., 2014). Consideration of highly related factors must include improved examination of menopausal symptoms, particularly those already known to be highly correlated with vascular disease. A longitudinal prospective design is necessary to allow insight into this dynamic interplay and to identify critical time periods when hormone exposures maximally impact later disease.

Chapter highlights

- Hormones play a key role at the intersection of vascular risk, inflammation, and neurodegenerative disease.
- Understanding the influence of this role across the 30-year prodrome of dementia, which aligns with the midlife to late-life period of estrogen decline in women, is crucial to identify potential therapeutics for this terminal disease.
- Timing of HT and patient selection will be crucial to determine the overall benefit of intervention. To determine these we need to expand available research on women's cognition across the menopausal transition and into aging.

References

Abu-Taha, M., Rius, C., Hermenegildo, C., Noguera, I., Cerda-Nicolas, J.-M., Issekutz, A. C., et al. (2009). Menopause and ovariectomy cause a low grade of systemic inflammation that may be prevented by chronic treatment with low doses of estrogen or losartan. *The Journal of Immunology*, *183*(2), 1393.

Almeida, O. P. (1999). Sex playing with the mind. Effects of oestrogen and testosterone on mood and cognition. *Arquivos de Neuro-Psiquiatria*, *57*(3A), 701–706.

Almeida, S., et al. (2006). ESR1 and APOE gene polymorphisms, serum lipids, and hormonal replacement therapy. *Maturitas*, *54*(2), 119–126.

Altmann, A., Tian, L., Henderson, V. W., & Greicius, M. D. (2014). Alzheimer's disease neuroimaging initiative I. Sex modifies the APOE-related risk of developing Alzheimer disease. *Annals of Neurology*, *75*(4), 563–573.

Alvarez-de-la-Rosa, M., Silva, I., Nilsen, J., Perez, M. M., Garcia-Segura, L. M., Avila, J., et al. (2005). Estradiol prevents neural tau hyperphosphorylation characteristic of Alzheimer's disease. *Annals of the New York Academy of Sciences*, *1052*, 210–224.

Alzheimer Association. (2014). *Alzheimer's disease facts and figures. Includes a special report on women and Alzheimer's disease*. Alzheimer Association.

American Heart Association. (2019). *Prevent heart disease and stroke*. Available from: https://www.heart.org/en/healthy-living/healthy-lifestyle/prevent-heart-disease-and-stroke.

Ammann, E. M., Pottala, J. V., Harris, W. S., Espeland, M. A., Wallace, R., Denburg, N. L., et al. (2013). Omega-3 fatty acids and domain-specific cognitive aging: Secondary analyses of data from WHISCA. *Neurology*, *81*(17), 1484–1491.

Anagnostis, P., Paschou, S. A., Katsiki, N., Krikidis, D., Lambrinoudaki, I., & Goulis, D. G. (2019). Menopausal hormone therapy and cardiovascular risk: Where are we now? *Current Vascular Pharmacology*, *17*(6), 564–572.

Anderson, G. L., Limacher, M., Assaf, A. R., Bassford, T., Beresford, S. A. A., Black, H., et al. (2004). Effects of conjugated equine estrogen in postmenopausal women with hysterectomy: The women's health initiative randomized controlled trial. *JAMA: The Journal of the American Medical Association*, *291*(14), 1701–1712.

Anstey, K. J., Cherbuin, N., Budge, M., & Young, J. (2011). Body mass index in midlife and late-life as a risk factor for dementia: A meta-analysis of prospective studies. *Obesity Reviews*, *12*(5), e426–e437.

Anstey, K. J., Cherbuin, N., & Herath, P. M. (2013). Development of a new method for assessing global risk of Alzheimer's disease for use in population health approaches to prevention. *Prevention Science: The Official Journal of the Society for Prevention Research*, *14*(4), 411–421.

Antov, M. I., & Stockhorst, U. (2018). Women with high estradiol status are protected against declarative memory impairment by pre-learning stress. *Neurobiology of Learning and Memory*, *155*, 403–411.

Bagger, Y. Z., Tanko, L. B., Alexandersen, P., Qin, G., Christiansen, C., & PERF Study Group. (2005). Early postmenopausal hormone therapy may prevent cognitive impairment later in life. *Menopause*, *12*(1), 12–17.

Baker, J. M., Al-Nakkash, L., & Herbst-Kralovetz, M. M. (2017). Estrogen-gut microbiome axis: Physiological and clinical implications. *Maturitas*, *103*, 45–53.

Barnes, D. E., & Yaffe, K. (2011). The projected effect of risk factor reduction on Alzheimer's disease prevalence. *Lancet Neurology*, *10*(9), 819–828.

Barnes, D. E., Yaffe, K., Byers, A. L., McCormick, M., Schaefer, C., & Whitmer, R. A. (2012). Midlife vs late-life depressive symptoms and risk of dementia: Differential effects for Alzheimer disease and vascular dementia. *Archives of General Psychiatry*, *69*(5), 493–498.

Barnett, K., Mercer, S. W., Norbury, M., Watt, G., Wyke, S., & Guthrie, B. (2012). Epidemiology of multimorbidity and implications for health care, research, and medical education: A cross-sectional study. *Lancet*, *380*(9836), 37–43.

Barrett-Connor, E., & Laughlin, G. A. (2009). Endogenous and exogenous estrogen, cognitive function, and dementia in postmenopausal women: Evidence from epidemiologic studies and clinical trials. *Seminars in Reproductive Medicine*, *27*(3), 275–282.

Barros, L. A., Tufik, S., & Andersen, M. L. (2015). The role of progesterone in memory: An overview of three decades. *Neuroscience and Biobehavioral Reviews*, *49*, 193–204.

Bateman, R. J., Xiong, C., Benzinger, T. L. S., Fagan, A. M., Goate, A., Fox, N. C., et al. (2012). Clinical and biomarker changes in dominantly inherited Alzheimer's disease. *The New England Journal of Medicine*, *367*(9), 795–804.

Bechlioulis, A., Kalantaridou, S. N., Naka, K. K., Chatzikyriakidou, A., Calis, K. A., Makrigiannakis, A., et al. (2010). Endothelial function, but not carotid intima-media thickness, is affected early in menopause and is associated with severity of hot flushes. *The Journal of Clinical Endocrinology and Metabolism*, *95*(3), 1199–1206.

Benson, V. S., Kirichek, O., Beral, V., & Green, J. (2015). Menopausal hormone therapy and central nervous system tumor risk: Large UK prospective study and meta-analysis. *International Journal of Cancer*, *136*(10), 2369–2377.

Biessels, G. J. (2014). Capitalising on modifiable risk factors for Alzheimer's disease. *Lancet Neurology*, *13*(8), 752–753.

Boardman, H. M., Hartley, L., Eisinga, A., Main, C., Roque i Figuls, M., Bonfill Cosp, X., et al. (2015). Hormone therapy for preventing cardiovascular disease in post-menopausal women. *Cochrane Database of Systematic Reviews*, *3*, CD002229.

Borshchev, Y. Y., Uspensky, Y. P., & Galagudza, M. M. (2019). Pathogenetic pathways of cognitive dysfunction and dementia in metabolic syndrome. *Life Sciences*, *237*, 116932.

Bove, R. M., Brick, D. J., Healy, B. C., Mancuso, S. M., Gerweck, A. V., Bredella, M. A., et al. (2013). Metabolic and endocrine correlates of cognitive function in healthy young women. *Obesity (Silver Spring)*, *21*(7), 1343–1349.

Bove, R., Secor, E., Chibnik, L. B., Barnes, L. L., Schneider, J. A., Bennett, D. A., et al. (2014). Age at surgical menopause influences cognitive decline and Alzheimer pathology in older women. *Neurology, 82*, 222–229.

Burkhardt, M. S., Foster, J. K., Laws, S. M., Baker, L. D., Craft, S., Gandy, S. E., et al. (2004). Oestrogen replacement therapy may improve memory functioning in the absence of APOE epsilon4. *Journal of Alzheimer's Disease, 6*(3), 221–228.

Cagnacci, A., & Venier, M. (2019). The controversial history of hormone replacement therapy. *Medicina, 55*(9), 602.

Calcoen, D., Elias, L., & Yu, X. (2015). What does it take to produce a breakthrough drug? *Nature Reviews. Drug Discovery, 14*(3), 161–162.

Caldwell, B. M. (1954). An evaluation of psychological effects of sex hormone administration in aged women: Result of therapy after eighteen months. *Journal of Gerontology, 9*(2), 168–174.

Canonico, M., Plu-Bureau, G., O'Sullivan, M. J., Stefanick, M. L., Cochrane, B., Scarabin, P. Y., et al. (2014). Age at menopause, reproductive history, and venous thromboembolism risk among postmenopausal women: The women's health initiative hormone therapy clinical trials. *Menopause, 21*(3), 214–220.

Cherrier, M. M., Rose, A. L., & Higano, C. (2003). The effects of combined androgen blockade on cognitive function during the first cycle of intermittent androgen suppression in patients with prostate cancer. *The Journal of Urology, 170*(5), 1808–1811.

Cherrier, M. M., Borghesani, P. R., Shelton, A. L., & Higano, C. S. (2010). Changes in neuronal activation patterns in response to androgen deprivation therapy: A pilot study. *BMC Cancer, 10*, 1.

Cioffi, M., Esposito, K., Vietri, M. T., Gazzerro, P., D'Auria, A., Ardovino, I., et al. (2002). Cytokine pattern in postmenopause. *Maturitas, 41*(3), 187–192.

Clark, I. A., & Vissel, B. (2014). Inflammation-sleep interface in brain disease: TNF, insulin, orexin. *Journal of Neuroinflammation, 11*, 51.

Coker, L. H., Espeland, M. A., Rapp, S. R., Legault, C., Resnick, S. M., Hogan, P., et al. (2010). Postmenopausal hormone therapy and cognitive outcomes: The Women's Health Initiative Memory Study (WHIMS). *The Journal of Steroid Biochemistry and Molecular Biology, 118*(4–5), 304–310.

Coker, L. H., Espeland, M. A., Hogan, P. E., Resnick, S. M., Bryan, R. N., Robinson, J. G., et al. (2014). Change in brain and lesion volumes after CEE therapies: The WHIMS-MRI studies. *Neurology, 82*(5), 427–434.

Collaborative Group on Hormonal Factors in Breast C. (2019). Type and timing of menopausal hormone therapy and breast cancer risk: Individual participant meta-analysis of the worldwide epidemiological evidence. *The Lancet, 394*(10204), 1159–1168.

Daviglus, M. L., Bell, C. C., Berrettini, W., Bowen, P. E., Connolly, E. S., Jr., Cox, N. J., et al. (2010). National Institutes of health state-of-the-science conference statement: Preventing Alzheimer disease and cognitive decline. *Annals of Internal Medicine, 153*(3), 176–181.

Davis, S., Panjari, M., & Stanczyk, F. (2011). DHEA replacement for postmenopausal women. *The Journal of Clinical Endocrinology & Metabolism, 96*(6), 1642–1653.

Davis, S. R., Jane, F., Robinson, P. J., Davison, S. L., Worsley, R., Maruff, P., et al. (2014). Transdermal testosterone improves verbal learning and memory in postmenopausal women not on oestrogen therapy. *Clinical Endocrinology, 81*(4), 621–628.

Davis, S. R., Bell, R. J., Robinson, P. J., Handelsman, D. J., Gilbert, T., Phung, J., et al. (2019). Testosterone and estrone increase from the age of 70 years: Findings from the sex hormones in older women study. *The Journal of Clinical Endocrinology and Metabolism, 104*(12), 6291–6300.

Davis, S. R., Baber, R., Panay, N., Bitzer, J., Perez, S. C., Islam, R. M., et al. (2019). Global consensus position statement on the use of testosterone therapy for women. *The Journal of Clinical Endocrinology and Metabolism, 104*(10), 4660–4666.

de la Torre, J. C. (2010a). Alzheimer's disease is incurable but preventable. *Journal of Alzheimer's Disease, 20*(3), 861–870.

de la Torre, J. C. (2010b). Vascular risk factor detection and control may prevent Alzheimer's disease. *Ageing Research Reviews, 9*(3), 218–225.

de Villiers, T. J., Hall, J. E., Pinkerton, J. V., Cerdas Perez, S., Rees, M., Yang, C., et al. (2016). Revised global consensus statement on menopausal hormone therapy. *Climacteric, 19*(4), 313–315.

Depypere, H., Vierin, A., Weyers, S., & Sieben, A. (2016). Alzheimer's disease, apolipoprotein E and hormone replacement therapy. *Maturitas, 94*, 98–105.

Disanto, G., & Ramagopalan, S. V. (2013). On the sex ratio of multiple sclerosis. *Multiple Sclerosis Journal, 19*(1), 3–4.

Eichner, J. E., Dunn, S. T., Perveen, G., Thompson, D. M., Stewart, K. E., & Stroehla, B. C. (2002). Apolipoprotein E polymorphism and cardiovascular disease: A HuGE review. *American Journal of Epidemiology, 155*(6), 487–495.

Eid, R. S., Gobinath, A. R., & Galea, L. A. M. (2019). Sex differences in depression: Insights from clinical and preclinical studies. *Progress in Neurobiology, 176*, 86–102.

Espeland, M. A., Rapp, S. R., Shumaker, S. A., Brunner, R., Manson, J. E., Sherwin, B. B., et al. (2004). Conjugated equine estrogens and global cognitive function in postmenopausal women: Women's health initiative memory study. *Journal of the American Medical Association, 291*(24), 2959–2968.

Espeland, M. A., Brunner, R. L., Hogan, P. E., Rapp, S. R., Coker, L. H., Legault, C., et al. (2010). Long-term effects of conjugated equine estrogen therapies on domain-specific cognitive function: Results from the Women's Health Initiative study of cognitive aging extension. *Journal of the American Geriatrics Society, 58*(7), 1263–1271.

Espeland, M. A., Shumaker, S. A., Leng, I., Manson, J. E., Brown, C. M., LeBlanc, E. S., et al. (2013). Long-term effects on cognitive function of postmenopausal hormone therapy prescribed to women aged 50 to 55 years. *JAMA Internal Medicine, 173*(15), 1429–1436.

Espeland, M. A., Brinton, R. D., Hugenschmidt, C., Manson, J. E., Craft, S., Yaffe, K., et al. (2015). Impact of type 2 diabetes and postmenopausal hormone therapy on incidence of cognitive impairment in older women. *Diabetes Care, 38*(12), 2316–2324.

France, E. F., Wyke, S., Gunn, J. M., Mair, F. S., McLean, G., & Mercer, S. W. (2012). Multimorbidity in primary care: A systematic review of prospective cohort studies. *The British Journal of General Practice, 62*(597), e297–e307.

Gartlehner, G., Patel, S. V., Feltner, C., Weber, R. P., Long, R., Mullican, K., et al. (2017). Hormone therapy for the primary prevention of chronic conditions in postmenopausal women: Evidence report and systematic review for the US preventive services task force. *Journal of the American Medical Association, 318*(22), 2234–2249.

Gleason, C. E., Dowling, N. M., Wharton, W., Manson, J. E., Miller, V. M., Atwood, C. S., et al. (2015). Effects of hormone therapy on cognition and mood in recently postmenopausal women: Findings from the randomized, controlled KEEPS-cognitive and affective study. *PLoS Medicine/Public Library of Science, 12*(6), e1001833.

Goveas, J. S., Rapp, S. R., Hogan, P. E., Driscoll, I., Tindle, H. A., Smith, J. C., et al. (2016). Predictors of optimal cognitive aging in 80 + women: The women's health initiative memory study. *The Journals of Gerontology. Series A, Biological Sciences and Medical Sciences, 71*(Suppl. 1), S62–S71.

Grady, D., Yaffe, K., Kristof, M., Lin, F., Richards, C., & Barrett-Connor, E. (2002). Effect of postmenopausal hormone therapy on cognitive function: The heart and estrogen/progestin replacement study. *The American Journal of Medicine*, *113*(7), 543–548.

Gregersen, I., et al. (2019). Effect of hormone replacement therapy on atherogenic lipid profile in postmenopausal women. *Thrombosis Research*, *184*, 1–7.

Grossman, D. C., Curry, S. J., Owens, D. K., Barry, M. J., Davidson, K. W., et al. (2017). Hormone therapy for the primary prevention of chronic conditions in postmenopausal women: US preventive services task force recommendation statement. *Journal of the American Medical Association*, *318*(22), 2224–2233.

Handelsman, D. J. (2017). Testosterone and male aging: Faltering hope for rejuvenation. *Journal of the American Medical Association*, *317*(7), 699–701.

Handelsman, D., Sikaris, K., & Ly, L. (2016). Estimating age-specific trends in circulating testosterone and sex hormone-binding globulin in males and females across the lifespan. *Annals of Clinical Biochemistry: International Journal of Laboratory Medicine*, *53*(3), 377–384.

Harrison, S. L., Ding, J., Tang, E. Y., Siervo, M., Robinson, L., Jagger, C., et al. (2014). Cardiovascular disease risk models and longitudinal changes in cognition: A systematic review. *PLoS One*, *9*(12), e114431.

Henderson, V. W., St John, J. A., Hodis, H. N., McCleary, C. A., Stanczyk, F. Z., Shoupe, D., et al. (2016). Cognitive effects of estradiol after menopause: A randomized trial of the timing hypothesis. *Neurology*, *87*(7), 699–708.

Hendrie, H. C., Albert, M. S., Butters, M. A., Gao, S., Knopman, D. S., Launer, L. J., et al. (2006). The NIH cognitive and emotional health project. Report of the critical evaluation study committee. *Alzheimer's & Dementia*, *2*(1), 12–32.

Herrera, A. Y., Hodis, H. N., Mack, W. J., & Mather, M. (2017). Estradiol therapy after menopause mitigates effects of stress on cortisol and working memory. *The Journal of Clinical Endocrinology and Metabolism*, *102*(12), 4457–4466.

Hickey, M., & Banks, E. (2016). NICE guidelines on the menopause. *BMJ*, *352*, i191.

Hodis, H. N., Mack, W. J., Henderson, V. W., Shoupe, D., Budoff, M. J., Hwang-Levine, J., et al. (2016). Vascular effects of early versus late postmenopausal treatment with estradiol. *The New England Journal of Medicine*, *374*(13), 1221–1231.

Hua, J. T., Hildreth, K. L., & Pelak, V. S. (2016). Effects of testosterone therapy on cognitive function in aging: A systematic review. *Cognitive and Behavioral Neurology*, *29*(3), 122–138.

Huhtaniemi, I. (2014). Late-onset hypogonadism: Current concepts and controversies of pathogenesis, diagnosis and treatment. *Asian Journal of Andrology*, *16*(2), 192–202.

IMS. (2019). *Testosterone and women*. Available from: https://www.menopause.org.au/health-info/resources/1484-testosterone-and-women.

Imtiaz, B., Taipale, H., Tanskanen, A., Tiihonen, M., Kivipelto, M., Heikkinen, A. M., et al. (2017). Risk of Alzheimer's disease among users of postmenopausal hormone therapy: A nationwide case-control study. *Maturitas*, *98*, 7–13.

Imtiaz, B., Tolppanen, A. M., Solomon, A., Soininen, H., & Kivipelto, M. (2017). Estradiol and cognition in the cardiovascular risk factors, aging and dementia (CAIDE) cohort study. *Journal of Alzheimer's Disease*, *56*(2), 453–458.

Jack, C. R., Jr., Knopman, D. S., Jagust, W. J., Petersen, R. C., Weiner, M. W., Aisen, P. S., et al. (2013). Tracking pathophysiological processes in Alzheimer's disease: An updated hypothetical model of dynamic biomarkers. *The Lancet Neurology*, *12*(2), 207–216.

Jacobs, E. G., Weiss, B., Makris, N., Whitfield-Gabrieli, S., Buka, S. L., Klibanski, A., et al. (2017). Reorganization of functional networks in verbal working memory circuitry in early midlife: The impact of sex and menopausal status. *Cerebral Cortex, 27*(5), 2857–2870.

Jacobsen, B. K., Nilssen, S., Heuch, I., & Kvale, G. (1997). Does age at natural menopause affect mortality from ischemic heart disease? *Journal of Clinical Epidemiology, 50*(4), 475–479.

Jameson, J. L., Fauci, A. S., Kasper, D. L., Hauser, S. L., Longo, D. L., & Loscalzo, J. (2018). In *Harrison's Principles of Internal Medicine* McGraw-Hill Education.

Jane, F. M., & Davis, S. R. (2014). A practitioner's toolkit for the management of the menopause. *Climacteric, 17*(5), 564–579.

Jayadevappa, R., Chhatre, S., Malkowicz, S. B., Parikh, R. B., Guzzo, T., & Wein, A. J. (2019). Association between androgen deprivation therapy use and diagnosis of dementia in men with prostate cancer. *JAMA Network Open, 2*(7), e196562.

Kampen, D. L., & Sherwin, B. B. (1994). Estrogen use and verbal memory in healthy postmenopausal women. *Obstetrics and Gynecology, 83*(6), 979–983.

Kanaya, A. M., Herrington, D., Vittinghoff, E., Lin, F., Grady, D., Bittner, V., et al. (2003). Glycemic effects of postmenopausal hormone therapy: The heart and estrogen/progestin replacement study. A randomized, double-blind, placebo-controlled trial. *Annals of Internal Medicine, 138*(1), 1–9.

Kantarci, K., Tosakulwong, N., Lesnick, T. G., Zuk, S. M., Lowe, V. J., Fields, J. A., et al. (2018). Brain structure and cognition 3 years after the end of an early menopausal hormone therapy trial. *Neurology, 90*(16). e1404–e12.

L'Hermite, M., Simoncini, T., Fuller, S., & Genazzani, A. R. (2008). Could transdermal estradiol + progesterone be a safer postmenopausal HRT? A review. *Maturitas, 60*(3–4), 185–201.

Labrie, F., Bélanger, A., Cusan, L., Gomez, J. L., & Candas, B. (1997). Marked decline in serum concentrations of adrenal C19 sex steroid precursors and conjugated androgen metabolites during aging. *The Journal of Clinical Endocrinology and Metabolism, 82*(8), 2396–2402.

Labrie, F., Luu-The, V., Labrie, C., Belanger, A., Simard, J., Lin, S.-X., et al. (2003). Endocrine and intracrine sources of androgens in women: Inhibition of breast cancer and other roles of androgens and their precursor dehydroepiandrosterone. *Endocrine Reviews, 24*(2), 152–182.

Laws, K. R., Irvine, K., & Gale, T. M. (2016). Sex differences in cognitive impairment in Alzheimer's Disease. *World Journal of Psychiatry, 6*(1), 54–65.

Lee, H. H., Park, S., Joung, J. Y., & Kim, S. H. (2020). How does androgen deprivation therapy affect mental health including cognitive dysfunction in patients with prostate cancer? *The World Journal of Men's Health, 38*.

Legault, C., Maki, P. M., Resnick, S. M., Coker, L., Hogan, P., Bevers, T. B., et al. (2009). Effects of tamoxifen and raloxifene on memory and other cognitive abilities: Cognition in the study of tamoxifen and raloxifene. *Journal of Clinical Oncology, 27*(31), 5144–5152.

Li, K., Huang, X., Han, Y., Zhang, J., Lai, Y., Yuan, L., et al. (2015). Enhanced neuroactivation during working memory task in postmenopausal women receiving hormone therapy: A coordinate-based meta-analysis. *Frontiers in Human Neuroscience, 9*.

Lithgow, B. J., & Moussavi, Z. (2017). Physiological differences in the follicular, luteal, and menstrual phases in healthy women determined by electrovestibulography: Depression, anxiety, or other associations? *Neuropsychobiology, 76*, 72–81.

Maki, P. M. (2015). Verbal memory and menopause. *Maturitas, 82*, 288–289.

Maki, P., Girard, L., & Manson, J. (2019). Menopausal hormone therapy and cognition. *BMJ: British Medical Journal, 364*, l877–1.

Manson, J. E., Chlebowski, R. T., Stefanick, M. L., Aragaki, A. K., Rossouw, J. E., Prentice, R. L., et al. (2013). Menopausal hormone therapy and health outcomes during the intervention and extended poststopping phases of the women's health initiative randomized trials. *Journal of the American Medical Association, 310*(13), 1353–1368.

Manson, J. E., Aragaki, A. K., Rossouw, J. E., Anderson, G. L., Prentice, R. L., LaCroix, A. Z., et al. (2017). Menopausal hormone therapy and long-term all-cause and cause-specific mortality: The women's health initiative randomized trials. *Journal of the American Medical Association, 318*(10), 927–938.

Matyi, J. M., Rattinger, G. B., Schwartz, S., Buhusi, M., & Tschanz, J. T. (2019). Lifetime estrogen exposure and cognition in late life: The cache county study. *Menopause, 26*(12), 1366–1374.

McEwen, B. S., & Milner, T. A. (2007). Hippocampal formation: Shedding light on the influence of sex and stress on the brain. *Brain Research Reviews, 55*(2), 343–355.

McEwen, B. S., Alves, S. E., Bulloch, K., & Weiland, N. G. (1998). Clinically relevant basic science studies of gender differences and sex hormone effects. *Psychopharmacology Bulletin, 34*(3), 251–259.

McEwen, B. S., Nasca, C., & Gray, J. D. (2016). Stress effects on neuronal structure: Hippocampus, amygdala, and prefrontal cortex. *Neuropsychopharmacology, 41*(1), 3–23.

Medicines and Healthcare Products Regulatory Agency. (2003). In *Vol. 29. Current problems in pharmacovigilance*. UK: Medicines and Healthcare Products Regulatory Agency.

Medicines and Healthcare Products Regulatory Agency. (2007). In *Vol. 1. Drug safety update*. UK: Medicines and Healthcare Products Regulatory Agency.

Mercer, S. W., Gunn, J., & Wyke, S. (2011). Improving the health of people with multimorbidity: The need for prospective cohort studies. *Journal of Comorbidity, 1*(1), 4–7.

Mikkola, T. S., Tuomikoski, P., Lyytinen, H., Korhonen, P., Hoti, F., Vattulainen, P., et al. (2015). Increased cardiovascular mortality risk in women discontinuing postmenopausal hormone therapy. *The Journal of Clinical Endocrinology and Metabolism, 100*(12), 4588–4594.

Mikkola, T. S., Savolainen-Peltonen, H., Tuomikoski, P., Hoti, F., Vattulainen, P., Gissler, M., et al. (2017). Lower death risk for vascular dementia than for Alzheimer's disease with postmenopausal hormone therapy users. *The Journal of Clinical Endocrinology and Metabolism, 102*(3), 870–877.

Miller, V. M., Naftolin, F., Asthana, S., Black, D. M., Brinton, E. A., Budoff, M. J., et al. (2019). The kronos early estrogen prevention study (KEEPS): What have we learned? *Menopause, 26*(9), 1071–1084.

Morales, A. (2004). Andropause (or symptomatic late-onset hypogonadism): Facts, fiction and controversies. *The Aging Male, 7*(4), 297–303.

Mosconi, L., & Brinton, R. D. (2018). How would we combat menopause as an Alzheimer's risk factor? *Expert Review of Neurotherapeutics, 18*(9), 689–691.

Mosconi, L., Berti, V., Guyara-Quinn, C., McHugh, P., Petrongolo, G., Osorio, R. S., et al. (2017). Perimenopause and emergence of an Alzheimer's bioenergetic phenotype in brain and periphery. *PLoS One, 12*(10), e0185926.

Mosconi, L., Berti, V., Quinn, C., McHugh, P., Petrongolo, G., Varsavsky, I., et al. (2017). Sex differences in Alzheimer risk: Brain imaging of endocrine vs chronologic aging. *Neurology, 89*(13), 1382–1390.

Mulligan, E. M., Hajcak, G., Klawohn, J., Nelson, B., & Meyer, A. (2019). Effects of menstrual cycle phase on associations between the error-related negativity and checking symptoms in women. *Psychoneuroendocrinology, 103*, 233–240.

Nead, K. T., Gaskin, G., Chester, C., Swisher-McClure, S., Dudley, J. T., Leeper, N. J., et al. (2016). Androgen deprivation therapy and future Alzheimer's disease risk. *Journal of Clinical Oncology, 34*(6), 566–571.

Nebel, R. A., Aggarwal, N. T., Barnes, L. L., Gallagher, A., Goldstein, J. M., Kantarci, K., et al. (2018). Understanding the impact of sex and gender in Alzheimer's disease: A call to action. *Alzheimer's & Dementia, 14*(9), 1171–1183.

Nelson, H. D. (2008). Menopause. *The Lancet, 371*(9614), 760–770.

Neves-e-Castro, M., Birkhauser, M., Samsioe, G., Lambrinoudaki, I., Palacios, S., Borrego, R. S., et al. (2015). EMAS postion statement: The ten point guide to the integral management of menopausal health. *Maturitas, 81*, 88–92.

Norton, S., Matthews, F. E., Barnes, D. E., Yaffe, K., & Brayne, C. (2014). Potential for primary prevention of Alzheimer's disease: An analysis of population-based data. *The Lancet Neurology, 13*(8), 788–794.

O'Brien, J., Jackson, J. W., Grodstein, F., Blacker, D., & Weuve, J. (2014). Postmenopausal hormone therapy is not associated with risk of all-cause dementia and Alzheimer's disease. *Epidemiologic Reviews, 36*, 83–103.

The North American Menopause Society (NAMS). (2017). The 2017 hormone therapy position statement of The North American Menopause Society. *Menopause, 24*(7), 728–753.

Pfeilschifter, J., Köditz, R., Pfohl, M., & Schatz, H. (2002). Changes in proinflammatory cytokine activity after menopause. *Endocrine Reviews, 23*(1), 90–119.

Phillips, S. M., & Sherwin, B. B. (1992). Variations in memory function and sex steroid hormones across the menstrual cycle. *Psychoneuroendocrinology, 17*(5), 497–506.

Pietrzak, R. H., Lim, Y. Y., Ames, D., Harrington, K., Restrepo, C., Martins, R. N., et al. (2015). Trajectories of memory decline in preclinical Alzheimer's disease: Results from the Australian imaging, biomarkers and lifestyle flagship study of ageing. *Neurobiology of Aging, 36*(3), 1231–1238.

Pike, C. J., Carroll, J. C., Rosario, E. R., & Barron, A. M. (2009). Protective actions of sex steroid hormones in Alzheimer's disease. *Frontiers in Neuroendocrinology, 30*(2), 239–258.

Pinkerton, J. V., & Stovall, D. W. (2010). Reproductive aging, menopause, and health outcomes. Reproductive aging. *Annals of the New York Academy of Sciences, 1204*, 169–178.

Rapp, S. R., Espeland, M. A., Shumaker, S. A., Henderson, V. W., Brunner, R. L., Manson, J. E., et al. (2003). Effect of estrogen plus progestin on global cognitive function in postmenopausal women: The women's health initiative memory study: A randomized controlled trial. *Journal of the American Medical Association, 289*(20), 2663–2672.

Reboussin, B. A., Greendale, G. A., & Espeland, M. A. (1998). Effect of hormone replacement therapy on self-reported cognitive symptoms: Results from the postmenopausal estrogen/progestin interventions (PEPI) trial. *Climacteric, 1*(3), 172–179.

Resnick, S. M., Coker, L. H., Maki, P. M., Rapp, S. R., Espeland, M. A., & Shumaker, S. A. (2004). The women's health initiative study of cognitive aging (WHISCA): A randomized clinical trial of the effects of hormone therapy on age-associated cognitive decline. *Clinical Trials, 1*(5), 440–450.

Resnick, S. M., Maki, P. M., Rapp, S. R., Espeland, M. A., Brunner, R., Coker, L. H., et al. (2006). Effects of combination estrogen plus progestin hormone treatment on cognition and affect. *The Journal of Clinical Endocrinology and Metabolism, 91*(5), 1802–1810.

Resnick, S. M., Espeland, M. A., Jaramillo, S. A., Hirsch, C., Stefanick, M. L., Murray, A. M., et al. (2009). Postmenopausal hormone therapy and regional brain volumes: The WHIMS-MRI Study. *Neurology, 72*(2), 135–142.

Resnick, S. M., Espeland, M. A., An, Y., Maki, P. M., Coker, L. H., Jackson, R., et al. (2009). Effects of conjugated equine estrogens on cognition and affect in postmenopausal women with prior hysterectomy. *The Journal of Clinical Endocrinology and Metabolism, 94*(11), 4152–4161.

Resnick, S. M., Matsumoto, A. M., Stephens-Shields, A. J., Ellenberg, S. S., Gill, T. M., Shumaker, S. A., et al. (2017). Testosterone treatment and cognitive function in older men with low testosterone and age-associated memory impairment. *Journal of the American Medical Association, 317*(7), 717–727.

Ritchie, C. W., Terrera, G. M., & Quinn, T. J. (2015). Dementia trials and dementia tribulations: Methodological and analytical challenges in dementia research. *Alzheimer's Research & Therapy, 7*(1), 31.

Rivera, C. M., Grossardt, B. R., Rhodes, D. J., Brown, R. D., Jr., Roger, V. L., Melton, L. J., 3rd, et al. (2009). Increased cardiovascular mortality after early bilateral oophorectomy. *Menopause, 16*(1), 15–23.

Rocca, W. A., Grossardt, B. R., & Maraganore, D. M. (2008). The long-term effects of oophorectomy on cognitive and motor aging are age dependent. *Neurodegenerative Diseases, 5*, 257–260.

Rosenson, R. S., Brewer, H. B., Barter, P. J., Bjorkegren, J. L. M., Chapman, M. J., Gaudet, D., et al. (2018). HDL and atherosclerotic cardiovascular disease: Genetic insights into complex biology. *Nature Reviews, 15*, 9–19.

Rossouw, J. E., Anderson, G. L., Prentice, R. L., LaCroix, A. Z., Kooperberg, C., Stefanick, M. L., et al. (2002). Risks and benefits of estrogen plus progestin in healthy postmenopausal women: Principal results from the women's health initiative randomized controlled trial. *Journal of the American Medical Association, 288*(3), 321–333.

Rossouw, J. E., Prentice, R. L., Manson, J. E., Wu, L., Barad, D., Barnabei, V. M., et al. (2007). Postmenopausal hormone therapy and risk of cardiovascular disease by age and years since menopause. *Journal of the American Medical Association, 297*(13), 1465–1477.

Roth, J. A., Etzioni, R., Waters, T. M., Pettinger, M., Rossouw, J. E., Anderson, G. L., et al. (2014). Economic return from the women's health initiative estrogen plus progestin clinical trial: A modeling study. *Annals of Internal Medicine, 160*(9), 594–602.

Ryan, J., Scali, J., Carriere, I., Amieva, H., Rouaud, O., Berr, C., et al. (2014). Impact of a premature menopause on cognitive function in later life. *BJOG : An International Journal of Obstetrics and Gynaecology*, 1729–1739.

Sachdev, P. S., Lipnicki, D. M., Crawford, J., Reppermund, S., Kochan, N. A., Trollor, J. N., et al. (2012). Risk profiles for mild cognitive impairment vary by age and sex: The Sydney memory and ageing study. *The American Journal of Geriatric Psychiatry, 20*(10), 854–865.

Salpeter, S. R., Walsh, J. M., Greyber, E., Ormiston, T. M., & Salpeter, E. E. (2004). Mortality associated with hormone replacement therapy in younger and older women: A meta-analysis. *Journal of General Internal Medicine, 19*(7), 791–804.

Salpeter, S. R., Walsh, J. M., Ormiston, T. M., Greyber, E., Buckley, N. S., & Salpeter, E. E. (2006). Meta-analysis: Effect of hormone-replacement therapy on components of the metabolic syndrome in postmenopausal women. *Diabetes, Obesity & Metabolism, 8*(5), 538–554.

Salpeter, S. R., Cheng, J., Thabane, L., Buckley, N. S., & Salpeter, E. E. (2009). Bayesian meta-analysis of hormone therapy and mortality in younger postmenopausal women. *The American Journal of Medicine, 122*(11). 1016–1022.e1.

Savolainen-Peltonen, H., Rahkola-Soisalo, P., Hoti, F., Vattulainen, P., Gissler, M., Ylikorkala, O., et al. (2019). Use of postmenopausal hormone therapy and risk of Alzheimer's disease in Finland: Nationwide case-control study. *BMJ (Clinical Research Ed), 364*, l665.

Schierbeck, L. L., Rejnmark, L., Tofteng, C. L., Stilgren, L., Eiken, P., Mosekilde, L., et al. (2012). Effect of hormone replacement therapy on cardiovascular events in recently postmenopausal women: Randomised trial. *BMJ, 345*, e6409.

Schmidt, R., Fazekas, F., Reinhart, B., Kapeller, P., Fazekas, G., Offenbacher, H., et al. (1996). Estrogen replacement therapy in older women: A neuropsychological and brain MRI study. *Journal of the American Geriatrics Society, 44*(11), 1307–1313.

Shao, H., Breitner, J. C., Whitmer, R. A., Wang, J., Hayden, K., Wengreen, H., et al. (2012). Hormone therapy and Alzheimer disease dementia: New findings from the Cache County Study. *Neurology, 79*(18), 1846–1852.

Sharma, S. (2003). Hormone replacement therapy in menopause: Current concerns and considerations. *Kathmandu University Medical Journal, 1*(4), 288–293.

Shepardson, N. E., Shankar, G. M., & Selkoe, D. J., et al. (2011). Cholesterol level and statin use in Alzheimer disease: I. Review of human trials and recommendations. *Archives of Neurology, 68*(10), 1239–1244.

Shlipak, M. G., Angeja, B. G., Go, A. S., Frederick, P. D., Canto, J. G., & Grady, D. (2001). Hormone therapy and in-hospital survival after myocardial infarction in postmenopausal women. *Circulation, 104*(19), 2300–2304.

Shumaker, S. A., Reboussin, B. A., Espeland, M. A., Rapp, S. R., McBee, W. L., Dailey, M., et al. (1998). The women's health initiative memory study (WHIMS): A trial of the effect of estrogen therapy in preventing and slowing the progression of dementia. *Controlled Clinical Trials, 19*, 604–621.

Shumaker, S. A., Legault, C., Kuller, L., Rapp, S. R., Thal, L., Lane, D. S., et al. (2004). Conjugated equine estrogens and incidence of probable dementia and mild cognitive impairment in postmenopausal women: Women's Health Initiative Memory Study. *Journal of the American Medical Association, 291*(24), 2947–2958.

Sitruk-Ware, R. (2007). New hormonal therapies and regimens in the postmenopause: Routes of administration and timing of initiation. *Climacteric, 10*(5), 358–370.

Snyder, H. M., Asthana, S., Bain, L., Brinton, R., Craft, S., Dubal, D. B., et al. (2016). Sex biology contributions to vulnerability to Alzheimer's disease: A think tank convened by the women's Alzheimer's research initiative. *Alzheimer's & Dementia, 12*(11), 1186–1196.

Sobhani, K., Nieves Castro, D. K., Fu, Q., Gottlieb, R. A., Van Eyk, J. E., & Noel Bairey Merz, C. (2018). Sex differences in ischemic heart disease and heart failure biomarkers. *Biology of Sex Differences, 9*(1), 43.

Sohrabji, F., & Bake, S. (2006). Age-related changes in neuroprotection: Is estrogen proinflammatory for the reproductive senescent brain? *Endocrine, 29*(2), 191–197.

Sperling, R. A., Aisen, P. S., Beckett, L. A., Bennett, D. A., Craft, S., Fagan, A. M., et al. (2011). Toward defining the preclinical stages of Alzheimer's disease: Recommendations from the National Institute on Aging-Alzheimer's Association workgroups on diagnostic guidelines for Alzheimer's disease. *Alzheimer's & Dementia, 7*(3), 280–292.

Speroff, L. (2010). Transdermal hormone therapy and the risk of stroke and venous thrombosis. *Climacteric, 13*(5), 429–432.

Stevens-Lapsley, J. E., & Kohrt, W. M. (2010). Osteoarthritis in women: Effects of estrogen, obesity and physical activity. *Women's Health (London, England), 6*(4), 601–615.

Szoeke, C., Cicuttini, F., Guthrie, J., & Dennerstein, L. (2008). The relationship of reports of aches and joint pains to the menopausal transition: A longitudinal study. *Climacteric*, *11*(1), 55–62.

Szoeke, C., Campbell, S., Chiu, E., & Ames, D. (2009). *Vascular cognitive disorder. Textbook of Alzheimer disease and other dementias. 1* (pp. 181–193). US (Arlington): American Psychiatric Publishing.

Tackett, A. H., Bailey, A. L., Foody, J. M., Miller, J. M., Apperson-Hansen, C., Ohman, E. M., et al. (2010). Hormone replacement therapy among postmenopausal women presenting with acute myocardial infarction: Insights from the GUSTO-III trial. *American Heart Journal*, *160*(4), 678–684.

Taylor, C. M., Pritschet, L., Yu, S., & Jacobs, E. G. (2019). Applying a women's health lens to the study of the aging brain. *Frontiers in Human Neuroscience*, *13*, 224.

Teodorescu, V. J., Vavra, A. K., & Kibbe, M. R. (2013). Peripheral arterial disease in women. *Journal of Vascular Surgery*, *57*(4 Suppl), 18S–26S.

The International Menopause Society's [IMS] response to The Lancet's publication of a report suggesting HRT substantially increases breast cancer risk [press release]. (2019).

The Women's Health Initiative Study Group. (1998). Design of the women's health initiative clinical trial and observational study. The Women's Health Initiative Study Group. *Controlled Clinical Trials*, *19*(1), 61–109.

Thurston, R. C., Kuller, L. H., Edmundowicz, D., & Matthews, K. A. (2010). History of hot flashes and aortic calcification among postmenopausal women. *Menopause*, *17*(2), 256–261.

Thurston, R. C., Sutton-Tyrrell, K., Everson-Rose, S. A., Hess, R., Powell, L. H., & Matthews, K. A. (2011). Hot flashes and carotid intima media thickness among midlife women. *Menopause*, *18*(4), 352–358.

Toodayan, N. (2016). Professor Alois Alzheimer (1864-1915): Lest we forget. *Journal of Clinical Neuroscience*, *31*, 47–55.

Tully, K. H., Nguyen, D. D., Herzog, P., Jin, G., Noldus, J., Nguyen, P. L., et al. (2021). Risk of dementia and depression in young and middle-aged men presenting with nonmetastatic prostate cancer treated with androgen deprivation therapy. *European Urology Oncology*, *4*(1), 66–72.

US Food & Drug Administration. (2015). *FDA Drug Safety Communication: FDA cautions about using testosterone products for low testosterone due to aging; requires labeling change to inform of possible increased risk of heart attack and stroke with use*. Washington, DC: US Food & Drug Administration.

van der Schouw, Y. T., van der Graaf, Y., Steyerberg, E. W., Eijkemans, M. J. C., & Banga, J. D. (1996). Age at menopause as a risk factor for cardiovascular mortallity. *The Lancet*, *347*(March 16), 714–718.

van der Voort, D. J. M., van der Weijer, P. H. M., & Barentsen, R. (2003). Early menopause: Increaed fracture risk at older age. *Osteoporosis International*, *14*, 525–530.

Vanhulle, G., & Demol, R. (1976). A double-blind study into the influence of estriol on a number of psychological tests in post-menopausal women. In P. A. van Keep, R. B Greenblatt, & M. Albeaux-Fernet (Eds.), *Consensus on menopause research* (pp. 94–99). Springer.

Vaughan, L., Espeland, M. A., Snively, B., Shumaker, S. A., Rapp, S. R., Shupe, J., et al. (2013). The rationale, design, and baseline characteristics of the women's health initiative memory study of younger women (WHIMS-Y). *Brain Research*, *1514*, 3–11.

Verdile, G., Laws, S. M., Henley, D., Ames, D., Bush, A. I., Ellis, K. A., et al. (2014). Associations between gonadotropins, testosterone and beta amyloid in men at risk of Alzheimer's disease. *Molecular Psychiatry*, *19*(1), 69–75.

Verghese, J., Lipton, R. B., Katz, M. J., Hall, C. B., Derby, C. A., Kuslansky, G., et al. (2003). Leisure activities and the risk of dementia in the elderly. *The New England Journal of Medicine*, *348*(25), 2508–2516.

Villemagne, V. L., Burnham, S., Bourgeat, P., Brown, B., Ellis, K. A., Salvado, O., et al. (2013). Amyloid beta deposition, neurodegeneration, and cognitive decline in sporadic Alzheimer's disease: A prospective cohort study. *Lancet Neurology*, *12*(4), 357–367.

Vinogradova, Y., Coupland, C., & Hippisley-Cox, J. (2019). Use of hormone replacement therapy and risk of venous thromboembolism: Nested case-control studies using the QResearch and CPRD databases. *BMJ*, *364*, k4810.

Vranic, A., & Hromatko, I. (2008). Content-specific activational effects of estrogen on working memory performance. *The Journal of General Psychology*, *135*(3), 323–336.

Wenger, N. K. (2013). Prevention of cardiovascular disease in women: Highlights for the clinician of the 2011 American Heart Association Guidelines. *Advances in Chronic Kidney Disease*, *20*(5), 419–422.

Wharton, W., Gleason, C. E., Miller, V. M., & Asthana, S. (2013). Rationale and design of the kronos early estrogen prevention study (KEEPS) and the KEEPS cognitive and affective sub study (KEEPS Cog). *Brain Research*, *1514*, 12–17.

Wiesmann, M., Kiliaan, A. J., & Claassen, J. A. (2013). Vascular aspects of cognitive impairment and dementia. *Journal of Cerebral Blood Flow and Metabolism*, *33*(11), 1696–1706.

Windler, E., Stute, P., Ortmann, O., & Mueck, A. O. (2015). Is postmenopausal hormone replacement therapy suitable after a cardio- or cerebrovascular event? *Archives of Gynecology and Obstetrics*, *291*(1), 213–217.

World Health Organization. (2019). *Risk reduction of cognitive-declline and dementia: WHO guidelines*. Geneva: World Health Organization (WHO).

Wu, M., Li, M., Yuan, J., Liang, S., Chen, Z., Ye, M., et al. (2020). Postmenopausal hormone therapy and Alzheimer's disease, dementia, and Parkinson's disease: A systematic review and time-response meta-analysis. *Pharmacological Research*, *155*, 104693.

Yaffe, K., Sawaya, G., Lieberburg, I., & Grady, D. (1998). Estrogen therapy in postmenopausal women. *Journal of the American Medical Association*, *279*(9), 688–695.

Yaffe, K., Haan, M., Byers, A., Tangen, C., & Kuller, L. (2000). Estrogen use, APOE, and cognitive decline: Evidence of gene-environment interaction. *Neurology*, *54*(10), 1949–1954.

Yan, H., et al. (2019). Estrogen improves insulin sensitivity and suppresses gluconeogenesis via the transcription factor Foxo1. *Diabetes*, *68*(2), 291–304.

Yue, X., Lu, M., Lancaster, T., Cao, P., Honda, S., Staufenbiel, M., et al. (2005). Brain estrogen deficiency accelerates Abeta plaque formation in an Alzheimer's disease animal model. *Proceedings of the National Academy of Sciences of the United States of America*, *102*(52), 19198–19203.

Zhang, Z., Kang, D., & Li, H. (2020). Testosterone and cognitive impairment or dementia in middle-aged or aging males: Causation and intervention, a systematic review and meta-analysis. *Journal of Geriatric Psychiatry and Neurology*, 0891988720933351.

Zhou, C., Wu, Q., Wang, Z., Wang, Q., Liang, Y., & Liu, S. (2020). The effect of hormone replacement therapy on cognitive function in female patients with Alzheimer's disease: A meta-analysis. *American Journal of Alzheimer's Disease and Other Dementias*, *35*, 1533317520938585.

CHAPTER

Sex and gender differences in genetic and lifestyle risk and protective factors for dementia

10

Shireen Sindi[a,b], Sima Toopchiani[b], Mariagnese Barbera[c], Krister Håkansson[a], Jenni Lehtisalo[c,d], Anna Rosenberg[c], Ruth Stephen[c], Chinedu Udeh-Momoh[b], and Miia Kivipelto[a,b,e,f]

[a]*Division of Clinical Geriatrics, Center for Alzheimer Research, Karolinska Institutet, Stockholm, Sweden*
[b]*Ageing Epidemiology (AGE) Research Unit, School of Public Health, Imperial College London, London, United Kingdom*
[c]*Institute of Clinical Medicine, Neurology, University of Eastern Finland, Kuopio, Finland*
[d]*Population Health Unit, Finnish Institute for Health and Welfare, Helsinki, Finland*
[e]*Theme Aging, Karolinska University Hospital, Stockholm, Sweden*
[f]*Institute of Public Health and Clinical Nutrition and Institute of Clinical Medicine, Neurology, University of Eastern Finland, Kuopio, Finland*

Introduction

Two-thirds of individuals diagnosed with Alzheimer's disease (AD) are women, and these differences in AD prevalence are observed in different regions of the world (Alzheimers Association Report, 2020). Estimates have shown that women have higher prevalence of dementia worldwide (Georges et al., 2020; Prince et al., 2013). In Europe, the incidence of dementia has been reported to be higher among women in the oldest old age group (age 80+ years) (Andersen et al., 1999; Chene et al., 2015; Fratiglioni et al., 1997). However, these findings have not been replicated in the USA, where studies report no significant differences in dementia incidence between men and women, including among the oldest old (Mielke, 2018), suggesting the existence of geographical differences that may be influenced by environmental factors.

Considering that age is the most important risk factor for dementia and AD, the higher life expectancy among women—which is consistent globally—has commonly been proposed as a reason underlying the differences in the prevalence of these diseases (Alzheimers Association Report, 2020). In 2016, global life expectancy at birth was 74.2 years for women and 69.8 years for men, and the sex difference in life expectancy was 4.4 years (World Health Organization, 2020). Some recent evidence suggests that while the life expectancy gap has been narrowing in some areas of the world (e.g., Europe and the Americas), other regions do not show similar patterns (Mateos et al., 2020). Although biological factors may play a role, emerging evidence suggests that socioeconomic and lifestyle factors may also influence such differences in life expectancy gaps across the globe.

Several lines of evidence have suggested that the higher prevalence of dementia in older women compared to older men is due to "selective survival," as men are more likely to die of cardiovascular disease in midlife. Those who survive past age 65 may have healthier cardiovascular risk profiles and different health characteristics than women (for a review, Ferretti et al., 2020). This may include better management of vascular and metabolic risk factors, better diet, more physical activity, more moderate alcohol consumption, and a lower likelihood of smoking. Women, on the other hand, tend to be at higher risk for other risk factors in late-life, such as depression (see Chapter 7) (Livingston et al., 2020) and changes in sex hormone levels (see Chapter 9) (Pertesi et al., 2019).

Cohort effects are also important to consider when investigating sex differences in dementia. For example, during recent decades, there have been significant increases in the opportunities available to women with regards to educational attainment and, consequently, occupational attainment and socioeconomic status (Subramaniapillai et al., 2020). Recent evidence has shown that the higher levels of education in more recent Swedish cohorts were associated with lower dementia prevalence among older adults aged 85 years (Skoog et al., 2017), which further confirms the changes in psychosocial and lifestyle factors over the years and how they may relate to dementia risk.

While some risk factors are unique to one sex (e.g., menopause in women), others may be relevant to both sexes, but may still be more prevalent among one of the sexes (e.g., depression in women) (Mielke, 2018). A more thorough understanding of such risk factors and how they can differentially impact the sexes is important for better tailoring of risk reduction guidelines and future interventions. The goal of this chapter is to summarize the current evidence on sex differences in genetic and modifiable lifestyle factors that are associated with dementia risk (schematic representation available in Fig. 1). The findings are further discussed in light of recent, multidomain lifestyle intervention trials (which included factors such as diet, exercise, cognitive training and vascular/metabolic risk management). Considerations for future research and risk reduction initiatives are also highlighted.

APOE allele

The apolipoprotein E gene (APOE) consists of three main alleles: Ɛ2, Ɛ3, and Ɛ4. The Ɛ4 allele has been identified as one of the leading genetic risk factors for AD (Harold et al., 2009). The APOE-4 allele is associated with clinical and/or biological hallmarks of AD such as accumulating levels of abnormal β-amyloid (Aβ) plaques, steeper falls in global cognition, and hippocampal atrophy (Jack et al., 2015;

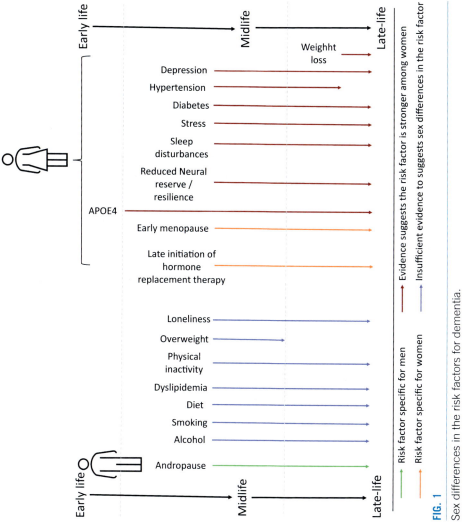

FIG. 1

Sex differences in the risk factors for dementia.

Lim et al., 2013). However, some studies have shown conflicting results and have not reported such associations (Landau et al., 2011; Lupton et al., 2016). Because these inconsistencies could be due to sex-related factors, it is important to evaluate probable sex differences in relation to the APOE-4 allele.

Despite the fact that women make up nearly two-thirds of AD cases, studies have yet to show sex differences in the prevalence of APOE-4 due to the small number of homozygotes (Sundermann et al., 2018). Several studies have reported an equal distribution of the allele but a stronger influence of the APOE-4 gene in women compared to men (Nebel et al., 2018; Neu et al., 2017). A meta-analysis by Neu and colleagues concluded that women with one copy of the APOE-4 allele have the same risk of AD as men, but are at increased risk of disease once they reach between 65 and 75 years of age (Neu et al., 2017). This suggests that APOE status and increased risk of AD in women are also age-dependent. A recent study also reported a significant interaction with other genes that was linked to increased AD risk among women who carried the APOE-4 allele (Hsu et al., 2019).

Studies on sex differences among APOE-4 carriers have reported an increased prevalence of AD, greater cognitive decline, severe memory loss, and faster AD progression among women (Altmann et al., 2014; Neu et al., 2017). Women are also known to experience higher rates of change in all brain regions (except the hippocampus) (Holland et al., 2013). Several studies have indicated higher tau burden in APOE-4 women as compared to men; for a discussion of sex differences among APOE-4 carriers in fluid and imaging biomarkers, we refer the reader to Chapters 4 and 5. Studies have looked at possible effects of sex and APOE status on the therapeutic response to interventions with cholinesterase inhibitors but found conflicting results: significant differences with APOE genotype were found among women, but no differences were seen in men (Farlow et al., 1998). Other studies reported no associations between APOE status, sex, and therapeutic responses (Rigaud et al., 2002; Winblad et al., 2001). Findings have indeed shown that changes in both brain structure and function were generally greater in magnitude among women. When developing potential treatments, it is important for clinical trials to consider both APOE status and sex, as biological and physical sex differences can influence pharmacokinetics and pharmacodynamics.

Hormones, menopause, and andropause

Sex hormones and the menopausal transition are key factors to consider when investigating sex differences in risk of AD and other forms of dementia. Findings from both in vitro and in vivo studies have established estrogen as having neuroprotective effects, which occur through various mechanisms (see Chapter 2). Estrogen may have the ability to block the harmful effects of the Aβ proteins by providing protection to brain cells and reducing the number of free radicals. It is thought that estrogen can trigger the brain into producing more antioxidants, which in turn protect brain cells (Zarate, Stevnsner, & Gredilla, 2017).

Hormone replacement therapy

Hormone replacement therapy (HRT) relieves the symptoms of menopause by replacing declining endogenous levels of estrogen and progesterone. Studies have investigated the association between HRT and dementia risk, but results from both observational and interventional studies to date have been inconclusive (see Chapter 9).

Observational studies—both case–control and retrospective—have shown that women who initiate HRT within the earlier stages of their menopausal transition or at a younger age have a lower risk of developing AD (Henderson et al., 2005; Nelson et al., 2002; Shao et al., 2012). This has been referred to as the "window of opportunity" hypothesis (Henderson et al., 2005; Whitmer et al., 2011; Zandi et al., 2002), which suggests that the effects of HRT depend on timing of initiation of treatment, such that beneficial effects are more likely when treatment is started closer to natural menopause. One study by Zandi et al. examined the influence of initiation timing, treatment duration, and treatment composition (estrogen alone or combined estrogen–progesterone therapy). This study found a significant reduction (by 30%) in AD risk in women who initiated HRT within 5 years of menopause onset (Zandi et al., 2002). The risk was even lower in women who not only initiated HRT early but continued its use for 10 years. Women who initiated therapy later than 5 years post-menopause showed no protective effect of HRT against AD risk (Zandi et al., 2002). The generalizability of these studies has been questioned due to their selection of participants: the majority of HRT users were relatively "healthy" in terms of cardiovascular factors and had higher educational status compared to women who had not used HRT. Furthermore, a recent Finnish study reported a 9%–17% increased AD risk among HRT users. However, in women who initiated HRT before the age of 60, this increase was only seen in users of the combined estrogen–progesterone therapy (Savolainen-Peltonen et al., 2019).

The window of opportunity hypothesis was not supported by some prospective studies examining HRT initiation timing and neuropsychological test performance. One study supported this hypothesis, but observed a positive impact of HRT on verbal fluency, working memory, and psychomotor speed regardless of timing (Ryan et al., 2009). The Nurses' Health Study, on the other hand, did not support the window of opportunity hypothesis, and showed that HRT users had slightly lower cognitive performance compared to non-users (Maki, 2013).

Earlier HRT trials reported a negative effect on cognition and other adverse events. Women aged 65+ years and randomized to the combined estrogen–progesterone arm had higher risk of cardiovascular and cancer events, as well as cognitive impairment and AD (Shumaker et al., 2003). Later analyses of these initial results showed more negative effects on cognition in women who had lower baseline cognitive function (Shumaker et al., 2004). These studies had several limitations as the majority of participants were older and on average 15 years out of menopause (65+), obese, and had prior HRT exposure. Indeed, these confounding variables are known to influence dementia risk. Another factor that was not accounted for in these trials was history of depression, another factor associated with increased risk of dementia (Goveas et al., 2011).

Findings from more recent and ongoing trials have placed great focus on the role of HRT initiation time in relation to the therapeutic benefits of estrogen-based HRT. Small trials failed to show HRT efficacy, although they emphasized the window of opportunity theory (Henderson et al., 2000; Mulnard et al., 2000; Wang et al., 2000). Neither benefits nor harm on global cognition and verbal memory were observed in women who initiated HRT between the ages of 50 and 54 years compared to controls (Miller et al., 2019). However, women with type-2 diabetes showed a higher risk of cognitive impairment (Henderson et al., 2013). These findings highlight the importance of considering timing of HRT initiation and comorbidities in HRT research. Another trial reported lower Aβ disposition in APOE-4 carriers who were randomized to the estradiol-only arm compared to those in the placebo arm (Kantarci et al., 2016). Several trials have observed improvements in verbal recall and verbal episodic memory among women younger than 65 years who received estrogen-only therapy (Baker et al., 2019; Joffe et al., 2006; Sherwin, 1988). A more recent study also confirmed benefits of estrogen-only therapy, showing a lower risk of death due to AD or dementia compared to women on placebo (Manson et al., 2017). Although these studies were conducted using small samples, they support the hypothesis that estrogen (alone) enhances cognition and may possess neuroprotective qualities.

Clinical trials have attempted to limit the selection bias and reduce the number of confounding factors encountered in observational studies. Nevertheless, the overall impact of HRT on dementia risk remains rather uncertain. Earlier trials provided useful data on the safety of HRT use, but failed to account for other dementia risk factors, such as cognitive performance, age, and history of depression, for instance. This could occur as a result of most trials reporting AD risk and cognition as a secondary outcome and other medical events such as stroke, cardiovascular, and cancer as primary outcomes, which themselves are dementia risk factors. More recent and ongoing studies have shown HRT to have no or positive effects on cognition and AD risk if not initiated too late after menopause onset.

To date, despite findings that have highlighted the importance of considering reproductive history, no studies have examined the relationship between lifetime exposure to synthetic hormones, the use of HRT, and their influence on AD risk. Future research should focus on gaining a better understanding of HRT efficacy, timing, type and modality of HRT (e.g., transdermal and cyclical hormone therapies), and sex-specific medical history.

Reproductive history and timing of menopause

The Alzheimer's Association International Conference (AAIC-2018) highlighted critical sex differences associated with dementia and AD risk throughout a woman's life course (Alzheimer's Association International Conference, 2018). When developing new treatments to prevent or delay the onset of AD, women's reproductive and pregnancy history should be strongly considered. Recent studies reported a 28%–33% elevated dementia risk in women who experienced natural menopause at aged 45 years or younger (Gilsanz et al., 2017). Another study suggested that the number of months a woman spends being pregnant is a significant predictor of AD, with a 20% reduced AD risk observed in women who spent 12.5% more months pregnant (Fox et al., 2018). Although the mechanisms whereby the number of miscarriages, pregnancy, and reproductive years would affect dementia risk have not been elucidated, it is possible that the process of pregnancy itself may have a neuroprotective ability to delay or reduce AD risk, and research focusing on such processes is ongoing.

Andropause

Recent studies have reported associations between hormonal changes and dementia and AD risk in men. Similar to women, men experience a depletion in free testosterone levels with increasing age as women do in estrogen levels. It has been suggested that the difference in AD risk between men and women is a result of men experiencing a depletion in testosterone levels at a more gradual pace compared to women who experience a more sudden, dramatic, and permanent decrease in estrogen levels in menopause (Feldman et al., 2002; Gray et al., 1991; Muller et al., 2003; Pike, 2017). The reductions in serum testosterone levels is a risk factor for AD (Rosario & Pike, 2008), a fact which has been confirmed by Holland, Bandelow, and Hogervorst (2011), who reported lower levels of testosterone in AD patients compared to healthy individuals (Holland et al., 2011). Several studies have also uncovered neuroprotective effects of testosterone on the brain and Aβ deposition (Bialek et al., 2004; Gouras et al., 2000; Pike, 2001; Thompson & Brenowitz, 2010).

Testosterone is much more abundant in men than in women (Clark et al., 1975). Observational studies have highlighted a link between a reduction in free testosterone and cognitive decline and increased AD risk (Hogervorst et al., 2004; Lv et al., 2016; Moffat et al., 2004). Interventional studies have also reported improved global cognition among participants who received testosterone treatment (Wahjoepramono et al., 2016). Animal studies have further confirmed the protective effects of testosterone on cognition in AD models (Jia et al., 2016; Jian-xin et al., 2015; Yan et al., 2019). Larger and more comprehensive trials with longer follow-up periods are needed to confirm these effects.

Cardiometabolic risk factors

Sex differences in the prevalence of cardiometabolic risk factors for AD have long been known (Azad, Al Bugami, & Loy-English, 2007) and have recently been confirmed (Peters, Muntner, & Woodward, 2019). Cardiovascular risk factors, especially in midlife, are more prevalent in men but affect women more severely, or at least in a different manner: women are more prone to microvascular disorders, and men to coronary artery disease (Leening et al., 2014). This could partly explain the differences in risk of AD (Seshadri et al., 1997) and vascular dementia (Ruitenberg et al., 2001) between men and women. However, the specific role of single risk factors in this complex picture has yet to be unraveled.

Hypertension is one of the most established risk factors for AD and a predictor of white matter lesions (Allan et al., 2015), which, together with the risk of MCI and dementia, can be significantly reduced by intensive blood pressure control (Nasrallah et al., 2019; Williamson et al., 2019). Although hypertension is reportedly more poorly managed in men than in women (Chudiak, Uchmanowicz, & Mazur, 2018), its impact on cognition (Gilsanz et al., 2017; Liu et al., 2018) and neurodegeneration (Cherbuin et al., 2015) seems stronger in women. Men's cognition may also benefit more from reductions in systolic blood pressure (Lacruz et al., 2016) compared to women's. One possible explanation may lie in the different factors affecting memory resilience, which is associated with blood pressure in women, but not in men (McDermott et al., 2017). Hypertension also seems to affect different cognitive domains based on sex (Kritz-Silverstein et al., 2017); nevertheless, women generally perform better on verbal ability tasks, and men on spatial ability tests, regardless of their blood pressure status (de Frias, Nilsson, & Herlitz, 2006; McCarrey et al., 2016).

The role of dyslipidemia in sex differences related to AD risk is less clear. Midlife hypercholesterolemia is associated with an increased risk of AD in late-life (Solomon et al., 2007), but the evidence on the efficacy of cholesterol-lowering treatment in risk-reduction is inconclusive (Geifman et al., 2017; McGuinness et al., 2016). Low triglycerides could be more protective in women (Ancelin et al., 2013; Lamar et al., 2019), whereas higher HDL serum level may be more beneficial in elderly men (Pancani et al., 2019). However, the evidence is inconsistent (Dufouil, Seshadri, & Chene, 2014) and, above all, indicates a complex, sex-specific pattern in which different dyslipidemia profiles are affected by genetic vulnerability (e.g., APOE) and hormone status, especially in women (Ancelin et al., 2014; Lu et al., 2017).

Diabetes is another well-established risk factor for AD, deemed by some as more relevant than hypertension (Fan et al., 2017); in fact, hyperglycemia without diabetes has also been shown to increase the risk of dementia (Crane et al., 2013). Previous studies looking at the association of diabetes with AD or dementia diagnosis did not report sex-specific differences (Dufouil et al., 2014). However, more recent findings point towards a larger impact of diabetes and hyperglycemia on dementia in women (Kim et al., 2017a) and confirm the results of a subgroup analysis which formally accounted for interaction by sex (Noale et al., 2013). In support of this, women with diabetes are also reported to be frailer (Nishimura et al., 2019), score lower on measures of health status and functioning factors (McCollum et al., 2005), and show more marked signs of neurodegeneration (Hempel, Onopa, & Convit, 2012) compared to their male counterparts. Nonetheless, the evidence is rather patchy, mostly from (albeit large) cross sectional cohorts, and a possible mediating role of depression and anxiety has been suggested (Trento et al., 2014).

Furthermore, understanding the sex-based differences in relation to overweight and obesity is complicated by its age-dependent correlation (Kivimaki et al., 2018) with the risk of AD and dementia, such that being overweight is a risk factor in midlife and a protective factor in late-life. Here, reverse causation has been proposed as an explanation (Kivimaki et al., 2018), and findings suggesting that weight loss precedes dementia diagnosis by several years in women but not in men (Knopman et al., 2007) could be particularly relevant in this regard.

Overall, evidence of sex differences related to overweight and obesity and AD risks are more robust and consistent in late-life, indicating not only that increased body mass index (Garcia-Ptacek et al., 2014) and central adiposity (Liu et al., 2018; West et al., 2016) would be more protective in older men than women, but also that overweight correlates with higher cortical thickness only in men (Kim et al., 2015a). However, this association could also be mediated by depression, which was reported to be more strongly associated with obesity in older women than men (Wild et al., 2012). Midlife findings are conflicting: overweight is more harmful for women in relation to dementia and AD diagnosis (Dufouil et al., 2014; Noale et al., 2013), but for men in relation to cognitive outcomes (Elias et al., 2005; Espeland et al., 2018). Collectively, although some findings suggest that sex modulates the associations between cardiometabolic risk factors and AD/dementia, more evidence is needed on sex differences in relation to specific AD pathology and from analyses accounting for formal interactions by sex.

Smoking and alcohol consumption

Smoking and alcohol consumption have also been implicated in the risk of AD and dementia (World Health Organization, 2019). Worldwide, smoking is still more prevalent among men (Giovino et al., 2012). However, in the Western world the gap has considerably narrowed over the last few decades (Higgins et al., 2015) due to sex differences in smoking patterns: women are less likely than men to quit smoking and more likely to relapse (Perkins, 2001; Piper et al., 2010; Wetter et al., 1999). Smoking affects brain and cognitive functions differently in both sexes (Hahn, Pogun, & Gunturkun, 2010); however, the limited evidence on the sex-stratified risk of AD and dementia due to smoking suggests no differences between men and women (Zhong et al., 2015).

Moreover, men consume larger amounts of alcohol than women, but excessive alcohol consumption is more detrimental to women's health (Agabio et al., 2017; Erol & Karpyak, 2015). Alcohol also triggers different neural responses (Seo et al., 2011) and affects different cognitive domains based on sex (Van den Berg et al., 2017). Current evidence indicates a U-shaped association between alcohol use and risk of AD, and it was suggested that women would benefit more from the "protective" effect of moderate alcohol intake (Dufouil, Ducimetiere, & Alperovitch, 1997; Yonker et al., 2005). However, moderate alcohol consumption in men was also associated with better outcomes related to AD pathology (Wardzala et al., 2018) and no clear sex-differences have emerged so far (Dufouil et al., 2014).

Physical activity and exercise

Physical inactivity has been associated with increased risk of developing cognitive decline and dementia (Santos-Lozano et al., 2016; World Health Organization, 2019). However, not much evidence is available on how it may differentially impact men and women. Physical inactivity seems to influence dementia risk, both directly as a risk factor and indirectly through other associated dementia risk factors such as obesity (Kim et al., 2017b), diabetes (Colberg et al., 2010), and cardiovascular disease (Carnethon, 2009).

Contrastingly, sustained exercise at midlife and possibly at late-life may be protective against dementia risk by decreasing obesity, diabetes, and cardiovascular risk (Livingston et al., 2020). Considering the direct effects of exercise, most of the available evidence points toward beneficial effects of exercise on the brain (World Health Organization, 2019). While exercise has been studied both in observational (Stephen et al., 2017) and interventional (Northey et al., 2018) studies, the recurrent question remains: what type, how much, and for whom is exercise most beneficial? Some studies have reported sex as a moderator between exercise and AD, implying that the effects of exercise in men and women may differ in the context of AD prevention (Kramer & Colcombe, 2018). Results across studies are mixed, and much evidence points to women's cognition benefiting more from exercise compared to men's (Barha et al., 2017; Dufouil et al., 2014; Kramer & Colcombe, 2018). However, some (albeit fewer) studies have also reported more exercise-related benefits in hippocampal volume (Carlson et al., 2015), global cognitive function, and executive functioning in men compared to women (Fallah et al., 2009; Lindwall, Rennemark, & Berggren, 2008; Tolppanen et al., 2015). While the pathological markers of AD (Aβ on brain imaging and in cerebrospinal fluid) may not consistently differ across the sexes, differential risk factors for AD and the response to interventions may indeed exist between men and women (Ferretti et al., 2018; Nebel et al., 2018). Markers of AD progression such as hippocampal atrophy rate show faster progression in women compared to men once AD pathology sets in (for a review, see Ferretti et al., 2018). However, women have been reported to benefit more from exercise interventions compared to men in multiple cognitive domains (Barha et al., 2017).

Aerobic exercise—the most widely studied form of exercise—has been associated with increased levels of brain derived neurotrophic factor (BDNF), insulin growth factor 1 (IGF-1), and calcium/calmodulin-dependent kinase II (Cassilhas et al., 2012). There are no studies to date that have directly investigated the interaction between sex and aerobic training. However, in subgroup analyses, studies may consider investigating the effect of exercise by sex (Baker et al., 2010). Resistance training is aimed at enhancing muscle mass, strength, and power, and is associated with improved executive functioning, especially in women with subjective cognitive decline, possibly due to the effect on IGF-1 and AKT (Cassilhas et al., 2012). Multimodal exercise incorporating both aerobic and resistance training has also been reported to benefit women more greatly than men, especially in the domain of executive functions (Barha et al., 2017).

Besides many potential physiological differences between the sexes (Barha & Liu-Ambrose, 2018), one mechanism underlying the above-mentioned effects may be sex-related differences in BDNF. For example, higher levels of estradiol have been associated with greater BDNF expression in the cortex and hippocampus of female rats (Barha & Liu-Ambrose, 2018; Scharfman et al., 2003; Singh, Meyer, & Simpkins, 1995; Sohrabji, Miranda, & Toran-Allerand, 1995). Estrogen levels are thought to moderate the association between higher fitness levels and better executive functioning as observed in postmenopausal women previously using hormone replacement therapy (Erickson et al., 2007). Furthermore, daily walking has been associated with structural benefits to the hippocampus in women (Varma, Tang, & Carlson, 2016).

The effect of sex remains understudied in the context of exercise and AD prevention. Recent research on genetic and phenotypic variability is helping the field gradually move away from a one-size-fits-all approach towards precision/personalized medicine (Ferretti et al., 2018). Increasing knowledge about possible moderators such as biological sex will aid future AD preventive interventions such as exercise to be more targeted and effective.

Nutrition

Perspectives to consider in evaluating the role of nutrition in the development of AD include food consumption, dietary intake, and dietary status. While it is well acknowledged that poor eating, malnutrition (low intake of energy and/or protein), and suboptimal biomarker levels of vitamins (e.g., B12, folate, vitamin D) are present in patients with AD, the direction of association between disease progression and nutritional changes is still unclear. Even more unclear in this relationship is the role of biological sex.

It is generally recognized that sex differences in dietary intake and dietary behavior exist, but the quality and quantity of these differences are not well characterized, particularly among older adults. On average, men have higher energy requirements at all ages because of higher energy expenditure, but this is mostly due to differences in body size and composition. Most general dietary guidelines recommend similar energy-adjusted dietary intake for men and women (e.g., macronutrients as percentage of energy, E%), but the absolute amount of some micronutrients (vitamins and minerals) may differ.

Most dietary surveys report healthier dietary patterns (Imamura et al., 2015) or more favorable food intake (Vitale et al., 2016) among women than among men, especially regarding the intake of fruits and vegetables (Nicklett & Kadell, 2013), including among older adults (Baker & Wardle, 2003). However, despite their generally higher intake of micronutrients, women may consume more fat and sugar compared to men (Bennett, Peters, & Woodward, 2018). The magnitude of such differences is moderate but consistent across studies, although there exists less evidence from studies in older adults. The differences seem evident at least up to 80 years of age

(Bates, Prentice, & Finch, 1999). There are also methodological concerns to consider when evaluating dietary intake and cognition. Validation studies have indicated that food frequency questionnaires may elicit more inaccurate responses from women compared to men (Lee et al., 2016) and women tend to underreport their energy intake more often (Archer, Hand, & Blair, 2013).

The majority of studies investigating the role of diet in AD or cognitive decline have reported their findings for both sexes combined, adjusting for sex. Two meta-analyses have assessed the sexes separately, concluding that for both the Mediterranean diet (Wu & Sun, 2017) and fruit and vegetable intake (Jiang et al., 2017), a protective association against developing cognitive disorders was only evident when the sexes were combined, without significant associations among men and women separately. Very few sex-specific studies are available, and these include smaller samples. At least one study has reported that adherence to the Mediterranean diet and dietary approaches to stop hypertension (DASH) pattern was higher among women, but still the association with cognitive decline was similar for both sexes (Wengreen et al., 2013). Additionally, no interaction was found for dietary inflammatory index (Frith et al., 2018). One systematic review suggested that the protective effect of caffeine may be stronger in women (Panza et al., 2015).

From a theoretical perspective, there are several mechanisms that could contribute to differential associations between diet and cognition. For example, microbiome profiles are suggested to differ between the sexes (Razavi et al., 2019), and sex hormones affect the metabolism of many nutrients such as glucose, amino acid, and protein (Comitato et al., 2015). Furthermore, differences in skeletal muscle metabolism have also been proposed (Gheller et al., 2016). This might be related to muscle wasting, which is evident in AD and aging in general. Lifelong differences in dietary intake are likely to contribute to many diet- and AD-related risk factors, such as hypertension or obesity. Hypothetically, the risk of dementia could be even higher among women without these differences in dietary intake. More evidence is needed on these potential mechanisms.

In summary, women tend to have healthier food habits than men, especially in terms of diet quality. The effect of these behavioral differences is confounded by biological differences (e.g., hormones) in the development of AD. While diet modification by sex should be studied in more detail, the current evidence suggests that similar dietary advice is beneficial for both sexes.

Sleep disturbances

Sleep disturbances are common among older adults, 50% of whom report insomnia symptoms (Li, Vitiello, & Gooneratne, 2018; Stone & Xiao, 2018). Accumulating evidence suggests that sleep disturbances are an important dementia risk factor (Shi et al., 2018; Sindi et al., 2018), and are associated with higher Aβ burden and inflammation (Irwin & Vitiello, 2019). Numerous studies have reported that a larger proportion of women report sleep disturbances compared to men, and these differences are greatest among older women (Aurora et al., 2010; Zhang & Wing, 2006) (see also Chapter 8). With regards to specific sleep disorders, although few studies have investigated sex differences among older adults, the evidence to date shows that women have a higher prevalence of insomnia, parasomnia (abnormal movements, behaviors, emotions, perceptions, and dreams occurring between sleep stages and when waking up), and sleep-related movement disorders (e.g., restless leg syndrome). Men, on the other hand, have a higher prevalence of sleep-related breathing disorders (Jee et al., 2020). Evidence on the sex differences in central disorders of hypersomnolence, which is characterized by excessive daytime sleepiness, is rather mixed (Crowley, 2011; Jee et al., 2020). Studies have also shown sex differences in the circadian period and melatonin regulation, with women having earlier sleep timing, more slow-wave sleep, and longer sleep duration (Santhi et al., 2016).

Sleep disturbances may be associated with dementia risk, due to their cooccurrence with multimorbidity (i.e., the simultaneous presence of two or more chronic conditions), including various vascular and metabolic risk factors, as well as depression, all of which are associated with increased dementia risk (Stone & Xiao, 2018). Sex differences have been reported regarding the associations between sleep disturbances and multimorbidity. For example, whereas short sleep duration is associated with multimorbidity among older women, short or long sleep duration are not associated with multimorbidity among men (Helbig et al., 2017). The relationship between sleep disturbances and multimorbidity may also be bidirectional, although the majority of studies on these associations have been cross-sectional (Helbig et al., 2017; Koyanagi et al., 2014; Nicholson et al., 2020; Ruiz-Castell et al., 2019) which limits the understanding of their temporality. One recent longitudinal study showed that sleep disturbances are associated with the speed of multimorbidity development after 9 years among older adults (Sindi et al., 2020). Further evidence is needed on the interplay between sleep disturbances, multimorbidity, and sex differences in dementia risk.

The role of sex hormones has recently gained significant attention in the field of sleep disturbances (Mong & Cusmano, 2016). Menopause is typically characterized by insomnia and poor sleep quality, with their prevalence ranging from 11.8% to 56.6% (Attarian et al., 2015). This may be due to changes is sex hormone levels (e.g., estrogen and progesterone) (Ameratunga, Goldin, & Hickey, 2012), in addition to vasomotor symptoms (e.g., hot flashes, night sweats). If left untreated, sleep disturbances are associated with higher prevalence of depression and anxiety, reduced productivity, low ratings of health-related quality of life, and higher healthcare utilization (Attarian et al., 2015; Baker et al., 2018). This suggests that postmenopausal sleep disturbances can, in some cases, remain chronic and warrant clinical attention. While several clinical trials have demonstrated that hormone therapy may improve sleep disturbances, others have shown mixed or negative results (Attarian et al., 2015; Cintron et al., 2017). Such trials also need to consider the increased risk of breast cancer associated with long-term hormone therapy usage (Proserpio et al., 2020).

Pharmacological treatments for insomnia (i.e., hypnotics) may exert different therapeutic and side effects on men and women due to sex differences in pharmacokinetic parameters, and thus caution is needed when prescribing such treatments (Jee et al., 2020). Evidence suggests that long-term usage of benzodiazepine is associated with poor cognitive performance among women but not men (Boeuf-Cazou et al., 2011), and the use of sedative-hypnotics has been associated with dementia risk (Ettcheto et al., 2020; Lee et al., 2018). Such treatments, therefore, need to be prescribed with caution, and further research is needed on whether sex differences exist in these associations. The American Academy of Sleep Medicine clinical guidelines recommend cognitive behavioral therapy for insomnia (CBTi) as the first-line treatment of chronic insomnia (Morgenthaler et al., 2006), as it has no adverse effects (Buysse et al., 2011). However, more trials targeting older adults are needed to identify those who may benefit from such accessible interventions. In conclusion, as highlighted by the recent Lancet Commission on dementia prevention, intervention, and care (2020), sleep disturbances are increasingly recognized as an important dementia risk factor, although further evidence is needed on their role (Livingston et al., 2020) and the mechanisms underlying their sex differences. Addressing sleep disturbances in multidomain dementia risk reduction initiatives may therefore further enhance their benefits.

Neural reserve and resilience

Of immense interest within different fields of medical research are the factors which render some individuals, and not others, resilient to the effects of disease and pathology. For instance, not all individuals who present with underlying pathology and/or multiple risk factors will go on to develop disease. Within the context of cognitive aging, reserve is a construct that explains the differences in clinical status and/or functional trajectories for individuals with comparable disease risk (Stern et al., 2018). Factors linked to reserve and resilience, such as premorbid etiological factors, may act to modify pathology and/or confer protection against the impact of underlying pathology, leading to preservation, or even improvement, of function, both cognitive and behavioral (Stern et al., 2018).

Sex and gender dichotomies in cognitive aging research

Cognitive capacity is represented by functional connectivity and synaptic plasticity, as well as structural attributes in the brain (Bastianello, Pezzella, & D'Angelo, 2008). There exist sex differences in brain anatomy and function with respect to age-related cognitive diseases (see also Chapter 6). At birth and in early life, girls are reported to have a larger head circumference than boys (Broere-Brown et al., 2016), though this trend reverses by age 4 (Jensen & Johnson, 1994). Larger head size alludes to greater structural capacity, evidenced by increased total cerebral volume and intracranial volumes (Tramo et al., 1998), thus suggestive of higher brain reserve. Indeed, postmortem studies have revealed that even with equivalent neurodegenerative pathology, women have a higher likelihood of attaining a more severe clinical state compared to men (Barnes et al., 2005). Further evidence supporting the higher capacity for pathology in men's brains and resultant impact on reserve was provided by Perneczky et al. in 2007 (Perneczky et al., 2007a, 2007b). Irrespective of dementia subtype, specific assessment of cerebral metabolism via FDG-PET in older men and women with clinical diagnosis revealed reduced cerebral blood flow in men (Perneczky et al., 2007a, 2007b). Thus, equivalent clinical states were evident despite greater levels of pathology in men, suggesting greater resilience to the consequences of more severe pathology. It is possible that gonadal factors are involved in conferring protection; however, conflicting evidence for the neuroprotective effects of HRT (Beauchet, 2006; Hogervorst et al., 2000; Shumaker et al., 2003; Siddiqui et al., 2016) shows the need for more research in this area. Furthermore, men have historically attained higher educational levels and engaged in more complex occupations (Russ et al., 2013), two factors linked to high cognitive reserve (Stern, 2012). Taken together, these findings may explain the sex differences with respect to resilience to pathologies and symptoms of age-related neurological diseases.

Although this area of scientific research is still largely unexplored, data from existing research imply that sex and gender differences in reserve and resilience mechanisms may be due to biochemical properties, as well as environmental exposures during development and across the life span. Research into the underlying mechanisms by which sex/gender attributes confer differences in preservation and maintenance of cognitive function is required, particularly to inform individualized strategies towards increasing resilience and delaying transitions to more severe clinical states.

The stress axes

The effects of stress on the body's physiological responses are primarily mediated through two known pathways: the hypothalamic–pituitary–adrenal (HPA) axis and the sympatho-adreno-medullary (SAM) axis) (Tsigos & Chrousos, 2002). The HPA axis, dually regulated by stress and circadian cues, plays a key role in modulation of the stress response (de Kloet, Joels, & Holsboer, 2005; Tsigos & Chrousos, 1994) via feedback and feed-forward processes across the brain and periphery. Such feedback loops are mediated by their effector hormones, which include corticotropin-releasing factor (CRF), adrenocorticotropic hormone (ACTH), and adrenal glucocorticoid (GC) hormones (see (Lightman et al., 2002; Young, Abelson, & Lightman, 2004) for review), released in the form of cortisol in humans and corticosterone in rodents (Kalafatakis et al., 2018; Spiga et al., 2011; Windle et al., 1998). The SAM axis is a rapid response pathway that mediates the immediacy of neuronal regulation during stress exposure and is an important regulator of the "fight or flight" response (reviewed in (Tsigos & Chrousos, 1994; Tsigos & Chrousos, 2002)).

Although both axes are activated by stress for both men and women, the sex-dimorphic nature of intrinsic biological processes in the body's response to stress is evident and may contribute to biases in sex-dependent manifestation of stress-related disorders. Such biological characteristics transcend cultural and societal influences on expression of the stress response, alluding to a higher impact of chromosomal/gonadal (sex) characteristics, in comparison to gender.

Implications of sex and gender differences in relation to stress

Aberrant stress response is implicated in the etiology and pathophysiology of various neuropsychiatric conditions, including major depressive disorder, post-traumatic stress disorder, and cognitive disorders such as AD. Interestingly, increased prevalence for these stress-related conditions have been reported in women (Verma, Balhara, & Gupta, 2011). Sex differences in the divergence in stress-response regulation and associated biological factors have also been reported, and are expected given the interplay between the stress and sex hormonal axes (Toufexis et al., 2014). Although the majority of stress-related studies have been done in animal models—with females noted to have higher circulatory stress hormone levels both at baseline (Bangasser & Wicks, 2017; Kitay, 1961) and in response to stress (Bangasser & Valentino, 2014; Weinstock et al., 1998)—clinical data are also available on biochemical properties of the sex dichotomy. These include differential HPA axis- and SAM axis-related responses, and function of the stress neuropeptide, corticotrophic-releasing factor (CRF) (HPA: Bangasser & Wiersielis, 2018; Yan et al., 2018; SAM: Bangasser, Wiersielis, & Khantsis, 2016; Curtis, Bethea, & Valentino, 2006), in relation to expression dynamics and downstream signaling actions, with women observed to be highly sensitive to increased CRF exposure, evident during stressful episodes (Heuser et al., 1994; Kunugi et al., 2006).

Sex-dependent differences in the modulation of the stress response by the stress hormone glucocorticoid are also evident. Although the response to acute stress is more robust in men, as evidenced by increased hormone levels (Kirschbaum et al., 1995a, 1995b; Reschke-Hernandez et al., 2017), the more detrimental chronic stress exposure has shown a more pronounced effect in women (Yan et al., 2018). In fact, a large-scale epidemiological study including 1671 Swedish mid-older adults has demonstrated higher cortisol levels in women compared to men, independent of age (Larsson et al., 2009). Indeed, imaging studies have revealed differences in neuroanatomy as well as brain circuitry that may impact the sex/gender-dependent stress response. For instance, a pioneering study on the neural correlates of stress-induced anxiety revealed hyperactivity in areas linked to cognitive awareness of emotive stimuli in women (Seo et al., 2017). Furthermore, parts of the limbic and frontal cortices sensitive to stressful stimuli have been reported to be larger in women compared to men (Ritchie et al., 2018). These reports suggest a greater propensity for women to over-utilize and engage cognitive processing brain centers during stressful events, potentially resulting in higher levels of anxiety. Nonetheless, scant information is available on sex dimorphisms in the contribution of stress-related mechanisms on etiopathogenesis of neurocognitive disorders such as AD and dementia. This is partly mediated by inconsistencies in reports on the dynamics of stress hormone intracellular signaling in human and animal research, as well as limited data on sex differences in basal levels of stress factors in AD patients versus controls (McEwen, Gray, & Nasca, 2015; Rasmuson, Nasman, & Olsson, 2011). Nevertheless, existing reports from both basic animal and human research on differential biological responses to stress for both sexes, alongside the notable interplay between the stress axes and molecular effectors of AD, with activation of amyloidogenic pathways found more prominently in females (Bangasser et al., 2017) allude to a higher propensity for increased AD risk in women compared to men, especially in view of their greater susceptibility to the effects of chronic stress, a major risk factor for dementia (reviewed extensively in (Yan et al., 2018)).

Observed differences may account for the reported susceptibility of women for stress-related neuro-psychiatric/psychosomatic conditions, although in-depth exploration into the biological processes that drive the noted sex differences is warranted (see also Chapter 7). Previous—and indeed current—research is limited by the paucity of data on sex-dependent regulation of the molecular mechanisms involved in regulating various functions related to the stress response. This is linked to classical use of male animals in stress experiments, given the largely accepted inference that the estrous cycle in female animals may pose a limitation for assessing effects of stress on physiological responses in health and disease paradigms (see also Chapter 1). Further preclinical and clinical research incorporating both sexes will inform our understanding of the role of sex- and gender-dependent physical, environmental, and biological attributes for development of stress-related conditions, thereby supporting more appropriate individualized and targeted interventions.

Loneliness and social isolation

Living alone has become increasingly common during the last half century, in almost all countries in the world (Ortiz-Ospina, 2019; Snell, 2017). Perhaps surprisingly, the trend of increasing proportions of single-person households does not necessarily correspond to increased feelings of loneliness (Hawkley et al., 2019; Nyqvist et al., 2017). This may be understood by two distinct concepts. The first, *social isolation*, refers to being alone in an objective sense. The second, *loneliness*, refers to a *perceived* social isolation (Cacioppo, Hawkley, & Bernston, 2003), or a perceived lack of a close friend, which causes distressing feelings due to one's social needs not being met by the quantity or quality of social relationships (Hawkley & Cacioppo, 2010). This implies that the presence of others does not alleviate these feelings.

For natural reasons, the sex difference is negligible in younger age but then accelerates with increasing age, with a progressively larger proportion of women living alone. Women tend to report feelings of loneliness, independent of their social networks, to a greater extent than men do, and this sex difference is more pronounced in old age (see Chapter 12) (Lim, Eres, & Vasan, 2020). This is due to the sex difference in life expectancy and additionally, because women in many cultures tend to marry older men. For example, in a population sample in Finland (the CAIDE study), the proportion of older participants who were widows was 40% among women and only

7% among men (Hakansson et al., 2009). The U.S. Bureau of Census reported that among older adults, widowhood was around three times as common for women as for men (Bureau, 2007). The shorter life expectancy for men also means that it is more difficult for an older widow to find a new partner, even more so in countries where cultural norms discourage remarriage for widows.

Many studies have shown that both loneliness and social isolation have detrimental health consequences (Courtin & Knapp, 2017) and increase the risk of developing neurocognitive disorders (Kuiper et al., 2015; Lara et al., 2019). Several studies have also indicated that being widowed may be especially detrimental to cognitive health (Gerritsen et al., 2017; Hakansson et al., 2009). In contrast, close relations, cohabiting, marriage, and proximity to a family network are protective (Desai et al., 2020; Håkansson, 2016; Hakansson et al., 2009; Kiecolt-Glaser & Newton, 2001; Rafnsson et al., 2020; Robles & Kiecolt-Glaser, 2003; van Gelder et al., 2006), and interactions, even if only with a few persons, are more important than the size of the social network (Pinquart & Sorensen, 2001). The evidence concerning the relative contribution of loneliness versus social isolation for the development of neurocognitive disorders is still inconclusive (Holwerda et al., 2014; Penninkilampi et al., 2018; Steptoe et al., 2013), and those exposed to both may have the highest risk (Håkansson, 2016; Shankar et al., 2013). It has been suggested that the objective condition of living alone and subjective feelings of loneliness impact health in their own independent ways through different biological mechanisms (Holwerda et al., 2012; Shankar et al., 2011).

While women more often report feelings of loneliness and live alone to a greater extent than men, there is no firm evidence that exposure of loneliness infers a higher dementia risk for women than for men (Holwerda et al., 2014; Luchetti et al., 2020; Sutin et al., 2020). In a Chinese population, men who reported loneliness were at higher risk for developing dementia than women who reported loneliness (Zhou, Wang, & Fang, 2018). To the best of our knowledge, no studies have reported sex differences in the associations between social isolation and dementia risk.

Some studies have indicated that cultural and socioeconomic conditions may affect sex differences in social networks and feelings of loneliness, including cultural differences in gender roles, norms against divorce or remarriage, acceptance of single life, access to material resources, and economic welfare. It will be important for future studies to further examine how such factors may modify the sex-specific associations with loneliness and social isolation. Feelings of loneliness may be regarded as an emotional dimension under the more general umbrella of depressive feelings, and also as a predictor of clinical depression (de la Torre-Luque et al., 2019; de la Torre-Luque & Ayuso-Mateos, 2020), which is a topic discussed in the next section.

Depression

Depression is defined as a syndrome characterized by sadness, loss of pleasure/interest, in addition to behavioral manifestations such as sleep disturbances, change in appetite, and psychomotor retardation or agitation, among other symptoms (American Psychiatric Association, 2013). Depressive disorders are classified into subtypes and degree of severity, as described in diagnostic guidelines (Vahia, 2013). Among 354 diseases, depression is one of the top three nonfatal diseases which globally contribute the most to years lost due to disability, and is surpassed only by lower back pain and headache disorders (GBD 2017 Disease and Injury Incidence and Prevalence Collaborators, 2018). The global prevalence of depression increased by 31.6% from 1990 to 2007, and by another 13.5% from 2007 to 2017, largely due to a combination of increasing global life expectancies in most parts of the world and given that the higher prevalence is elevated in old age. The increase in prevalence over the last 20 years is very similar in men and women. Today, around 250 million persons in the world have a diagnosis of major depression (GBD 2017 Disease and Injury Incidence and Prevalence Collaborators, 2018).

Depression is around twice as common among women compared to men, and this sex difference exists starting from the age of 12, widens during adolescence, and is then reduced in old age (see Chapter 7) (Salk, Hyde, & Abramson, 2017). Several explanations have been proposed, including a bias in reporting, as well as differences in the number of adverse life events over the life course, social support, and in genetics. However, none of these have received convincing empirical support (Piccinelli & Wilkinson, 2000). Other theories have highlighted the role of hormones and especially the changes during important transitions in the female reproductive lifecycle such as puberty, the postpartum period, and menopause (Eid, Gobinath, & Galea, 2019; Labaka et al., 2018). Building on the fact that the sex difference develops so early in life, recent models highlight the role of early adversity and stressors, which may be more commonly experienced by young girls (Hyde & Mezulis, 2020). One example is the "ABC" model put forth by Hyde et al. (Piccinelli & Wilkinson, 2000), which integrates the impact of childhood stressors with proposed sex differences in biological, affective, and cognitive vulnerabilities to account for the sex differences in depression (Piccinelli & Wilkinson, 2000).

The reported sex differences in depression suggest that women are not only more vulnerable to developing a depressive disorder, but also tend to develop other negative health consequences that could follow from depression (Brandao et al., 2019; Gan et al., 2014; Wang et al., 2020). There is substantial evidence for an association between depression and dementia (Chan et al., 2019), and the two conditions may also result in similar symptoms; the notion of *pseudodementia* has been used to describe cognitive deficits that resemble dementia among older adults with depression (Brodaty & Connors, 2020). The main controversy in the field concerns the type of relationship; that is, whether it is causal, prodromal, or even bidirectional (Byers & Yaffe, 2011). While some studies suggest that depression develops as a consequence of an underlying cognitive disorder (i.e., a prodromal relationship), the evidence today points toward depression does indeed contributing to an increased risk of dementia (Livingston et al., 2020). A few studies have followed trajectories of depressive feelings during the prodromal phase and, interestingly, they did not observe any noticeable changes in symptoms (Wilson et al., 2008, 2010). One study on hopelessness—known to be both a predictor of depression (Abramson, Metalsky, & Alloy, 1989) and a central dimension in depression (American Psychiatric Association, 2013; Hamilton, 1960; Steer et al., 1999; World Health Organization, 2004b; Yesavage et al., 1982)—has found that, at the time of dementia diagnosis, participants had significantly higher levels of hopelessness compared to participants who were still cognitively healthy at follow-up, but that these differences already existed two decades prior to diagnosis at baseline, and without noticeable increases between the two time points (Hakansson et al., 2015a, 2015b). Collectively, such results form a strong argument against the depression-dementia association being mainly prodromal in nature.

As depression is a risk factor for dementia, and because women are more likely to develop a depressive disorder during their life course, it may seem likely that depression could be a more important risk factor for dementia in women than in men. This notion has been brought up by several studies (Kim et al., 2015b; Sachdev et al., 2012; Sundermann, Katz, & Lipton, 2017), which also indicated that the driving force behind the sex difference in neurocognitive disorders may not only be about numbers: depression might affect women differently than men, thereby magnifying the risk of developing dementia as a consequence of depression. If there does in fact exists such an exacerbated sex difference in the risk linked to depression—both in the prevalence of depression and in its impact on cognitive health—then the extent to which these factors, in combination, account for the sex difference in dementia remains to be determined.

Response and adherence to multidomain lifestyle interventions

Three large, long-term, multidomain lifestyle randomized controlled trials (RCTs) aiming at preventing cognitive decline among cognitively unimpaired older adults have been completed to date: the Finnish Geriatric Intervention Study to Prevent Cognitive Impairment and Disability (FINGER) (Ngandu et al., 2015), the French Multidomain Alzheimer Preventive Trial (MAPT) (Andrieu et al., 2017), and the Dutch Prevention of Dementia by Intensive Vascular Care (PreDIVA) (Moll van Charante et al., 2016). Prespecified subgroup analyses by sex were conducted in the FINGER and PreDIVA RCTs, by studying the interaction of sex with intervention effects (FINGER) or stratifying the results by sex (PreDIVA). In FINGER, the overall beneficial effects of the 2-year lifestyle intervention did not vary by sex: benefits on all cognitive outcomes (i.e., global cognition, executive functioning, memory, and processing speed) were evident among both men and women (Rosenberg et al., 2018). The 6-year PreDIVA intervention did not have an impact on dementia incidence (primary endpoint), and the effects were nonsignificant in both sexes (Moll van Charante et al., 2016). With respect to sex differences in other outcomes, a pooled post hoc analysis of the FINGER, PreDIVA, and MAPT RCTs showed that the multidomain lifestyle interventions had a more pronounced effect on the CAIDE dementia risk score among women, meaning that the risk reduction was greater in women than in men (Barbera et al., 2020).

Regarding the overall adherence to the multidomain lifestyle interventions, no sex differences were observed in any of the three abovementioned trials (Beishuizen et al., 2017; Coley et al., 2019). Women adhered better to the FINGER dietary intervention, but sex was not associated with participation in the other individual FINGER intervention components (cardiovascular consultations, physical activity, cognitive training) (Coley et al., 2019).

In addition to the FINGER and PreDIVA RCTs, subgroup analyses by sex were also reported in the recently completed, large, multinational, 18-month-long eHealth RCT Healthy Aging Through Internet Counseling in the Elderly (HATICE) study, which investigated the efficacy of an online-based multidomain lifestyle intervention in improving older adults' cardiovascular risk profile and preventing cognitive decline as a secondary outcome (Richard et al., 2019). Compared to the control group, the intervention group had a modest but significant improvement in the cardiovascular risk profile, but there was no sex-related heterogeneity in the response to the intervention (Richard et al., 2019). Some other large lifestyle trials, such as Look AHEAD (Action for Health in Diabetes) (Espeland et al., 2017; Hayden et al., 2018) and the Diabetes Prevention Program Outcomes Study (Luchsinger et al., 2017), also reported largely similar intervention effects on cognitive outcomes among men and women.

In many small and/or short-term multidomain prevention trials, as well as in large single-domain prevention trials, either the effect modification by sex has not been examined (Bae et al., 2019; Barnes et al., 2013; Blumenthal et al., 2019; Diamond et al., 2015; Ihle-Hansen et al., 2014; Lam et al., 2015; Matz et al., 2015; Smith et al., 2010), or the main analyses have been adjusted for sex (Ball et al., 2002; Dangour et al., 2010; Martinez-Lapiscina et al., 2013; McEwen et al., 2018; Rebok et al., 2014; Romera-Liebana et al., 2018). Pooled analyses of two lifestyle interventions to prevent cognitive decline after stroke showed that sex was not associated with intervention effects (Teuschl et al., 2018). Similarly, sex did not modify the response to intervention in the large Lifestyle Interventions and Independence for Elders (LIFE) physical activity trial (Sink et al., 2015), nor in the Systolic Blood Pressure Intervention Trial—Memory and Cognition in Decreased Hypertension (SPRINT-MIND), which investigated the efficacy of intensive blood pressure control in reducing the risk of mild cognitive impairment and dementia (Williamson et al., 2019).

Taken together, there is little evidence for sex differences in the response and adherence to multidomain preventive interventions. Nevertheless, given that RCTs are rarely powered to detect subgroup differences and only a few large long-term dementia prevention RCTs have been completed so far, it remains relevant for future RCTs to investigate potential sex differences. Trials are currently planned or ongoing worldwide, for example within the World-Wide (WW) FINGERS global network, which now includes 30+ countries on all continents (Kivipelto et al., 2020). Harmonizing the methodology and outcomes of new RCTs, as done in the WW-FINGERS project, provides a unique opportunity to study sex differences in diverse populations and settings and to investigate which subgroups might benefit more from the interventions, as it allows data pooling and analyses of much larger samples. This increases the likelihood of detecting sex-specific differences and identifying the factors underlying such differences.

Discussion

In summary, during recent decades, several studies have reported sex differences in lifestyle risk factors that are associated with an increased risk for dementia and AD. In midlife, cardiovascular risk factors are more prevalent in men but have more detrimental AD-related effects in women. Hypertension is prevalent in both men and women, and although its management is worse among men, it has more harmful effects on cognition and neurodegeneration in women. Similarly, among older adults with diabetes, women generally tend to be frailer and have poorer health status. Smoking is more prevalent among men, and although this gap has been reduced over the years, sex differences still remain. Long-term consumption of excessive quantities of alcohol has been reported to have more negative effects on women's health, but it is unclear if this evidence extends to dementia risk. In late-life, higher body mass index may be more protective among older men, although being overweight in midlife has negative effects for both sexes. Physical exercise may also have more beneficial effects among women, however, physical inactivity is an important risk factor in both sexes. Despite lifelong differences in dietary intake, only minor sex differences have been reported regarding the associations between diet and development of AD. With regards to stress, while the response to acute stress is higher among men, exposure to chronic stress has more deleterious effects in women. Although the overall prevalence of sleep disturbances may be higher among women, men and women tend to suffer from different types of sleep disturbances and may respond differently to pharmacological treatments. Women are also more likely than men to live alone, suffer from depression, and experience social isolation. There are also differences in the influence of the APOE-4 allele between the sexes. Further research is needed on how these different factors interact and differentially impact the risk for dementia and AD in men and women.

The recent Lancet Commission on Dementia Prevention, Intervention, and Care (2020) outlines a range of modifiable risk factors which collectively account for 40% of the overall dementia risk (Livingston et al., 2020). The authors have also highlighted that our current knowledge does not allow for an in-depth understanding of the sex differences in these risk factors, nor their geographical influences. With no disease-modifying drugs for AD, great emphasis has been placed on primary and secondary prevention. The development of "personalized" interventions to prevent or postpone disease onset is crucial, considering that AD and dementia are multifactorial conditions consisting of numerous risk and protective factors. Although it is promising that several lifestyle intervention trials to date have not found modification effects by sex, it is important that future trials be sufficiently powered to assess these effects. It will also be important for future trials to collect detailed information allowing for the characterization of hormonal status, hormone replacement therapy use, and reproductive history. Such information may inform investigators on the influence of such factors on adherence and response to interventions.

While the current evidence has focused on biological sex differences in the risk factors for dementia and AD, further insight into the contribution of gender aspects, including gender roles and psychosocial factors, may inform us on how these factors influence older adults' engagement in healthy lifestyle behaviors, as well as their social resources and networks. This may also impact their health-seeking behaviors and healthcare utilization (Mauvais-Jarvis et al., 2020). In addition to the aforementioned risk factors, women often take on the role of caregivers, which is associated with various health, psychiatric, psychosocial, and economic burdens. Importantly, caregiving is also associated with an increased risk for dementia (Norton et al., 2010) (see also Chapter 14). Moreover, it has been shown that caregiver burden is higher among women, who may have to reduce or discontinue their employment and often suffer from various physical and mental health consequences including physical comorbidities, depression, and sleep disturbances (Xiong et al., 2020). Collectively, this evidence suggests that a better understanding of risk factors which exacerbate caregiver burden can better inform the provision of resources and policies, in order to reduce dementia incidence among caregivers.

In conclusion, although the evidence to date suggests that there are sex differences in several dementia risk factors, further knowledge is needed on how these factors interact and influence dementia risk. Knowledge about sex differences in these risk factors can contribute positively to individually-tailored interventions and risk reduction guidelines, as well as enhance the motivation to participate in, and increase the adherence and response to, novel interventions.

Chapter highlights

- While the evidence is strong for sex differences in certain dementia risk factors (e.g., depression), it also is the case that, for others, there are either no sex differences or more evidence is needed to inform potential differences (e.g., diet).
- Lifestyle factors may have different roles if present in early-, mid-, or late-life depending on their chronicity, which emphasizes the importance of a life course approach.
- Sex differences may be influenced by the use of hormones at different life stages, timing of menopause, and history of pregnancy and miscarriage, and the collection of such data in future studies will aid in understanding these mechanisms.
- Sufficiently powered studies will allow for the investigation of sex differences and interactions with various lifestyle factors and how they may influence the response to pharmacological/lifestyle interventions.
- Further evidence is needed on the role of gender and other psychosocial factors which may modify the observed sex differences in lifestyle factors and their association with dementia risk.

Funding

Shireen Sindi receives support from the Swedish Research Council, Alzheimerfonden, Demensförbundet, Karolinska Institute Foundation and Funds (KI Stiftelser och Fonder) and Loo and Hans Osterman Foundation for Medical Research. Miia Kivipelto receives research support from the Alzheimer's Research and Prevention Foundation, Academy of Finland (SALVE and 278457, 305810, 317465), Finnish Social Insurance Institution, Finnish Ministry of Education and Culture, Juho Vainio Foundation (Finland), Joint Programme—Neurodegenerative Disease Research (MIND-AD and EURO-FINGERS), Alzheimerfonden (Sweden), Swedish Research Council, Center for Innovative Medicine (CIMED) at Karolinska Institutet, Region Stockholm (ALF, NSV), AXA Research Fund, Knut and Alice Wallenberg Foundation (Sweden), Stiftelsen Stockholms sjukhem (Sweden), Konung Gustaf V:s och Drottning Victorias Frimurarstiftelse (Sweden), and Swedish Research Council for Health, Working Life, and Welfare (FORTE).

References

Abramson, L. Y., Metalsky, G. I., & Alloy, L. B. (1989). Hopelessness depression: A theory-based subtype of depression. *Psychological Review*, *96*(2), 358–372.

Agabio, R., et al. (2017). Sex differences in alcohol use disorder. *Current Medicinal Chemistry*, *24*(24), 2661–2670.

Allan, C. L., et al. (2015). Lifetime hypertension as a predictor of brain structure in older adults: Cohort study with a 28-year follow-up. *The British Journal of Psychiatry*, *206*(4), 308–315.

Altmann, A., et al. (2014). Sex modifies the APOE-related risk of developing Alzheimer disease. *Annals of Neurology*, *75*(4), 563–573.

Alzheimer's Association International Conference. (2018). *Pregnancy and reproductive history may impact dementia risk plus, the move to re-think the impact of hormone therapy on cognition.* AAIC.

Alzheimers Association Report. (2020). *2020 Alzheimer's disease facts and figures.* Alzheimers Dement.

Ameratunga, D., Goldin, J., & Hickey, M. (2012). Sleep disturbance in menopause. *Internal Medicine Journal*, *42*(7), 742–747.

American Psychiatric Association. (2013). *Diagnostic and statistical manual of mental disorders* (5th ed.). Washington, DC: American Psychiatric Publishing.

Ancelin, M. L., et al. (2013). Sex differences in the associations between lipid levels and incident dementia. *Journal of Alzheimer's Disease*, *34*(2), 519–528.

Ancelin, M. L., et al. (2014). Gender-specific associations between lipids and cognitive decline in the elderly. *European Neuropsychopharmacology*, *24*(7), 1056–1066.

Andersen, K., et al. (1999). Gender differences in the incidence of AD and vascular dementia: The EURODEM studies. EURODEM incidence research group. *Neurology*, *53*(9), 1992–1997.

Andrieu, S., et al. (2017). Effect of long-term omega 3 polyunsaturated fatty acid supplementation with or without multidomain intervention on cognitive function in elderly adults with memory complaints (MAPT): A randomised, placebo-controlled trial. *Lancet Neurology*, *16*(5), 377–389.

Archer, E., Hand, G. A., & Blair, S. N. (2013). Validity of U.S. nutritional surveillance: National Health and Nutrition Examination Survey caloric energy intake data, 1971-2010. *PLoS One*, *8*(10), e76632.

Attarian, H., et al. (2015). Treatment of chronic insomnia disorder in menopause: Evaluation of literature. *Menopause*, *22*(6), 674–684.

Aurora, R. N., et al. (2010). Best practice guide for the treatment of REM sleep behavior disorder (RBD). *Journal of Clinical Sleep Medicine*, *6*(1), 85–95.

Azad, N. A., Al Bugami, M., & Loy-English, I. (2007). Gender differences in dementia risk factors. *Gender Medicine*, *4*(2), 120–129.

Bae, S., et al. (2019). The effect of a multicomponent intervention to promote community activity on cognitive function in older adults with mild cognitive impairment: A randomized controlled trial. *Complementary Therapies in Medicine*, *42*, 164–169.

Baker, A. H., & Wardle, J. (2003). Sex differences in fruit and vegetable intake in older adults. *Appetite*, *40*(3), 269–275.

Baker, L. D., et al. (2010). Effects of aerobic exercise on mild cognitive impairment: A controlled trial. *Archives of Neurology*, *67*(1), 71–79.

Baker, F. C., et al. (2018). Sleep problems during the menopausal transition: Prevalence, impact, and management challenges. *Nature and Science of Sleep*, *10*, 73–95.

Baker, F. C., et al. (2019). Impact of sex steroids and reproductive stage on sleep-dependent memory consolidation in women. *Neurobiology of Learning and Memory*, *160*, 118–131.

Ball, K., et al. (2002). Effects of cognitive training interventions with older adults: A randomized controlled trial. *JAMA*, *288*(18), 2271–2281.

Bangasser, D. A., & Valentino, R. J. (2014). Sex differences in stress-related psychiatric disorders: Neurobiological perspectives. *Frontiers in Neuroendocrinology*, *35*(3), 303–319.

Bangasser, D. A., & Wicks, B. (2017). Sex-specific mechanisms for responding to stress. *Journal of Neuroscience Research*, *95*(1–2), 75–82.

Bangasser, D. A., & Wiersielis, K. R. (2018). Sex differences in stress responses: A critical role for corticotropin-releasing factor. *Hormones (Athens, Greece)*, *17*(1), 5–13.

Bangasser, D. A., Wiersielis, K. R., & Khantsis, S. (2016). Sex differences in the locus coeruleus-norepinephrine system and its regulation by stress. *Brain Research*, ***1641***(Pt. B), 177–188.

Bangasser, D. A., et al. (2017). Corticotropin-releasing factor overexpression gives rise to sex differences in Alzheimer's disease-related signaling. *Molecular Psychiatry*, *22*(8), 1126–1133.

Barbera, M., Ngandu, T., Levälahti, E., Coley, N., Mangialasche, F., Hoevenaar-Blom, M., et al. (2020). Effect of multidomain interventions on estimated dementia and cardiovascular risk reduction: An individual-participant data meta-analysis from FINGER, MAPT, and Pre-DIVA. *Alzheimer's & Dementia: The Journal of the Alzheimer's Association*.

Barha, C. K., & Liu-Ambrose, T. (2018). Exercise and the aging brain: Considerations for sex differences. *Brain Plast*, *4*(1), 53–63.

Barha, C. K., et al. (2017). Sex differences in exercise efficacy to improve cognition: A systematic review and meta-analysis of randomized controlled trials in older humans. *Frontiers in Neuroendocrinology*, *46*, 71–85.

Barnes, L. L., et al. (2005). Sex differences in the clinical manifestations of Alzheimer disease pathology. *Archives of General Psychiatry*, *62*(6), 685–691.

Barnes, D. E., et al. (2013). The mental activity and exercise (max) trial: A randomized controlled trial to enhance cognitive function in older adults. *JAMA Internal Medicine, 173*(9), 797–804.

Bastianello, S., Pezzella, F. R., & D'Angelo, E. (2008). Non-invasive imaging of brain structure and function in neural connectivity analysis. *Functional Neurology, 23*(4), 169–170.

Bates, C. J., Prentice, A., & Finch, S. (1999). Gender differences in food and nutrient intakes and status indices from the National Diet and Nutrition Survey of people aged 65 years and over. *European Journal of Clinical Nutrition, 53*(9), 694–699.

Beauchet, O. (2006). Testosterone and cognitive function: Current clinical evidence of a relationship. *European Journal of Endocrinology, 155*(6), 773–781.

Beishuizen, C. R. L., et al. (2017). Determinants of dropout and nonadherence in a dementia prevention randomized controlled trial: The prevention of dementia by intensive vascular care trial. *Journal of the American Geriatrics Society, 65*(7), 1505–1513.

Bennett, E., Peters, S. A. E., & Woodward, M. (2018). Sex differences in macronutrient intake and adherence to dietary recommendations: Findings from the UK Biobank. *BMJ Open, 8*(4), e020017.

Bialek, M., et al. (2004). Neuroprotective role of testosterone in the nervous system. *Polish Journal of Pharmacology, 56*(5), 509–518.

Blumenthal, J. A., et al. (2019). Lifestyle and neurocognition in older adults with cognitive impairments: A randomized trial. *Neurology, 92*(3), e212–e223.

Boeuf-Cazou, O., et al. (2011). Impact of long-term benzodiazepine use on cognitive functioning in young adults: The VISAT cohort. *European Journal of Clinical Pharmacology, 67*(10), 1045–1052.

Brandao, D. J., et al. (2019). Depression and excess mortality in the elderly living in low- and middle-income countries: Systematic review and meta-analysis. *International Journal of Geriatric Psychiatry, 34*(1), 22–30.

Brodaty, H., & Connors, M. H. (2020). Pseudodementia, pseudo-pseudodementia, and pseudodepression. *Alzheimers Dement, 12*(1), e12027.

Broere-Brown, Z. A., et al. (2016). Sex-specific differences in fetal and infant growth patterns: A prospective population-based cohort study. *Biology of Sex Differences, 7*, 65.

Bureau, U. S. C. (2007). *Older Americans month celebrated in May*. Washington, D.C: U.S. Census Bureau.

Buysse, D. J., et al. (2011). Efficacy of brief behavioral treatment for chronic insomnia in older adults. *Archives of Internal Medicine, 171*(10), 887–895.

Byers, A. L., & Yaffe, K. (2011). Depression and risk of developing dementia. *Nature Reviews. Neurology, 7*(6), 323–331.

Cacioppo, J., Hawkley, L. C., & Bernston, G. (2003). The anatomy of loneliness. *Current Directions in Psychological Science, 12*, 71–74.

Carlson, M. C., et al. (2015). Impact of the Baltimore Experience Corps Trial on cortical and hippocampal volumes. *Alzheimers Dement, 11*(11), 1340–1348.

Carnethon, M. R. (2009). Physical activity and cardiovascular disease: How much is enough? *American Journal of Lifestyle Medicine, 3*(1 Suppl), 44S–49S.

Cassilhas, R. C., et al. (2012). Spatial memory is improved by aerobic and resistance exercise through divergent molecular mechanisms. *Neuroscience, 202*, 309–317.

Chan, J. Y. C., et al. (2019). Depression and antidepressants as potential risk factors in dementia: A systematic review and meta-analysis of 18 longitudinal studies. *Journal of the American Medical Directors Association, 20*(3), 279–286 e1.

Chene, G., et al. (2015). Gender and incidence of dementia in the Framingham Heart Study from mid-adult life. *Alzheimers Dement, 11*(3), 310–320.

Cherbuin, N., et al. (2015). Blood pressure, brain structure, and cognition: Opposite associations in men and women. *American Journal of Hypertension, 28*(2), 225–231.

Chudiak, A., Uchmanowicz, I., & Mazur, G. (2018). Relation between cognitive impairment and treatment adherence in elderly hypertensive patients. *Clinical Interventions in Aging, 13*, 1409–1418.

Cintron, D., et al. (2017). Efficacy of menopausal hormone therapy on sleep quality: Systematic review and meta-analysis. *Endocrine, 55*(3), 702–711.

Clark, A. F., et al. (1975). Plasma testosterone free index: A better indicator of plasma androgen activity? *Fertility and Sterility, 26*(10), 1001–1005.

Colberg, S. R., et al. (2010). Exercise and type 2 diabetes: The american college of sports medicine and the American Diabetes Association: Joint position statement. *Diabetes Care, 33*(12), e147–e167.

Coley, N., et al. (2019). Adherence to multidomain interventions for dementia prevention: Data from the FINGER and MAPT trials. *Alzheimers Dement, 15*(6), 729–741.

Comitato, R., et al. (2015). Sex hormones and macronutrient metabolism. *Critical Reviews in Food Science and Nutrition, 55*(2), 227–241.

Courtin, E., & Knapp, M. (2017). Social isolation, loneliness and health in old age: A scoping review. *Health & Social Care in the Community, 25*(3), 799–812.

Crane, P. K., et al. (2013). Glucose levels and risk of dementia. *The New England Journal of Medicine, 369*(6), 540–548.

Crowley, K. (2011). Sleep and sleep disorders in older adults. *Neuropsychology Review, 21*(1), 41–53.

Curtis, A. L., Bethea, T., & Valentino, R. J. (2006). Sexually dimorphic responses of the brain norepinephrine system to stress and corticotropin-releasing factor. *Neuropsychopharmacology, 31*(3), 544–554.

Dangour, A. D., et al. (2010). Effect of 2-y n-3 long-chain polyunsaturated fatty acid supplementation on cognitive function in older people: A randomized, double-blind, controlled trial. *The American Journal of Clinical Nutrition, 91*(6), 1725–1732.

de Frias, C. M., Nilsson, L. G., & Herlitz, A. (2006). Sex differences in cognition are stable over a 10-year period in adulthood and old age. *Neuropsychology, Development, and Cognition. Section B, Aging, Neuropsychology and Cognition, 13*(3–4), 574–587.

de Kloet, E. R., Joels, M., & Holsboer, F. (2005). Stress and the brain: From adaptation to disease. *Nature Reviews. Neuroscience, 6*(6), 463–475.

de la Torre-Luque, A., & Ayuso-Mateos, J. L. (2020). The course of depression in late life: A longitudinal perspective. *Epidemiology and Psychiatric Sciences, 29*, e147.

de la Torre-Luque, A., et al. (2019). Stability of clinically relevant depression symptoms in old-age across 11 cohorts: A multi-state study. *Acta Psychiatrica Scandinavica, 140*(6), 541–551.

Desai, R., et al. (2020). Living alone and risk of dementia: A systematic review and meta-analysis. *Ageing Research Reviews, 62*, 101122.

Diamond, K., et al. (2015). Randomized controlled trial of a healthy brain ageing cognitive training program: Effects on memory, mood, and sleep. *Journal of Alzheimer's Disease, 44*(4), 1181–1191.

Dufouil, C., Ducimetiere, P., & Alperovitch, A. (1997). Sex differences in the association between alcohol consumption and cognitive performance. EVA Study Group. Epidemiology of vascular aging. *American Journal of Epidemiology, 146*(5), 405–412.

Dufouil, C., Seshadri, S., & Chene, G. (2014). Cardiovascular risk profile in women and dementia. *Journal of Alzheimer's Disease, 42*(Suppl. 4), S353–S363.

Eid, R. S., Gobinath, A. R., & Galea, L. A. M. (2019). Sex differences in depression: Insights from clinical and preclinical studies. *Progress in Neurobiology*, *176*, 86–102.

Elias, M. F., et al. (2005). Obesity, diabetes and cognitive deficit: The Framingham Heart Study. *Neurobiology of Aging*, *26*(Suppl. 1), 11–16.

Erickson, K. I., et al. (2007). Interactive effects of fitness and hormone treatment on brain health in postmenopausal women. *Neurobiology of Aging*, *28*(2), 179–185.

Erol, A., & Karpyak, V. M. (2015). Sex and gender-related differences in alcohol use and its consequences: Contemporary knowledge and future research considerations. *Drug and Alcohol Dependence*, *156*, 1–13.

Espeland, M. A., et al. (2017). Effect of a long-term intensive lifestyle intervention on prevalence of cognitive impairment. *Neurology*, *88*(21), 2026–2035.

Espeland, M. A., et al. (2018). Sex-related differences in the prevalence of cognitive impairment among overweight and obese adults with type 2 diabetes. *Alzheimers Dement*, *14*(9), 1184–1192.

Ettcheto, M., Olloquequi, J., Sánchez-López, E., Busquets, O., Cano, A., Manzine, P. R., ... Camins, A. (2020). Benzodiazepines and related drugs as a risk factor in Alzheimer's disease dementia. *Frontiers in Aging Neuroscience*, *11*, 344.

Fallah, N., et al. (2009). Modeling the impact of sex on how exercise is associated with cognitive changes and death in older Canadians. *Neuroepidemiology*, *33*(1), 47–54.

Fan, Y. C., et al. (2017). Increased dementia risk predominantly in diabetes mellitus rather than in hypertension or hyperlipidemia: A population-based cohort study. *Alzheimer's Research & Therapy*, *9*(1), 7.

Farlow, M. R., et al. (1998). Treatment outcome of tacrine therapy depends on apolipoprotein genotype and gender of the subjects with Alzheimer's disease. *Neurology*, *50*(3), 669–677.

Feldman, H. A., et al. (2002). Age trends in the level of serum testosterone and other hormones in middle-aged men: Longitudinal results from the Massachusetts male aging study. *The Journal of Clinical Endocrinology and Metabolism*, *87*(2), 589–598.

Ferretti, M. T., et al. (2018). Sex differences in Alzheimer disease—The gateway to precision medicine. *Nature Reviews. Neurology*, *14*(8), 457–469.

Ferretti, M. T., et al. (2020). Sex and gender differences in Alzheimer's disease: Current challenges and implications for clinical practice: Position paper of the Dementia and Cognitive Disorders Panel of the European Academy of Neurology. *European Journal of Neurology*, *27*(6), 928–943.

Fox, M., et al. (2018). Women's pregnancy life history and alzheimer's risk: Can immunoregulation explain the link? *American Journal of Alzheimer's Disease and Other Dementias*, *33*(8), 516–526.

Fratiglioni, L., et al. (1997). Very old women at highest risk of dementia and Alzheimer's disease: Incidence data from the Kungsholmen Project, Stockholm. *Neurology*, *48*(1), 132–138.

Frith, E., et al. (2018). Dietary inflammatory index and memory function: Population-based national sample of elderly Americans. *The British Journal of Nutrition*, *119*(5), 552–558.

Gan, Y., et al. (2014). Depression and the risk of coronary heart disease: A meta-analysis of prospective cohort studies. *BMC Psychiatry*, *14*, 371.

Garcia-Ptacek, S., et al. (2014). Body-mass index and mortality in incident dementia: a cohort study on 11,398 patients from SveDem, the Swedish Dementia Registry. *Journal of the American Medical Directors Association*, *15*(6), 447.e1-7.

GBD 2017 Disease and Injury Incidence and Prevalence Collaborators. (2018). Global, regional, and national incidence, prevalence, and years lived with disability for 354 diseases and injuries for 195 countries and territories, 1990-2017: A systematic analysis for the Global Burden of Disease Study 2017. *Lancet, 392*(10159), 1789–1858.

Geifman, N., et al. (2017). Evidence for benefit of statins to modify cognitive decline and risk in Alzheimer's disease. *Alzheimer's Research & Therapy, 9*(1), 10.

Georges, J., Miller, O., & Bintener, C. (2020). *Estimating the prevalence of dementia in Europe*. Alzheimer Europe.

Gerritsen, L., et al. (2017). Influence of negative life events and widowhood on risk for dementia. *The American Journal of Geriatric Psychiatry, 25*(7), 766–778.

Gheller, B. J., et al. (2016). Understanding age-related changes in skeletal muscle metabolism: Differences between females and males. *Annual Review of Nutrition, 36*, 129–156.

Gilsanz, P., et al. (2017). Association between birth in a high stroke mortality state, race, and risk of dementia. *JAMA Neurology, 74*(9), 1056–1062.

Giovino, G. A., et al. (2012). Tobacco use in 3 billion individuals from 16 countries: An analysis of nationally representative cross-sectional household surveys. *Lancet, 380*(9842), 668–679.

Gouras, G. K., et al. (2000). Testosterone reduces neuronal secretion of Alzheimer's beta-amyloid peptides. *Proceedings of the National Academy of Sciences of the United States of America, 97*(3), 1202–1205.

Goveas, J. S., et al. (2011). Depressive symptoms and incidence of mild cognitive impairment and probable dementia in elderly women: The Women's Health Initiative Memory Study. *Journal of the American Geriatrics Society, 59*(1), 57–66.

Gray, A., et al. (1991). Age, disease, and changing sex hormone levels in middle-aged men: Results of the Massachusetts Male Aging Study. *The Journal of Clinical Endocrinology and Metabolism, 73*(5), 1016–1025.

Hahn, C., Pogun, S., & Gunturkun, O. (2010). Smoking modulates language lateralization in a sex-specific way. *Neuropsychologia, 48*(14), 3993–4002.

Håkansson, K. (2016). *The role of socio-emotional factors for cognitive health in later life (Thesis)*. Karolinska Institutet.

Hakansson, K., et al. (2009). Association between mid-life marital status and cognitive function in later life: Population based cohort study. *BMJ, 339*, b2462.

Hakansson, K., et al. (2015a). Feelings of hopelessness in midlife and cognitive health in later life: A prospective population-based cohort study. *PLoS One, 10*(10), e0140261.

Hakansson, K., et al. (2015b). Correction: Feelings of hopelessness in midlife and cognitive health in later life: A prospective population-based cohort study. *PLoS One, 10*(11), e0142465.

Hamilton, M. (1960). A rating scale for depression. *Journal of Neurology, Neurosurgery, and Psychiatry, 23*, 56–62.

Harold, D., et al. (2009). Genome-wide association study identifies variants at CLU and PICALM associated with Alzheimer's disease. *Nature Genetics, 41*(10), 1088–1093.

Hawkley, L. C., & Cacioppo, J. T. (2010). Loneliness matters: A theoretical and empirical review of consequences and mechanisms. *Annals of Behavioral Medicine, 40*(2), 218–227.

Hawkley, L. C., et al. (2019). Are U.S. older adults getting lonelier? Age, period, and cohort differences. *Psychology and Aging, 34*(8), 1144–1157.

Hayden, K.M., et al., LLong-term impact of intensive lifestyle intervention on cognitive function assessed with the National Institutes of Health Toolbox: The Look AHEAD study. Alzheimers Dement, 2018. 10: p. 41-48.

Helbig, A. K., et al. (2017). Relationship between sleep disturbances and multimorbidity among community-dwelling men and women aged 65-93 years: Results from the KORA Age Study. *Sleep Medicine, 33*, 151–159.

Hempel, R., Onopa, R., & Convit, A. (2012). Type 2 diabetes affects hippocampus volume differentially in men and women. *Diabetes/Metabolism Research and Reviews, 28*(1), 76–83.

Henderson, V. W., et al. (2000). Estrogen for Alzheimer's disease in women: Randomized, double-blind, placebo-controlled trial. *Neurology, 54*(2), 295–301.

Henderson, V. W., et al. (2005). Postmenopausal hormone therapy and Alzheimer's disease risk: Interaction with age. *Journal of Neurology, Neurosurgery, and Psychiatry, 76*(1), 103–105.

Henderson, V. W., et al. (2013). Cognition, mood, and physiological concentrations of sex hormones in the early and late postmenopause. *Proceedings of the National Academy of Sciences of the United States of America, 110*(50), 20290–20295.

Heuser, I. J., et al. (1994). Age-associated changes of pituitary-adrenocortical hormone regulation in humans: Importance of gender. *Neurobiology of Aging, 15*(2), 227–231.

Higgins, S. T., et al. (2015). A literature review on prevalence of gender differences and intersections with other vulnerabilities to tobacco use in the United States, 2004-2014. *Preventive Medicine, 80*, 89–100.

Hogervorst, E., et al. (2000). The nature of the effect of female gonadal hormone replacement therapy on cognitive function in post-menopausal women: A meta-analysis. *Neuroscience, 101*(3), 485–512.

Hogervorst, E., et al. (2004). Low free testosterone is an independent risk factor for Alzheimer's disease. *Experimental Gerontology, 39*(11–12), 1633–1639.

Holland, J., Bandelow, S., & Hogervorst, E. (2011). Testosterone levels and cognition in elderly men: A review. *Maturitas, 69*(4), 322–337.

Holland, D., et al. (2013). Higher rates of decline for women and apolipoprotein E epsilon4 carriers. *AJNR. American Journal of Neuroradiology, 34*(12), 2287–2293.

Holwerda, T. J., et al. (2012). Increased risk of mortality associated with social isolation in older men: only when feeling lonely? Results from the Amsterdam Study of the Elderly (AMSTEL). *Psychological Medicine, 42*(4), 843–853.

Holwerda, T. J., et al. (2014). Feelings of loneliness, but not social isolation, predict dementia onset: Results from the Amsterdam Study of the Elderly (AMSTEL). *Journal of Neurology, Neurosurgery, and Psychiatry, 85*(2), 135–142.

Hsu, M., et al. (2019). Sex differences in gene expression patterns associated with the APOE4 allele. *F1000Res, 8*, 387.

Hyde, J. S., & Mezulis, A. H. (2020). Gender differences in depression: Biological, affective, cognitive, and sociocultural factors. *Harvard Review of Psychiatry, 28*(1), 4–13.

Ihle-Hansen, H., et al. (2014). Multifactorial vascular risk factor intervention to prevent cognitive impairment after stroke and TIA: A 12-month randomized controlled trial. *International Journal of Stroke, 9*(7), 932–938.

Imamura, F., et al. (2015). Dietary quality among men and women in 187 countries in 1990 and 2010: A systematic assessment. *The Lancet Global Health, 3*(3), e132–e142.

Irwin, M. R., & Vitiello, M. V. (2019). Implications of sleep disturbance and inflammation for Alzheimer's disease dementia. *Lancet Neurology, 18*(3), 296–306.

Jack, C. R., Jr., et al. (2015). Different definitions of neurodegeneration produce similar amyloid/neurodegeneration biomarker group findings. *Brain, 138*(Pt. 12), 3747–3759.

Jee, H. J., et al. (2020). Impact of sleep disorder as a risk factor for dementia in men and women. *Biomolecules & Therapeutics, 28*(1), 58–73.

Jensen, A. R., & Johnson, F. W. (1994). Race and sex-differences in head size and Iq. *Intelligence, 18*(3), 309–333.

Jia, J. X., et al. (2016). Effects of testosterone on synaptic plasticity mediated by androgen receptors in male SAMP8 mice. *Journal of Toxicology and Environmental Health. Part A, 79*(19), 849–855.

Jiang, X., et al. (2017). Increased consumption of fruit and vegetables is related to a reduced risk of cognitive impairment and dementia: Meta-analysis. *Frontiers in Aging Neuroscience, 9*, 18.

Jian-xin, J., et al. (2015). Effects of testosterone treatment on synaptic plasticity and behavior in senescence accelerated mice. *Journal of Toxicology and Environmental Health. Part A, 78*(21–22), 1311–1320.

Joffe, H., et al. (2006). Estrogen therapy selectively enhances prefrontal cognitive processes: A randomized, double-blind, placebo-controlled study with functional magnetic resonance imaging in perimenopausal and recently postmenopausal women. *Menopause, 13*(3), 411–422.

Kalafatakis, K., et al. (2018). Ultradian rhythmicity of plasma cortisol is necessary for normal emotional and cognitive responses in man. *Proceedings of the National Academy of Sciences of the United States of America, 115*(17), E4091–E4100.

Kantarci, K., et al. (2016). Early postmenopausal transdermal 17beta-estradiol therapy and amyloid-beta deposition. *Journal of Alzheimer's Disease, 53*(2), 547–556.

Kiecolt-Glaser, J. K., & Newton, T. L. (2001). Marriage and health: His and hers. *Psychological Bulletin, 127*(4), 472–503.

Kim, H., et al. (2015a). Association between body mass index and cortical thickness: Among elderly cognitively normal men and women. *International Psychogeriatrics, 27*(1), 121–130.

Kim, S., et al. (2015b). Gender differences in risk factors for transition from mild cognitive impairment to Alzheimer's disease: A CREDOS study. *Comprehensive Psychiatry, 62*, 114–122.

Kim, Y. H., et al. (2017a). Sex differences in metabolic risk indicator of dementia in an elderly urban Korean population: A community-based cross-sectional study. *Geriatrics & Gerontology International, 17*(11), 2136–2142.

Kim, B. Y., et al. (2017b). Obesity and physical activity. *Journal of Obesity & Metabolic Syndrome, 26*(1), 15–22.

Kirschbaum, C., et al. (1995a). Sex-specific effects of social support on cortisol and subjective responses to acute psychological stress. *Psychosomatic Medicine, 57*(1), 23–31.

Kirschbaum, C., et al. (1995b). Persistent high cortisol responses to repeated psychological stress in a subpopulation of healthy men. *Psychosomatic Medicine, 57*(5), 468–474.

Kitay, J. I. (1961). Sex differences in adrenal cortical secretion in the rat. *Endocrinology, 68*, 818–824.

Kivimaki, M., et al. (2018). Body mass index and risk of dementia: Analysis of individual-level data from 1.3 million individuals. *Alzheimers Dement, 14*(5), 601–609.

Kivipelto, M., et al. (2020). World-Wide FINGERS Network: A global approach to risk reduction and prevention of dementia. *Alzheimers Dement, 16*(7), 1078–1094.

Knopman, D. S., et al. (2007). Incident dementia in women is preceded by weight loss by at least a decade. *Neurology, 69*(8), 739–746.

Koyanagi, A., et al. (2014). Chronic conditions and sleep problems among adults aged 50 years or over in nine countries: A multi-country study. *PLoS One, 9*(12), e114742.

Kramer, A. F., & Colcombe, S. (2018). Fitness effects on the cognitive function of older adults: A meta-analytic study-revisited. *Perspectives on Psychological Science, 13*(2), 213–217.

Kritz-Silverstein, D., et al. (2017). Sex and age differences in the association of blood pressure and hypertension with cognitive function in the elderly: The rancho bernardo study. *The Journal of Prevention of Alzheimer's Disease, 4*(3), 165–173.

Kuiper, J. S., et al. (2015). Social relationships and risk of dementia: A systematic review and meta-analysis of longitudinal cohort studies. *Ageing Research Reviews, 22*, 39–57.

Kunugi, H., et al. (2006). Assessment of the dexamethasone/CRH test as a state-dependent marker for hypothalamic-pituitary-adrenal (HPA) axis abnormalities in major depressive episode: A multicenter study. *Neuropsychopharmacology, 31*(1), 212–220.

Labaka, A., et al. (2018). Biological sex differences in depression: A systematic review. *Biological Research for Nursing, 20*(4), 383–392.

Lacruz, M. E., et al. (2016). Association of late-life changes in blood pressure and cognitive status. *Journal of Geriatric Cardiology, 13*(1), 37–43.

Lam, L. C., et al. (2015). Would older adults with mild cognitive impairment adhere to and benefit from a structured lifestyle activity intervention to enhance cognition?: A cluster randomized controlled trial. *PLoS One, 10*(3), e0118173.

Lamar, M., et al. (2019). Associations of lipid levels and cognition: Findings from the hispanic community health study/study of latinos. *Journal of the International Neuropsychological Society*, 1–12.

Landau, S. M., et al. (2011). Associations between cognitive, functional, and FDG-PET measures of decline in AD and MCI. *Neurobiology of Aging, 32*(7), 1207–1218.

Lara, E., et al. (2019). Does loneliness contribute to mild cognitive impairment and dementia? A systematic review and meta-analysis of longitudinal studies. *Ageing Research Reviews, 52*, 7–16.

Larsson, C. A., et al. (2009). Salivary cortisol differs with age and sex and shows inverse associations with WHR in Swedish women: A cross-sectional study. *BMC Endocrine Disorders, 9*, 16.

Lee, H., et al. (2016). Gender analysis in the development and validation of FFQ: A systematic review. *The British Journal of Nutrition, 115*(4), 666–671.

Lee, J., et al. (2018). Use of sedative-hypnotics and the risk of Alzheimer's dementia: A retrospective cohort study. *PLoS One, 13*(9), e0204413.

Leening, M. J., et al. (2014). Sex differences in lifetime risk and first manifestation of cardiovascular disease: Prospective population based cohort study. *BMJ, 349*, g5992.

Li, J., Vitiello, M. V., & Gooneratne, N. S. (2018). Sleep in normal aging. *Sleep Medicine Clinics, 13*(1), 1–11.

Lightman, S. L., et al. (2002). Hypothalamic-pituitary-adrenal function. *Archives of Physiology and Biochemistry, 110*(1-2), 90–93.

Lim, M. H., Eres, R., & Vasan, S. (2020). Understanding loneliness in the twenty-first century: An update on correlates, risk factors, and potential solutions. *Social Psychiatry and Psychiatric Epidemiology, 55*(7), 793–810.

Lim, Y. Y., et al. (2013). Abeta amyloid, cognition, and APOE genotype in healthy older adults. *Alzheimers Dement, 9*(5), 538–545.

Lindwall, M., Rennemark, M., & Berggren, T. (2008). Movement in mind: The relationship of exercise with cognitive status for older adults in the Swedish National Study on Aging and Care (SNAC). *Aging & Mental Health, 12*(2), 212–220.

Liu, W., et al. (2018). Sex differences in the prevalence of and risk factors for nonvascular cognitive function in rural, low-income elderly in Tianjin, China. *Neuroepidemiology, 51*(3–4), 138–148.

Livingston, G., et al. (2020). Dementia prevention, intervention, and care: 2020 report of the Lancet Commission. *Lancet, 396*(10248), 413–446.

Lu, Y., et al. (2017). Sex-specific nonlinear associations between serum lipids and different domains of cognitive function in middle to older age individuals. *Metabolic Brain Disease*, *32*(4), 1089–1097.

Luchetti, M., et al. (2020). Loneliness is associated with risk of cognitive impairment in the Survey of Health, Ageing and Retirement in Europe. *International Journal of Geriatric Psychiatry*, *35*(7), 794–801.

Luchsinger, J. A., et al. (2017). Metformin, lifestyle intervention, and cognition in the diabetes prevention program outcomes study. *Diabetes Care*, *40*(7), 958–965.

Lupton, M. K., et al. (2016). The effect of increased genetic risk for Alzheimer's disease on hippocampal and amygdala volume. *Neurobiology of Aging*, *40*, 68–77.

Lv, W., et al. (2016). Low testosterone level and risk of Alzheimer's disease in the elderly men: A systematic review and meta-analysis. *Molecular Neurobiology*, *53*(4), 2679–2684.

Maki, P. M. (2013). Critical window hypothesis of hormone therapy and cognition: A scientific update on clinical studies. *Menopause*, *20*(6), 695–709.

Manson, J. E., et al. (2017). Menopausal hormone therapy and long-term all-cause and cause-specific mortality: The women's health initiative randomized trials. *JAMA*, *318*(10), 927–938.

Martinez-Lapiscina, E. H., et al. (2013). Mediterranean diet improves cognition: The PREDIMED-NAVARRA randomised trial. *Journal of Neurology, Neurosurgery, and Psychiatry*, *84*(12), 1318–1325.

Mateos, J. T., Fernández-Sáez, J., Marcos-Marcos, J., Álvarez-Dardet, C., Bambra, C., Popay, J., … Baum, F. (2020). Gender equality and the global gender gap in life expectancy: an exploratory analysis of 152 countries. *International Journal of Health Policy and Management*. https://doi.org/10.34172/ijhpm.2020.192.

Matz, K., et al. (2015). Multidomain lifestyle interventions for the prevention of cognitive decline after ischemic stroke: Randomized trial. *Stroke*, *46*(10), 2874–2880.

Mauvais-Jarvis, F., et al. (2020). Sex and gender: Modifiers of health, disease, and medicine. *Lancet*, *396*(10250), 565–582.

McCarrey, A. C., et al. (2016). Sex differences in cognitive trajectories in clinically normal older adults. *Psychology and Aging*, *31*(2), 166–175.

McCollum, M., et al. (2005). Gender differences in diabetes mellitus and effects on self-care activity. *Gender Medicine*, *2*(4), 246–254.

McDermott, K. L., et al. (2017). Memory resilience to Alzheimer's genetic risk: Sex effects in predictor profiles. *The Journals of Gerontology. Series B, Psychological Sciences and Social Sciences*, *72*(6), 937–946.

McEwen, B. S., Gray, J. D., & Nasca, C. (2015). 60 YEARS OF NEUROENDOCRINOLOGY: Redefining neuroendocrinology: Stress, sex and cognitive and emotional regulation. *The Journal of Endocrinology*, *226*(2), T67–T83.

McEwen, S. C., et al. (2018). Simultaneous aerobic exercise and memory training program in older adults with subjective memory impairments. *Journal of Alzheimer's Disease*, *62*(2), 795–806.

McGuinness, B., et al. (2016). Statins for the prevention of dementia. *Cochrane Database of Systematic Reviews*, (1), Cd003160.

Mielke, M. M. (2018). Sex and gender differences in Alzheimer's disease dementia. *Psychiatric Times*, *35*(11), 14–17.

Miller, V. M., et al. (2019). The Kronos early estrogen prevention study (keeps): What have we learned? *Menopause*, *26*, 1071–1084.

Moffat, S. D., et al. (2004). Free testosterone and risk for Alzheimer disease in older men. *Neurology*, *62*(2), 188–193.

Moll van Charante, E. P., et al. (2016). Effectiveness of a 6-year multidomain vascular care intervention to prevent dementia (preDIVA): A cluster-randomised controlled trial. *Lancet, 388*(10046), 797–805.

Mong, J. A., & Cusmano, D. M. (2016). Sex differences in sleep: Impact of biological sex and sex steroids. *Philosophical Transactions of the Royal Society of London. Series B, Biological Sciences, 371*(1688), 20150110.

Morgenthaler, T., et al. (2006). Practice parameters for the psychological and behavioral treatment of insomnia: An update. An american academy of sleep medicine report. *Sleep, 29*(11), 1415–1419.

Muller, M., et al. (2003). Endogenous sex hormones in men aged 40-80 years. *European Journal of Endocrinology, 149*(6), 583–589.

Mulnard, R. A., et al. (2000). Estrogen replacement therapy for treatment of mild to moderate Alzheimer disease: A randomized controlled trial. Alzheimer's Disease Cooperative Study. *JAMA, 283*(8), 1007–1015.

Nasrallah, I. M., et al. (2019). Association of intensive vs standard blood pressure control with cerebral white matter lesions. *JAMA, 322*(6), 524–534.

Nebel, R. A., et al. (2018). Understanding the impact of sex and gender in Alzheimer's disease: A call to action. *Alzheimers Dement, 14*(9), 1171–1183.

Nelson, H. D., et al. (2002). Postmenopausal hormone replacement therapy: Scientific review. *JAMA, 288*(7), 872–881.

Neu, S. C., et al. (2017). Apolipoprotein E genotype and sex risk factors for Alzheimer disease: A meta-analysis. *JAMA Neurology, 74*(10), 1178–1189.

Ngandu, T., et al. (2015). A 2 year multidomain intervention of diet, exercise, cognitive training, and vascular risk monitoring versus control to prevent cognitive decline in at-risk elderly people (FINGER): A randomised controlled trial. *Lancet, 385*(9984), 2255–2263.

Nicholson, K., et al. (2020). Sleep behaviours and multimorbidity occurrence in middle-aged and older adults: Findings from the Canadian Longitudinal Study on Aging (CLSA). *Sleep Medicine, 75*, 156–162.

Nicklett, E. J., & Kadell, A. R. (2013). Fruit and vegetable intake among older adults: A scoping review. *Maturitas, 75*(4), 305–312.

Nishimura, A., et al. (2019). Sex-related differences in frailty factors in older persons with type 2 diabetes: A cross-sectional study. *Therapeutic Advances in Endocrinology and Metabolism, 10*, 2042018819833304.

Noale, M., et al. (2013). Incidence of dementia: Evidence for an effect modification by gender. The ILSA study. *International Psychogeriatrics, 25*(11), 1867–1876.

Northey, J. M., et al. (2018). Exercise interventions for cognitive function in adults older than 50: A systematic review with meta-analysis. *British Journal of Sports Medicine, 52*(3), 154–160.

Norton, M. C., et al. (2010). Greater risk of dementia when spouse has dementia? The Cache County study. *Journal of the American Geriatrics Society, 58*(5), 895–900.

Nyqvist, F., et al. (2017). Prevalence of loneliness over ten years among the oldest old. *Scandinavian Journal of Public Health, 45*(4), 411–418.

Ortiz-Ospina, E. (2019). *The rise of living alone: How one-person households are becoming increasingly common around the world*. Available from: https://ourworldindata.org/living-alone.

Pancani, S., et al. (2019). HDL cholesterol is independently associated with cognitive function in males but not in females within a cohort of nonagenarians: The MUGELLO Study. *The Journal of Nutrition, Health & Aging, 23*(6), 552–557.

Panza, F., et al. (2015). Coffee, tea, and caffeine consumption and prevention of late-life cognitive decline and dementia: A systematic review. *The Journal of Nutrition, Health & Aging, 19*(3), 313–328.

Penninkilampi, R., et al. (2018). The association between social engagement, loneliness, and risk of dementia: A systematic review and meta-analysis. *Journal of Alzheimer's Disease, 66*(4), 1619–1633.

Perkins, K. A. (2001). Smoking cessation in women. Special considerations. *CNS Drugs, 15*(5), 391–411.

Perneczky, R., et al. (2007a). Male gender is associated with greater cerebral hypometabolism in frontotemporal dementia: Evidence for sex-related cognitive reserve. *International Journal of Geriatric Psychiatry, 22*(11), 1135–1140.

Perneczky, R., et al. (2007b). Gender differences in brain reserve: An (18)F-FDG PET study in Alzheimer's disease. *Journal of Neurology, 254*(10), 1395–1400.

Pertesi, S., et al. (2019). Menopause, cognition and dementia—A review. *Post Reproductive Health, 25*(4), 200–206.

Peters, S. A. E., Muntner, P., & Woodward, M. (2019). Sex differences in the prevalence of, and trends in, cardiovascular risk factors, treatment, and control in the United States, 2001 to 2016. *Circulation, 139*(8), 1025–1035.

Piccinelli, M., & Wilkinson, G. (2000). Gender differences in depression. Critical review. *The British Journal of Psychiatry, 177*, 486–492.

Pike, C. J. (2001). Testosterone attenuates beta-amyloid toxicity in cultured hippocampal neurons. *Brain Research, 919*(1), 160–165.

Pike, C. J. (2017). Sex and the development of Alzheimer's disease. *Journal of Neuroscience Research, 95*(1–2), 671–680.

Pinquart, M., & Sorensen, S. (2001). Influences on loneliness in older adults: A meta-analysis. *Basic and Applied Social Psychology, 23*(4), 245–266.

Piper, M. E., et al. (2010). Gender, race, and education differences in abstinence rates among participants in two randomized smoking cessation trials. *Nicotine & Tobacco Research, 12*(6), 647–657.

Prince, M., et al. (2013). The global prevalence of dementia: a systematic review and meta-analysis. *Alzheimers Dement, 9*(1), 63–75 e2.

Proserpio, P., et al. (2020). Insomnia and menopause: A narrative review on mechanisms and treatments. *Climacteric*, 1–11.

Rafnsson, S. B., et al. (2020). Loneliness, social integration, and incident dementia over 6 years: Prospective findings from the english longitudinal study of ageing. *The Journals of Gerontology. Series B, Psychological Sciences and Social Sciences, 75*(1), 114–124.

Rasmuson, S., Nasman, B., & Olsson, T. (2011). Increased serum levels of dehydroepiandrosterone (DHEA) and interleukin-6 (IL-6) in women with mild to moderate Alzheimer's disease. *International Psychogeriatrics, 23*(9), 1386–1392.

Razavi, A. C., et al. (2019). Sex, gut microbiome, and cardiovascular disease risk. *Biology of Sex Differences, 10*(1), 29.

Rebok, G. W., et al. (2014). Ten-year effects of the advanced cognitive training for independent and vital elderly cognitive training trial on cognition and everyday functioning in older adults. *Journal of the American Geriatrics Society, 62*(1), 16–24.

Reschke-Hernandez, A. E., et al. (2017). Sex and stress: Men and women show different cortisol responses to psychological stress induced by the Trier social stress test and the Iowa singing social stress test. *Journal of Neuroscience Research, 95*(1-2), 106–114.

Richard, E., Moll van Charante, E. P., Hoevenaar-Blom, M. P., Coley, N., Barbera, M., van der Groep, A., et al. (2019). Healthy ageing through internet counselling in the elderly (HATICE): A multinational, randomised controlled trial. *The Lancet*.

Rigaud, A. S., et al. (2002). Presence or absence of at least one epsilon 4 allele and gender are not predictive for the response to donepezil treatment in Alzheimer's disease. *Pharmacogenetics, 12*(5), 415–420.

Ritchie, S. J., et al. (2018). Sex differences in the adult human brain: Evidence from 5216 UK biobank participants. *Cerebral Cortex, 28*(8), 2959–2975.

Robles, T. F., & Kiecolt-Glaser, J. K. (2003). The physiology of marriage: Pathways to health. *Physiology & Behavior, 79*(3), 409–416.

Romera-Liebana, L., et al. (2018). Effects of a primary care-based multifactorial intervention on physical and cognitive function in frail, elderly individuals: A randomized controlled trial. *The Journals of Gerontology. Series A, Biological Sciences and Medical Sciences, 73*(12), 1668–1674.

Rosario, E. R., & Pike, C. J. (2008). Androgen regulation of beta-amyloid protein and the risk of Alzheimer's disease. *Brain Research Reviews, 57*(2), 444–453.

Rosenberg, A., et al. (2018). Multidomain lifestyle intervention benefits a large elderly population at risk for cognitive decline and dementia regardless of baseline characteristics: The FINGER trial. *Alzheimers Dement, 14*(3), 263–270.

Ruitenberg, A., et al. (2001). Incidence of dementia: Does gender make a difference? *Neurobiology of Aging, 22*(4), 575–580.

Ruiz-Castell, M., et al. (2019). Sleep duration and multimorbidity in Luxembourg: Results from the European Health Examination Survey in Luxembourg, 2013-2015. *BMJ Open, 9*(8), e026942.

Russ, T. C., et al. (2013). Socioeconomic status as a risk factor for dementia death: Individual participant meta-analysis of 86 508 men and women from the UK. *The British Journal of Psychiatry, 203*(1), 10–17.

Ryan, J., et al. (2009). Characteristics of hormone therapy, cognitive function, and dementia: The prospective 3C Study. *Neurology, 73*(21), 1729–1737.

Sachdev, P. S., et al. (2012). Risk profiles for mild cognitive impairment vary by age and sex: The Sydney Memory and Ageing study. *The American Journal of Geriatric Psychiatry, 20*(10), 854–865.

Salk, R. H., Hyde, J. S., & Abramson, L. Y. (2017). Gender differences in depression in representative national samples: Meta-analyses of diagnoses and symptoms. *Psychological Bulletin, 143*(8), 783–822.

Santhi, N., et al. (2016). Sex differences in the circadian regulation of sleep and waking cognition in humans. *Proceedings of the National Academy of Sciences of the United States of America, 113*(19), E2730–E2739.

Santos-Lozano, A., et al. (2016). Physical activity and alzheimer disease: A protective association. *Mayo Clinic Proceedings, 91*(8), 999–1020.

Savolainen-Peltonen, H., et al. (2019). Use of postmenopausal hormone therapy and risk of Alzheimer's disease in Finland: Nationwide case-control study. *BMJ, 364*, l665.

Scharfman, H. E., et al. (2003). Hippocampal excitability increases during the estrous cycle in the rat: A potential role for brain-derived neurotrophic factor. *The Journal of Neuroscience, 23*(37), 11641–11652.

Seo, D., et al. (2011). Sex differences in neural responses to stress and alcohol context cues. *Human Brain Mapping, 32*(11), 1998–2013.

Seo, D., et al. (2017). Gender differences in neural correlates of stress-induced anxiety. *Journal of Neuroscience Research, 95*(1–2), 115–125.

Seshadri, S., et al. (1997). Lifetime risk of dementia and Alzheimer's disease. The impact of mortality on risk estimates in the Framingham Study. *Neurology, 49*(6), 1498–1504.

Shankar, A., et al. (2011). Loneliness, social isolation, and behavioral and biological health indicators in older adults. *Health Psychology, 30*(4), 377–385.

Shankar, A., et al. (2013). Social isolation and loneliness: Relationships with cognitive function during 4 years of follow-up in the English Longitudinal Study of Ageing. *Psychosomatic Medicine, 75*(2), 161–170.

Shao, H., et al. (2012). Hormone therapy and Alzheimer disease dementia: New findings from the cache county study. *Neurology, 79*(18), 1846–1852.

Sherwin, B. B. (1988). Estrogen and/or androgen replacement therapy and cognitive functioning in surgically menopausal women. *Psychoneuroendocrinology, 13*(4), 345–357.

Shi, L., et al. (2018). Sleep disturbances increase the risk of dementia: A systematic review and meta-analysis. *Sleep Medicine Reviews, 40*, 4–16.

Shumaker, S. A., et al. (2003). Estrogen plus progestin and the incidence of dementia and mild cognitive impairment in postmenopausal women: the Women's Health Initiative Memory Study: A randomized controlled trial. *JAMA, 289*(20), 2651–2662.

Shumaker, S. A., et al. (2004). Conjugated equine estrogens and incidence of probable dementia and mild cognitive impairment in postmenopausal women: Women's Health Initiative Memory Study. *JAMA, 291*(24), 2947–2958.

Siddiqui, A. N., et al. (2016). Neuroprotective role of steroidal sex hormones: An overview. *CNS Neuroscience & Therapeutics, 22*(5), 342–350.

Sindi, S., et al. (2018). Sleep disturbances and dementia risk: A multicenter study. *Alzheimers Dement, 14*(10), 1235–1242.

Sindi, S., et al. (2020). Sleep disturbances and the speed of multimorbidity development in old age: Results from a longitudinal population-based study. *BMC Medicine, 18*(1), 382.

Singh, M., Meyer, E. M., & Simpkins, J. W. (1995). The effect of ovariectomy and estradiol replacement on brain-derived neurotrophic factor messenger ribonucleic acid expression in cortical and hippocampal brain regions of female Sprague-Dawley rats. *Endocrinology, 136*(5), 2320–2324.

Sink, K. M., et al. (2015). Effect of a 24-month physical activity intervention vs health education on cognitive outcomes in sedentary older adults: The life randomized trial. *JAMA, 314*(8), 781–790.

Skoog, I., et al. (2017). Decreasing prevalence of dementia in 85-year olds examined 22 years apart: The influence of education and stroke. *Scientific Reports, 7*(1), 6136.

Smith, P. J., et al. (2010). Effects of the dietary approaches to stop hypertension diet, exercise, and caloric restriction on neurocognition in overweight adults with high blood pressure. *Hypertension, 55*(6), 1331–1338.

Snell, K. D. M. (2017). The rise of living alone and loneliness in history. *Social History, 42*(1), 2–28.

Sohrabji, F., Miranda, R. C., & Toran-Allerand, C. D. (1995). Identification of a putative estrogen response element in the gene encoding brain-derived neurotrophic factor. *Proceedings of the National Academy of Sciences of the United States of America, 92*(24), 11110–11114.

Solomon, A., et al. (2007). Serum cholesterol changes after midlife and late-life cognition: Twenty-one-year follow-up study. *Neurology, 68*(10), 751–756.

Spiga, F., et al. (2011). ACTH-dependent ultradian rhythm of corticosterone secretion. *Endocrinology, 152*(4), 1448–1457.

Steer, R. A., et al. (1999). Dimensions of the beck depression inventory-II in clinically depressed outpatients. *Journal of Clinical Psychology, 55*(1), 117–128.

Stephen, R., et al. (2017). Physical activity and Alzheimer's disease: A systematic review. *The Journals of Gerontology. Series A, Biological Sciences and Medical Sciences, 72*(6), 733–739.

Steptoe, A., et al. (2013). Social isolation, loneliness, and all-cause mortality in older men and women. *Proceedings of the National Academy of Sciences of the United States of America, 110*(15), 5797–5801.

Stern, Y. (2012). Cognitive reserve in ageing and Alzheimer's disease. *Lancet Neurology, 11*(11), 1006–1012.

Stern, Y., et al. (2018). Whitepaper*: Defining and investigating cognitive reserve, brain reserve, and brain maintenance. Alzheimers Dement, 16*, 1305–1311.

Stone, K. L., & Xiao, Q. (2018). Impact of poor sleep on physical and mental health in older women. *Sleep Medicine Clinics, 13*(3), 457–465.

Subramaniapillai, S., et al. (2020). Sex and gender differences in cognitive and brain reserve: Implications for Alzheimer's disease in women. *Frontiers in Neuroendocrinology*, 100879.

Sundermann, E. E., Katz, M. J., & Lipton, R. B. (2017). Sex differences in the relationship between depressive symptoms and risk of amnestic mild cognitive impairment. *The American Journal of Geriatric Psychiatry, 25*(1), 13–22.

Sundermann, E. E., et al. (2018). Sex differences in the association between apolipoprotein E epsilon4 allele and Alzheimer's disease markers. *Alzheimers Dement, 10*, 438–447.

Sutin, A. R., et al. (2020). Loneliness and risk of dementia. *The Journals of Gerontology. Series B, Psychological Sciences and Social Sciences, 75*(7), 1414–1422.

Teuschl, Y., et al. (2018). Multidomain intervention for the prevention of cognitive decline after stroke—A pooled patient-level data analysis. *European Journal of Neurology, 25*(9), 1182–1188.

Thompson, C. K., & Brenowitz, E. A. (2010). Neuroprotective effects of testosterone in a naturally occurring model of neurodegeneration in the adult avian song control system. *The Journal of Comparative Neurology, 518*(23), 4760–4770.

Tolppanen, A. M., et al. (2015). Leisure-time physical activity from mid- to late life, body mass index, and risk of dementia. *Alzheimers Dement, 11*(4), 434–443 e6.

Toufexis, D., et al. (2014). Stress and the reproductive axis. *Journal of Neuroendocrinology, 26*(9), 573–586.

Tramo, M. J., et al. (1998). Brain size, head size, and intelligence quotient in monozygotic twins. *Neurology, 50*(5), 1246–1252.

Trento, M., et al. (2014). Depression, anxiety, cognitive impairment and their association with clinical and demographic variables in people with type 2 diabetes: A 4-year prospective study. *Journal of Endocrinological Investigation, 37*(1), 79–85.

Tsigos, C., & Chrousos, G. P. (1994). Physiology of the hypothalamic-pituitary-adrenal axis in health and dysregulation in psychiatric and autoimmune disorders. *Endocrinology and Metabolism Clinics of North America, 23*(3), 451–466.

Tsigos, C., & Chrousos, G. P. (2002). Hypothalamic-pituitary-adrenal axis, neuroendocrine factors and stress. *Journal of Psychosomatic Research, 53*(4), 865–871.

Vahia, V. N. (2013). Diagnostic and statistical manual of mental disorders 5: A quick glance. *Indian Journal of Psychiatry, 55*(3), 220–223.

Van den Berg, J. F., et al. (2017). Gender differences in cognitive functioning in older alcohol-dependent patients. *Substance Use & Misuse, 52*(5), 574–580.

van Gelder, B. M., et al. (2006). Marital status and living situation during a 5-year period are associated with a subsequent 10-year cognitive decline in older men: The FINE study.

The Journals of Gerontology. Series B, Psychological Sciences and Social Sciences, 61(4), P213–P219.

Varma, V. R., Tang, X., & Carlson, M. C. (2016). Hippocampal sub-regional shape and physical activity in older adults. *Hippocampus, 26*(8), 1051–1060.

Verma, R., Balhara, Y. P., & Gupta, C. S. (2011). Gender differences in stress response: Role of developmental and biological determinants. *Industrial Psychiatry Journal, 20*(1), 4–10.

Vitale, M., et al. (2016). Sex differences in food choices, adherence to dietary recommendations and plasma lipid profile in type 2 diabetes–The TOSCA.IT study. *Nutrition, Metabolism, and Cardiovascular Diseases, 26*(10), 879–885.

Wahjoepramono, E. J., et al. (2016). The effects of testosterone supplementation on cognitive functioning in older men. *CNS & Neurological Disorders Drug Targets, 15*(3), 337–343.

Wang, P. N., et al. (2000). Effects of estrogen on cognition, mood, and cerebral blood flow in AD: A controlled study. *Neurology, 54*(11), 2061–2066.

Wang, Y. H., et al. (2020). Depression and anxiety in relation to cancer incidence and mortality: A systematic review and meta-analysis of cohort studies. *Molecular Psychiatry, 25*(7), 1487–1499.

Wardzala, C., et al. (2018). Sex differences in the association of alcohol with cognitive decline and brain pathology in a cohort of octogenarians. *Psychopharmacology, 235*(3), 761–770.

Weinstock, M., et al. (1998). Gender differences in sympathoadrenal activity in rats at rest and in response to footshock stress. *Neuroscience Letters*, S43–S44.

Wengreen, H., et al. (2013). Prospective study of Dietary Approaches to Stop Hypertension- and Mediterranean-style dietary patterns and age-related cognitive change: The Cache County Study on Memory, Health and Aging. *The American Journal of Clinical Nutrition, 98*(5), 1263–1271.

West, R. K., et al. (2016). Waist circumference is correlated with poorer cognition in elderly type 2 diabetes women. *Alzheimers Dement, 12*(8), 925–929.

Wetter, D. W., et al. (1999). Gender differences in smoking cessation. *Journal of Consulting and Clinical Psychology, 67*(4), 555–562.

Whitmer, R. A., et al. (2011). Timing of hormone therapy and dementia: The critical window theory revisited. *Annals of Neurology, 69*(1), 163–169.

Wild, B., et al. (2012). Gender specific temporal and cross-sectional associations between BMI-class and symptoms of depression in the elderly. *Journal of Psychosomatic Research, 72*(5), 376–382.

Williamson, J. D., et al. (2019). Effect of intensive vs standard blood pressure control on probable dementia: A randomized clinical trial. *JAMA, 321*(6), 553–561.

Wilson, R. S., et al. (2008). Change in depressive symptoms during the prodromal phase of Alzheimer disease. *Archives of General Psychiatry, 65*(4), 439–445.

Wilson, R. S., et al. (2010). Temporal course of depressive symptoms during the development of Alzheimer disease. *Neurology, 75*(1), 21–26.

Winblad, B., et al. (2001). A 1-year, randomized, placebo-controlled study of donepezil in patients with mild to moderate AD. *Neurology, 57*(3), 489–495.

Windle, R. J., et al. (1998). Ultradian rhythm of basal corticosterone release in the female rat: Dynamic interaction with the response to acute stress. *Endocrinology, 139*(2), 443–450.

World Health Organization. (2004b). *ICD-10: International statistical classification of diseases and related health problems: Tenth revision.* WHO IRIS. Retrieved from https://apps.who.int/iris/handle/10665/42980.

World Health Organization. (2019). *Risk reduction of cognitive decline and dementia.* Geneva: WHO Guidelines.

World Health Organization. (2020). *The global health observatory. Life expectancy and Healthy life expectancy. World Health Statistics*. Accessed 27 October 2020. Available from: https://www.who.int/data/gho/data/themes/topics/indicator-groups/indicator-group-details/GHO/life-expectancy-and-healthy-life-expecancy.

Wu, L., & Sun, D. (2017). Adherence to Mediterranean diet and risk of developing cognitive disorders: An updated systematic review and meta-analysis of prospective cohort studies. *Scientific Reports*, *7*, 41317.

Xiong, C., et al. (2020). Sex and gender differences in caregiving burden experienced by family caregivers of persons with dementia: A systematic review. *PLoS One*, *15*(4), e0231848.

Yan, Y., et al. (2018). Sex differences in chronic stress responses and Alzheimer's disease. *Neurobiology of Stress*, *8*, 120–126.

Yan, X. S., et al. (2019). Protective mechanism of testosterone on cognitive impairment in a rat model of Alzheimer's disease. *Neural Regeneration Research*, *14*(4), 649–657.

Yesavage, J. A., et al. (1982). Development and validation of a geriatric depression screening scale: A preliminary report. *Journal of Psychiatric Research*, *17*(1), 37–49.

Yonker, J. E., et al. (2005). Sex differences in spatial visualization and episodic memory as a function of alcohol consumption. *Alcohol and Alcoholism*, *40*(3), 201–207.

Young, E. A., Abelson, J., & Lightman, S. L. (2004). Cortisol pulsatility and its role in stress regulation and health. *Frontiers in Neuroendocrinology*, *25*(2), 69–76.

Zandi, P. P., et al. (2002). Hormone replacement therapy and incidence of Alzheimer disease in older women: The Cache County Study. *JAMA*, *288*(17), 2123–2129.

Zarate, S., Stevnsner, T., & Gredilla, R. (2017). Role of estrogen and other sex hormones in brain aging. Neuroprotection and DNA repair. *Frontiers in Aging Neuroscience*, *9*, 430.

Zhang, B., & Wing, Y. K. (2006). Sex differences in insomnia: A meta-analysis. *Sleep*, *29*(1), 85–93.

Zhong, G., et al. (2015). Smoking is associated with an increased risk of dementia: A meta-analysis of prospective cohort studies with investigation of potential effect modifiers. *PLoS One*, *10*(3), e0118333.

Zhou, Z., Wang, P., & Fang, Y. (2018). Loneliness and the risk of dementia among older Chinese adults: Gender differences. *Aging & Mental Health*, *22*(4), 519–525.

CHAPTER 11

Sex and gender considerations in clinical trials for Alzheimer's disease: Current state and recommendations

Maitee Rosende-Roca[a], Carla Abdelnour[a,b], Ester Esteban[a], Mercè Boada Rovira[a,b], Julie N. Martinkova[c,d], Simona Mellino[d], and Antonella Santuccione Chadha[d]

[a]*Research Center and Memory Clinic, Fundació ACE, Institut Català de Neurociències Aplicades, Universitat Internacional de Catalunya, Barcelona, Spain*
[b]*Networking Research Center on Neurodegenerative Diseases (CIBERNED), Instituto de Salud Carlos III, Madrid, Spain*
[c]*Memory Clinic, Department of Neurology, Second Faculty of Medicine, Charles University and Motol University Hospital, Prague, Czech Republic*
[d]*Women's Brain Project, Guntershausen, Switzerland*

Introduction

The US National Institute of Health defines clinical trials as: "A research study in which one or more human subjects are prospectively assigned to one or more interventions (which may include placebo or other control) to evaluate the effects of those interventions on health-related biomedical or behavioral outcomes" (National Institute of Health, 2014). In other words, a clinical trial is an experiment in which the efficacy, safety, tolerability, and other properties of investigational drugs or devices are determined. Clinical trials represent an essential tool in discovering new medicines and new approaches to treatment. Given sex and gender differences described throughout this volume, as well as the importance of clinical trials, it is all the more striking that for much of our history, sex and gender were not considered as a critical variable to include in the characterization of the efficacy and safety profile of treatment interventions. In this section, we provide a general overview of sex and gender differences in clinical trials, describe the current state of sex and gender differences in Alzheimer's disease (AD), and provide recommendations for considering sex and gender in clinical trials.

Table 1 Overview of clinical trial stages.

Stage	Population	Goal
Preclinical	Cells, tissues, laboratory animals	- Efficacy of the drug in vitro and in vivo - Pharmacokinetics and pharmacodynamics in laboratory animals
Phase I	Healthy volunteers or end-stage patients for highly toxic substances, n = approx. 10–100	- Pharmacokinetics and pharmacodynamics in human subjects - Safety/toxicity assessment - Determine appropriate dosing
Phase II	Patients with target disease, n = approx. 50 to several hundreds	- Safety and tolerability of the medication (primary) - Preliminary efficacy in human subjects (secondary)
Phase III	Patients with target disease, n = several hundreds to thousands	- Determine long-term efficacy (primary goal) - Long-term safety and tolerability
Phase IV (post-marketing)	Patients with target disease, medicated with investigated drug	- Long-term safety (and possibly effectiveness) in routine use, pharmacovigilance

Typically, drug development process consists of five stages: the preclinical phase, which utilizes in vitro research or laboratory animals, and clinical phases I, II, III, and IV, which involve human subjects. An overview of the basic characteristics of clinical trial stages is provided in Table 1. Clinical trials are typically controlled: some enrolled subjects are assigned to the treatment arm, while others are assigned to the control arm, which usually involves placebo or gold standard treatment; arm assignment is usually randomized to ensure the comparability of treatment arms. Clinical trials with these characteristics (or randomized clinical trials, RCTs), augmented by double or triple-blinding involved parties (the subjects, the treatment-givers and the assessors) are, with some reservations (Kaptchuk, 2001), considered the gold standard for clinical research.

Sex considerations in preclinical stages of clinical trials

The preclinical stage involves laboratory animals, usually mice, rats, or primates. Historically, female rodents were often excluded for fear of variations introduced by their relatively short estrous cycle (reviewed in Shansky, 2019). This, among other factors, led to the underrepresentation of female animals presented in some publications; according to Beery et al., this phenomenon is particularly prevalent in neuroscience, where studies conducted solely on males outnumbered studies on females 5.5:1 (Beery & Zucker, 2011). Other reviews revealed different problematic tendencies, where a significant number of reported preclinical studies neglected to note the animals' sex and/or age (Flórez-Vargas et al., 2016).

Since the preclinical phase forms the basis for future clinical phases (see Chapter 1), improving sex representation and reporting could prevent future complications, as well as the economic burden presented by withdrawing medications later in development, by considering female-specific pharmacokinetics and pharmacodynamics in the early stages of the process. It must be noted that this opinion is not universally shared. For example, Richardson et al. argue that many discrepancies present in latter stages of trials (in human subjects) are actually not related to sex, but caused by other variables, such as body weight. They express concerns that including both sexes of laboratory animals would introduce other issues, such as reduced statistical power or ignoring other variations besides those introduced by sex (Richardson et al., 2015). Indeed, Prendergast et al. noted that the estrous cycle caused little variation in animal traits (and surprisingly, variation was higher for males in several traits), while group housing introduced much more variability (Prendergast, Onishi, & Zucker, 2014). It seems that minimizing bias (including balancing of animal sex) and reporting all relevant variables will be crucial for both preclinical and clinical studies, and this is reflected in several current recommendations (Clayton & Collins, 2014; Franconi, Rosano, & Campesi, 2015; Kilkenny et al., 2010).

Sex and gender considerations in clinical trial stages involving human subjects

In phases I–III, sex/gender bias was probably in part directly introduced by regulatory agency recommendations, at least in the United States of America. The US Food and Drug Administration (FDA) recommended that women of reproductive age should not be included in phase I–II clinical trials due to fears of possible teratogenic effects in light of the thalidomide scandal (Food and Drug Administration, 1977). Although this guidance specified exclusion only from the earliest phases, it was often interpreted more broadly and led to the underrepresentation of women in RCTs in general, which later resulted in the decision to overturn this recommendation (Food and Drug Administration, 1993). In the year preceding the reversal, General Accounting Office noted insufficient participation of women in clinical trials (General Accounting Office, 1992; reviewed in Liu & Dipietro Mager, 2016).

Recent investigations differ in their view on sex/gender representation in clinical trials; some posit that most RCTs and nonrandomized trials still include more men than women (Prakash et al., 2018), while others report the opposite in certain RCT phases (Labots et al., 2018). The difference is most marked in phase I, which includes 22%–36% women depending on the publication, while phase II and III involve approximately 48% and 49% women, respectively. However, it must be considered that many clinical trials are allowed to forgo phase II and enter phase III directly from phase I; underrepresentation of women in phase I trials then represents a significant issue in terms of missing information about pharmacokinetics and pharmacodynamics. Interestingly, according to the latter publication, gender was not reported at all for 9% of participants.

Agencies such as the US National Institutes of Health (NIH) recommend using RCT design "in a manner sufficient to provide for valid analysis of whether the variables being studied in the trial affect women or members of minority groups" (National Institute of Health, 2001). Despite this, reports of such analyses are still sedlom published (Phillips & Hamberg, 2016). A European review study showed that 17.9% of trials evaluated study population by sex/gender, while 3.6% published sex/gender-disaggregated data, i.e., data collected and analyzed separately by sex (Laguna-Goya & De Andres-Trelles, 2014). A Canadian study found only 6% of RCTs performed subgroup comparison, while 4% reported sex-disaggregated data (Welch et al., 2017). Differences in definition and methodology may have contributed to the significant geographic difference.

In terms of neurologic and psychiatric diseases specifically, a recent review of large-scale RCTs in stroke reported that 40% of enrolled patients were women (Carcel et al., 2019). In this particular study, 36% of trials stratified results by sex/gender, of which 33% were prespecified subgroup analyses. Although inclusion of stratified data showed a positive temporal trend, the authors commented that this was likely a reflection of the overall increase in the number of studies rather than an actual increase in sex/gender-stratified reporting.

Sex and gender considerations in Alzheimer's disease clinical trials

Prevalence and pathophysiology of the disease in men and women

AD is a multifactorial disease where patient's sex and gender plays a crucial role. Women represent the majority of AD patients; in the dementia phase of the disease, as many as two-thirds of AD patients are women (Alzheimer Association, 2019). It has been reported than the progression of cognitive decline is faster in women (Tifratene et al., 2015), a possible result of a delayed diagnosis compared to men (reviewed in Ferretti et al., 2018) (see Chapter 6). Autopsy studies further discovered than women more often than men progress to more severe cognitive dysfunction, higher levels of AD pathology, and greater gross atrophy (Filon et al., 2016; Liesinger et al., 2018).

The examples above illustrate that sex (and gender) is one of the drivers of AD heterogeneity. Since AD is currently neither curable nor effectively controllable by medications, there is an urgent need for effective medications besides currently available cholinesterase inhibitors and memantine. In the following sections, we summarize how clinical trials can be augmented by including sex (and gender) considerations to better reflect AD heterogeneity.

Differences in AD biomarkers between men and women

In the last 10 years, biomarkers have acquired an important role in understanding the causality of AD. Several biomarkers have also been explored for their potential role in indicating early stages of Alzheimer's disease. Guidelines published by the US Food and Drugs Administration (FDA), recommend the usage of biomarkers as an aid to diagnosis. Further, biomarkers can aid the development of novel drug candidates for Alzheimer's disease (Blennow & Zetterberg, 2018; Budelier & Bateman, 2020).

In April 2011, the National Institute of Aging and the Alzheimer's Association (NIA-AA) published the updated diagnostic criteria for AD dementia, which included the use of biomarkers, and were further updated in 2018. Amyloid, tau, and neurodegeneration (ATN) biomarkers have been proposed by the NIA-AA research framework for supporting AD diagnosis (Albert et al., 2011; Jack Jr. et al., 2018).

Generally, the measurement of biomarkers relies on imaging, cerebrospinal fluid, blood, and genetic testing techniques. Brain scans using CT or MRI are generally conducted in the standard evaluation for Alzheimer,s and other forms of dementia. These reveal the anatomic structure of the brain and can rule out other conditions that can masquerade as AD (e.g., tumor, hemorrhage, stroke). Additionally, they can pick up brain mass loss in the form of disproportionate hippocampus atrophy and other more minute changes in other areas (including those assessed by more complicated methods such as volumetry) that suggest AD dementia. If CT and MRI scans prove inconclusive, positron emission tomography (PET), and single-photon emission computed tomography (SPECT) can be used to assess brain activity based on blood flow, oxygen consumption, and glucose use. Additionally, CSF (cerebrospinal fluid) measurements can be conducted to assess phosphorylated tau levels as well as amyloid-beta 1–42.

However, the described brain imaging techniques are expensive and CSF measurements are invasive as they require a lumbar puncture; thus, novel approaches using blood biomarkers have been explored recently. For example, phospho-tau217 (p-tau217) is one of the tau proteins found in tangles and is suggested to be a relatively sensitive indicator of both plaques and tangles, which are predictive for AD. Even if more validation work is required, there are some promising results. In a large study of 1402 cognitively impaired and unimpaired individuals, the p-tau217 blood test was able to distinguish those with and without "high likelihood of Alzheimer's disease" (based on traditional diagnosis techniques including CSF, PET, and MRI) with high accuracy. (Palmqvist et al., 2020).

Literature on sex and gender differences in AD biomarkers is still scarce. For a comprehensive review on sex/gender differences in CSF and imaging biomarkers we refer the reader to Chapters 4 and 5. However, we summarize here some studies that highlight some interesting findings in both diagnostic biomarkers and markers of disease progression.

Amyloid-beta

Controversial results have been shown in amyloid-beta. In mild cognitive impairment (MCI) and AD, no clear sex/gender differences in amyloid-beta burden have been reported. Using either CSF or PET techniques, no consistent results have been reported in global and absolute levels of amyloid in patients with MCI or AD in large cross-sectional studies (Ferretti et al., 2018). Studies on the uptake of Pittsburgh compound B (PiB) also present diverse results, with some studies reporting higher uptake in women and other reporting higher uptake in men.

A recent study by Mosconi et al. explored the impact of menopause on Alzheimer's disease biomarkers changes in a 3-year brain imaging study. The study included pre-, peri- and postmenopausal women as well as men. The authors found that the postmenopausal group showed higher rates of amyloid-beta deposition than men. Over the period of observation of 3 years, frontal PiB increased by an average of 6.3% in the postmenopausal group (Mosconi et al., 2018).

Tau

Tau levels can be monitored both via imaging techniques (PET) and by CSF measures of total and phosphorylated tau (p-tau). In individuals with MCI, higher CSF tau levels have been observed in females with ApoE-4 carriers as compared with male carriers.

Cross-sectional imaging studies have not reported significant sex/gender differences in global tau load. However, there is evidence of potential regional differences, especially in AD-affected regions. Buckley et al. reported that cognitively normal women showed more tau tangles in entorhinal cortices compared to men; this was associated with an increased amyloid deposition. (Buckley et al., 2019) Another recent study examined, among other things, the associations between CSF biomarkers (tau, p-tau, neurogranin—marker of synaptic dysfunction) and two AD imaging signatures. The associations between p-tau and neurogranin and the imaging signatures were stronger among female participants; according to the authors, this means that tau phosphorylation and synaptic dysfunction may be more prominent in AD-affected regions among females. (Moore et al., 2020).

Notably, sex/gender differences may exist in longitudinal associations. For example, Smith et al. reported that tau accumulation rate is greater in females and younger amyloid-beta-positive individuals (Smith et al., 2020). Further studies can elucidate the reasons and enhance our understanding of the determinants of faster tau aggregation and spread.

Furthermore, there is emerging evidence of possible sex/gender differences in tau accumulation associated with the presence of the strongest genetic risk factor of AD, the ApoE-4 allele. Evaluating CSF tau and p-tau, Mofrad et al. concluded that among ApoE-4 carriers, sex-differences in CSF p-Tau are more evident in early disease stages (subjective cognitive decline), whereas among ApoE-4 noncarriers, they are more evident in advanced disease stages (mild cognitive decline and dementia) (Babapour Mofrad et al., 2020).

Neurodegenerative markers

Common biomarkers for neurodegeneration include structural MRI and fluorine-18 fluorodeoxyglucose PET (FDG-PET) hypometabolism. Studies attempting to understand sex differences have largely explored structural MRI. Some structural MRI studies found higher atrophy in elderly men as compared to women (Jack et al., 2017). However, independent analyses of data, such as the MIRIAD database analysis of patients with probable AD, found that the rate of hippocampus atrophy as measured by structural MRI is instead significantly faster in women as compared to men. (Ardekani, Convit, & Bachman, 2016).

In FDG-PET, sex and gender differences have been explored more sparingly. There have been reports of differences in glucose uptake in certain cerebral regions; for example, Cavedo et al. posit that in cognitively intact individuals with subjective memory complaints, regional glucose metabolism may be more active or preserved in women than in men, and that men may exhibit higher resilience to AD neuropathological processes than women (Cavedo et al., 2018). An interesting study in cognitively intact women revealed that cerebral glucose metabolism in AD vulnerable regions, represented by a decrease of glucose uptake in FDG-PET, decreases with menopause progression and is most significant in postmenopausal women (Mosconi et al., 2017). This further highlights the need for adequate hormonal history in female patients.

We can conclude that biomarkers have become an essential tool in early diagnosis as well as in clinical research and trials, where they can ensure homogeneity among study participants by improving the reliability of clinical diagnoses. They also allow precise target engagement and proof-of-pharmacology, demonstration of disease-modification, and monitoring side effects. However, a better understanding of underlying sex/gender differences is required. Furthermore, the use of biomarkers of hormone function should be considered to improve the characterization of trial participants and sex-specific effects.

Efficacy of AD drugs in men and women

Since 1993, when the FDA approved Tacrine as the first treatment for AD, only four drugs have been authorized and are currently available to be used in patients with AD. Unfortunately, sex/gender-specific effects were on the whole under-addressed during the clinical development of AD medications. To our knowledge, these effects have also been largely ignored in real-world evidence studies performed after the drugs were introduced. As a result, whether these drugs have different effects in men and women remains largely unknown.

In the first systematic review looking at sex and gender considerations in clinical trials for cholinesterase inhibitors and memantine, Canevelli et al. (2017) found that none of the trials considered for the review reported data on safety, tolerability, or efficacy separately for men and women. Moreover, only 2 out of the 48 trials took into account potential sex and gender differences in efficacy; no difference was reported. None of the 48 trials considered potential sex and gender differences in safety or tolerability.

Since the majority of the trials presented in Canevelli et al were conducted in previous decades, the lack of sex and gender considerations is likely influenced by the overall lack of knowledge on sex and gender differences; more recent trials on not yet approved pharmaceuticals did report certain sex and gender effects, as described below.

The GuidAge prospective RCT on the efficacy of a ginkgo biloba extract called Egb 761 studied conversion to AD in a cohort of elderly adults with subjective memory complaints. Although the compound was not found effective overall, in an exploratory prespecified subgroup analysis including males only, Egb 761 was found effective with a hazard ratio of 0.43 (0.23–0.80, 95% confidence interval, $p = 0.011$). However, due to the absence of adjustment for multiple testing, these results should be interpreted with caution and studied further in appropriately powered studies (Vellas et al., 2012).

A publication by Claxton et al reported the results of a post-hoc analysis on a trial of intranasal insulin for AD or MCI, which focused on studying potential ApoE ε4 and sex effects. The report concluded that sex differences were present, with more memory improvement in men. The sex effect was especially pronounced in the ApoE ε4 negative group (Claxton et al., 2013).

A non-RCT observational study on AD incidence in statin users reported a negative association between AD and statin use, with a slightly lower incidence in women. The study also defined subgroups by sex and ethnicity; the most prominent association between lower AD incidence and statin use was noted in white women, while there was no significant association in black men. These results should be further confirmed in an RCT (Zissimopoulos et al., 2017).

We have conducted a pilot study on sex and gender considerations in AD clinical trials of nonapproved drugs, which was, to our knowledge, the first such study to be performed. We collected data on which of the 22 recent publications of 16 compounds took into account potential sex or gender difference (Ferretti et al., 2020). Only three publications presented the results of such an analysis. One of the three publications, an RCT of nilvadipine, reported an effect present in men but not in women, although the results did not reach statistical significance and should be interpreted with caution (Lawlor et al., 2018).

AD patients often receive additional symptomatic treatment, especially for behavioral symptoms (see Chapter 7). Interestingly, women are more frequently prescribed antipsychotic drugs, which are a proxy indicator of poor care (Health at a Glance, 2019).

Safety and pharmacokinetics of AD drugs in men and women

Drug pharmacokinetics also differs between men and women. Thus, differences in weight, body structure, liver metabolism, and elimination pathways, as well as hormonal changes can interfere and lead to women having more side effects than men using the same dose of the same component. (Ferretti et al., 2020).

While Canevelli et al. reported in their systematic review that sex and gender differences in safety profile were not analyzed during clinical development of currently approved drugs, interestingly, the FDA medical review that led to the approval of the anticholinesterase drug rivastagmine and of memantine identified a sex/gender difference in the incidence of adverse events.

For rivastigmine, the incidence rate of vomiting was higher in women than in men during the clinical development of its oral formulation. Also, approximately 26% of women on high doses of rivastigmine (brand name Exelon, doses greater than 9 mg/day) had weight loss equal to or greater than 7% of their baseline weight compared to 6% in the placebo-treated patients in these trials. In contrast, only about 18% of the males in the high dose group experienced a similar degree of weight loss compared to 4% in placebo-treated patients. It is not clear how much of the weight loss was associated with anorexia, nausea, vomiting, and diarrhea associated with the drug (Food and Drug Administration, 2000).

According to the FDA medical review that led to approval of memantine, this compound showed a sex difference in clinical pharmacology: following multiple dose administration of Namenda 20 mg daily, females had about 45% higher exposure than males, but there was no difference in exposure when body weight was taken into account. This finding should be further explored, as there were other sex and gender differences described in memantine response. The clinical reviewer who assessed the safety profile of the drug based on the safety data related to the drug clinical developmental program found a higher relative risk of certain adverse events in the female population, such as hallucinations and asthenia. In men, the risk was relatively higher for eye abnormalities and hyperuricemia (Food and Drug Administration, 2003).

Demographic factors in the efficacy and safety assessment or the subgroup analysis by sex/gender or age are not included in the majority of clinical studies or trials, despite evident differences by sex/gender and age having been demonstrated (Ferretti et al., 2018).

Participation of women in AD clinical trials

The sex and gender ratio in clinical trials of Alzheimer's has not been extensively studied. Even though women represent two-thirds of the total number of patients affected by AD (62%–67% depending on the region), we have recently reported that many large phase III trials for experimental drugs included a comparable number of men and women, with women ranging from 45.9% to 63% of all participants (Ferretti et al., 2020). This underrepresentation of women might indicate issues with inclusion and exclusion criteria, or retention and drop out, which are worth discussing. These preliminary findings will be further discussed in a systematic review and metaanalysis (Martinkova et al., manuscript in preparation).

The reason for this discrepancy has not been fully elucidated; we provide possible explanations below.

Inclusion and exclusion criteria—Screening

The screening protocols built to support enrolment of patients into clinical trials aim to obtain a homogeneous sample to reduce variability. This means that at this point, the trial participants selected are homogenous in terms of age range, educational level or years of schooling, cognitive performance, and comorbidities, which democratizes the sample. In our experience, at the Fundació ACE, we have not observed differences between men and women at the screening stage.

However, the clinical trials unit at Fundació ACE has introduced an additional step, called a prescreening protocol, in order to improve the quality of the screening process and predict and prevent dropouts that can take place during the clinical trial. A preliminary analysis revealed that differences between men and women, while absent after screening, can be found in the previous step of the selection process, the prescreening (Boada, 2019). These data suggest that the main determinant of the observed reduced eligibility in women was the difference in completed years of schooling. Thus, although these differences tend to disappear in younger generations, the large differences that persist among the elderly induce the exclusion of many otherwise eligible women from participating in clinical trials. Interestingly, although earlier AD trials did not require a minimum number of years of formal schooling (Boada, 2019), it is a common practice nowadays, which hampers the inclusion of elderly women in RCTs.

In fact, in our experience in Fundació ACE, based in Barcelona, Spain (Boada et al., 2014), a public-private, nonprofit institution dedicated to diagnosis, treatment and research of dementia under a holistic approach, up to 52% of the patients (Cañabate et al., 2017) had less than 6 years of schooling and of these, 60% were women. This study was carried out in our memory unit and included 5792 patients with Alzheimer's disease and their families.

It is worth noting that sex and gender differences in trial participation might also differ by disease stage; in this regard, it is important to analyze separately data on MCI trials. Preliminary study conducted on the data from FACE suggest that specific sex and gender differences are present in MCI trials (Boada, 2019).

AD trial duration and its socioeconomic implications

Another element that might influence access of women to CTs is the duration and economic burden of participating in such trials. This is becoming increasingly relevant as current clinical trials in AD tend to have a duration of 2 years or longer. In contrast, previous CTs, such as those which led to the approval of the currently available cognition-enhancing treatments, typically lasted 6 months (Espinosa et al., 2013). This generates a problem in patient retention, which could affect female participants more. These long trials rely on the presence of a caregiver, a role traditionally played by women (Cañabate et al., 2017). However, cognitively impaired women often lack a caregiver: women are more likely to be widowed and are more often institutionalized (Organization for Economic Co-operation and Development, no date) (see Chapter 12). Long-term participation in a lengthy trial is also an economic burden for the patient; women are known to have lower income due to generally lower or nonexistent pensions—this is highly dependent on the region of the world were the trial is be conducted (Cañabate et al., 2017). All these factors could prevent women from participating in trials and could also lead to higher dropout rates among them. (Boada, 2019) The occurrence of side effects is also an important cause of dropouts. While these intended effects could occur more frequently among women, there are currently not enough data to draw definite conclusions on this. We do know, however, that the participation and retention in clinical trials is proportional to the socioeconomic conditions of the family (Cañabate et al., 2017); therefore, women might be particularly exposed to this specific issue.

The role of biomarkers in selection/stratification of men/women

A body of evidence hints at potential sex and gender differences in risk factors for AD that are relevant for selection and stratification in clinical trials. For example, education level has been associated with the incidence of AD, and reduced access to education for women in the past might represent an important socioeconomic factor influencing the epidemiology of AD. The role of hormones has also been investigated (Ferretti et al., 2018). Considering the hormonal history of the subject as another biomarker seems reasonable, due to the clear evidence of its involvement in the pathophysiology of AD differences between sexes. Conditions such as early menopause or hypertensive pregnancy disorders are also associated with higher AD risk in women (Mauvais-Jarvis et al., 2020).

As mentioned in previous chapters of this book (Chapters 4 and 5), the role of sex/gender in biomarkers for diagnostic purposes such as beta-amyloid and tau requires further investigation. Women, particularly ApoE-4 carriers, can be more vulnerable to accumulation of tau in the presence of β-amyloid (Mauvais-Jarvis et al., 2020). Even when no absolute differences in these biomarkers are found, their effect on disease trajectories has been shown to be modified by sex/gender (reviewed in Ferretti et al., 2018, 2020). Biomarkers are thus essential to monitor cognitive decline and better understand these differences.

Recent research in AD has focused on preventative measures, early intervention, and predementia stages of the disease. The importance of preventative strategies can be explained by drawing parallels from other diseases, such as cardiovascular diseases (CVD). Improvements in death rates in the US (between 1980 and 2002) were associated with effective control of risk factors and were reported to be better in men (Ford & Capewell, 2007). However, it was just recently that the first guidelines for CVD prevention were tailored to women and published first in 2004 and later corrected in 2011 (Mosca, Barrett-Connor, & Wenger, 2011).

Inclusion of sex and gender might improve these strategies in AD:

1. Even before mild cognitive impairment, preventative campaigns specific and targeted to individual subgroups of patients might be beneficial. A report published in 2020, showed that that 35% of the risk of Alzheimer's is modifiable via lifestyle changes. As risk factors might differ, it is important to consider the right subgroup of patients (Livingston et al., 2020) (see Chapter 10).
2. Stratification of high-risk patients with MCI might allow for earlier interventions and planning strategies for patients and caregivers (Michaud et al., 2015).

Greater attention to sex and gender differences might offer improvement for clinical trials research. For example, the effect of biomarkers on disease trajectories might suggest the need to have different cut-offs, which are adjusted according to sex/gender.

Even if, taken in isolation, sex/gender differences might be small or moderate, population screening should take into consideration all the relevant factors including demographic, clinical, genetic, biomarker, and other relevant data to identify subsets of patients at risk and move towards precision medicine approaches (Ferretti et al., 2020).

Digital biomarkers

Digital biomarkers are defined as objective, quantifiable physiological and behavioral data that are collected and measured by means of portable, wearables, implantable, or digestible digital devices. The data collected is typically used to explain, influence, and/or predict health-related outcomes (Babrak et al., 2019). Some digital biomarkers have been developed starting from improvement of traditional biomarkers, whilst others provide a higher degree of novelty, both in type of measurement and in outcomes (Wang, Azad, & Rajan, n.d.).

The opportunities for digital biomarkers are very evident in neurological disorders, where several limitations exist: traditional clinical scales might be susceptible to inter- and intra-rater variability and might take a long time to administer, with clinical appointments possibly being infrequent, occurring just once or twice a year. Additionally, in diseases such as Alzheimer's, a wide spectrum of changes (sensory, motor) might precede clinical manifestations, and thus, it could be of great help to capture those changes early on (Kourtis et al., 2019). An interesting application is the use of digital vocal biomarkers as a predictor for cognitive function. Several studies have been published in this field (Robin et al., 2020). For example, a study conducted by Evidation Health analyzed recordings from the Framingham Heart Study between 2005 and 2016 to identify individuals at risk of dementia (Stück et al., 2018).

The use of digital biomarkers has gained interest in recent years, and they have been increasingly deployed in clinical trials as well as in real-world settings. Collecting frequent and objective information on patient status might help to better understand individual changes in disease and personalize therapeutic intervention. Digital biomarkers might aid internal decision-making in drug development and even serve as a primary or secondary endpoint in trials (Dockendorf et al., 2020). Additionally, the usage of digital biomarkers might offer flexibility to clinical trials participants by reducing the number of in-clinic visits, collecting information remotely, and measuring what matters most to patients (Coravos, Khozin, & Mandl, 2019).

An interesting example is Altoida, a predictive digital biomarker company. Its Neuro Monitor Index (NMI) is a class II medical device (FDA classification) that can predict patients at risk of developing MCI due to 6–10 CE years prior to the onset of symptoms with a 94% accuracy. The device tests the functional and cognitive aptitude of a patient with the help of a gamified 10-min assessment, which can be performed on a tablet or computer. In a longitudinal, multisite, 40-month prospective study collecting data in memory clinics, GP offices, and home environments, the assessment has been shown to accurately discriminate between healthy subjects and individuals at risk to progress to dementia within 3 years. Notably, the assessment was able to distinguish between individuals who progress rapidly to dementia (i.e., within 18 months of diagnosis) and those who decline slowly (i.e., after 36 months). The predictive performance was high at ROC-AUC 91% (Buegler et al., 2020).

Despite the fact that sex and gender differences in this field have not been fully examined, the Women's Brain Project recently published a review paper in Nature Partner Journal (Npj) Digital Medicine highlighting the need to include these considerations in developing digital biomarkers (Cirillo et al., 2020). As an example, it is crucially important that the algorithms are trained on a representative sample of patients, especially in those diseases where symptoms can be different between males and females (for example in Parkinson's disease). If an algorithm is overtrained on males, it might lead to a better accuracy to detect male symptoms only (Cirillo et al., 2020). Fundació ACE has also recently started to investigate this field and participated in the RAMCI project (robot research to help people with mild cognitive impairment) and in several clinical trials of monitoring devices.

Conclusion

The FDA has made great efforts to promote inclusion of women in clinical trials. The aim is to protect specific needs of men and women and encourage drug developers to consider specific clinical outcomes and drug-safety profiles in terms of gender and sex. AD affects predominantly women, who represent two-thirds of the AD population. Through these efforts, the medical field will be able to identify sex/gender differences, which includes assessing the safety and efficacy of medications, thereby allowing careful direction of clinical decisions. While there are still barriers and questions that need to be addressed, women's health research continues to advance.

We should rethink clinical trial design in general and eligibility criteria in particular to avoid elements that favor the underrepresentation of women. Thus, efforts should be taken to formulate inclusion and exclusion criteria so they do not lead to unnecessary exclusion of women, either by the persisting educational gap or due to socioeconomic considerations such as the absence of a caregiver. Investigators should design their investigations so they appropriately address the gender issue, including estimating and reporting sex-disaggregated data.

While the use of biomarkers improves the validity and reproducibility of clinical diagnoses, we should guarantee that their use does not introduce new biases in representation of women in research by acknowledging existing sex/gender differences in these biomarkers. Thus, sex/gender differences should be explored and considered in the study design.

Recommendations for considering sex and gender in clinical trials

We present detailed recommendations for AD in the aforementioned review (Ferretti et al., 2020). Main considerations include:

1. Aim for adequate representation of men and women in clinical trials. If possible, avoid the exclusion of phase II to combat the unequal representation in phase I of the trials.
2. Consider sex in the design of clinical trials. Design and publish prespecified analysis of results by sex/gender (even if no difference was noted). If possible, especially if a sex-effect was seen in previous analyses, subjects should be stratified into experimental groups by sex.
3. Ideally, note if sex (biologic characteristics) or gender (influence of social factors, role in society) was recorded, and present the method for determining sex and/or gender.
4. Design and implement large-scale metaanalyses and reviews determining role of sex and gender in past clinical trials.
5. If developing algorithms for patient enrolment into clinical trials, consider sex/gender among other clinically relevant variables.
6. Carry out a preselection process (prescreening) of possible candidates for clinical trials to reduce screening and drop-out failures, taking into account the differences that exist according to sex/gender.
7. Adapt the scales to be used in clinical trials in terms of educational level and age so as not to exclude women in the selection and assessment stages of the inclusion.
8. Adapt the functionality scales according to sex and gender.
9. Add data on the subject's hormonal history to the screening for future clinical trials.
10. Take into account stratification by sex/gender in the risk factors for future studies and clinical trials.

Chapter highlights

- To our knowledge, published clinical trials have not consistently reported sex/gender-disaggregated data. Not considering sex and gender in clinical trials could lead to unnecessary exclusion of compounds that could be effective or safe for only one of the sexes.
- Clinical trials should consider known and emerging sex/gender differences in relevant areas such as AD biomarkers (including digital biomarkers), pharmacokinetics, or pharmacodynamics, and include female-specific data such as hormonal status. These potential differences should be considered not only in the design and implementation of clinical trials, but also in daily clinical practice.
- Women comprise two-thirds of the AD population, however, preliminary data suggest that the proportion of women is lower in current clinical trials. The underrepresentation of women in clinical trials could be caused by numerous factors such as inappropriate inclusion/exclusion criteria

omitting those with lower educational levels, socioeconomic considerations, including absence of a caregiver, comorbidities, or excluding drugs. The selection of subjects to take part in clinical trials can be improved by including a prescreening phase.

References

Albert, M. S., et al. (2011). The diagnosis of mild cognitive impairment due to Alzheimer's disease: Recommendations from the National Institute on Aging-Alzheimer's association workgroups on diagnostic guidelines for Alzheimer's disease. *Alzheimer's & Dementia, 7*(3), 270–279. https://doi.org/10.1016/j.jalz.2011.03.008.

Alzheimer Association. (2019). Alzheimer disease facts and figures 2019. *Alzheimer's & Dementia*, 1–88. Available at: https://www.alz.org/alzheimers-dementia/10_signs.

Ardekani, B. A., Convit, A., & Bachman, A. H. (2016). Analysis of the MIRIAD data shows sex differences in hippocampal atrophy progression. *Journal of Alzheimer's Disease, 50*(3), 847–857. https://doi.org/10.3233/JAD-150780. Netherlands.

Babapour Mofrad, R., et al. (2020). Sex differences in CSF biomarkers vary by Alzheimer disease stage and APOE ε4 genotype. *Neurology, 95*(17), e2378–e2388. https://doi.org/10.1212/WNL.0000000000010629. NLM (Medline).

Babrak, L. M., et al. (2019). Traditional and digital biomarkers: Two worlds apart? *Digital Biomarkers, 3*(2), 92–102. https://doi.org/10.1159/000502000. S. Karger AG.

Beery, A. K., & Zucker, I. (2011). Sex bias in neuroscience and biomedical research. *Neuroscience and Biobehavioral Reviews*, 565–572. https://doi.org/10.1016/j.neubiorev.2010.07.002. NIH Public Access.

Blennow, K., & Zetterberg, H. (2018). Biomarkers for Alzheimer's disease: Current status and prospects for the future. *Journal of Internal Medicine*, 643–663. https://doi.org/10.1111/joim.12816. Blackwell Publishing Ltd.

Boada, M. (2019). Gender and sex bias in clinical trials, recruitment in Alzheimer's disease: Findings from Fundacio ACE. In *Presentation in Clinical Trials on Alzheimer's Disease (CTAD) 2019 and Alzheimer Association International Conference (AAIC) 2020*.

Boada, M., et al. (2014). Design of a comprehensive Alzheimer's disease clinic and research center in Spain to meet critical patient and family needs. *Alzheimer's & Dementia, 10*(3), 409–415. https://doi.org/10.1016/j.jalz.2013.03.006. Elsevier Inc.

Buckley, R. F., et al. (2019). Sex differences in the association of global amyloid and regional tau deposition measured by positron emission tomography in clinically normal older adults. *JAMA Neurology*. https://doi.org/10.1001/jamaneurol.2018.4693.

Budelier, M. M., & Bateman, R. J. (2020). Biomarkers of Alzheimer disease. *The Journal of Applied Laboratory Medicine, 5*(1), 194–208. https://doi.org/10.1373/jalm.2019.030080. Oxford Academic.

Buegler, M., et al. (2020). Digital biomarker-based individualized prognosis for people at risk of dementia. *Alzheimer's & Dementia: Diagnosis, Assessment & Disease Monitoring, 12*(1), e12073. https://doi.org/10.1002/dad2.12073. Wiley.

Cañabate, P., et al. (2017). Social representation of dementia: An analysis of 5,792 consecutive cases evaluated in a memory clinic. *Journal of Alzheimer's Disease, 58*(4), 1099–1108. https://doi.org/10.3233/JAD-161119. IOS Press.

Canevelli, M., et al. (2017). Sex and gender differences in the treatment of Alzheimer's disease: A systematic review of randomized controlled trials. *Pharmacological Research*, *115*, 218–223. https://doi.org/10.1016/j.phrs.2016.11.035. Academic Press.

Carcel, C., et al. (2019). Sex differences in treatment and outcome after stroke: Pooled analysis including 19,000 participants. *Neurology*, *93*(24), e2170–e2180. https://doi.org/10.1212/WNL.0000000000008615. NLM (Medline).

Cavedo, E., et al. (2018). Sex differences in functional and molecular neuroimaging biomarkers of Alzheimer's disease in cognitively normal older adults with subjective memory complaints. *Alzheimer's & Dementia*, *14*(9), 1204–1215. https://doi.org/10.1016/j.jalz.2018.05.014. Elsevier.

Cirillo, D., et al. (2020). Sex and gender differences and biases in artificial intelligence for biomedicine and healthcare. *npj Digital Medicine*, 1–11. https://doi.org/10.1038/s41746-020-0288-5. Nature Research.

Claxton, A., et al. (2013). Sex and ApoE genotype differences in treatment response to two doses of intranasal insulin in adults with mild cognitive impairment or alzheimer's disease. *Journal of Alzheimer's Disease*, 789–797. https://doi.org/10.3233/JAD-122308.

Clayton, J. A., & Collins, F. S. (2014). NIH to balance sex in cell and animal studies. *Nature*, 282–283. https://doi.org/10.1038/509282a. Nature Publishing Group.

Coravos, A., Khozin, S., & Mandl, K. D. (2019). Developing and adopting safe and effective digital biomarkers to improve patient outcomes. *npj Digital Medicine*, 1–5. https://doi.org/10.1038/s41746-019-0090-4. Nature Publishing Group.

Dockendorf, M. F., et al. (2020). Digitally enabled, patient-centric clinical trials: Shifting the drug development paradigm. *Clinical and Translational Science*, 1–15. https://doi.org/10.1111/cts.12910.

Espinosa, A., Alegret, M., Valero, S., Vinyes-Junqué, G., Hernández, I., Mauleón, A., … Boada, M. (2013). A longitudinal follow-up of 550 mild cognitive impairment patients: evidence for large conversion to dementia rates and detection of major risk factors involved. *Journal of Alzheimer's Disease*, *34*, 769–780. https://doi.org/10.3233/JAD-122002.

Ferretti, M. T., et al. (2018). Sex differences in Alzheimer disease—The gateway to precision medicine. *Nature Reviews Neurology*, *14*(8), 457–469. https://doi.org/10.1038/s41582-018-0032-9. Nature Publishing Group.

Ferretti, M. T., et al. (2020). Sex and gender differences in Alzheimer's disease: Current challenges and implications for clinical practice: Position paper of the dementia and cognitive disorders panel of the European academy of neurology. *European Journal of Neurology*, *27*, 928–943. https://doi.org/10.1111/ene.14174.

Filon, J. R., et al. (2016). Gender differences in Alzheimer disease: Brain atrophy, histopathology burden, and cognition. *Journal of Neuropathology and Experimental Neurology*, *75*(8), 748–754. https://doi.org/10.1093/jnen/nlw047.

Flórez-Vargas, O., et al. (2016). Bias in the reporting of sex and age in biomedical research on mouse models. *eLife*. https://doi.org/10.7554/eLife.13615. eLife sciences publications ltd, 5(MARCH2016).

Food and Drug Administration. (1977). *General considerations for the clinical evaluation of drugs*. Available at: https://www.fda.gov/regulatory-information/search-fda-guidance-documents/general-considerations-clinical-evaluation-drugs. (Accessed 23 February 2020).

Food and Drug Administration. (1993). *Study and evaluation of gender differences in the clinical evaluation of drugs*. Available at: https://www.fda.gov/regulatory-information/search-fda-guidance-documents/study-and-evaluation-gender-differences-clinical-evaluation-drugs.

Food and Drug Administration. (2000). *EXELON (rivastigmine tartrate) draft package insert*. Available at: https://www.accessdata.fda.gov/drugsatfda_docs/label/2000/20823lbl.pdf. (Accessed 24 July 2020).

Food and Drug Administration. (2003). *Namenda (Memantine HCI) tablets medical review, Part 4*. Available at: https://www.accessdata.fda.gov/drugsatfda_docs/nda/2003/21-487_Namenda_Medr_P4.pdf. (Accessed 24 July 2020).

Ford, E. S., & Capewell, S. (2007). Coronary heart disease mortality among young adults in the U.S. From 1980 through 2002. Concealed leveling of mortality rates. *Journal of the American College of Cardiology*, *50*(22), 2128–2132. https://doi.org/10.1016/j.jacc.2007.05.056.

Franconi, F., Rosano, G., & Campesi, I. (2015). Need for gender-specific pre-analytical testing: The dark side of the moon in laboratory testing. *International Journal of Cardiology*, 514–535. https://doi.org/10.1016/j.ijcard.2014.11.019. Elsevier Ireland ltd.

General Accounting Office. (1992). *Women's health: FDA needs to ensure more study of gender differences in prescription drug testing, Women's Health: FDA needs to ensure more study of gender differences in prescription drug testing*. Available at: https://www.gao.gov/products/hrd-93-17. (Accessed 23 February 2020).

Health at a Glance. (2019). *OECD (Health at a Glance)*. https://doi.org/10.1787/4dd50c09-en.

Jack, C. R., Jr., et al. (2018). NIA-AA research framework: Toward a biological definition of Alzheimer's disease. *Alzheimer's & Dementia: The Journal of the Alzheimer's Association*, *14*(4), 535–562. https://doi.org/10.1016/j.jalz.2018.02.018. United States: Elsevier.

Jack, C. R., et al. (2017). Age-specific and sex-specific prevalence of cerebral β-amyloidosis, tauopathy, and neurodegeneration in cognitively unimpaired individuals aged 50–95 years: A cross-sectional study. *The Lancet Neurology*, *16*(6), 435–444. https://doi.org/10.1016/S1474-4422(17)30077-7. Lancet Publishing Group.

Kaptchuk, T. J. (2001). The double-blind, randomized, placebo-controlled trial: Gold standard or golden calf? *Journal of Clinical Epidemiology*, 541–549. https://doi.org/10.1016/S0895-4356(00)00347-4. Elsevier Inc.

Kilkenny, C., et al. (2010). Improving bioscience research reporting: The arrive guidelines for reporting animal research. *PLoS Biology*, *8*(6). https://doi.org/10.1371/journal.pbio.1000412.

Kourtis, L. C., et al. (2019). Digital biomarkers for Alzheimer's disease: The mobile/wearable devices opportunity. *npj Digital Medicine*, *2*(1), 1–9. https://doi.org/10.1038/s41746-019-0084-2. Springer Science and Business Media LLC.

Labots, G., et al. (2018). Gender differences in clinical registration trials: Is there a real problem? *British Journal of Clinical Pharmacology*, *84*(4), 700–707. https://doi.org/10.1111/bcp.13497. Blackwell Publishing Ltd.

Laguna-Goya, N., & De Andres-Trelles, F. (2014). Sex as a variable in medicines assessment reports for licensing in the European Union. Can gender bias be excluded? *European Journal of Clinical Pharmacology*, 519–525. https://doi.org/10.1007/s00228-014-1646-5. Springer Verlag.

Lawlor, B., et al. (2018). Nilvadipine in mild to moderate Alzheimer disease: A randomised controlled trial. *PLoS Medicine*, *15*(9), 1–20. https://doi.org/10.1371/journal.pmed.1002660. United States.

Liesinger, A. M., et al. (2018). Sex and age interact to determine clinicopathologic differences in Alzheimer's disease. *Acta Neuropathologica*, *136*(6), 873–885. https://doi.org/10.1007/s00401-018-1908-x. Springer Berlin Heidelberg.

Liu, K. A., & Dipietro Mager, N. A. (2016). Women's involvement in clinical trials: Historical perspective and future implications. *Pharmacy Practice*. https://doi.org/10.18549/PharmPract.2016.01.708. Grupo de Investigacion en Atencion Farmaceutica.

Livingston, G., et al. (2020). Dementia prevention, intervention, and care: 2020 report of the lancet commission. *The Lancet*, 413–446. https://doi.org/10.1016/S0140-6736(20)30367-6. Lancet Publishing Group.

Mauvais-Jarvis, F., et al. (2020). Sex and gender: Modifiers of health, disease, and medicine. *The Lancet*, 565–582. https://doi.org/10.1016/S0140-6736(20)31561-0. Lancet Publishing Group.

Michaud, T. L., et al. (2015). 'Risk stratification using cerebrospinal fluid biomarkers in patients with mild cognitive impairment: An exploratory analysis. *Journal of Alzheimer's Disease*, *47*(3), 729–740. https://doi.org/10.3233/JAD-150066. IOS Press.

Moore, E. E., et al. (2020). Cerebrospinal fluid biomarkers of neurodegeneration, synaptic dysfunction, and axonal injury relate to atrophy in structural brain regions specific to Alzheimer's disease. *Alzheimer's & Dementia*, *16*(6), 883–895. https://doi.org/10.1002/alz.12087. John Wiley and Sons Inc.

Mosca, L., Barrett-Connor, E., & Wenger, N. K. (2011). *Sex/gender differences in cardiovascular disease prevention what a difference a decade makes*. https://doi.org/10.1161/CIRCULATIONAHA.110.968792.

Mosconi, L., et al. (2017). Perimenopause and emergence of an Alzheimer's bioenergetic phenotype in brain and periphery. *PLoS One*, *12*(10), e0185926. https://doi.org/10.1371/journal.pone.0185926. Public library of science.

Mosconi, L., et al. (2018). Increased Alzheimer's risk during the menopause transition: A 3-year longitudinal brain imaging study. *PLoS One*, *13*(12). https://doi.org/10.1371/journal.pone.0207885. Public Library of Science.

National Institute of Health. (2001). *NIH policy on the inclusion of women and minorities as subjects in clinical research*. https://doi.org/10.1016/b978-012274065-7/50013-7.

National Institute of Health. (2014). *NOT-OD-15-015: Notice of Revised NIH Definition of Clinical Trial*.

Palmqvist, S., et al. (2020). Discriminative accuracy of plasma Phospho-tau217 for Alzheimer disease vs other neurodegenerative disorders. *JAMA*, *324*(8), 772–781. https://doi.org/10.1001/jama.2020.12134.

Phillips, S. P., & Hamberg, K. (2016). Doubly blind: A systematic review of gender in randomised controlled trials. *Global Health Action*, *9*(1). https://doi.org/10.3402/gha.v9.29597. Co-Action Publishing.

Prakash, V. S., et al. (2018). Sex Bias in interventional clinical trials. *Journal of Women's Health*, *27*(11), 1342–1348. https://doi.org/10.1089/jwh.2017.6873. Mary Ann Liebert Inc.

Prendergast, B. J., Onishi, K. G., & Zucker, I. (2014). Female mice liberated for inclusion in neuroscience and biomedical research. *Neuroscience and Biobehavioral Reviews*, 1–5. https://doi.org/10.1016/j.neubiorev.2014.01.001. Pergamon.

Richardson, S. S., et al. (2015). Opinion: Focus on preclinical sex differences will not address women's and men's health disparities. *Proceedings of the National Academy of Sciences of the United States of America*, 13419–13420. https://doi.org/10.1073/pnas.1516958112. National Academy of Sciences.

Robin, J., et al. (2020). Evaluation of speech-based digital biomarkers: Review and recommendations. *Digital Biomarkers*, *4*(3), 99–108. https://doi.org/10.1159/000510820. S. Karger AG.

Shansky, R. M. (2019). Are hormones a "female problem" for animal research? *Science*, *364*(6443), 825–826. https://doi.org/10.1126/science.aaw7570.

Smith, R., et al. (2020). The accumulation rate of tau aggregates is higher in females and younger amyloid-positive subjects. *Brain*. https://doi.org/10.1093/brain/awaa327. Oxford University Press (OUP).

Stück, D., et al. (2018). Novel digital voice biomarkers of dementia from the framingham study. In *ALzheimer's Association International Conference*. Available at: https://evidation.com/research/novel-digital-voice-biomarkers-of-dementia-from-the-framingham-study/.

Tifratene, K., et al. (2015). Progression of mild cognitive impairment to dementia due to AD in clinical settings. *Neurology*, *85*(4), 331–338. https://doi.org/10.1212/WNL.0000000000001788. Lippincott Williams and Wilkins.

Vellas, B., et al. (2012). Long-term use of standardised ginkgo biloba extract for the prevention of Alzheimer's disease (GuidAge): A randomised placebo-controlled trial. *The Lancet Neurology*, *11*(10), 851–859. https://doi.org/10.1016/S1474-4422(12)70206-5. Elsevier.

Wang, T., Azad, T. and Rajan, R. (n.d.) The emerging influence of digital biomarkers on healthcare. Available at https://rockhealth.com/reports/the-emerging-influence-of-digital-biomarkers-on-healthcare/ (Accessed 15 February 2021).

Welch, V., et al. (2017). Reporting of sex and gender in randomized controlled trials in Canada: A cross-sectional methods study. *Research Integrity and Peer Review*, *2*(1). https://doi.org/10.1186/s41073-017-0039-6. Springer Science and Business Media LLC.

Zissimopoulos, J. M., et al. (2017). Sex and race differences in the association between statin use and the incidence of Alzheimer disease. *JAMA Neurology*, *74*(2), 225–232. https://doi.org/10.1001/jamaneurol.2016.3783. American Medical Association.

Further reading

Organisation for Economic Co-operation and Development (n.d.) Women and men in OECD countries. Available at: http://www.oecd.org/sdd/womenandmeninoecdcountries.htm (Accessed 24 July 2020).

Rahman, A., et al. (2020). Sex-driven modifiers of Alzheimer risk: A multimodality brain imaging study. *Neurology*, *95*(2), E166–E178. https://doi.org/10.1212/WNL.0000000000009781. Lippincott Williams and Wilkins.

SECTION 3

Gender differences in the socio-economic factors linked to Alzheimer's disease

Maria Teresa Ferretti[a], Annemarie Schumacher Dimech[a,b], and Antonella Santuccione Chadha[a]

[a]*Women's Brain Project, Guntershausen, Switzerland*
[b]*Program Manager, Palliative Care, University of Lucerne, Lucerne, Switzerland*

Alzheimer's disease (AD) is mostly associated with neurological changes in the brain and with its main symptom, memory loss. Nevertheless, the impact of this disease goes beyond neurological symptoms. Socioeconomic factors have been linked to AD and other dementias, both as risk factors and in the study of the disease's impact on an individual as well as a familial and societal level.

Hence, the interest and study in the socioeconomic and psychological factors linked with AD and other dementias are increasing. Indeed, findings in this field of study have led to important observations that have contributed to various aspects of AD and dementia, including drug development, prevention and intervention strategies, and policy. Furthermore, a gender imbalance is observed in many socioeconomic factors, which, as a consequence, contributes to gender differences observed in AD and other dementias. The study of socioeconomic factors is thus relevant, both when investigating risk factors of AD and other dementias, and in consideration of the impact of this disease.

Various socioeconomic factors have been identified as risk factors for AD and other dementias. This knowledge has a very important implication: most, if not all, of these risk factors are modifiable, meaning that addressing and considering them in policy and preventive strategies can actively lead to reducing risk of AD and other dementias. Moreover, various socioeconomic factors, such as education and income, are related to our general health or specific aspects thereof, thus underlining the importance of addressing the gender inequity in these areas. In this section, we focus on the imbalance observed between men and women and how this affects women's brain and mental health. The gender differences observed in various socioeconomic risk factors of AD and other dementias are discussed in detail in Chapter 12, where Ilinca and Suzuki present a comprehensive picture describing the current imbalance and how this is linked to risk of AD.

A second approach in the consideration of socioeconomic factors related to AD and other dementias is understanding the socioeconomic impact of this disease for the person directly affected, as well as that on the individual's family and society in general. Moreover, individual characteristics including gender must be taken into account when considering socioeconomic factors. These considerations contribute to a better understanding of the effects of this disease on the individual and their families, as well as helping develop effective and sustainable policy and strategies to support and empower families living with AD.

In Chapter 13, C. Scerri, Abela and A. Scerri present a broad overview of the psychosocial considerations of living with AD and other dementias. In this chapter, they discuss psychosocial aspects of AD and dementia from a gender perspective in various social contexts, ranging from the family to formal caregivers, and psychosocial interventions.

In Chapter 14, Lorenz-Dant and Mittelman focus on the impact of AD and other dementias on caregivers, providing a comprehensive overview of gender differences observed in AD caregivers. The gender differences presented are not solely linked to the fact that the majority of unpaid caregivers are female, but also to the fact that various studies show that women report more negative outcomes related to their caregiver role.

The last two chapters consider both the preventive aspect of socioeconomic factors and the impact of AD and other dementias. In Chapter 15, Rubinelli and Diviani discuss the significance of communication in AD and dementia, and how individual characteristics such as gender combined with the communication challenges posed by this disease influence the communication process. Ethical aspects of communication with persons living with AD are also addressed in this chapter.

In Chapter 16, Weidner, Barbarino and Lynch discuss the consideration of gender in policy related to AD, where they also put forward concrete proposals for addressing gender inequities. This chapter gives a comprehensive overview of current policies from an international perspective and discusses gender-transformational dementia policies for more effective and sustainable AD and dementia strategies.

In this section, the focus mainly lies on gender, rather than sex, differences. The term "gender" is based on the World Health Organisation's definition referring to the socially constructed characteristics attributed to the male or female sex, including learned behavior, societal expectations, norms, and roles. In this book, we focus on gender differences relating to men and women. This does not signify a lack of recognition of transgender and nonbinary identities. We encourage more inclusive research and data to provide an informed and evidence-based discussion toward an all-inclusive precision medicine approach.

CHAPTER 12

Gender and socioeconomic differences in modifiable risk factors for Alzheimer's disease and other types of dementia throughout the life course

Stefania Ilinca[a] and Elina Suzuki[b]

[a]*European Centre for Social Welfare Policy and Research, Vienna, Austria*
[b]*Organization for Economic Co-operation and Development, Directorate for Employment, Labour and Social Affairs, Paris, France*

In recent years, a growing body of evidence has begun to demonstrate that many risk factors for Alzheimer's disease (AD) and other forms of dementia[a] are modifiable (Livingston et al., 2017, 2020; Sindi, Mangialasche, & Kivipelto, 2015). For many of these risk factors, behavioral changes across the life course could have a positive impact on risk reduction for the onset of AD and dementia in later life. Many potentially modifiable risk factors demonstrate strong socioeconomic inequalities, with people of lower socioeconomic status manifesting a higher prevalence of risk factors including lower educational attainment and physical activity, as well as higher rates of hypertension, diabetes, social isolation, and depression (Fig. 1). Throughout this chapter we focus on some (marked in black in Fig. 1), although not all, risk factors at each life stage, recognizing that their effect is more often than not felt throughout an individual's life course (as represented by the horizontal arrows).

While awareness of the role of behavioral risk factors for AD and other dementias has grown, there has been less attention paid to the sex and gender dimensions of many of these risk factors, as well as how gender inequalities may interact with and exacerbate socioeconomic inequalities in risk factor prevalence. This oversight is particularly notable given the significant differences in dementia prevalence between men and women: women make up two-thirds of people living with AD (Andrew & Tierney, 2018). Furthermore, recent research has investigated the possibility that risk

---

[a] This chapter discusses the impact of modifiable risk factors on dementia, including Alzheimer's disease and other forms, such as vascular dementia.

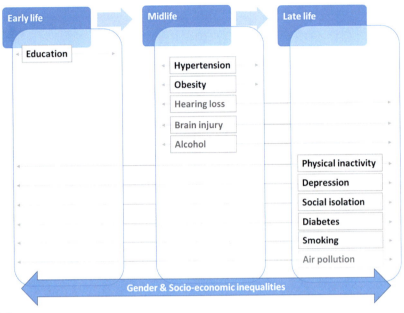

FIG. 1

Risk factors for dementia and Alzheimer's disease across the lifespan. Note: Own elaboration based on Livingston et al. (2020), and Sindi et al. (2015).

factors for dementia are different for women as compared to men and that their relative relevance varies according to sex (Choi, Kwon, Lim, & Chun, 2020).

As populations age and the number of people living with AD and other dementias is set to climb even further, addressing modifiable risk factors for these diseases will be critical in reducing prevalence. Ensuring the gendered dimensions of these risk factors are adequately addressed is fundamental—not only to reducing the sex and gender gap in dementia prevalence, but to reducing the risk of developing this condition.

Recent decades have seen significant progress in reducing gender-based inequalities. Nevertheless, these inequalities persist and can compound over their life course, with attendant effects particularly visible during middle and late adulthood. Strategies that take a life course approach, beginning in early life, are needed to help prevent inequalities from developing in the first place, while policies that address existing inequalities at all life stages can help reduce their impact on health and life outcomes for women.

Sex differences in lifestyle and genetic risk factors are discussed in Chapter 10; the roles of psychiatric comorbidities in Alzheimer's risk (Chapter 7) and of sleep disorders (Chapter 8) are also specifically addressed elsewhere in the book. This chapter examines how gender—that is, the socially constructed characteristics ascribed to being male or female—impacts exposure to modifiable risk factors for AD and dementia throughout the life course, focusing on early life education, behavioral risk factors, socioeconomic aspects of clinical risk factors, mental health, and social contact. It considers how gender and socioeconomic inequalities may intersect, and compound over people's lives, to exacerbate differences in risk factor exposure, and evaluates how these inequalities can impact women's risk of developing AD and other dementias later in life. The impact of socioeconomic determinants is considered both at the individual and the community-level (Brown et al., 2004). We conclude with a consideration of how attenuating these sex and gender differences in modifiable risk factors can be achieved, and what the implications of doing so would be.

Inequality in early educational achievement
Cognitive resilience and dementia risk are associated with early childhood outcomes

Lower educational attainment is robustly associated with a higher risk of developing dementia (Choi et al., 2020), even when individuals achieve higher socioeconomic status in adulthood (Karp et al., 2004). A metaanalysis of available evidence suggests each additional year of education reduces the risk of developing AD by 8% and the risk of developing dementia by 7% (Maccora, Peters, & Anstey, 2020). The relative risk of developing dementia has been found to be quite similar between people with high and medium levels of educational attainment, underscoring the impact that low educational attainment can have across the life course (Karp et al., 2004; Livingston et al., 2017). Moreover, even with the same diagnosis of AD or other dementias, not all individuals follow the same functional trajectory, even with similar changes to the brain (Stern, 2012).

There is a growing consensus that some of these differences may be related to differences in the level of people's cognitive reserve, which may help to protect against some of the biological changes to the brain that occur with the onset of AD and other dementias (Livingston et al., 2017; Stern, 2012; Chapter 6 on neuropsychological symptoms). Low educational attainment has been associated with a lower level of cognitive resilience, indicating that, in addition to a higher likelihood of developing dementia in the first place, individuals with lower levels of educational attainment may be less protected from the biological changes caused by AD and other dementias (Karp et al., 2004). Some of this may be driven by the association between educational attainment and lifelong occupational attainment. Among individuals with high occupational attainment, the risk of developing dementia has been found to be 2.25 times lower than among those with low occupational attainment (Stern, 2012).

Gender and socioeconomic inequalities in educational attainment

Educational attainment has increased considerably in recent decades. Gains have been particularly impressive for women, with gender-based inequalities in educational attainment disappearing or even reversing in many countries (Riphahn & Schwientek,

2015). This is particularly true among middle- and upper-income countries. Among women aged 25–34 in OECD countries, for example, a higher proportion of women (86.7%) than men (83.3%) completed at least upper secondary education. Among those aged 55–64, fewer women than men had completed at least upper secondary education. Across G20 countries, the trend toward higher educational attainment for women than men is even stronger: while nearly three-quarters of women aged 25–34 have at least upper secondary educational attainment, just over half of men have achieved the same level of education (Fig. 2).

While significant gains to education attainment have been made across the board in recent years, gender inequalities in quality and attainment persist. A strong association between parental educational attainment and children's educational attainment continues to be observed. Even though intergenerational educational mobility is largely positive—that is, children who complete a different level of education than their parents are more likely to have completed more schooling rather than less—family background continues to strongly influence educational outcomes (see Fig. 3). Across OECD countries, for example, 42% of children whose parents did not finish upper secondary schooling complete lower secondary schooling or less, compared with just 7% of children where at least one parent attained tertiary education (OECD, 2018). From the other side of the inequality lens, just 13% of children whose parents did not complete upper secondary school attain tertiary education, compared with more than three-fifths (63%) of children where at least one parent had also finished tertiary education (OECD, 2018).

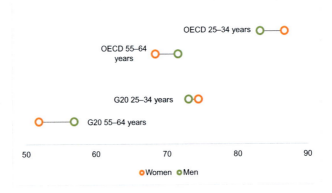

FIG. 2

Percentage of population with upper secondary educational attainment or higher, by gender and age group (2018).

Source: OECD Statistics—Educational attainment and labour-force status database.

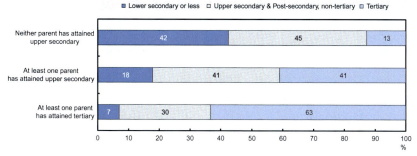

FIG. 3

Likelihood of educational attainment by parental education background—OECD average percentage.

Source: OECD (2018). A broken social elevator? How to promote social mobility. Paris: OECD Publishing. https://doi.org/10.1787/9789264301085-en.

Reducing inequalities in cognitive reserve

The absolute gains to educational attainment made across many countries in recent decades reflect a major global achievement. As women continue to make strides in educational and occupational attainment, it appears likely that at least some of the modifiable, gender-based differences in dementia rates will be reduced, if not eliminated. Given the association between low educational attainment and dementia risk, these educational gains may also have longer-term positive impacts on reducing the number of people who develop dementia in the years to come. At the same time, further research is needed to understand how educational attainment and occupational attainment interact to impact the accumulation of cognitive reserve. For example, while current inconsistencies in the operationalization and measurement of lower education across studies limits comparability and the formulation of precise recommendations (Maccora, Peters, & Anstey, 2020), nevertheless, large gains in dementia prevention can be made by further improving access to education across the globe (Montero-Odasso, Ismail, & Livingston, 2020).

Inequality in behavioral risk factors: Obesity and physical activity

Obesity in midlife represents a major risk factor for developing Alzheimer's disease and other dementias. Overweight and obesity, and in particular obesity in middle age, have been found to dramatically increase the risk of AD and dementia (Beydoun, Beydoun, & Wang, 2008; Fitzpatrick et al., 2009; Kivipelto, Ngandu, Fratiglioni, et al., 2005; Ma, Ajnakina, Steptoe, & Cadar, 2020; Whitmer, Gunderson, Barrett-Connor, Quesenberry, & Yaffe, 2005). Research suggests that individuals with a body mass index (BMI) over 30 (the clinical classification for obesity) are at a 74% higher risk of developing dementia compared with those with a normal BMI, while people with a BMI of 25–30 (the clinical definition of overweight) are 35% more likely to develop dementia, compared with individuals with a normal BMI. Moreover, obesity itself represents a major risk factor for developing other diseases, including vascular diseases and diabetes, which themselves increase the risk of developing dementia (Kivipelto et al., 2005).

The prevalence of obesity has increased rapidly in recent years. Since 1975, obesity has almost tripled around the world, to 650 million adults in 2016 (World Health Organization, 2020). Close to 2 billion adults globally are now overweight (World Health Organization, 2020) (Fig. 4).

In Chapter 10, sex differences in obesity and lack of physical exercise are discussed from a physiological perspective. Additionally, there are strong socioeconomic inequalities in rates of overweight and obesity. Across 27 OECD countries, for example, adults with low educational attainment were 24% more likely to be overweight than those who had completed tertiary schooling (OECD, 2019a). While rates of obesity among men and women are largely similar in high-income countries, the prevalence of obesity is higher among women than men in G20 countries (OECD, 2019a). Moreover, socioeconomic disparities in obesity rates are higher among women than men, highlighting how the intersection of socioeconomic and gender disparities can exacerbate gender-based inequalities. Women have much higher rates of income-based inequality in obesity rates compared with men (Bilger, Kruger, & Finkelstein, 2017; Lakdawalla & Philipson, 2009). Compared with those in the highest income quintile, men in the bottom income quintile are 50% more likely to be obese, while women are 90% more likely to be obese (OECD, 2019a). While more than half (52%) of women who have not completed high school are overweight or obese in OECD countries, just over one-third (36%) of those with tertiary education

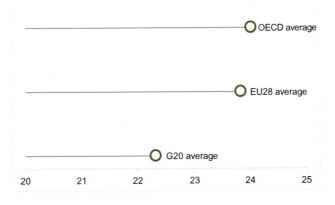

FIG. 4

Percentage prevalence of morbid obesity among adults, 2016.

Source: OECD (2019). The heavy burden of obesity: The economics of prevention, OECD health policy studies. Paris: OECD Publishing. https://doi.org/10.1787/67450d67-en.

are overweight or obese (OECD, 2019a). This gap is much smaller among men: 54% of men with tertiary educational attainment are overweight or obese, compared with 58% of men who did not complete high school (OECD, 2019a).

An unhealthy diet and poor nutritional status are closely linked with sedentary behaviors and levels of physical activity throughout the life course. Physical activity not only determines one's ability to maintain a healthy weight but represents a further independent behavioral risk factor that has been associated with the risk of developing AD and other dementias, with higher levels of physical activity linked with lower risks of dementia onset and cognitive decline among people with dementia (Blondell, Hammersley-Mather, & Veerman, 2014; Buchman et al., 2012; Groot et al., 2016; Laurin, Verreault, Lindsay, Macpherson, & Rockwood, 2001; Podewils et al., 2005; Rovio et al., 2005). In a metaanalysis of studies on physical activity and cognitive decline, Blondell et al. (2014) found higher physical activity to be associated with an 18% reduction in dementia risk. Studies suggest that there may be a dose response to the relationship between physical activity and reductions in dementia risk, with higher levels of physical activity associated with lower risk of developing dementia (Blondell et al., 2014; Buchman et al., 2012; Xu et al., 2017). A further metaanalysis of 18 cohort studies investigating the association between sedentary behavior and cognitive decline has recently established the risk of developing dementia is 30% higher among individuals with sedentary lifestyles (Yan et al., 2020).

There are significant gender- and socioeconomic-based inequalities in physical activity rates. Physical activity is lower overall among women compared with men, and particularly low among women of low socioeconomic status (Weiss, Puterman, Prather, Ware, & Rehkopf, 2020) (Fig. 5).

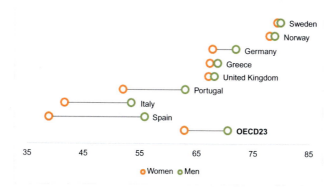

FIG. 5

Percentage of adults who reported moderate weekly physical activity (more than 150 min per week) in 2014.

Source: OECD (2019). The heavy burden of obesity: The economics of prevention, OECD health policy studies. Paris: OECD Publishing. https://doi.org/10.1787/67450d67-en.

Many of the behavioral risk factors for obesity are unequally distributed across populations, with higher rates of unhealthy diet and lower rates of physical activity found among people of lower socioeconomic status (OECD, 2019a). The socioeconomic gradient is steeper for women and children, who are particularly vulnerable to suffering a higher burden of obesity (World Health Organization, 2014). Expanding access to healthy nutrition should be considered a key policy priority for reducing inequalities in obesity based on socioeconomic status. Interventions to maintain a healthy weight targeted at pregnant women and young mothers and those supporting adolescent girls to increase their participation in organized physical activities can also lead to important gains (World Health Organization, 2014). As individuals age, their rates of physical activity decline, while sedentary behaviors become more frequent, with important consequences for their health-related quality of life. High quality impact studies on policy interventions in this field are lacking, but the well documented increase in sedentary behaviors over the last decade in Europe (López-Valenciano et al., 2020) suggests more decisive interventions are needed across gender and throughout the life course.

Inequality in clinical risk factors: Hypertension and diabetes

As for many other chronic conditions, socioeconomic status is recognized as a risk factor for both hypertension and diabetes (Neufcourt, Deguen, Bayat, Zins, & Grimaud, 2020), which in turn are associated with an increased likelihood of developing AD and other dementias in later life (Biessels, Staekenborg, Brunner, Brayne, & Scheltens, 2006; Nagai, Hoshide, & Kario, 2010). An individual's social position and access to economic and social resources impacts cardiovascular and metabolic health both directly and indirectly, through a complex web of interactions between biological, behavioral, and systemic factors. These often include, but are not restricted to, ability to access needed care, quality of care processes, and likelihood of compliance with treatment and lifestyle recommendations (Brown et al., 2004). Although most available research focuses on socioeconomic-related inequalities in chronic conditions during adulthood or later life, there is a growing understanding of the detrimental impact of the accumulation of disadvantage over the life course on cardiovascular health (Pollitt, Rose, & Kaufman, 2005). The available evidence points to large gender and socioeconomic inequalities in both the prevalence and the management of hypertension and diabetes, with considerable heterogeneity between countries and global regions. In the remainder of this chapter we focus on hypertension and diabetes as risk factors from a socioeconomic perspective. A detailed treatment of both risk factors from a physiological perspective is available in Chapter 10.

Gender and socioeconomic inequalities in hypertension among current adult cohorts

Recent data from Europe reveal a small gender gap in the prevalence of hypertension, with women more likely to report high blood pressure (a 2 percentage point—hereafter pp—difference averaged across the EU28), although there is high variability between countries (European Core Health Indicators database). Whereas in Germany, Ireland, the United Kingdom, and Norway, men are at a disadvantage, prevalence is higher among women in most EU countries, with marked gender differences in some Eastern European (Bulgaria 7 pp, Hungary 5 pp) and Baltic countries (Lithuania 11 pp., Latvia 12 pp) (Fig. 6).

Gender differences in hypertension prevalence are closely paralleled by socio-economic inequalities. An overall increased risk of hypertension among low SES individuals is confirmed, irrespective of whether one uses income, occupational, or educational achievement, with more robust associations for women (Leng, Jin, Li, Chen, & Jin, 2015). Recent data from Europe confirms low educational achievement in early life is strongly associated with higher rates of hypertension in all surveyed countries. On average, the proportion of individuals with low educational achievement reporting hypertension across the EU28 is 27.6%, 12 percentage points higher than the share reported among higher educated groups. Confirming previous results (Von dem Knesebeck, Verde, & Dragano, 2006), large variations in the level of educational inequalities in health are apparent between European countries, ranging from 5 pp between the highest and lowest education groups in Norway to 20 pp in Lithuania. While the determinants of these differences are not fully understood, cultural, political, and contextual factors are known to contribute to the patterning and magnitude of social inequalities in health (Eikemo, Huisman, Bambra, & Kunst, 2008) (Fig. 7).

Further complexity is added by a differentiated impact of SES by gender, although evidence is scarce. While some studies find stronger associations of low SES with hypertension among women (Baek, Lee, Lim, & Park, 2015—South Korea; Van Minh, Byass, Chuc, et al., 2006—Vietnam; Veenstra, 2013—Canada), others have failed to identify a significant gender difference (de Gaudemaris et al., 2002—France). Despite

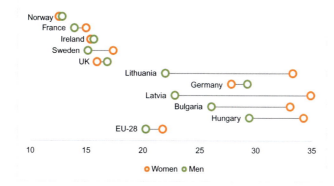

FIG. 6

Share of population reporting high blood pressure: percentage by gender (2014). Note: Own elaboration based on data from the ECHI database. Selected countries include those with the highest and lowest shares of people reporting high blood pressure.

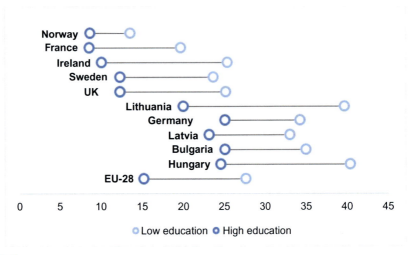

FIG. 7

Proportion of population reporting high blood pressure, by educational attainment (2014). Note: Own elaboration based on data from the ECHI database, collected in 2014. Selected countries include those with the highest and lowest shares of people reporting high blood pressure. Low educational attainment corresponds to less than primary, primary, or lower secondary education, in accordance with ISCED codes; high educational attainment corresponds to tertiary education, in accordance with ISCED codes.

these divergences, at the intersection of gender and socioeconomic disadvantage, lower educated and lower income women represent a group with increased vulnerability and higher likelihood to report high blood pressure, and should be particularly targeted by health promotion and prevention initiatives.

Scarcity of data from low- and middle-income countries renders the assessment of gender and socioeconomic inequalities in prevalence of hypertension in these settings very difficult. This gap in knowledge urgently needs to be addressed, as the prevalence and burden of hypertension is significantly higher in the developing world (two out of every three people with hypertension live in low- or middle-income countries). While insufficient to draw any definitive conclusions, available evidence points to a positive association of hypertension with socioeconomic status in some developing countries, although results are mixed on whether this gradient is significant in both urban and rural settings (Busingye et al., 2014) and in different geographical regions (Leng et al., 2015).

Gender and socioeconomic inequalities in diabetes among current adult cohorts

The number of adults with diabetes in the world increased from 108 million in 1980 to 422 million in 2014, as the global age-standardized diabetes prevalence rose from

4.3% in 1980 to 9.0% in 2014 in men, and from 5.0% to 7.9% in women. Diabetes prevalence has risen during this period in all countries (albeit at various rates), an increase which can only partly be accounted for by population aging (NCD RisC, 2016). In close connection with obesity patterns, diabetes incidence rises with age in both sexes and reaches the highest rates among very old women (Kautzky-Willer, Harreiter, & Pacini, 2016), although diabetes tends to be diagnosed at earlier ages and lower BMI for men. Sex differences in diabetes as a risk factor for AD and other dementias are discussed in Chapter 10. While gender differences in prevalence of diabetes are pervasive, their size varies significantly across countries, partly reflecting differences in population structure but also cultural, lifestyle, and environmental differences.

Similarly to hypertension, socioeconomic status is inversely associated with diabetes prevalence in both sexes (Agardh, Allebeck, Hallqvist, Moradi, & Sidorchuk, 2011), but the strength of the association has been found to be higher for women, after controlling for other known risk factors (Kautzky-Willer, Dorner, Jensby, & Rieder, 2012). Confirming this pattern, recent data from Europe points to consistently higher diabetes prevalence among lower income older age groups (lowest income quintile), while those at the top of the income distribution fare much better. The largest differences are observed in Southern European countries, while relatively lower differences are registered in Eastern and Western Europe. The impact of SES on diabetes prevalence is stronger for women as compared to men, as evidenced by higher absolute differences between the poorest and richest groups of older women (Fig. 8).

More individuals live with diabetes in low- and middle-income countries than in the developed world. China and India alone account for almost one third of all individuals living with diabetes globally. Nonetheless, age-standardized prevalence rates tend to be lower in low- and middle-income countries, whereas in high-income countries, diabetes is disproportionately concentrated among lower socioeconomic groups (Kautzky-Willer et al., 2016). Further research is needed in order to identify the patterns of association and establish links between the risk of developing diabetes and socioeconomic status in low- and middle-income countries. Current evidence is equivocal with some studies identifying an inverse association (Agardh et al., 2011) while others point to a positive relationship (Mutyambizi, Booysen, Stokes, Pavlova, & Groot, 2019).

As evidence accumulates, it becomes increasingly evident that not only is diabetes associated with a considerable increase in the risk of developing AD and other types of dementia (Gudala, Bansal, Schifano, & Bhansali, 2013), but that the strength of this association differs between men and women (Choi et al., 2020). The incidence and prevalence of dementia are considerably higher among women diagnosed with diabetes with respect to men, with both showing an increasing trend over recent decades (Alsharif et al., 2020).

Inequalities in awareness, access to care, and rate of complications

Inequalities in outcomes and health status are determined not only by the distribution of socioeconomic risk factors but also by inequitable access to care and

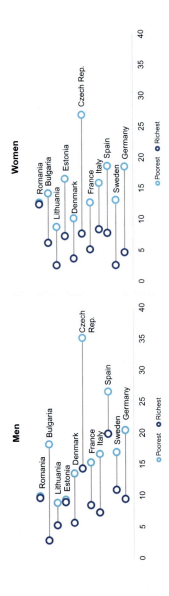

FIG. 8

Percentage prevalence of diabetes and high blood sugar by gender and income quintile in Europe, 2016. Note: Own elaborations based on data from SHARE wave 7 for individuals aged 50 and above in 2016. The richest group refers to people in the top income quintile (20% of the population with the highest income), while the poorest group refers to people in the bottom income quintile (20% of the population with the lowest income). Weighted, not age-standardized. Country subsample selected to maximize geographical coverage.

support services, by levels of health literacy, and different treatment adherence patterns between groups. Consistent with a large body of research on gender differences in awareness and health-seeking behavior, women and individuals with higher educational achievement were shown to be more likely to control and manage hypertension, once diagnosed (Chow et al., 2013). No gender differences in access to care and treatment of diabetes were found in OECD countries (Ricci-Cabello, Ruiz-Perez, De Labry-Lima, & Marquez-Calderon, 2010). However, low socioeconomic status is associated with lower rates of effective disease management and higher probability of complications. Low-income individuals and those from minority ethnic groups were found to be less likely to receive a timely diabetes diagnosis and access appropriate treatment, leading to lower rates of diabetes control in these groups (Ricci-Cabello et al., 2010). Higher barriers to accessing care and lower care quality in deprived areas contribute to these negative outcomes and have been directly linked to higher risk of developing complications in people living in poorly served communities (Grintsova, Maier, & Mielck, 2014). (Gender differences in communication relating to AD is discussed in detail in Chapter 15)

From a global perspective, awareness, treatment, and management of hypertension and diabetes are lower in the developing world as compared with high-income countries (Chow, Teo, Rangarajan, et al., 2013; De Silva et al., 2016). Sustained investment in awareness-raising and management programs have led to increases in the rates of hypertension treatment and control in high-income countries, gains that were not replicated in lower-resource settings where parallel investment has, by and large, been missing (Mills et al., 2016). Similarly, higher rates of complications can be traced back to poor diabetes management in low- and middle-income countries. An integrated prevention and management approach for cardiovascular and metabolic health is essential for improving health outcomes and reducing inequalities in health, particularly in the developing world, where the burden of disease is higher. In turn, improvements in prevention and management strategies would contribute to lower risk for AD and other dementias, in particular, in high-risk groups including women and other minorities.

Social support, social isolation, and depression

Depressive symptoms and social isolation occur so commonly in the clinical presentation of dementia that they are recognized as prodromal symptoms (Livingston et al., 2017) (see Chapter 7 on psychiatric symptoms). However, evidence is accumulating that both depression and social isolation also act as independent risk factors for dementia, particularly when they occur in later life. Depression can influence cognitive function by triggering changes in stress hormones, neuronal growth factors, and hippocampal volume (Livingston, 2017), while social isolation can lead to cognitive inactivity, lack of stimulation, and decline in cognitive function (Evans, Martyr, Collins, Brayne, & Clare, 2019; Kuiper et al., 2015). In a complex pattern of interactions, social isolation and loneliness contribute to increases in dementia-risk through their association with higher risk of hypertension, heart disease, and depression (Courtin & Knapp, 2017). The lack of social support and small social networks in old age are known to be associated with excess mortality risk, early mortality, and generally lower physical and psychological health (Coyle & Dugan, 2012; Mund, Freuding, Möbius, Horn, & Neyer, 2019).

Social isolation and poor mental health are deeply rooted in socioeconomic circumstances in all age groups, but are particularly pertinent for older individuals, who are more exposed and more susceptible to the detrimental effects of poverty, loss of independence, and "trigger events" such as bereavement and severe health shocks (Yasamy, Dua, Harper, & Saxena, 2013). While the size of gender and socioeconomic differences in depression varies substantially across countries, reflecting large discrepancies in social environments (Richardson, Keyes, Medina, & Calvo, 2020), women are consistently found to experience depression more frequently over the life course, and to be more susceptible to it in old age as well (OECD/EU, 2018). They are also more likely to live alone, in isolation, or in poverty, placing them at considerable disadvantage for poor mental and cognitive health outcomes.

Old-age poverty

Material deprivation and poverty are key determinants of wellbeing for older people and have been found to predict incident dementia in this age group, with a strength of association comparable with that of low educational achievement (Samuel et al., 2020). Financial distress in old age is amenable to policy intervention and closely linked to the generosity and breadth of pension systems. In 15 OECD countries, poverty rates are higher in older age groups (65 years and above) than in the general population, exposing them to insecurity, distress, and increased risk of poor mental health (OECD, 2019b). Furthermore, poverty, social exclusion, and isolation mutually reinforce each other, placing those groups that find themselves at the intersection of multiple sources of disadvantage (e.g., older women, minority ethnic groups, migrants) in positions of extreme vulnerability (WHO, 2016).

A review of empirical research on old age poverty found higher prevalence of poverty among women and higher vulnerability to its detrimental effects on mental health. Older women who experience deprivation and poverty are more likely to report negative mental health outcomes and psychological distress than men with low SES. This is especially the case for older women who live alone. At the intersection of gender discrimination, isolation, and deprivation they are subjected to a complex interplay of economic, social, and cultural disadvantage, which reflects in high rates of adverse physical and mental health outcomes (Kwan & Walsh, 2018).

In OECD countries, older women are at considerably greater risk of poverty than men (Fig. 9). The average old age poverty rate for women across OECD countries was 15.7% in 2016, as compared to 10.3% for older men (data from 2016 or latest available). Korea, Sweden, and the United States had the largest gender gaps in old age poverty rates, while countries where old age poverty is less prevalent also tend to fare better in terms of gender equality in old age poverty.

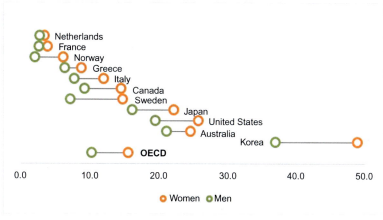

FIG. 9

Percentage poverty rates by gender in selected OECD countries, 2016. Note: Poverty rate calculated as a percentage with incomes less than 50% of median household disposable income at country level. Based on data from OECD (2019b)—Pensions at a glance.

Data scarcity and differences in measurement and reporting practice make a comparison across world regions difficult. However, older age groups are more likely to be exposed and vulnerable to poverty in the developing world. The World Ageing Report 2015 concludes that older persons in most sub-Saharan African countries are at a considerable socioeconomic disadvantage and experience poverty more often than other age groups. In Asian countries, differences in poverty rates between age groups remain small, while in most Latin American countries, older people fare better than younger age groups (World Health Organization, 2015). Poverty rates are higher among older women globally, partly due to systematically lower pension coverage, as women are more heavily involved in informal or unpaid family work (International Labour Organization, 2014).

Prevailing rates of old age poverty around the world are hampering ongoing dementia prevention efforts, placing millions of older individuals at higher risk of developing the disease. It is essential to complement public health initiatives toward dementia prevention-targeted policies that improve access to economic opportunity throughout the life course and strengthen safety net programs (Samuel et al., 2020).

Gender and socioeconomic inequalities in clinical depression among current adult cohorts

Globally, the total number of people with depression was estimated to exceed 300 million in 2015 (equivalent to 4.4% of the world's population), with enormous consequences for societies. Depression is ranked by the WHO as the single largest contributor to global disability, accounting for 7.5% of all years lived with disability in 2015, and contributing considerably to preventable mortality statistics (World Health

Organization, 2017a). The staggering economic and social costs of depression worldwide are primarily associated with impaired human capital development and productivity losses, which weigh heavily on communities in developed and developing countries, and slow economic growth. Depression affects all population groups but prevalence rates increase with age, peaking in older adulthood (55–74 years), in disadvantaged and deprived communities and among groups exposed to violence and displacement (World Health Organization, 2017b). The total number of people living with depression globally continues to increase. It is estimated that depression prevalence worldwide rose by 18.4% between 2005 and 2015. The increase is partly a reflection of demographic growth and a failure to address the determinants of depression and contain the number of those affected, particularly in late adulthood (Global Burden of Disease, 2015), although it could also be associated with increased diagnosis rates as awareness of mental health issues increases around the world.

Depressive disorders (as well as anxiety and bipolar disorders) are known to be more common among women (OECD/EU, 2018) (see also Chapter 7 on psychiatric symptoms). As a result, the burden of depression and its economic, social, and health-related consequences disproportionately affect women, in all age groups (Ferrari et al., 2013). Analyses of data from 10 European countries found rates of depression to be more than twice as high among older women (60–80 years old) than among men, and showing a pronounced educational gradient. Differences in later life depression were larger in countries with lower economic development and weaker welfare systems, showing a clear East-West divide (Hansen, Slagsvold, & Veenstra, 2017).

Estimates of chronic depression prevalence in European countries show depression rates are higher among women (8.8%, averaged over all age groups) than men (5.3%) and prevalence increases steadily with age. Older women (75+) report the highest rates of any gender-age group (12.4%) (OECD/EU, 2018) (Fig. 10).

Across gender and age groups, depression is more commonly reported by people with lower socioeconomic status, be it measured by education level or income. In the EU, those living in the lowest income group are more than two times as likely to report chronic depression than those at the top of the income distribution (OECD/EU, 2018). Income inequalities are more pronounced among women in all countries, suggesting they are more vulnerable to the detrimental mental health effects of poverty and deprivation (Box 1; Fig. 11).

Depression and dementia are the most common mental and neurological disorders among older individuals at a global level and account for a considerable proportion of years lived with disability in this age group (World Health Organization, 2017b). By reducing the prevalence of depression in the general population and particularly among vulnerable groups, significant gains in dementia risk reduction can be expected. It is therefore important to continue combating the stigma associated with mental disorders, and to train and support care professionals in primary care settings in order to increase diagnosis and improve care options for older people with depression. At the same time, effective dementia and depression prevention strategies must emphasize the development of age-friendly environments and communities, ensuring

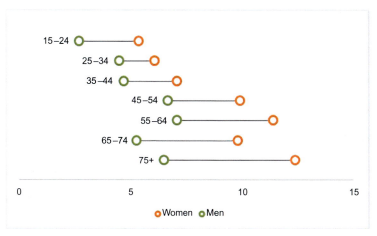

FIG. 10

Percentage prevalence of depression (self-reported) in the EU by age group and gender, 2018.

Source: Own elaboration based on data from Eurostat Database (based on European Health Interview Survey, 2014), as reported in Health at a Glance: Europe 2018.

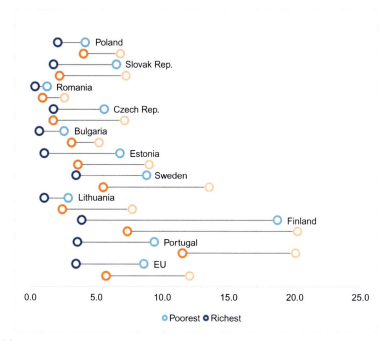

FIG. 11

Percentage prevalence of depression in selected EU countries by gender and income, 2018.

Source: Own elaboration based on data from Eurostat Database (based on European Health Interview Survey collected in 2014), as reported in Health at a Glance: Europe 2018. The richest group refers to people in the top income quintile (20% of the population with the highest income), while the poorest group refers to people in the bottom income quintile (20% of the population with the lowest income).

> **Box 1 Late life depression—misdiagnosis and under-recognition**
> - Depression in late life co-occurs with mild cognitive impairment in an estimated 32% of cases and is associated with higher relative risk of progressing to dementia, lower quality of life, and reduced functioning (Ismail et al., 2017). It is often associated with risk factors that become significantly more prevalent in late life: chronic somatic illness, functional impairment, lack of close social contacts, stressful life-events, and bereavement (Girgus, Yang, & Ferri, 2017).
> - Depression remains underdiagnosed and undertreated in older age groups. Older people are less likely to identify symptoms as related to a depressive mood but rather as physical complaints such as fatigue, weight loss, and social withdrawal. It is therefore left to clinicians, often primary care professionals, to identify the underlying cause (Allen, Balfour, Bell, & Marmot, 2014). Diagnosis is further complicated by widespread stigma related to depression and a common belief among older people that depression symptoms are a normal consequence of distressing events related to aging and physical ill health. This often leads to avoidance of mentioning symptoms in medical consultations, particularly by older men (Murray et al., 2006).
> - Care professionals are more likely to overlook depression symptoms in older adults as compared to younger patients. Some care professionals still hold normalizing attitudes toward late life depression, which is seen as a justifiable and understandable consequence of distress related to aging, social isolation, and loneliness (Barley, Murray, Walters, et al., 2011). They are prone to undertreat and might be reluctant to consider pharmacological treatment to address a problem they perceive as deriving primarily from social circumstances (Murray et al., 2006). Limited availability of psychosocial interventions to prevent and to address late life depression and the reluctance of care professionals to prescribe pharmacological treatment leads to considerable rates of undertreatment, likely to be higher in more deprived areas and in care systems with gaps in coverage and development of mental health services.

living conditions that support wellbeing and that all older people have the necessary resources for a dignified and decent standard of living.

Gender and socioeconomic inequalities in social isolation and loneliness

Loneliness and social isolation are closely related but separate concepts that are often cited among the risk factors for AD and other dementias (Adolfsson, Nordin, Adolfsson, & Anderson, 2020; Rafnsson, Orrell, d'Orsi, Hogervorst, & Steptoe, 2020; Sutin, Stephan, Luchetti, & Terracciano, 2020). While loneliness describes a subjective feeling of unfulfilled need for social and intimate connections (sometimes referred to as painful isolation), it is conceptually distinct from solitude or aloneness, which refer to objective physical isolation (McHugh, Kenny, Lawlor, Steptoe, & Kee, 2017). While a positive correlation exists between loneliness and social isolation, this overlap is limited, with survey data showing diverging response patterns on the two measures of social connectedness (Coyle & Dugan, 2012). People can feel lonely even if they have extensive social contacts, just as many people who live relatively isolated lives do not experience loneliness—a concept described as social asymmetry (McHugh et al., 2017). Social connections and companionship are as fundamental for psychological wellbeing in old age as they are in all life stages. However, concerns have been mounting over a potential public health crisis of loneliness and isolation in old age accentuated by demographic aging, as well as changing cultural and living arrangement patterns.

Changing patterns of living arrangements and marital status

Mental distress, loneliness, and isolation in older adults are closely linked to their living arrangements. As compared to those living in larger households, older people living alone are significantly more likely to report feeling sad or depressed and might face more barriers to maintaining good health and independence (OECD, 2019b). Living arrangements among older age groups have shifted considerably over recent decades, increasingly moving away from a high prevalence of large families co-residing in intergenerational households to smaller households and nuclear families. Globally, co-residence with children among older adults has declined from 65% in 1990 to approximately 53% in 2010 (United Nations, 2017).

Living arrangements patterns differ markedly across countries and regions, reflecting differences in family sizes and demographic structure, as well as cultural norms, social dynamics, and economic conditions. Older adults in advanced economies are more likely to live alone, while co-residence with children was a common household living arrangement for older persons in developing regions (OECD, 2019c; United Nations, 2017).

Cultural differences notwithstanding, the degree of independence individuals can maintain in old age and their ability to continue to live alone, in the community, is linked to accessibility of financial and community-based support systems (United Nations, 2017). In this sense, higher rates of older people living alone in high-income countries are a reflection of considerable achievements in social protection and support systems, allowing financial and functional independence to be maintained long after working age. At the same time, the trend toward independent living has exposed many older adults to isolation and loneliness, particularly women and those relying on limited material resources, and as a result, to increased health risks related to loneliness.

The share of older people living alone increases with age and is considerably higher among women in all world regions. In 2010, 15% of older women aged 60–79 and 32% of those aged 80 and above lived alone. These rates are twice as high as those registered for older men. Gender differences are widest in Europe and North America, irrespective of age, and smallest in Asian countries. While older men are less likely to live alone than women, some evidence suggests those who do so are at higher risk of experiencing loneliness and lack of social contacts (World Health Organization, 2018) (Fig. 12).

A pronounced income gradient is apparent in the living arrangements of older persons, irrespective of gender. Poorer older individuals are more likely to live alone across European countries, while those as the top of the income distribution more often live in larger households. Similarly to the case of depression and clinical risk factors, income gaps are relatively larger for older women as compared to men, suggesting older women living alone are particularly vulnerable to deprivation and economic hardship (Box 2; Fig. 13).

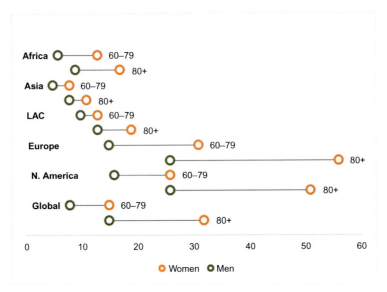

FIG. 12

Percentage share of older people living alone by gender, age group, and geographical region, 2017. *LAC*, Latin American countries; *N. America*, North America.

Source: Own elaboration based on data from the United Nations Database on the Living Arrangements of Older Persons 2017 (United Nations, 2017).

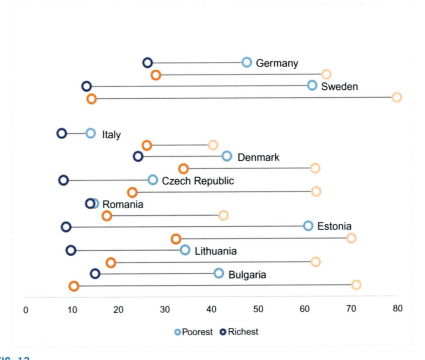

FIG. 13

Percentage share of older people in Europe living alone, by gender and income quintile, 2016. Note: Elaborations based on SHARE wave 7 for individuals aged 60 and above in 2016. Weighted data. *Orange circles* represent women, while *blue circles* represent men.

Box 2 Combating social isolation and loneliness—lessons for policy-making

Several European countries have launched public awareness campaigns, implemented support measures to reduce social isolation, and increased targeting of social support programs toward groups at risk of social isolation and exclusion. In 2018, the UK famously launched a national strategy to address loneliness and appointed a Minister for Loneliness. By that time, many other European countries had explicitly identified reducing loneliness and social exclusion as part of their national health and aging strategies (e.g., Portugal, Finland, Czech Republic, France, Poland) and were implementing peer-to-peer, group, and community-level interventions to support older people at risk of loneliness (Zolyomi, 2019).

To date, a comprehensive evaluation of their impact is lacking but some lessons for policy-making can be identified:

- Effective interventions for promoting mentally healthy aging emphasize adaptability, and focus on community-wide approaches and on productive engagement. Older adults can be encouraged to remain socially engaged through organizing community arts and cultural activities as well as friendship building programs. Signposting services and ensuring accessibility of activities to older people with functional limitations can improve take-up and promote equity in access (McDaid, Hewlett, & Park, 2017).
- Policies focused on empowering older people are effective in challenging ageist attitudes and combating isolation. In Europe, the share of people who volunteer among older age groups (65+) is comparable to that in the general population (Eurofound, EQLS 2016). Older volunteers report the main benefits they derive are the opportunity to use existing skills, develop social contacts, reduce isolation, and build self-esteem. All countries can and should invest in developing the necessary social infrastructure to allow older people to remain active and contribute to their communities (EUROFOUND European Foundation for the Improvement of Living and Working Conditions, 2011).
- Universally delivered interventions should be supplemented by specific initiatives targeted at vulnerable groups of older people. As the experience and challenges of aging vary widely for those placed at the intersection of different sources of vulnerability, a focus on tailoring support services to the specific needs of users and ensuring one-to-one support is available when needed is essential for effectiveness and impact.

Discussion

Gender differences in the prevalence of AD and dementia are large and ubiquitous. Two-thirds of people with dementia living in the United States are women and the most recent European estimates suggest that out of the 8.8 million people living with dementia in Europe, over 6 million are women (Alzheimer Europe, 2019). These statistics are often explained by the survival advantage of women: dementia prevalence increases markedly with age and women live longer than men. It is, in fact, the case that in the oldest age group (85+), where dementia prevalence is highest, women outnumber men 2 to 1 in Europe. Throughout this chapter we have summarized the growing evidence for a complementary, although not competing, explanation: that there are pervasive inequalities in risk factors, which systematically place certain population groups, including women, at increased risk of dementia. In so doing, we are hoping to contribute to a growing literature that explores factors other than age and survival advantage in explaining sex and gender differences in dementia (Ferretti et al., 2018). Importantly, all AD and dementia risk factors we have considered are modifiable. So, while the evidence we collected is cause for alarm, it also offers a direct pathway to the prevention of millions of dementia cases worldwide, while reducing inequity in health.

Women are placed at considerable disadvantage with respect to both behavioral and clinical risk factors, and they experience worse mental health and social isolation than men. Put simply, women belonging to old age cohorts today have been more exposed to risk throughout the life course. Similarly, people with low socioeconomic status, be it measured by income, or by educational or occupational attainment, show higher exposure to all risk factors and limited opportunity to mitigate their effects. What is more, women are systematically more vulnerable to the detrimental impacts of low SES on health outcomes, highlighting the vulnerability to adverse health outcomes of those groups that find themselves at the intersection of gender, social class, and other sources of disadvantage.

Progress on reducing prevalence and inequalities in modifiable risk factors for dementia can be and has been made. Large gains in educational attainment in early life for women across the world will likely contribute to reducing the number of dementia cases for future cohorts. Similarly, disease management programs and better access to preventive and curative care have helped to address the high prevalence of clinical risk factors in those developed countries that have invested in health promotion efforts. If similar gains can be made in the developing world, where the majority of people with dementia live today, one can expect a relevant reduction in prevalence for future old age cohorts. It remains however the case that reducing inequality in modifiable risk factors for dementia will hinge on countries' ability to reduce levels of gender and socioeconomic inequality more generally; because, while some facets of inequality in health and access to care can be improved through sustained action within health systems and the purposive targeting of preventive health programs to women and lower SES groups, the majority of differences we have described have deep roots that must be addressed through more comprehensive, society-wide approaches.

It is, therefore, crucial that researchers increase their efforts to identify differences between groups not only in AD and dementia prevalence but also in the risk factors they are exposed to. The data they collect should be regularly questioned on group specific effects, both for sex and socioeconomic status, rather than assuming people living with or at risk of developing AD and dementia are a homogeneous group. It is only through understanding and addressing the gendered and unequal nature of modifiable risk factors that we can ensure that more effective and sustainable prevention strategies are put in place.

Chapter highlights

- There are pervasive gender inequalities in modifiable risk factors for Alzheimer's disease and dementia, which place women at a disadvantage throughout the life course.
- Gender and social class inequality intersect, rendering women more vulnerable to the detrimental impacts of low SES on health outcomes.

- Some gender differences in risk factors will be attenuated as more recent cohorts move toward old age (e.g., education) showing important progress can be made by addressing the social determinants of health.
- Systematic failures to identify and properly address modifiable risk factors for dementia (e.g., chronic disease management), particularly among disadvantaged groups, have put considerable numbers of people at increased risk for developing the condition.
- A successful prevention strategy for dementia must take a population health approach and build on reducing inequalities in risk factors and access to treatment and care.

References

Adolfsson, A. N., Nordin, M., Adolfsson, R., & Anderson, N. C. (2020). Loneliness increases the risk of all-cause dementia and Alzheimer's disease. *Journals of Gerontology. Series B, Psychological Sciences and Social Sciences*, 75(5), 919–926.

Agardh, E., Allebeck, P., Hallqvist, J., Moradi, T., & Sidorchuk, A. (2011). Type 2 diabetes incidence and socio-economic position: A systematic review and meta-analysis. *International Journal of Epidemiology*, 40, 804–818.

Allen, J., Balfour, R., Bell, R., & Marmot, M. (2014). Social determinants of mental health. *International Review of Psychiatry*, 26(4), 392–407. https://doi.org/10.3109/09540261.2014.928270.

Alsharif, A. A., Wei, L., Ma, T., Man, K. K., Lau, W. C., Brauer, R., … Wong, I. C. (2020). Prevalence and incidence of dementia in people with diabetes mellitus. *Journal of Alzheimer's Disease*, 75(2), 607–615.

Alzheimer Europe. (2019). *Dementia in Europe yearbook 2019: Estimating the prevalence of dementia in Europe*. Available from https://www.alzheimer-europe.org/content/download/195515/1457520/file/FINAL%2005707%20Alzheimer%20Europe%20yearbook%202019.pdf.

Andrew, M. K., & Tierney, M. C. (2018). The puzzle of sex, gender and Alzheimer's disease: Why are women more often affected than men? *Women's Health*, 14, 1745506518817995.

Baek, T. H., Lee, H. Y., Lim, N. K., & Park, H. Y. (2015). Gender differences in the association between socioeconomic status and hypertension incidence: The Korean Genome and Epidemiology Study (KoGES). *BMC Public Health*, 15(1), 852.

Barley, E. A., Murray, J., Walters, P., et al. (2011). Managing depression in primary care: A meta-synthesis of qualitative and quantitative research from the UK to identify barriers and facilitators. *BMC Family Practice*, 12. https://doi.org/10.1186/1471-2296-12-47.

Beydoun, M., Beydoun, H., & Wang, Y. (2008). Obesity and central obesity as risk factors for incident dementia and its subtypes: A systematic review and meta-analysis. *Obesity Reviews*, 9(3), 204–218.

Biessels, G. J., Staekenborg, S., Brunner, E., Brayne, C., & Scheltens, P. (2006). Risk of dementia in diabetes mellitus: A systematic review. *Lancet Neurology*, 5(1), 64–74.

Bilger, M., Kruger, E. J., & Finkelstein, E. A. (2017). Measuring socioeconomic inequality in obesity: Looking beyond the obesity threshold. *Health Economics*, 26(8), 1052–1066.

Blondell, S. J., Hammersley-Mather, R., & Veerman, J. L. (2014). Does physical activity prevent cognitive decline and dementia?: A systematic review and meta-analysis of longitudinal studies. *BMC Public Health*, 14(1), 510.

Brown, A. F., Ettner, S. L., Piette, J., Weinberger, M., Gregg, E., Shapiro, M. F., et al. (2004). Socioeconomic position and health among persons with diabetes mellitus: A conceptual framework and review of the literature. *Epidemiologic Reviews*, *26*(1), 63–77.

Buchman, A. S., Boyle, P. A., Yu, L., Shah, R. C., Wilson, R. S., & Bennett, D. A. (2012). Total daily physical activity and the risk of AD and cognitive decline in older adults. *Neurology*, *78*(17), 1323–1329.

Businger, D., Arabshahi, S., Subasinghe, A. K., Evans, R. G., Riddell, M. A., & Thrift, A. G. (2014). Do the socioeconomic and hypertension gradients in rural populations of low- and middle-income countries differ by geographical region? A systematic review and meta-analysis. *International Journal of Epidemiology*, *43*(5), 1563–1577. https://doi.org/10.1093/ije/dyu112.

Choi, J., Kwon, L. N., Lim, H., & Chun, H. W. (2020). Gender-based analysis of risk factors for dementia using senior cohort. *International Journal of Environmental Research and Public Health*, *17*(19), 7274.

Chow, C. K., Teo, K. K., Rangarajan, S., et al. (2013). Prevalence, awareness, treatment, and control of hypertension in rural and urban communities in high-, middle-, and low-income countries. *JAMA*, *310*(9), 959–968. https://doi.org/10.1001/jama.2013.184182.

Courtin, E., & Knapp, M. (2017). Social isolation, loneliness and health in old age: A scoping review. *Health & Social Care in the Community*, *25*(3), 799–812.

Coyle, C. E., & Dugan, E. (2012). Social isolation, loneliness and health among older adults. *Journal of Aging and Health*, *24*(8), 1346–1363.

de Gaudemaris, R., Lang, T., Chatellier, G., Larabi, L., Lauwers-Cances, V., Maitre, A., & Diene, E. (2002). Socioeconomic inequalities in hypertension prevalence and care: The IHPAF Study. *Hypertension*, *39*(6), 1119–1125. https://doi.org/10.1161/01.HYP.0000018912.05345.55.

De Silva, A. P., De Silva, S. H., Haniffa, R., Liyanage, I. K., Jayasinghe, K. S., Katulanda, P., ... Rajapakse, L. C. (2016). A survey on socioeconomic determinants of diabetes mellitus management in a lower middle income setting. *International Journal for Equity in Health*, *15*, 74. https://doi.org/10.1186/s12939-016-0363-3.

Eikemo, T. A., Huisman, M., Bambra, C., & Kunst, A. E. (2008). Health inequalities according to educational level in different welfare regimes: A comparison of 23 European countries. *Sociology of Health & Illness*, *30*(4), 565–582.

EUROFOUND European Foundation for the Improvement of Living and Working Conditions. (2011). *Participation in volunteering and unpaid work*. Luxembourg: Second European Quality of Life Survey.

Evans, I. E., Martyr, A., Collins, R., Brayne, C., & Clare, L. (2019). Social isolation and cognitive function in later life: A systematic review and meta-analysis. *Journal of Alzheimer's Disease*, *70*(s1), S119–S144.

Ferrari, A. J., Charlson, F. J., Norman, R. E., Patten, S. B., Freedman, G., Murray, C. J., ... Whiteford, H. A. (2013). Burden of depressive disorders by country, sex, age, and year: Findings from the global burden of disease study 2010. *PLoS Medicine*, *10*(11). https://doi.org/10.1371/journal.pmed.1001547, e1001547.

Ferretti, M. T., Iulita, M. F., Cavedo, E., Chiesa, P. A., Schumacher Dimech, A., Chadha, A. S., ... Depypere, H. (2018). Sex differences in Alzheimer disease—The gateway to precision medicine. *Nature Reviews Neurology*, *14*(8), 457–469.

Fitzpatrick, A. L., Kuller, L. H., Lopez, O. L., Diehr, P., O'Meara, E. S., Longstreth, W. T., & Luchsinger, J. A. (2009). Midlife and late-life obesity and the risk of dementia: Cardiovascular health study. *Archives of Neurology*, *66*(3), 336–342.

Girgus, J. S., Yang, K., & Ferri, C. V. (2017). The gender difference in depression: Are elderly women at greater risk for depression than elderly men? *Geriatrics*, *2*(4), 35.

Global Burden of Disease. (2015). Disease and Injury Incidence and Prevalence Collaborators, and others. Global, regional, and national incidence, prevalence, and years lived with disability for 310 diseases and injuries, 1990–2015: A systematic analysis for the Global Burden of Disease Study 2015. *Lancet*, *388*, 10053.

Grintsova, O., Maier, W., & Mielck, A. (2014). Inequalities in health care among patients with type 2 diabetes by individual socio-economic status (SES) and regional deprivation: A systematic literature review. *International Journal for Equity in Health*, *13*, 43. https://doi.org/10.1186/1475-9276-13-43.

Groot, C., Hooghiemstra, A. M., Raijmakers, P. G. H. M., Van Berckel, B. N. M., Scheltens, P., Scherder, E. J. A., ... Ossenkoppele, R. (2016). The effect of physical activity on cognitive function in patients with dementia: A meta-analysis of randomized control trials. *Ageing Research Reviews*, *25*, 13–23.

Gudala, K., Bansal, D., Schifano, F., & Bhansali, A. (2013). Diabetes mellitus and risk of dementia: A meta-analysis of prospective observational studies. *Journal of Diabetes Investigation*, *4*, 640–650.

Hansen, T., Slagsvold, B., & Veenstra, M. (2017). Educational inequalities in late-life depression across Europe: Results from the generations and gender survey. *European Journal of Ageing*, *14*(4), 407–418.

International Labour Organization. (2014). *Social protection for older persons: Key policy trends and statistics*. Geneva: International Labour Office, Social Protection Department. Social Protection Policy Paper; No. 11, ISSN: 1020-9581; 1020-959X (web pdf).

Ismail, Z., Elbayoumi, H., Fischer, C. E., Hogan, D. B., Millikin, C. P., Schweizer, T., ... Fiest, K. M. (2017). Prevalence of depression in patients with mild cognitive impairment: a systematic review and meta-analysis. *JAMA Psychiatry*, *74*(1), 58–67.

Karp, A., Kårehold, I., Qiu, C., Bellander, T., Winblad, B., & Fratiglioni, L. (2004). Relation to education and occupation-based socioeconomic status to incident Alzheimer's disease. *American Journal of Epidemiology*, *159*(2), 175–183.

Kautzky-Willer, A., Dorner, T., Jensby, A., & Rieder, A. (2012). Women show a closer association between educational level and hypertension or diabetes mellitus than males: A secondary analysis from the Austrian HIS. *BMC Public Health*, *12*, 392.

Kautzky-Willer, A., Harreiter, J., & Pacini, G. (2016). Sex and gender differences in risk, pathophysiology and complications of type 2 diabetes mellitus. *Endocrine Reviews*, *37*(3), 278–316. https://doi.org/10.1210/er.2015-1137.

Kivipelto, M., Ngandu, T., Fratiglioni, L., et al. (2005). Obesity and vascular risk factors at midlife and the risk of dementia and Alzheimer disease. *Archives of Neurology*, *62*, 1556–1560.

Kuiper, J. S., Zuidersma, M., Voshaar, R. C. O., Zuidema, S. U., van den Heuvel, E. R., Stolk, R. P., & Smidt, N. (2015). Social relationships and risk of dementia: A systematic review and meta-analysis of longitudinal cohort studies. *Ageing Research Reviews*, *22*, 39–57.

Kwan, C., & Walsh, C. A. (2018). Old age poverty: A scoping review of the literature. *Cogent Social Sciences*, *4*(1), 1478479.

Lakdawalla, D., & Philipson, T. (2009). The growth of obesity and technological change. *Economics & Human Biology*, *7*(3), 283–293.

Laurin, D., Verreault, R., Lindsay, J., Macpherson, K., & Rockwood, K. (2001). Physical activity and risk of cognitive impairment and dementia in elderly persons. *Archives of Neurology*, *58*, 498–504.

Leng, B., Jin, Y., Li, G., Chen, L., & Jin, N. (2015). Socioeconomic status and hypertension: A meta-analysis. *Journal of Hypertension*, *33*(2), 221–229.

Livingston, G., Sommerlad, A., Orgeta, V., Costafreda, S. G., Huntley, J., Ames, D., et al. (2017). Dementia prevention, intervention, and care. *Lancet, 390*(10113), 2673–2734.

Livingston, G., Huntley, J., Sommerlad, A., Ames, D., Ballard, C., Banerjee, S., et al. (2020). Dementia prevention, intervention, and care: 2020 report of the Lancet Commission. *Lancet, 396*(10248), 413–446.

López-Valenciano, A., Mayo, X., Liguori, G., Copeland, R. J., Lamb, M., & Jimenez, A. (2020). Changes in sedentary behaviour in European Union adults between 2002 and 2017. *BMC Public Health, 20*(1), 1–10.

Ma, Y., Ajnakina, O., Steptoe, A., & Cadar, D. (2020). Higher risk of dementia in English older individuals who are overweight or obese. *International Journal of Epidemiology, 49*(4), 1353–1365. https://doi.org/10.1093/ije/dyaa099.

Maccora, J., Peters, R., & Anstey, K. J. (2020). What does (low) education mean in terms of dementia risk?: A systematic review and meta-analysis highlighting inconsistency in measuring and operationalising education. *SSM-Population Health, 12*, 100654.

McDaid, D., Hewlett, E., & Park, A. (2017). *Understanding effective approaches to promoting mental health and preventing mental illness*. OECD Health Working Papers, No. 97 Paris: OECD Publishing. https://doi.org/10.1787/bc364fb2-en.

McHugh, J. E., Kenny, R. A., Lawlor, B. A., Steptoe, A., & Kee, F. (2017). The discrepancy between social isolation and loneliness as a clinically meaningful metric: Findings from the Irish and English longitudinal studies of ageing (TILDA and ELSA). *International Journal of Geriatric Psychiatry, 32*(6), 664–674.

Mills, K. T., Bundy, J. D., Kelly, T. N., Reed, J. E., Kearney, P. M., Reynolds, K., … He, J. (2016). Global disparities of hypertension prevalence and control: A systematic analysis of population-based studies from 90 countries. *Circulation, 134*(6), 441–450. https://doi.org/10.1161/CIRCULATIONAHA.115.018912.

Montero-Odasso, M., Ismail, Z., & Livingston, G. (2020). One third of dementia cases can be prevented within the next 25 years by tackling risk factors. The case "for" and "against". *Alzheimer's Research & Therapy, 12*(1), 1–5.

Mund, M., Freuding, M. M., Möbius, K., Horn, N., & Neyer, F. J. (2019). The stability and change of loneliness across the life span: A meta-analysis of longitudinal studies. *Personality and Social Psychology Review, 24*(1), 24–52.

Murray, J., Banerjee, S., Byng, R., Tylee, A., Bhugra, D., & Macdonald, A. (2006). Primary care professionals' perceptions of depression in older people: A qualitative study. *Social Science & Medicine, 63*(5), 1363–1373.

Mutyambizi, C., Booysen, F., Stokes, A., Pavlova, M., & Groot, W. (2019). Lifestyle and socio-economic inequalities in diabetes prevalence in South Africa: A decomposition analysis. *PLoS One, 14*(1). https://doi.org/10.1371/journal.pone.0211208, e0211208.

Nagai, M., Hoshide, S., & Kario, K. (2010). Hypertension and dementia. *American Journal of Hypertension, 23*(2), 116–124.

NCD Risk Factor Collaboration (NCD-RisC). (2016). Worldwide trends in diabetes since 1980: A pooled analysis of 751 population-based studies with 4.4 million participants. *Lancet, 387*(10027), 1513–1530. https://doi.org/10.1016/S0140-6736(16)00618-8.

Neufcourt, L., Deguen, S., Bayat, S., Zins, M., & Grimaud, O. (2020). Gender differences in the association between socioeconomic status and hypertension in France: A cross-sectional analysis of the CONSTANCES cohort. *PLoS One, 15*(4), e0231878.

OECD. (2018). *A broken social elevator? How to promote social mobility*. Paris: OECD Publishing. https://doi.org/10.1787/9789264301085-en.

OECD. (2019a). *The heavy burden of obesity: The economics of prevention, OECD health policy studies*. Paris: OECD Publishing. https://doi.org/10.1787/67450d67-en.

OECD. (2019b). *Pensions at a glance 2019: OECD and G20 indicators*. Paris: OECD Publishing. https://doi.org/10.1787/b6d3dcfc-en.

OECD. (2019c). *Promoting Healthy Ageing Background report for the 2019 Japanese G20 Presidency*. Available from https://www.oecd.org/g20/topics/global-health/G20-report-promoting-healthy-ageing.pdf.

OECD/EU. (2018). *Health at a glance: Europe 2018: State of health in the EU cycle*. Paris: OECD Publishing. https://doi.org/10.1787/health_glance_eur-2018-4-en. Available from.

Podewils, L. J., Guallar, E., Kuller, L. H., Fried, L. P., Lopez, O. L., Carlson, M., & Lyketsos, C. G. (2005). Physical activity, APOE genotype, and dementia risk: Findings from the Cardiovascular Health Cognition Study. *American Journal of Epidemiology*, *161*(7), 639–651.

Pollitt, R. A., Rose, K. M., & Kaufman, J. S. (2005). Evaluating the evidence for models of life course socioeconomic factors and cardiovascular outcomes: A systematic review. *BMC Public Health*, *5*(7). https://doi.org/10.1186/1471-2458-5-7.

Rafnsson, S. B., Orrell, M., d'Orsi, E., Hogervorst, E., & Steptoe, A. (2020). Loneliness, social integration, and incident dementia over 6 years: Prospective findings from the English Longitudinal Study of Ageing. *Journals of Gerontology. Series B, Psychological Sciences and Social Sciences*, *75*(1), 114–124.

Ricci-Cabello, I., Ruiz-Perez, I., De Labry-Lima, A. O., & Marquez-Calderon, S. (2010). Do social inequalities exist in terms of the prevention, diagnosis, treatment, control and monitoring of diabetes? A systematic review. *Health & Social Care in the Community*, *18*(6), 572–587.

Richardson, R. A., Keyes, K. M., Medina, J. T., & Calvo, E. (2020). Sociodemographic inequalities in depression among older adults: Cross-sectional evidence from 18 countries. *Lancet Psychiatry*, *7*(8), 673–681.

Riphahn, R. T., & Schwientek, C. (2015). What drives the reversal of the gender education gap? Evidence from Germany. *Applied Economics*, *47*(53), 5748–5775.

Rovio, S., Kåreholt, I., Helkala, E. L., Viitanen, M., Winblad, B., Tuomilehto, J., … Kivipelto, M. (2005). Leisure-time physical activity at midlife and the risk of dementia and Alzheimer's disease. *Lancet Neurology*, *4*(11), 705–711.

Samuel, L. J., Szanton, S. L., Wolff, J. L., Ornstein, K. A., Parker, L. J., & Gitlin, L. N. (2020). Socioeconomic disparities in six-year incident dementia in a nationally representative cohort of US older adults: An examination of financial resources. *BMC Geriatrics*, *20*, 1–9.

Sindi, S., Mangialasche, F., & Kivipelto, M. (2015). Advances in the prevention of Alzheimer's disease. *F1000prime Reports*, *7*, 50.

Stern, Y. (2012). Cognitive reserve in ageing and Alzheimer's disease. *Lancet Neurology*, *11*, 1006–1012.

Sutin, A. R., Stephan, Y., Luchetti, M., & Terracciano, A. (2020). Loneliness and risk of dementia. *Journals of Gerontology. Series B, Psychological Sciences and Social Sciences*, *75*(7), 1414–1422.

United Nations, Department of Economic and Social Affairs, Population Division. (2017). *World population ageing 2017 (ST/ESA/SER.A/408)*.

Van Minh, H., Byass, P., Chuc, N., et al. (2006). Gender differences in prevalence and socioeconomic determinants of hypertension: Findings from the WHO STEPs survey in a rural community of Vietnam. *Journal of Human Hypertension*, *20*, 109–115. https://doi.org/10.1038/sj.jhh.1001942.

Veenstra, G. (2013). Race, gender, class, sexuality (RGCS) and hypertension. *Social Science & Medicine*, *89*, 16–24.

Von dem Knesebeck, O., Verde, P. E., & Dragano, N. (2006). Education and health in 22 European countries. *Social Science & Medicine*, *63*(5), 1344–1351.

Weiss, J., Puterman, E., Prather, A. A., Ware, E. B., & Rehkopf, D. H. (2020). A data-driven prospective study of dementia among older adults in the United States. *PLoS One*, *15*(10). https://doi.org/10.1371/journal.pone.0239994, e0239994.

Whitmer, R., Gunderson, E., Barrett-Connor, E., Quesenberry, C., & Yaffe, K. (2005). Obesity in middle age and future risk of dementia: A 27 year longitudinal population-based study. *BMJ*, *330*(7504), 1360–1364.

World Health Organization. (2014). *Obesity and inequities: Guidance for addressing inequities in overweight and obesity*. Copenhagen: World Health Organization Regional Office for Europe.

World Health Organization. (2015). *World report on ageing and health*. Geneva: World Health Organization.

World Health Organization. (2016). *Women's health and well-being in Europe: Beyond the mortality advantage*. Copenhagen: World Health Organization. Regional Office for Europe.

World Health Organization. (2017a). *Depression and other common mental disorders: Global health estimates*. Geneva: World Health Organization.

World Health Organization. (2017b). *Mental health of older adults. Factsheets*. World Helath Organization. Available from https://www.who.int/news-room/fact-sheets/detail/mental-health-of-older-adults.

World Health Organization. (2018). *The health and well-being of men in the WHO European Region: Better health through a gender approach*. Available from http://www.euro.who.int/__data/assets/pdf_file/0007/380716/mhr-report-eng.pdf.

World Health Organization. (2020). *Obesity and overweight*. Factsheet April 2020. Available from https://www.who.int/news-room/fact-sheets/detail/obesity-and-overweight.

Xu, W., Wang, H. F., Wan, Y., Tan, C. C., Yu, J. T., & Tan, L. (2017). Leisure time physical activity and dementia risk: A dose-response meta-analysis of prospective studies. *BMJ Open*, *7*(10), e014706.

Yan, S., Fu, W., Wang, C., Mao, J., Liu, B., Zou, L., & Lv, C. (2020). Association between sedentary behavior and the risk of dementia: A systematic review and meta-analysis. *Translational Psychiatry*, *10*(1), 1–8.

Yasamy, M. T., Dua, T., Harper, M., & Saxena, S. (2013). *Mental health of older adults, addressing a growing concern*. Vol. 10 (pp. 4–9). World Health Organization, Department of Mental Health and Substance Abuse.

Zolyomi, E. (2019). *Strategies for supporting social inclusion at older age*. Thematic discussion paper European Commission—DG for Employment, Social Affairs and Inclusion. Available from https://ec.europa.eu/social/main.jsp?langId=en&catId=1024&furtherNews=yes&newsId=9418.

CHAPTER 13

Living with dementia and caregiving: Psychosocial considerations through the gender lens

Charles Scerri[a,b], Angela Abela[c], and Anthony Scerri[d]

[a]*Department of Pathology, Faculty of Medicine and Surgery, University of Malta, Msida, Malta*
[b]*Alzheimer Europe, Luxembourg*
[c]*Department of Family Studies, Faculty for Social Wellbeing, University of Malta, Msida, Malta*
[d]*Department of Nursing, Faculty of Health Sciences, University of Malta, Msida, Malta*

Introduction

Looking after an individual living with dementia has become a common occurrence across families worldwide. According to the World Health Organization (WHO, 2017), dementia is a major cause of disability, with more women than men being affected (Prince et al., 2015). Diagnosis of dementia is set to increase exponentially over the years. It reached 47 million individuals in 2015 and is expected to rise to 75 million in 2030 and then experience a dramatic increase to 132 million in 2050. The first section of this chapter will discuss the family context surrounding caregiving in dementia. In the second part of the chapter, a number of psychosocial interventions aimed at improving the quality of life in these individuals will be reviewed. The last section will be dedicated to the influence of gender on psychosocial interventions for behavioral and psychological symptoms in dementia.

Family dynamics in the context of caregiving in individuals living with dementia

A diagnosis of dementia does not only impact the individual in question but also affects his or her family and friends. Indeed, the emergence and progression of this disease, the challenges encountered, and the new tasks and roles required often change the family dynamic (e.g., Teel & Carson, 2003). This change has an effect on both the person living with dementia and on immediate family and friends.

Tatangelo, McCabe, Macleod, and Konis (2018) note that the family context is not given much importance when researching on the care of individuals living with dementia, in spite of the fact that it plays an important role in the wellbeing of all persons concerned. Usually, it is the spouse who cares for the individual living with dementia (Schultz & Martire, 2004). Many caregiving spouses do not feel comfortable burdening their adult children with this responsibility (Fenech & Scerri, 2014) as they know that they have a family of their own to look after. Others do not seek help, to avoid conflict about health decisions (Cooper, Katona, Orrell, & Livingston, 2008). At the same time, practical help and support from family members is often expected and considered to be an important coping strategy. In those circumstances where the spouse has passed away or is unable to provide care, the children often step in to help (Tatangelo et al., 2018).

Spouses as caregivers of individuals living with dementia

Dementia caregiving, whether provided by the spouse, the children, or any other family members, is usually considered as a very stressful experience and has been linked with various physical, psychological, and emotional symptoms, and poorer health in general (Roth, Fredman, & Haley, 2015) (Box 1).

As dementia progresses, caregivers tend to experience the impact of the illness and the burden on them according to the stage their family member is in. A recent systematic review (Egilstrod, Bay Ravn, & Schultz Petersen, 2019) covering 15 qualitative studies provided a thematic synthesis of the lived experiences of spouses of individuals living with dementia. The authors highlighted the sense of loss of a close relationship, and grief and uncertainty engulfing the spouse during the onset of dementia. This observation was echoed in another systematic metasynthesis of qualitative studies that looked into the experiences, quality of life, and psychosocial impact of caregiving (Cross, Garip, & Sheffield, 2018). In a study included in the latter metasynthesis,

Box 1

Viola, a social worker, got married and continued to live in the city of Dresden in Germany, visiting her parents regularly. When both parents were in their 70s, she started to notice that her mother was no longer as well-kept as she used to be. The house was becoming untidy. She even abandoned the plants she loved so much. Alarm bells started to ring when she started getting lost on her way back home from church. The doctor diagnosed her with dementia. Her husband tried to support her; however, her angry outbursts became very upsetting for him. He was feeling physically weak and she would resist his help even as he tried to assist her with basic activities of daily living. With time, Viola's mother started to become confused and it was impossible for Viola's father to leave her alone, even for a short period of time. Viola was unable to visit her parents on a daily basis as she had her own family to look after. It was a time of intense grief for her and her father. When her brother visited from the United States, he was shocked to witness the deterioration his mum was going through. As a family, they knew that finding a good nursing home was an inevitable and painful decision they had to take. They found one that was about an hour's drive away from Viola's parents' residence. Viola's mother now had difficulty swallowing and started to lose weight. She also stopped recognizing her loved ones. Going to visit her was extremely painful for both the father and her children. On his return to the States, Viola's brother found it difficult to talk about his mother's illness and avoided the topic with his sister or father whenever they met online.

Livingston et al. (2010) reported that misunderstandings sometimes ensue when consulting health professionals, either due to the overload of information spouses receive at the point of diagnosis and/or the denial they experience. Nevertheless, various studies report that spouses and other family caregivers are relieved to discover that there is a diagnosis explaining the symptoms their spouses are experiencing (Chan et al., 2010; Ducharme, Kergoa, Antoine, Pasquier, & Coulombe, 2013; Quinn, Clare, Pearce, & van Dijkhuizen, 2008; Teel & Carson, 2003).

A whole gamut of feelings is depicted, as caregivers' transition from a relative or family member identity to a caregiver identity, in the metasynthesis by Cross et al. (2018) and that by Egilstrod et al. (2019). These feelings include, among others, shock, responsibility, and worry. Caregivers who look after spouses with early-onset dementia feel psychologically distraught and grieved about the plans they would have made for their retirement as a couple, whereas spouses of partners with late-onset dementia tend to accept the situation more. In the later stages of the illness, individuals living with dementia may fail to recognize their caregivers, which is a painful loss for the latter, who keep searching for such signs.

In the early stages of dementia, caregivers try to adjust to a new reality by attempting to find a balance between helping their spouse and keeping in touch with the outside world. However, caregiving becomes increasingly time-consuming because of increased dependence, such as difficulties in eating and loss of physical and communicative abilities that dementia can bring with it. In spite of the high level of stress and burden, O'Dwyer, Moyle, Taylor, Creese, and Zimmer-Gembeck (2016) reported that self-determination helps caregiving family members to cope better. The participants interviewed by Quinn et al. (2008) gave importance to the acceptance of the illness and the ability of taking it day by day. For many, the act of caregiving becomes a meaningful endeavor and a sense of satisfaction at being so supportive toward their loved one is experienced. In these circumstances, spouses feel greater closeness and intimacy with the individual living with dementia (Bergman, Graff, Eriksdotter, Fugl-Meyer, & Schuster, 2016). For others, the difficulty in or lack of meaningful communication (Hellström, Håkanson, Eriksson, & Sandberg, 2017) contributes to a loss of intimacy (Boylstein & Hayes, 2012; Quinn et al., 2008).

Some spousal caregivers experience an irreconcilable difference between their needs and those of their spouses. When trying to meet their own needs, a number of caregivers feel guilty (O'Shaunessy, Lee, & Lintern, 2010). Frustrations are experienced, which in turn influence their mood and that of the individual living with dementia (Vikstrom, Josephsson, Stigsdotter-Neely, & Nygard, 2008). Discord may also be present in a number of cases and may even include physical and/or verbal abuse (O'Dwyer et al., 2016). Some spouses may also have thoughts of harm toward the care recipient or passive death wishes, which in turn make them feel guilty. Women, in particular, are reported to feel evil for having such thoughts (Madsen & Birkelund, 2013) (more on gender differences in caregiving in Chapter 14). Usually, caregivers do not disclose any of these thoughts and keep them to themselves (Madsen & Birkelund, 2013; O'Dwyer et al., 2016). Having someone to talk to is, nevertheless, very therapeutic for caregivers. Family members are not always the preferred first port of call as caregivers would rather open up with someone who is going through a similar situation (Quinn et al., 2008). Practical support, rather than emotional support, is preferred for some family members (Donnellan, Bennett, & Soulsby, 2015).

Ashley and Kleinpeter (2002) and Pöysti et al. (2012) reported that female spouses of individuals living with dementia report feeling more depressed than men. Rose-Rego, Strauss, and Smyth (1998) and Swinkels, Tilburg, Verbakel, and Broese van Groenou (2019) noted that the depression experienced by women could be explained by the fact that women tend to spend more time on caregiving, be more emotion-focused in their care, and invest more energy on caring and nurturing. Furthermore, whilst women tend to be more self-reliant, men are more likely to seek external help (Rose-Rego et al., 1998). In a study by Russel (2001), carried out with an all-male sample of caregivers, it emerged that male caregivers were more pragmatic in their caring approach and tended to be more accepting of difficult situations. Furthermore, male spouses who sought social support experienced less depression, though this was not the case for female spouses. Both male and female spouses who were socially avoidant were more likely to be depressed. Pretorius, Walker, and Heyns (2009) reported that, in South Africa, men preferred to seek support from their daughters or housekeepers, as they experienced support groups to be mostly attended by females and highly charged emotionally.

The adult child caregiver of a parent living with dementia and the effect of gender on expectations

According to Hwang et al. (2017), adult children and adult children-in-law form the largest group of informal dementia caregivers in Canada and the United States, reaching almost half of all caregivers. Tatangelo et al. (2018) pointed out that family dynamics are different when the caregivers are adult children rather than the partners of individuals living with dementia. Adult child caregivers have to handle a much more complex relationship system and this can cause significant conflict (Kwak, Ingersoll-Dayton, & Kim, 2012) starting from that of their own nuclear family. In a number of cases, these caregivers are in midlife and are bringing up their own children. This is a very stressful time for them and many would complain that they do not have enough time for their own family (Kjallman-Alm, Norbergh, & Hellzen, 2013). In addition, adult children who take the role of the primary caregiver have to tend to the relationship with their siblings, if any, and be sensitive to the needs of their siblings' families as well as the position that the partners of their siblings take vis-à-vis the caregiving of the parent. At the same time, they expect greater support from their siblings than what spousal caregivers normally expect from their children (Kwak et al., 2012). Hwang et al. (2017) mention how primary caregivers sometimes come into conflict with their siblings over support, whereas others resign themselves to the situation so as not to create further difficulties. Good family functioning, especially with regard to sibling relationships, is therefore crucial for the smooth running of this collaborative endeavor and this necessitates skillful interaction. Tatangelo et al. (2018) interviewed an extensive number of adult child caregivers who were all (but one) caring for their own parents with dementia in a community in Melbourne, Australia. The authors reported four particularly distressing situations that unfolded in the context of caregiving.

One of these is how the caregiver, usually a woman, is "designated." In fact, it is estimated that, globally, 71% of informal caregiving is provided by women (Wimo, Gauthier, & Prince, 2018). Usually this is the person perceived to be more available and/or living closest to the parent or perhaps having more aptitude for care. Such an expectation may fill the identified person with a sense of unwelcome and unexpected obligation and could create a certain degree of resentment and pressure on the person concerned. Romero-Moreno et al. (2014) reported that daughters, in particular, feel obliged to fulfill the role and experience guilt if they do not, to the extent that they may even refrain from seeking support when looking after their parents. Tatangelo et al. (2018) highlight how beliefs around gendered roles hinder brothers from supporting their sisters in the care of the parents, as they do not feel it is their role as males to, for instance, wash their mother "and do those things that you would as a girl" (p. 374). On the other hand, two individuals in the study sample who were sons and had no sisters to count on had no issue with being primary caregivers to their mothers. Interestingly, this situation actually prompted them to take up this role. Morgan, Williams, Trussardi, and Gott (2016) highlight the importance of moving away from perceiving caregiving as designated for females, thus ensuring that any family caregiver, irrespective of gender, would take the role. This would allow for better sharing of responsibility, leading to an increased sense of wellbeing among family members.

Hwang et al. (2017) reported that a number of daughters in their sample did not expect any help from their brothers as their values around gender prescribed caring as a daughter's responsibility. Cultural expectations with regards to caregiving are, in some countries, stronger than in others and have a strong mandate on one's gendered behavior. Tatangelo et al. (2018) pointed out that more research is needed on how gendered expectations contribute to care burden, especially when other siblings do not or cannot offer help for one reason or another. Innes, Abela, and Scerri (2011) reported how family members in Malta looked after parents or parents-in-law living with dementia by developing "innovative rotating care patterns to accommodate individual family members, social and working lives while maintaining their responsibilities" (p. 181). The authors further highlighted that this way of looking after one of their parents presented its own difficulties, especially the fact that the parent living with dementia had to relocate from one home to another every few days. Furthermore, siblings did not always agree on how the obligation of care was to be shared and male siblings tended to shirk this responsibility. However, family members preferred this care arrangement rather than placing their parent living with dementia in institutional care. Such an arrangement was only possible given the small size of the island and close proximity of the households. At the other end of the spectrum, Bei, Rotem-Mindali, and Vilchinsky (2020) alert us to the fact that a considerable number of caregivers, ranging from 15% to 20%, are distance caregivers and their experience is largely understudied.

According to Tatangelo et al. (2018), siblings who encounter tangible difficulties are usually more willing to discuss them with the adult child caregiver. These may include resistance from the sibling's partner, who opposes to the idea that the sibling dedicates time for the care of their ill parent when this resource is already in short supply within the nuclear family. Other siblings may have to cope with a sick or disabled child or live at a considerable distance away from the residence of the family of origin. Furthermore, some of the siblings are ruled out because they may not be considered to be competent enough to look after the sick parent. These kinds of conversations are usually experienced as helpful, as caregivers of individuals living with dementia feel particularly frustrated and isolated when siblings fail to show their appreciation for the effort and dedication that they are contributing. This lack of appreciation probably occurs because the noncommitted siblings feel that such conversations would weaken their position of power, especially in a context where they are not willing to offer their support.

Denial and poor understanding of dementia is also considered a stumbling block among siblings. Stokes, Combes, and Stokes (2015) pointed out that there is insufficient knowledge on dementia among the general public. This isolates caregivers even from friends who have little insight regarding the situation and do not offer their support as normally the case with other conditions such as cancer (Bramble, Moyle, & McAllister, 2009). Moreover, siblings who spend very little time with the individual living with dementia probably have the least understanding of what the illness entails. Another scenario that creates friction is one where siblings have different views about caregiving. This is exacerbated during the time when the parent living with dementia may need more intensive care (Bramble et al., 2009). According to the latter authors, it took around 4 years of care at home for the participants forming part of their study before care in an institution was considered. In most cases, the person caring for the parent prolongs the decision and this strains the relationship among siblings. The primary caregiver finds it hard and agonizing to take such a critical decision, with the result that such decisions are often delayed (Butcher, Holkup, Park, & Maas, 2001).

Contrasting views about caregiving may even lead to breakdown in communication between siblings. Legal and financial arrangements, including caregivers having powers of attorney, create a lot of conflict, with some siblings who are not appointed withdrawing their support (Hwang et al., 2017). Serious disagreement among siblings is devastating and further increases the distress on the caregiver and that of the other family members, besides impacting on the care of the parent living with dementia. Tatangelo et al. (2018) reported that most of the caregivers they interviewed felt that they were incapable of resolving such differences on their own.

In light of the complexity of such situations, many siblings need support in the community. Efforts at providing such support are becoming more common in many countries. For example, in Melbourne, Australia, communication between siblings is facilitated by a family care worker who calls meetings every 2 or 3 months, where siblings including the primary caregiver touch base on the needs of the parent living with dementia being cared for in the community. Such meetings can prevent breakdown of the sibling relationship and provide timely support for the primary caregiver. Such interventions could also include partners and spouses of caregivers, especially in a context where in-laws are being looked after. Looking after in-laws with dementia is an under-researched area (Tatangelo et al., 2018) and it would be interesting to study family dynamics in this context whilst taking gender into account.

Family dynamics and residential long-term care for persons living with dementia

As Gaugler (2005) pointed out in a synthesis and critical review of family involvement in residential long-term care, many family members remain involved when their relatives with dementia enter into long-term care. Out of the 29 family members of individuals living with dementia, 37.9% visited several times per week (Monahan, 1995). In another study by Tornatore and Grant (2002), 76% visited once a week or more. When they visited, they helped in keeping the identity of the individual living with dementia alive, helped the person eat, or assisted in other activities of daily living. Above all, they kept a very good relationship with the staff. Numerous authors consider this relationship to be important for the wellbeing of all the family members, including the caregivers themselves (Bramble et al., 2009; Robinson, Reid, & Cooke, 2010).

Not all individuals living with dementia move to institutional care. Some seek public homecare services, whereas those who are more economically advantaged hire private care for greater flexibility and individualized care. For example, in Malta, the Carer at Home Scheme (enabling senior citizens to employ a caregiver of their choice to assist them at home in their daily needs) is financially supported from public funds. As Abela (2016) pointed out, most of the caregivers are foreign women who come and live with the individual living with dementia in their home setting. Family caregivers then visit their relative at their convenience. This arrangement may be considered to be a more convenient one for adult child caregivers to that reported by Innes et al. (2011).

Robinson et al. (2010) also mentioned the transition into cottages rather than institutional care for individuals living with dementia in Canada. These residences, which are smaller in size compared to traditional institutional settings with around-the-clock professional care being provided by a nonprofit organization, are homelier and more inviting to such individuals, particularly in the later stages of the disease. Some of the participants in the study noted that the relative living with dementia seemed much happier in such settings and this helped caregivers feel less anxious about this living arrangement, with visits becoming more enjoyable. Some of the participants mentioned how their own children accompanied when visiting their grandparents. During the visit, the children drew pictures that were later hung in their relative's room. Such an interesting observation provided yet another family dynamic in the area of caregiving for individuals living with dementia.

Although caring for an individual living with dementia can be challenging and stressful, a number of interventions have been developed with the aim of supporting caregivers and family members in enhancing the level of care and management of these individuals. The next section will give an overview of psychosocial interventions that are currently available, putting particular emphasis on their effectiveness for improving dementia-related behavioral symptoms and quality of life.

Psychosocial interventions for individuals living with dementia and their caregivers

In the absence of effective pharmacotherapeutic agents able to halt the neurodegenerative decline that is characteristic to diseases that lead to the major forms of dementia, nonpharmacological interventions have lately been given considerable importance. This is due to their reported positive outcomes in terms of improvement in behavioral symptoms and quality of life for individuals living with dementia, their caregivers, and family members. Among the most commonly used nonpharmacological approaches, one finds psychosocial interventions, with literature increasingly pointing toward their positive impact on the behavioral and psychological symptoms of dementia (BPSD), cognitive function, and quality of life, especially in mild to moderate AD (Epperly, Dunay, & Boice, 2017). However, the type of intervention considered to be the most effective is still debatable, with outcomes resting on a number of factors including the setting, disease progression, individual needs and preferences, together with the goal behavior of the individual living with dementia (Dröes, van Mierlo, van der Roest, & Meiland, 2010). Furthermore, differences between countries exist, with low- to middle-income countries not routinely offering such interventions compared to high-income countries (Stoner, Lakshminarayanan, Durgante, & Spector, 2019).

According to Kitwood (1997), supporting individuals living with dementia should be based on a person-centered care approach, in which personhood should occupy center stage during the whole course of the dementia process. This entails the identification of behaviors that undermine or enhance a person's wellbeing, thus enabling health and social care professionals to deliver the optimum level of care. A person's level of ill-being is often expressed through a change in behavior, due to an inability to meet that person's needs. The "Unmet Needs Model" (Cohen-Mansfield & Werner, 1995) postulates that unmet needs arise because of dementia-related impairments in both communication and the ability to utilize the environment appropriately to accommodate needs. Understanding unmet needs in individuals living with dementia is central in the provision of quality care and should form the basis of nonpharmacological interventions in these individuals (Kolanowski, Litaker, Buettner, Moeller, & Costa, 2011). The introduction of such an approach in the management of behavioral manifestations in dementia has been instrumental in reducing the use of antipsychotic prescribing (Banerjee, 2009) and nowadays is considered to be the first line of intervention in the management of BPSD.

Over the years, a number of psychosocial interventions have been heralded as effective in improving the quality of life in individuals living with dementia and their caregivers. Quality of life has often been identified as a primary goal in dementia management and is regarded as an important indicator of the impact of psychosocial interventions on the overall wellbeing of these individuals (Logsdon, McCurry, & Teri, 2007). Factors that are associated with quality of life in dementia are various and include maintenance of cognitive and physical functions, engaging in pleasurable activities, and sensory stimulation.

Psychosocial interventions targeting cognitive function
Cognitive stimulation therapy

Cognitive stimulation therapy is one of the most widely used psychosocial interventions in individuals living with dementia (Spector, Thorgrimsen, Woods, & Orrell, 2006). An intervention using cognitive stimulation therapy is carried out in groups, in which a number of sessions involving themed activities, such as current affairs, are used to engage participants by seeking their opinions. The session is conducted by a trained individual, using a manual, with the theme being selected by the participants. In a metaanalysis of randomized controlled trials on the efficacy of cognitive stimulation therapy in individuals living with dementia, Kim et al. (2017) found that participants receiving cognitive stimulation therapy performed better on the Mini Mental State Examination (MMSE) test and the Alzheimer's Disease Assessment Scale-Cognitive Subscale (ADAS-Cog). In addition to this, Hall, Orrell, Stott, and Spector (2013) reported an improvement in memory, orientation, and syntax in individuals living with dementia undergoing cognitive stimulation therapy.

Significant improvement in cognition was also reported by Aguirre et al. (2013), with increasing age and female gender acting as predictors for higher MMSE and ADAS-Cog scores. The authors argued that the greater improvement in cognition reported with the female gender was possibly due to females significantly outnumbering males in the study and that female-dominated groups are generally more conversational and interactive. Cognitive stimulation therapy has also been found to improve the quality of life in individuals living with dementia, possibly through an improvement in cognition and communication and a reduction in depressive symptoms (Woods, Thorgrimsen, Spector, Royan, & Orrell, 2006).

Cognitive rehabilitation therapy

Originally developed for individuals with cognitive impairment due to brain injury, cognitive rehabilitation therapy is a personalized approach that uses problem-solving techniques to enable individuals living with dementia to engage and manage everyday activities in order to maintain their independence for as long as possible (Kudlicka, Martyr, Bahar-Fuchs, Woods, & Clare, 2019). Cognitive rehabilitation therapy's main objective is to improve function in areas that the individual identifies as relevant to them. Using a single-blind randomized controlled trial, Clare et al. (2010) found that, in comparison to the control group, individuals who had received cognitive rehabilitation therapy rated themselves as more satisfied with their ability to carry out meaningful activities of daily living immediately after therapy completion. Furthermore, participants in the therapy group rated their overall quality of life as higher than that of participants in the control condition at 6 months' post intervention.

Reminiscence therapy
Reminiscence therapy involves the discussion of past events and experiences with the use of aids such as items from the past, photographs, video recordings, or any other means that prompts personal memories. Although such a technique has been found to be particularly useful in enhancing mood and quality of life in individuals with depression (Bohlmeijer, Smit, & Cuijpers, 2003), a recent Cochrane review found that the effects of reminiscence interventions in individuals living with dementia are inconsistent, often small in size, and can differ considerably across settings (Woods, O'Philbin, Farrell, Spector, & Orrell, 2018).

Validation therapy
Validation therapy involves communicating with individuals living with dementia by acknowledging their actions through empathy. Most commonly, validation therapy is used in moderate to severe dementia, where the individual is driven by basic needs that are difficult to express due to disease progression. Examples of such an intervention include making eye contact, not arguing, turning the conversation toward a positive experience from the past, and listening carefully to what the individual is saying. Regrettably, there is a dearth in literature about the efficacy of validation therapy in individuals living with dementia. Neil and Wright (2009), in reviewing a number of randomized controlled trials, concluded that insufficient evidence exists to allow any conclusion about the efficacy of validation therapy for individuals living with dementia or cognitive impairment.

Activity-based psychosocial interventions
Exercise
Physical exercise has been touted as a protective factor in a number of disease processes, including those involved in dementia. Numerous studies suggest that exercise has a protective effect on the brain, possibly through an increase in hippocampal volume (Den Ouden et al., 2018). Apart from benefits on physical health, exercise has also been shown to alleviate low mood and improve quality of life (Chan et al., 2019; Wipfli, Rethorst, & Landers, 2008). Individuals living with dementia may benefit from physical exercise in a number of ways, even though most evidence for this comes from animal studies. Various hypotheses have been put forward, including the role of physical exercise in improving blood circulation, enhancing cognitive reserve, and reducing stress. As a result, a number of physical activity programs have been developed to alleviate the symptoms of dementia. For example, Hauer et al. (2012) reported that regular exercise improved functional ability, whereas in a systematic review by Law, Lam, Chung, and Pang (2020), exercise was found to reduce global cognitive decline and lessen behavioral challenges in individuals with mild cognitive impairment or dementia. Since exercise is often conducted as a group

activity, it may also play an important role in reducing loneliness and social isolation (Cohen-Mansfield & Perach, 2015). Despite the potential of physical exercise in ameliorating the symptoms of dementia, more research is needed, in particular on its long-term effects following exercise completion.

Dance/movement therapy

A number of studies have investigated the effects of dance/movement therapy on social, behavioral, and cognitive symptoms in individuals living with dementia. According to the UK Association of Dance Movement Psychotherapy, dance/movement therapy "is the psychotherapeutic use of movement and dance through which a person can engage creatively in a process to further their emotional, cognitive, physical and social integration" (Association of Dance Movement Psychotherapy UK, 2020, p. 1). The moderate physical activity involved in such therapy would be expected to stimulate brain areas engaged in cognition and motor and executive functions. However, despite evidence from existing studies about the beneficial role of dance/movement therapy in dementia, including a positive effect on quality of life (Hameed et al., 2018), a recent Cochrane review (Karkou & Meekums, 2017) found that none of the identified studies met the inclusion criteria, with the authors highlighting the need to conduct trials of high methodological quality, large sample sizes, and clarity in the way the intervention is planned and delivered.

Music therapy

Compared to other psychosocial interventions, the effects of music therapy use in individuals living with dementia has been extensively studied, with the majority of results pointing toward positive outcomes through reducing BPSD and enhancing quality of life (Cooke, Moyle, Shum, Harrison, & Murfield, 2010; Gallego & Garcia, 2017). Music therapy is usually delivered in groups or tailored to a specific individual and can be either active (in which the participant engages in singing or instrument-playing) or passive (listening to music). Analyzing a number of randomized controlled trials of music-based therapeutic interventions for individuals living with dementia, van der Steen et al. (2018) found that providing institutionalized individuals with dementia with at least five music sessions helped in reducing depressive symptoms, improved overall behavior and quality of life, but had little effect on agitation, aggression, or cognition.

Visual art-based therapy

The overarching aim of art-based therapy in individuals living with dementia is to act as a leisure activity. Historically, the use of painting and drawing has been recognized as a therapeutic intervention in a number of neurological conditions including depression and schizophrenia (Chiang, Reid-Varley, & Fan, 2019). The theoretical basis is still not fully understood but visual art can engage participants in abstract thinking, creativity, and communication, all of which stimulate cognition and promote general wellbeing. Through visual arts, participants can also express their inner feelings. A number of studies have investigated the role of visual art therapy on cognitive decline, BPSD, and quality of life. It has been found to improve working memory and attention (Mahendran et al., 2018), episodic memory (Pongan et al., 2017), and protected against cognitive decline (Cetinkaya, Duru Asiret, Direk, & Özkanli, 2019), with the latter mostly encountered in the case of tasks that stimulate creativity. Furthermore, visual art-based therapy has been associated with a positive impact on the quality of life in cognitively impaired individuals (Im & Lee, 2014). Notwithstanding such positive outcomes, adequately-powered and high-quality studies are needed to provide further evidence about the efficacy of art therapy for individuals living with dementia (Deshmukh, Holmes, & Cardno, 2018).

Life story work

According to Dementia UK, life story work is an activity in which the individual living with dementia is supported by staff and family members to gather and review their past life events and build a personal biography. Rooted in reminiscence therapy, life story work has a relatively long history in geriatric studies, where the main objective is not to determine whether the individual's storytelling is true, but rather to attempt to understand why the person is sharing that particular story at that particular time (Kindell, Burrow, Wilkinson, & Keady, 2014). In individuals living with dementia, especially in the later stages, storytelling turns out to be difficult, as chronological order becomes compromised, with events in the past and present becoming intertwined. Furthermore, the progressive development of dementia-related communication impairments makes this task even more challenging. A number of studies have evaluated the role of life story work as a psychosocial intervention in individuals living with dementia. For example, Moos and Björn (2006) found that life story work increased self-esteem, whereas Gridley, Brooks, Birks, Baxter, and Parker (2016) reported improvement in quality of life and positive changes in staff attitudes toward dementia. Although, in general, life story work is recognized as helpful for both individuals living with dementia and their caregivers, the varying nature of its implementation, the outcomes sought, and the need of having trained staff warrants further investigation.

Other nonpharmacological therapies for dementia

Light therapy

In the last two decades, a significant number of studies have been conducted on the role of light therapy in the management of dementia. Among the first reports to be published, 4 weeks of morning bright therapy was found to improve sleep and BPSD in individuals living with dementia (Mishima et al., 1994). The biological basis of light therapy intervention lies in the premise that such individuals show circadian dysregulation leading to an abnormal sleep/wake cycle. This is often accompanied by changes in behavior, such as confusion and increased agitation, often referred to as "sundowning" (Khachiyants, Trinkle, Son, & Kim, 2011). A recent systematic review involving 31 studies reported promising results on the effect of light therapy on sleep, circadian rhythmicity, and behavioral symptoms in individuals living with dementia (Hjetland et al., 2020). However, the authors noted that the different study designs and interventions used may have resulted in inconsistent results, thus recommending that future light therapy studies should use a randomized placebo-controlled design for a period of not less than 2 months.

Aromatherapy

Over the years, there has been a growing interest in the use of aromatherapy in individuals living with dementia to manage BPSD. In essence, aromatherapy uses plant-extracted essential oils that are applied via inhalation or directly to the skin. In particular, the essential oils of lavender and lemon balm have been extensively studied with promising results. For example, lemon balm oil applied as a massage for 4 weeks resulted in a reduction in agitation (Ballard, O'Brien, Reichelt, & Perry, 2002). Similarly, in a placebo-controlled study, lavender oil was found to reduce agitation in individuals living with dementia (Holmes et al., 2002). However, a Cochrane review aimed at assessing the efficacy of aromatherapy as a psychosocial intervention for individuals living with dementia found that the benefits of aromatherapy are equivocal (Forrester et al., 2014). The authors noted several methodological inconsistencies in the studies they examined and thus recommended that, in order to reach a clear conclusion on the effect of such therapy in individuals living with dementia, more well-designed, large-scale randomized controlled trials are needed.

Animal-assisted therapy

Animal-assisted therapy is used as a psychosocial intervention on the premise that animals could help individuals living with dementia by providing sensory stimulation and companionship, leading to better cognition and mood, as well as reduced behavioral symptoms. The majority of animals used are those that are normally associated with pets, such as cats, dogs, rabbits, and birds, however "pet" robots are also becoming popular. Although a number of studies have investigated the effectiveness of conventional pets and robot therapies in dementia, validated scientific data remains scarce and the underlying mechanisms for its benefit remain unclear (Peluso et al., 2018). Studies that are currently available are weak in design and methodology. A recent Cochrane review that analyzed nine randomized controlled trials conducted in Europe and the United States found that, although animal-assisted therapy may reduce the symptoms of depression in individuals living with dementia, no conclusions could be drawn about the overall benefits of this intervention in such individuals (Lai et al., 2019). Furthermore, the use of robot devices has been questioned by formal dementia caregivers in terms of their acceptability, adoption, and routine use in practice (Scerri, Sammut, & Scerri, 2021).

Multisensory stimulation therapy

Multisensory stimulation has become increasing popular in recent years to manage BPSD in individuals living with dementia. Such therapy involves the stimulation of more than one human sensory system—sight, smell, taste, touch, and hearing. Popular among such interventions is Snoezelen therapy, in which the individual is placed in a calming and stimulating environment, called the "Snoezelen room," specifically designed to deliver a number of stimuli using colors, sounds, scents, etc. A number of studies have found evidence where multisensory stimulation interventions improved BPSD, had a positive impact on mood, and also reduced caregiver stress (Sánchez, Millán-Calenti, Lorenzo-López, & Maseda, 2013). However, although such therapy is extensively utilized worldwide, limited evidence exists to support its use in individuals living with dementia.

Doll therapy

The use of dolls as a psychosocial intervention in individuals living with dementia is based on the attachment theory, which rests on the individual's lifelong need for protection and security (Shin, 2015). According to Miesen (1993), dementia-related challenging behaviors such as wandering, crying, shadowing, and agitation are all representative of attachment requests. A systematic review by Ng, Ho, Koh, Tan, and Chan (2017) found that doll therapy enhanced communication skills and improved social behavior. More recently, Yilmaz and Aşiret (2020) reported that, in a randomized controlled study, doll therapy was found to be effective in decreasing BPSD in individuals with moderate to severe dementia. Notwithstanding the reported therapeutic effectiveness of doll therapy, ethical concerns associated with its use remain, especially in healthcare professionals. However, the application of a "rights-based approach" should empower such professionals in resolving ethical issues that may arise with the use of this therapy (Mitchell & Templeton, 2014).

The list of psychosocial interventions described above is not exhaustive. The ones highlighted in this section are those in which the most research work has been conducted to date. Other interventions include occupational therapy, play/drama therapy, the use of assistive technologies, and touch therapy, to mention a few. Although significant progress has been made in rigorous evaluation of the outcomes of psychosocial interventions in individuals living with dementia, more high-powered studies are needed. Furthermore, future research should focus on interventions that add dignity, purpose, and autonomy of individuals living with dementia, and ways with which their wider implementation can be achieved (Oyebode & Parveen, 2019).

The influence of gender on psychosocial interventions for behavioral and psychological symptoms in dementia and Alzheimer's disease

The previous section highlighted a number of psychosocial interventions that have been developed, implemented, and evaluated, targeting individuals living with dementia. The first part of this section will give a brief overview of gender differences on the incidence of BPSD in such individuals. It will then seek to critically appraise whether and how gender differences influence psychosocial interventions for individuals living with dementia and their formal and informal caregivers.

Gender differences in behavioral and psychological symptoms of individuals living with dementia

Behavioral and psychological symptoms of dementia (BPSD), also referred to as neuropsychiatric symptoms, is an umbrella term that describes a heterogeneous group of noncognitive psychological symptoms and observed behaviors that commonly occur in individuals living with dementia at any moment during the course of the condition. Symptoms include anxiety, agitation, abnormal motor behavior, euphoria, irritability, depression, apathy, disinhibition, delusions, paranoia, hallucinations, and appetite and sleep disorders (Cerejeira, Lagarto, & Mukaetova-Ladinska, 2012). Kales, Gitlin, and Lyketsos (2015) conceptualized three factors that determine BPSD, including patient factors (e.g., personality, presence of acute medical conditions, unmet needs, and disease progression), caregiver factors (e.g., stress, caregiver burden, lack of communication skills, and dementia training), and environmental factors (e.g., overstimulation, understimulation, safety issues, and lack of activity or routines). Whilst these factors have been associated with BPSD, it is still unclear whether gender plays a significant role (Lee, Lee, & Kim, 2017). Studies comparing prevalence of BPSD between male and female individuals with cognitive impairment show differing findings. For example, Kitamura, Kitamura, Hino, Tanaka, and Kurata (2012) reported significant gender differences in clinical manifestations of hospitalized patients with BPSD. Men were more likely to exhibit aggressiveness and sleeping disorders, whereas females had significantly more affective disorders, paranoia, and hallucinations. Similar findings were also reported in patients with mild but not moderate AD (Lee et al., 2017) and in cognitively impaired individuals residing in geriatric settings (Lövheim, Sandman, Karlsson, & Gustafson, 2009). The fact that men tend to exhibit more aggressive behavior may be the result of hereditary, endocrine, or learned behaviors. On the contrary, Lee, Im, Kim, and Lee (2014) did not find any significant gender differences in BPSD of AD patients, whilst female patients with dementia were not more depressed than male dementia patients in the Prado-Jean et al. (2010) study. However, factors such as personality, caregiving, and the environment may play a more important role than gender in causing BPSD in individuals living with AD.

Gender differences in BPSD have also been found in dementia types other than AD. For example, Xing et al. (2012) found that women with mild vascular dementia exhibited significantly more delusions, depression, and hallucinations, whilst men with moderate-severe stage vascular dementia were significantly more apathetic. Similarly, a retrospective study comparing the initial symptoms of persons with probable Lewy body dementia (DLB) on diagnosis found significant gender differences in the symptomatology (Utsumi et al., 2020). Whilst psychiatric symptoms and auditory hallucinations were more common in women with DLB in this cohort, men exhibited more sleep disorders, Parkinsonism, hyposmia, and syncope. There is still limited evidence about gender differences in BPSD for other rarer types of dementia.

Gender differences in psychosocial interventions for individuals living with dementia

Gender differences can have a significant impact on the effectiveness of psychosocial interventions for behavioral and psychological symptoms and psychosocial domains in individuals living with dementia and cognitive impairment. Moreover, in general, women seem to benefit more than men from supportive therapy rather than interpretative psychotherapy, especially when group therapy is used (Ogrodniczuk, 2006). In individuals with cognitive impairment, there is some evidence that gender influences the outcome of psychosocial interventions (Van Mierlo, Van der Roest, Meiland, & Dröes, 2010). Kurz et al. (2012) showed that cognitive rehabilitation in individuals with early AD reduced self-reported depressive symptoms in women more than in men. Similarly, cognitive stimulation therapy was found to have a stronger effect on quality of life (Spector et al., 2003) in female participants with dementia. Better cognitive improvement following cognitive training was also reported in female compared to male patients (Rahe et al., 2015).

Whilst the female gender seems to benefit more from these interventions (Baron, Ulstein, & Werheid, 2015), a number of studies have indicated otherwise, with male participants benefitting the most in managing behavioral symptoms and in particular, psychosocial domains. For instance, release from mandatory confinement was associated with a significant reduction in aggressive behavior in male residents when compared to female residents (McMinn & Hinton, 2000). Similarly, the mental component of health-related quality of life improved only in male community-dwelling adults with mild cognitive impairment following a walking program (van Uffelen, Paw, Hopman-Rock, & van Mechelen, 2007).

These studies provide some initial indications of gender differences on the effect of psychosocial interventions for individuals living with dementia and mild cognitive impairment and highlight the importance of considering these differences when selecting the most appropriate psychosocial interventions. However, Baron et al. (2015) found that there is evidence for gender and reporting bias in these investigations, with females being underrepresented, especially on considering the gender ratio and the dementia prevalence rates. Consequently, this review (Baron et al., 2015) concluded that further research is needed to address the influence of gender on the effect of psychosocial interventions for individuals living with dementia, whilst gender bias needs to be considered when developing such studies.

Gender differences in psychosocial interventions for informal caregivers

It has long been established that psychosocial interventions, especially psychoeducational, multicomponent supportive interventions, have a positive effect on informal caregivers and significantly reduce psychological distress (Brodaty, Green, & Koschera, 2003). Such interventions may be more beneficial for female caregivers who often report higher levels of burden and depression compared to male caregivers (Pillemer, Davis, & Tremont, 2018). In fact, a metaanalysis of psychosocial interventions for informal caregivers found that caregiver gender could have a strong influence on the effect size of these interventions (Pinquart & Sörensen, 2006). The authors of this study indicated that the higher the proportion of women participating in the study, the stronger was the effect of the intervention, especially on their depressive symptoms and ability/knowledge. This difference could be attributed to the fact that female caregivers start off with more depressive symptoms than male caregivers. Another reason could be that male and female caregivers tend to use different coping strategies, with women most likely adopting emotion-focused strategies that are less effective than men's problem-focused strategies (Tamres, Janicki, & Helgeson, 2002).

The reason why male caregivers are less likely to decline in depressive symptoms following such interventions could be associated with their general lack of attentiveness in recognizing and reporting caregiver distress (Lutzky & Knight, 1994). Similarly, Van Mierlo, Meiland, Van der Roest, and Dröes (2012), on reviewing the effectiveness of psychosocial interventions in subgroups of caregivers, concluded that these interventions had a more positive effect in reducing depression and enhancing self-efficacy in female caregivers, especially in wives of individuals living with dementia. However, since most of the informal caregivers are women (Erol, Brooker, & Peel, 2015), studies evaluating psychosocial interventions tend to be gender biased (Dickinson et al., 2017). Consequently, more research work is needed that includes both male and female informal caregivers in order to shed more light on what works for specific subgroups of caregivers. Erol et al. (2015) argued that healthcare professionals and researchers need to better understand these gender differences in order to develop and implement interventions that are targeted to the specific needs of male and female caregivers.

There are various reasons for the difficulty in measuring gender differences in psychosocial research. Male caregivers are difficult to recruit and obtain in sufficient number for comparative purposes. Secondly, McFarland and Sanders (2000) argued that male caregivers may be reluctant to express their stress and emotional reactions to caregiving, making it difficult to report and measure self-reported psychosocial outcomes. In accordance with this, Gant, Steffen, and Lauderdale (2007) found that two distance-based psychosocial interventions for male caregivers did not achieve the desired results, especially when comparing the two interventions. The authors suggested that one of the reasons for such an observation could be due to the reluctance of male caregivers in reporting caregiver distress.

Although there are significant challenges in measuring gender differences in informal caregiving, there is evidence indicating that these differences are underreported in studies evaluating the effectiveness of informal caregiver support interventions (Gilmore-Bykovskyi, Johnson, Walljasper, Block, & Werner, 2018). The authors argued that the reason for this can be attributed to the researchers' lack of appreciation of the importance of measuring gender differences when evaluating the impact of such interventions. One solution could be to stratify the targeted population based on gender and prior randomization when planning studies evaluating psychosocial interventions (Ulstein, Sandvik, Wyller, & Engedal, 2007). Increasing awareness of the importance of measuring gender differences when evaluating such interventions will help in tailoring the specific needs of informal caregivers of individuals living with dementia.

Gender differences in psychosocial interventions for formal caregivers

Similar to informal caregivers, formal caregivers such as nurses, care assistants, dementia care staff and other healthcare professionals are at an increased risk of caregiver burden (Miyamoto, Tachimori, & Ito, 2010) and psychological distress (Zwijsen et al., 2014) especially when caring for individuals living with dementia who exhibit BPSD. Psychosocial domains of the dementia care workforce such as staff knowledge, attitudes toward individuals with dementia, perceived self-efficacy, perceived empathy, and emotional exhaustion have been extensively studied as they are associated with a decrease in staff burnout, increased resilience, psychological coping, and emotional wellbeing (Alidosti, Delaram, Dehgani, & Maleki Moghadam, 2016; Bassal, Czellar, Kaiser, & Dan-Glauser, 2016; Kokkonen, Cheston, Dallos, & Smart, 2014). Psychoeducational interventions such as staff training and support programs not only positively influence these domains (Spector, Revolta, & Orrell, 2016) but can also reduce BPSD in individuals living with dementia (Spector, Orrell, & Goyder, 2013). Nevertheless, there is little evidence indicating whether staff training has a similar effect on male and female care staff. Moreover, it is also unclear whether there are significant gender differences in the staff domains of formal dementia caregivers in cross-sectional studies. This section will seek to critically discuss the limited evidence available.

One of the psychosocial domains that has been most commonly related to gender is empathy. Females report being more empathic than males, although such difference is not always significant and could be related to gender-related stereotypes (Baez et al., 2017). Similarly, Gilson and Moyer (2000) found significantly different levels of empathy between male and female caregivers of individuals living with dementia, with female caregivers reporting a generally higher degree of empathy compared to their male counterparts.

With respect to cross-sectional studies that measured attitudes toward individuals living with dementia, the influence of gender is still unclear. Brodaty, Draper, and Low (2003) found no association between the attitudes of Australian nursing home staff and gender. Similarly, a Norwegian cross-sectional study did not find any significant differences in hope attitude scores or person-centered attitude scores between male and female care staff (Kada, Nygaard, Mukesh, & Geitung, 2009). Such a finding was also reported in a similar cross-sectional study that sought to measure this association in residential homes in Hong Kong (Leung et al., 2013). On the contrary, Scerri and Scerri (2019) demonstrated that there were significant gender differences in dementia attitude scores of nursing staff working in residential homes in Malta with female nurses reporting more positive attitudes. This gender difference was also found in Maltese nurses working in acute hospital wards (Scerri, Innes, &

Scerri, 2020). A plausible reason for the different findings in these studies could be attributed to the fact that, unlike the Maltese studies, in which the male population constituted around a third of the sample for both studies, male care staff were heavily underrepresented in the other studies (Brodaty, Draper, et al., 2003—8%; Kada et al., 2009—3%; Leung et al., 2013—8%).

No significant gender difference in dementia knowledge was found in residential staff (Attard, Sammut, & Scerri, 2020), healthcare staff (Smyth et al., 2013), nursing students (Scerri & Scerri, 2013), and acute hospital nurses (Lin, Hsieh, Chen, Yang, & Lin, 2018; Scerri et al., 2020). This could be explained by the fact that both the male and female care workforce are provided with the same staff training and continuous professional development programs. With regard to the training needs required between male and female care staff, although very limited evidence exists, female nursing students reported the need for more training in how to deal with BPSD compared to male nursing students (Scerri & Scerri, 2013). This gender difference could be attributed to the fact that male student nurses identified themselves to be more confident than female students in maintaining their safety and in their personal practical ability to deal with aggressive behavior, as demonstrated during an aggression prevention training program (Beech, 2008).

Psychosocial and communication skills/person-centered dementia care training programs for health and social care staff working in residential homes (Kuske et al., 2007; Spector et al., 2016) and in acute care settings (Scerri, Innes, & Scerri, 2017; Surr & Gates, 2017) seem to have a positive effect on staff and patient outcomes, although the extent of such evidence is still considered poor (Elliott, Scott, Stirling, Martin, & Robinson, 2012). The characteristics of these programs have been clearly described (Surr et al., 2017), nevertheless, there seems to be a lack of empirical research on the characteristics of the participants who generally participate in these programs, especially in terms of gender. This could be partly due to the fact that researchers do not consider this variable as important in evaluating whether it has an impact on these programs even though, as highlighted above, there are significant gender differences at baseline in a number of psychological domains such as attitudes and perceived empathy. Another possible reason could be that the majority of these training programs are developed for a population who, in many countries, is predominantly composed of women. In fact, a secondary analysis of a dataset for the English dementia social care workforce found that it is female dominated, with 87% of the workforce being women and an odds ratio of 1.77 of being female and working in a dementia workforce when compared to other workers (Hussein & Manthorpe, 2012). This resonates with a worldwide report (World Health Organization, 2019), which showed that, currently, women account for the majority of the global health and social care workforce. Moreover, Hussein and Manthorpe (2012) also found that the female healthcare workers in their study had little to no qualifications and therefore required considerable dementia care training. Therefore, gender differences in the composition of dementia care workforce need to considered when developing dementia training programs, for example by ensuring an adequate sex ratio when taking weighed samples of participants in randomized controlled trials to study such programs. On the other hand, the specific training needs of male dementia care workers need to be taken into consideration and significant differences, if any, in the psychosocial domains of male versus female caregivers should be measured before and after the training program delivery.

In summary, this section has sought to provide a comprehensive critical appraisal of the current literature with regards to the effect of gender on psychosocial interventions for individuals living with dementia and their formal and informal caregivers. Although there is some evidence of their effectiveness, more research needs to be conducted in the development of these studies in order to avoid gender bias. This can be achieved by ensuring that both men and women adequately represent the ratios of the targeted populations, report all findings by gender, and develop gender-specific interventions. Moreover, further, adequately powered, cross-sectional studies need to be designed to understand better the gender differences of behavioral and psychological symptoms in individuals living with dementia and the differences in the psychosocial domains of male and female informal and formal caregivers.

Conclusion

This chapter highlighted the family dynamics in the context of caregiving of individuals living with dementia with particular reference to spouses and adult child caregivers. An overview of the effectiveness of psychosocial interventions targeting individuals living with dementia and their caregivers was also provided. The last section sought to critically appraise whether and how gender differences influence these psychosocial factors, especially for formal and informal caregivers. This contribution showed that whilst numerous psychosocial interventions in dementia care have been developed and implemented, their effect, especially the influence of gender, needs to be further studied.

Chapter highlights

- Female spouses tend to be more prone to depression in their role as caregivers. This is explained by the fact that they spend longer hours, use more emotion-focused coping strategies, and invest more energy in caring and nurturing. Male spouses are more pragmatic and accepting in their role as caregiver and are more willing to ask for outside help when caring for their ill spouse.
- Family caregiving, especially when managed by siblings, can be complicated, and fraught with conflict and resentment. Moreover, beliefs and expectations influenced by gender stereotypes and gendered roles also have an impact on decision making, expectations, and support related to caregiving. Family care workers can help manage such conflict in a constructive manner, leading to shared responsibility and an increased sense of wellbeing among family members.

- Male caregivers may prefer the support of their daughters or other relatives rather than that of support groups that are female dominated. Gender-specific support groups may be better suited for male and female caregivers as they tend to have different needs.
- Nonpharmacological interventions have been reported to improve behavioral symptoms and quality of life in individuals living with dementia, their caregivers, and family members.
- Studies that include developing and evaluating psychosocial interventions for formal and informal caregivers should take into consideration gender differences to avoid gender bias.

References

Abela, A. (2016). Family life. In M. Briguglio, & M. Brown (Eds.), *Sociology of the Maltese islands* (pp. 17–46). Malta: Miller Publishing.

Aguirre, E., Hoare, Z., Streater, A., Spector, A., Woods, B., Hoe, J., et al. (2013). Cognitive stimulation therapy (CST) for people with dementia-who benefits most? *International Journal of Geriatric Psychiatry*, 28(3), 284–290. https://doi.org/10.1002/gps.3823.

Alidosti, M., Delaram, M., Dehgani, L., & Maleki Moghadam, M. (2016). Relationship between self-efficacy and burnout among nurses in Behbahan City, Iran. *Women's Health Bulletin*, 3(4), 1–5.

Ashley, N. R., & Kleinpeter, C. (2002). Gender differences in coping strategies of spousal dementia caregivers. *Journal of Human Behavior in the Social Environment*, 6(2), 29–46. https://doi.org/10.1300/J137v06n02_03.

Association of Dance Movement Psychotherapy UK. (2020). *What is dance movement psychotherapy?*. http://www.admt.org.uk/whatis.html2016.

Attard, R., Sammut, R., & Scerri, A. (2020). Exploring the knowledge, attitudes and perceived learning needs of formal carers of people with dementia. *Nursing Older People*, 32(3). https://doi.org/10.7748/nop.2020.e1225.

Baez, S., Flichtentrei, D., Prats, M., Mastandueno, R., García, A. M., Cetkovich, M., et al. (2017). Men, women … who cares? A population-based study on sex differences and gender roles in empathy and moral cognition. *PLoS One*, 12(6). https://doi.org/10.1371/journal.pone.0179336, e0179336.

Ballard, C. G., O'Brien, J. T., Reichelt, K., & Perry, E. K. (2002). Aromatherapy as a safe and effective treatment for the management of agitation in severe dementia: The results of a double-blind, placebo-controlled trial with Melissa. *Journal of Clinical Psychiatry*, 63(7), 553–558. https://doi.org/10.4088/jcp.v63n0703.

Banerjee, S. (2009). *The use of antipsychotic medication for people with dementia: Time for action (A report for the Minister of State for Care Services)*. UK Department of Health.

Baron, S., Ulstein, I., & Werheid, K. (2015). Psychosocial interventions in Alzheimer's disease and amnestic mild cognitive impairment: Evidence for gender bias in clinical trials. *Aging & Mental Health*, 19(4), 290–305. https://doi.org/10.1080/13607863.2014.938601.

Bassal, C., Czellar, J., Kaiser, S., & Dan-Glauser, E. S. (2016). Relationship between emotions, emotion regulation, and well-being of professional caregivers of people with dementia. *Research on Aging*, 38(4), 477–503. https://doi.org/10.1177/0164027515591629.

Beech, B. (2008). Aggression prevention training for student nurses: Differential responses to training and the interaction between theory and practice. *Nurse Education in Practice*, *8*(2), 94–102. https://doi.org/10.1016/j.nepr.2007.04.004.

Bei, E., Rotem-Mindali, O., & Vilchinsky, N. (2020). Providing care from afar: A growing yet understudied phenomenon in the caregiving field. *Frontiers in Psychology*, *11*, 681. https://doi.org/10.3389/fpsyg.2020.00681.

Bergman, M., Graff, C., Eriksdotter, M., Fugl-Meyer, K. S., & Schuster, M. (2016). The meaning of living close to a person with Alzheimer disease. *Medicine, Health Care, and Philosophy*, *19*(3), 341–349. https://doi.org/10.1007/s11019-016-9696-3.

Bohlmeijer, E., Smit, F., & Cuijpers, P. (2003). Effects of reminiscence and life review on late-life depression: A meta-analysis. *International Journal of Geriatric Psychiatry*, *18*, 1088–1094. https://doi.org/10.1002/gps.1018.

Boylstein, C., & Hayes, J. (2012). Reconstructing marital closeness while caring for a spouse with Alzheimer's. *Journal of Family Issues*, *33*(5), 584–612. https://doi.org/10.1177/0192513X11416449.

Bramble, M., Moyle, W., & McAllister, M. (2009). Seeking connection: Family care experiences following long-term dementia care placement. *Journal of Clinical Nursing*, *18*(22), 3118–3125. https://doi.org/10.1111/j.1365-2702.2009.02878.x.

Brodaty, H., Draper, B., & Low, L. F. (2003). Nursing home staff attitudes towards residents with dementia: Strain and satisfaction with work. *Journal of Advanced Nursing*, *44*(6), 583–590. https://doi.org/10.1046/j.0309-2402.2003.02848.x.

Brodaty, H., Green, A., & Koschera, A. (2003). Meta-analysis of psychosocial interventions for caregivers of people with dementia. *Journal of the American Geriatrics Society*, *51*(5), 657–664. https://doi.org/10.1034/j.1600-0579.2003.00210.x.

Butcher, H. K., Holkup, P. A., Park, M., & Maas, M. (2001). Thematic analysis of the experience of making a decision to place a family member with Alzheimer's disease in a special care unit. *Research in Nursing & Health*, *24*(6), 470–480. https://doi.org/10.1002/nur.10005.

Cerejeira, J., Lagarto, L., & Mukaetova-Ladinska, E. (2012). Behavioral and psychological symptoms of dementia. *Frontiers in Neurology*, *3*, 73. https://doi.org/10.3389/fneur.2012.00073.

Cetinkaya, F., Duru Asiret, G., Direk, F., & Özkanli, N. N. (2019). The effect of ceramic painting on the life satisfaction and cognitive status of older adults residing in a nursing home. *Topics in Geriatric Rehabilitation*, *35*(2), 108–112. https://doi.org/10.1097/TGR.0000000000000208.

Chan, W. C., Ng, C., Mok, C. C., Wong, F. L., Pang, S. L., & Chiu, H. F. (2010). Lived experience of caregivers of persons with dementia in Hong Kong: A qualitative study. *East Asian Archives of Psychiatry*, *20*(4), 163–168.

Chan, J. S., Liu, G., Liang, D., Deng, K., Wu, J., & Yan, J. H. (2019). Special issue–therapeutic benefits of physical activity for mood: A systematic review on the effects of exercise intensity, duration, and modality. *Journal of Psychology*, *153*(1), 102–125.

Chiang, M., Reid-Varley, W. B., & Fan, X. (2019). Creative art therapy for mental illness. *Psychiatry Research*, *275*, 129–136. https://doi.org/10.1016/j.psychres.2019.03.025.

Clare, L., Linden, D. E., Woods, R. T., Whitaker, R., Evans, S. J., Parkinson, C. H., et al. (2010). Goal-oriented cognitive rehabilitation for people with early-stage Alzheimer disease: A single-blind randomized controlled trial of clinical efficacy. *American Journal of Geriatric Psychiatry*, *18*(10), 928–939. https://doi.org/10.1097/JGP.0b013e3181d5792a.

Cohen-Mansfield, J., & Perach, R. (2015). Interventions for alleviating loneliness among older persons: A critical review. *American Journal of Health Promotion*, *29*(3), e109–e125. https://doi.org/10.4278/ajhp.130418-LIT-182.

Cohen-Mansfield, J., & Werner, P. (1995). Environmental influences on agitation: An integrative summary of an observational study. *American Journal of Alzheimer's Disease & Other Dementias, 10*, 32–39. https://doi.org/10.1177/153331759501000108.

Cooke, M. L., Moyle, W., Shum, D. H. K., Harrison, S. D., & Murfield, J. E. (2010). A randomized controlled trial exploring the effect of music on agitated behaviours and anxiety in older people with dementia. *Aging & Mental Health, 14*, 905–916. https://doi.org/10.1080/13607861003713190.

Cooper, C., Katona, C., Orrell, M., & Livingston, G. (2008). Coping strategies, anxiety and depression in caregivers of people with Alzheimer's disease. *International Journal of Geriatric Psychiatry, 23*, 929–936. https://doi.org/10.1002/gps.2007.

Cross, A. J., Garip, C., & Sheffield, D. (2018). The psychosocial impact of caregiving in dementia and quality of life: A systematic review and meta-synthesis of qualitative research. *Psychology & Health, 33*(11), 1321–1342. https://doi.org/10.1080/08870446.2018.1496250.

Den Ouden, L., Kandola, A., Suo, C., Hendrikse, J., Costa, R., Watt, M. J., et al. (2018). The influence of aerobic exercise on hippocampal integrity and function: Preliminary findings of a multi-modal imaging analysis. *Brain Plasticity (Amsterdam, Netherlands), 4*(2), 211–216. https://doi.org/10.3233/BPL-170053.

Deshmukh, S. R., Holmes, J., & Cardno, A. (2018). Art therapy for people with dementia. *Cochrane Database of Systematic Reviews, 9*(9). https://doi.org/10.1002/14651858.CD011073.pub2, CD011073.

Dickinson, C., Dow, J., Gibson, G., Hayes, L., Robalino, S., & Robinson, L. (2017). Psychosocial intervention for carers of people with dementia: What components are most effective and when? A systematic review of systematic reviews. *International Psychogeriatrics, 29*(1), 31–43. https://doi.org/10.1017/S1041610216001447.

Donnellan, W. J., Bennett, K. M., & Soulsby, L. K. (2015). What are the factors that facilitate or hinder resilience in older spousal dementia carers? A qualitative study. *Aging & Mental Health, 19*(10), 932–939. https://doi.org/10.1080/13607863.2014.977771.

Dröes, R. M., van Mierlo, L. D., van der Roest, H. G., & Meiland, F. J. M. (2010). Focus and effectiveness of psychosocial interventions for people with dementia in institutional care settings from the perspective of coping with disease. *Non-Pharmacological Therapies in Dementia, 1*(2), 139–161.

Ducharme, F., Kergoa, M. J., Antoine, P., Pasquier, F., & Coulombe, R. (2013). The unique experience of spouses in early-onset dementia. *American Journal of Alzheimer's Disease & Other Dementias, 28*(6), 634–641. https://doi.org/10.1177/1533317513494443.

Egilstrod, B., Bay Ravn, M., & Schultz Petersen, K. (2019). Living with a partner with dementia: A systematic review and thematic synthesis of spouses' lived experiences of changes in their everyday lives. *Aging & Mental Health, 23*(5), 541–550. https://doi.org/10.1080/13607863.2018.1433634.

Elliott, K. E. J., Scott, J. L., Stirling, C., Martin, A. J., & Robinson, A. (2012). Building capacity and resilience in the dementia care workforce: A systematic review of interventions targeting worker and organizational outcomes. *International Psychogeriatrics, 24*(6), 882–894. https://doi.org/10.1017/S1041610211002651.

Epperly, T., Dunay, M. A., & Boice, J. L. (2017). Alzheimer disease: Pharmacologic and nonpharmacologic therapies for cognitive and functional symptoms. *American Family Physician, 95*(12), 771–778.

Erol, R., Brooker, D., & Peel, E. (2015). *Women and dementia: A global research review*. Alzheimer Disease International. https://www.alz.co.uk/women-and-dementia.

Fenech, M., & Scerri, J. (2014). The impact of providing care to the relatives with a severe illness: The caregivers' experience. *Malta Journal of Health Sciences, 1*(1), 19–23. http://dx.medra.org/10.14614/SMICARE.1.19.

Forrester, L. T., Maayan, N., Orrell, M., Spector, A. E., Buchan, L. D., & Soares-Weiser, K. (2014). Aromatherapy for dementia. *Cochrane Database of Systematic Reviews, 2*. https://doi.org/10.1002/14651858.CD003150.pub2, CD003150.

Gallego, M. G., & Garcia, J. G. (2017). Music therapy and Alzheimer's disease: Cognitive, psychological, and behavioural effects. *Neurología, 32*(5), 300–308. https://doi.org/10.1016/j.nrl.2015.12.003.

Gant, J. R., Steffen, A. M., & Lauderdale, S. A. (2007). Comparative outcomes of two distance-based interventions for male caregivers of family members with dementia. *American Journal of Alzheimer's Disease & Other Dementias, 22*(2), 120–128. https://doi.org/10.1177/1533317506298880.

Gaugler, J. E. (2005). Family involvement in residential long-term care: A synthesis and critical review. *Aging & Mental Health, 9*(2), 105–118. https://doi.org/10.1080/13607860412331310245.

Gilmore-Bykovskyi, A., Johnson, R., Walljasper, L., Block, L., & Werner, N. (2018). Underreporting of gender and race/ethnicity differences in NIH-funded dementia caregiver support interventions. *American Journal of Alzheimer's Disease & Other Dementias, 33*(3), 145–152. https://doi.org/10.1177/1533317517749465.

Gilson, A. M., & Moyer, D. M. (2000). Predictors of empathy in dementia care staff. *American Journal of Alzheimer's Disease, 15*(4), 239–251. https://doi.org/10.1177/153331750001500403.

Gridley, K., Brooks, J., Birks, Y., Baxter, K., & Parker, G. (2016). *Improving care for people with dementia: Development and initial feasibility study for evaluation of life story work in dementia care*. NIHR Journals Library.

Hall, L., Orrell, M., Stott, J., & Spector, A. (2013). Cognitive stimulation therapy (CST): Neuropsychological mechanisms of change. *International Psychogeriatrics, 25*(3), 479–489. https://doi.org/10.1017/S1041610212001822.

Hameed, S., Shah, J. M., Ting, S., Gabriel, C., Tay, S. Y., Chotpoksap, U., et al. (2018). Improving the quality of life in persons with dementia through a pilot study of a creative dance movement programme in an Asian setting. *International Journal of Neurorehabilitation, 5*, 334. https://doi.org/10.4172/2376-0281.1000334.

Hauer, K., Schwenk, M., Zieschang, T., Essig, M., Becker, C., & Oster, P. (2012). Physical training improves motor performance in people with dementia: A randomized controlled trial. *Journal of the American Geriatric Society, 60*, 8–15. https://doi.org/10.1111/j.1532-5415.2011.03778.x.

Hellström, I., Håkanson, C., Eriksson, H., & Sandberg, J. (2017). Development of older men's caregiving roles for wives with dementia. *Scandinavian Journal of Caring Sciences, 31*(4), 957–964. https://doi.org/10.1111/scs.12419.

Hjetland, G. J., Pallesen, S., Thun, E., Kolberg, E., Nordhus, I. H., & Flo, E. (2020). Light interventions and sleep, circadian, behavioral, and psychological disturbances in dementia: A systematic review of methods and outcomes. *Sleep Medicine Reviews, 52*, 101310. https://doi.org/10.1016/j.smrv.2020.101310.

Holmes, C., Hopkins, V., Hensford, C., MacLaughlin, V., Wilkinson, D., & Rosenvinge, H. (2002). Lavender oil as a treatment for agitated behaviour in severe dementia: A placebo controlled study. *International Journal of Geriatric Psychiatry, 17*(4), 305–308. https://doi.org/10.1002/gps.593.

Hussein, S., & Manthorpe, J. (2012). The dementia social care workforce in England: Secondary analysis of a national workforce dataset. *Aging & Mental Health*, *16*(1), 110–118. https://doi.org/10.1080/13607863.2011.596808.

Hwang, A. S., Rosenberg, L., Kontos, P., Cameron, J. I., Mihailidis, A., & Nygård, L. (2017). Sustaining care for a parent with dementia: An indefinite and intertwined process. *International Journal of Qualitative Studies on Health and Well-Being*, *12*(Suppl. 2), 1389578. https://doi.org/10.1080/17482631.2017.1389578.

Im, M. L., & Lee, J. I. (2014). Effects of art and music therapy on depression and cognitive function of the elderly. *Technology & Health Care*, *22*(3), 453–458. https://doi.org/10.3233/THC-140803.

Innes, A., Abela, S., & Scerri, C. (2011). The organisation of dementia care by families in Malta: The experiences of family caregivers. *Dementia*, *10*(2), 165–184. https://doi.org/10.1177/1471301211398988.

Kada, S., Nygaard, H. A., Mukesh, B. N., & Geitung, J. T. (2009). Staff attitudes towards institutionalised dementia residents. *Journal of Clinical Nursing*, *18*(16), 2383–2392. https://doi.org/10.1111/j.1365-2702.2009.02791.x.

Kales, H. C., Gitlin, L. N., & Lyketsos, C. G. (2015). Assessment and management of behavioral and psychological symptoms of dementia. *British Medical Journal*, *350*, h369. https://doi.org/10.1136/bmj.h369.

Karkou, V., & Meekums, B. (2017). Dance movement therapy for dementia. *Cochrane Database of Systematic Reviews*, *2*. https://doi.org/10.1002/14651858.CD011022.pub2, CD011022.

Khachiyants, N., Trinkle, D., Son, S. J., & Kim, K. Y. (2011). Sundown syndrome in persons with dementia: An update. *Psychiatry Investigation*, *8*, 275–287. https://doi.org/10.4306/pi.2011.8.4.275.

Kim, K., Han, J. W., So, Y., Seo, J., Kim, Y. J., Park, J. H., et al. (2017). Cognitive stimulation as a therapeutic modality for dementia: A meta-analysis. *Psychiatry Investigation*, *14*(5), 626–639. https://doi.org/10.4306/pi.2017.14.5.626.

Kindell, J., Burrow, S., Wilkinson, R., & Keady, J. D. (2014). Life story resources in dementia care: A review. *Quality in Ageing and Older Adults*, *15*(3), 151–161. https://doi.org/10.1108/QAOA-02-2014-0003.

Kitamura, T., Kitamura, M., Hino, S., Tanaka, N., & Kurata, K. (2012). Gender differences in clinical manifestations and outcomes among hospitalized patients with behavioral and psychological symptoms of dementia. *Journal of Clinical Psychiatry*, *73*(12), 1548–1554. https://doi.org/10.4088/JCP.11m07614.

Kitwood, T. (1997). *Dementia reconsidered: The person comes first*. Open University Press.

Kjallman-Alm, A., Norbergh, K., & Hellzen, O. (2013). What it means to be an adult child of a person with dementia. *International Journal of Qualitative Studies in Health and Well-being*, *8*, 21676. https://doi.org/10.3402/qhw.v8i0.21676.

Kokkonen, T. M., Cheston, R. I., Dallos, R., & Smart, C. A. (2014). Attachment and coping of dementia care staff: The role of staff attachment style, geriatric nursing self-efficacy, and approaches to dementia in burnout. *Dementia*, *13*(4), 544–568. https://doi.org/10.1177/1471301213479469.

Kolanowski, A., Litaker, M., Buettner, L., Moeller, J., & Costa, P. T., Jr. (2011). A randomized clinical trial of theory-based activities for the behavioral symptoms of dementia in nursing home residents. *Journal of American Geriatrics Society*, *59*, 1032–1041. https://doi.org/10.1111/j.1532-5415.2011.03449.x.

Kudlicka, A., Martyr, A., Bahar-Fuchs, A., Woods, B., & Clare, L. (2019). Cognitive rehabilitation for people with mild to moderate dementia. *Cochrane Database of Systematic Reviews*, 8. https://doi.org/10.1002/14651858.CD013388, CD013388.

Kurz, A., Thöne-Otto, A., Cramer, B., Egert, S., Frölich, L., Gertz, H. J., et al. (2012). CORDIAL: Cognitive rehabilitation and cognitive-behavioral treatment for early dementia in Alzheimer disease: A multicenter, randomized, controlled trial. *Alzheimer Disease and Associated Disorders*, 26(3), 246–253. https://doi.org/10.1097/WAD.0b013e318231e46e.

Kuske, B., Hanns, S., Luck, T., Angermeyer, M. C., Behrens, J., & Riedel-Heller, S. G. (2007). Nursing home staff training in dementia care: A systematic review of evaluated programs. *International Psychogeriatrics*, 19(5), 818–841. https://doi.org/10.1017/S1041610206004352.

Kwak, M., Ingersoll-Dayton, B., & Kim, J. (2012). Family conflict from the perspective of adult child caregivers: The influence of gender. *Journal of Social and Personal Relationships*, 29, 470–487. https://doi.org/10.1177/0265407511431188.

Lai, N. M., Chang, S., Ng, S. S., Tan, S. L., Chaiyakunapruk, N., & Stanaway, F. (2019). Animal-assisted therapy for dementia. *Cochrane Database of Systematic Reviews*, 11. https://doi.org/10.1002/14651858.CD013243.pub2, CD013243.

Law, C. K., Lam, F. M., Chung, R. C., & Pang, M. Y. (2020). Physical exercise attenuates cognitive decline and reduces behavioural problems in people with mild cognitive impairment and dementia: A systematic review. *Journal of Physiotherapy*, 66(1), 9–18. https://doi.org/10.1016/j.jphys.2019.11.014.

Lee, J. Y., Im, W. Y., Kim, H., & Lee, K. J. (2014). Gender differences in behavioral psychological symptoms of dementia in patients with Alzheimer's disease. *Korean Journal of Psychosomatic Medicine*, 22(2), 71–78. https://doi.org/10.0000/kjpm.2014.22.2.71.

Lee, J., Lee, K. J., & Kim, H. (2017). Gender differences in behavioral and psychological symptoms of patients with Alzheimer's disease. *Asian Journal of Psychiatry*, 26, 124–128. https://doi.org/10.1016/j.ajp.2017.01.027.

Leung, J. L. M., Sezto, N. W., Chan, W. C., Cheng, S. P., Tang, S. H., & Lam, L. C. W. (2013). Attitudes and perceived competence of residential care homes staff about dementia care. *Asian Journal of Gerontology and Geriatrics*, 8(1), 21–28.

Lin, P. C., Hsieh, M. H., Chen, M. C., Yang, Y. M., & Lin, L. C. (2018). Knowledge gap regarding dementia care among nurses in Taiwanese acute care hospitals: A cross-sectional study. *Geriatrics & Gerontology International*, 18(2), 276–285. https://doi.org/10.1111/ggi.13178.

Livingston, G., Leavey, G., Manela, M., Livingston, D., Rait, G., Sampson, E., et al. (2010). Making decisions for people with dementia who lack capacity: Qualitative study of family carers in UK. *British Medical Journal (Clinical Research Ed.)*, 341, c4184. https://doi.org/10.1136/bmj.c4184.

Logsdon, R. G., McCurry, S. M., & Teri, L. (2007). Evidence-based interventions to improve quality of life for individuals with dementia. *Alzheimer's Care Today*, 8(4), 309–318.

Lövheim, H., Sandman, P. O., Karlsson, S., & Gustafson, Y. (2009). Sex differences in the prevalence of behavioral and psychological symptoms of dementia. *International Psychogeriatrics*, 21(3), 469–475. https://doi.org/10.1017/S1041610209008497.

Lutzky, S. M., & Knight, B. G. (1994). Explaining gender differences in caregiver distress: The roles of emotional attentiveness and coping styles. *Psychology and Aging*, 9(4), 513–519. https://doi.org/10.1037//0882-7974.9.4.513.

Madsen, R., & Birkelund, R. (2013). 'The path through the unknown': The experience of being a relative of a dementia-suffering spouse or parent. *Journal of Clinical Nursing*, 22(21–22), 3024–3031. https://doi.org/10.1111/jocn.12131.

Mahendran, R., Gandhi, M., Moorakonda, R. B., Wong, J., Kanchi, M. M., Fam, J., et al. (2018). Art therapy is associated with sustained improvement in cognitive function in the elderly with mild neurocognitive disorder: Findings from a pilot randomized controlled trial for art therapy and music reminiscence activity versus usual care. *Trials*, *19*(1), 615. https://doi.org/10.1186/s13063-018-2988-6.

McFarland, P. L., & Sanders, S. (2000). Educational support groups for male caregivers of individuals with Alzheimer's disease. *American Journal of Alzheimer's Disease*, *15*(6), 367–373. https://doi.org/10.1177/153331750001500608.

McMinn, B. G., & Hinton, L. (2000). Confined to barracks: The effects of indoor confinement on aggressive behavior among inpatients of an acute psychogeriatric unit. *American Journal of Alzheimer's Disease*, *15*(1), 36–41. https://doi.org/10.1177/2F153331750001500106.

Miesen, B. (1993). Alzheimer's disease, the phenomenon of parent fixation and Bowlby's attachment theory. *International Journal of Geriatric Psychiatry*, *8*(5), 147–153. https://doi.org/10.1002/gps.930080207.

Mishima, K., Okawa, M., Hishikawa, Y., Hozumi, S., Hori, H., & Takahashi, K. (1994). Morning bright light therapy for sleep and behavior disorders in elderly patients with dementia. *Acta Psychiatrica Scandinavica*, *89*(1), 1–7. https://doi.org/10.1111/j.1600-0447.1994.tb01477.x.

Mitchell, G., & Templeton, M. (2014). Ethical considerations of doll therapy for people with dementia. *Nursing Ethics*, *21*(6), 720–730. https://doi.org/10.1177/0969733013518447.

Miyamoto, Y., Tachimori, H., & Ito, H. (2010). Formal caregiver burden in dementia: Impact of behavioral and psychological symptoms of dementia and activities of daily living. *Geriatric Nursing*, *31*(4), 246–253. https://doi.org/10.1016/j.gerinurse.2010.01.002.

Monahan, D. J. (1995). Informal caregivers of institutionalized dementia residents: Predictors of burden. *Journal of Gerontological Social Work*, *23*(3–4), 65–82. https://doi.org/10.1300/J083V23N03_05.

Moos, I., & Björn, A. (2006). Use of the life story in the institutional care of people with dementia: A review of intervention studies. *Ageing and Society*, *26*(3), 431–454. https://doi.org/10.1017/S0144686X06004806.

Morgan, T., Williams, L. A., Trussardi, G., & Gott, M. (2016). Gender and family caregiving at the end-of-life in the context of old age: A systematic review. *Palliative Medicine*, *30*(7), 616–624. https://doi.org/10.1177/0269216315625857.

Neil, M., & Wright, P. B. (2009). Validation therapy for dementia (update). *Cochrane Database of Systematic Reviews*, *1*, CD001394.

Ng, Q. X., Ho, C. Y., Koh, S. S., Tan, W. C., & Chan, H. W. (2017). Doll therapy for dementia sufferers: A systematic review. *Complementary Therapies in Clinical Practice*, *26*, 42–46. https://doi.org/10.1016/j.ctcp.2016.11.007.

O'Dwyer, S. T., Moyle, W., Taylor, T., Creese, J., & Zimmer-Gembeck, M. J. (2016). Homicidal ideation in family carers of people with dementia. *Aging & Mental Health*, *20*(11), 1174–1181. https://doi.org/10.1080/13607863.2015.1065793.

O'Shaunessy, M., Lee, K., & Lintern, T. (2010). Changes in the couple relationship in dementia care: Spouse carers experiences. *Dementia*, *9*(2), 237–258. https://doi.org/10.1177/1471301209354021.

Ogrodniczuk, J. S. (2006). Men, women, and their outcome in psychotherapy. *Psychotherapy Research*, *16*(4), 453–462. https://doi.org/10.1080/10503300600590702.

Oyebode, J. R., & Parveen, S. (2019). Psychosocial interventions for people with dementia: An overview and commentary on recent developments. *Dementia*, *18*(1), 8–35. https://doi.org/10.1177/1471301216656096.

Peluso, S., De Rosa, A., De Lucia, N., Antenora, A., Illario, M., Esposito, M., et al. (2018). Animal-assisted therapy in elderly patients: Evidence and controversies in dementia and psychiatric disorders and future perspectives in other neurological diseases. *Journal of Geriatric Psychiatry and Neurology, 31*(3), 149–157. https://doi.org/10.1177/0891988718774634.

Pillemer, S., Davis, J., & Tremont, G. (2018). Gender effects on components of burden and depression among dementia caregivers. *Aging & Mental Health, 22*(9), 1162–1167. https://doi.org/10.1080/13607863.2017.1337718.

Pinquart, M., & Sörensen, S. (2006). Helping caregivers of persons with dementia: Which interventions work and how large are their effects? *International Psychogeriatrics, 18*(4), 577–595. https://doi.org/10.1017/S1041610206003462.

Pongan, E., Tillmann, B., Leveque, Y., Trombert, B., Getenet, J. C., Auguste, N., et al. (2017). Can musical or painting interventions improve chronic pain, mood, quality of life and cognition in patients with mild Alzheimer's disease? Evidence from a randomized controlled trial. *Journal of Alzheimer's Disease, 60*(2), 663–677. https://doi.org/10.3233/JAD-170410.

Pöysti, M. M., Laakkonen, M. L., Strandberg, T., Savikko, N., Tilvis, R. S., Eloniemi-Sulkava, U., et al. (2012). Gender differences in dementia spousal caregiving. *International Journal of Alzheimer's Disease, 2012*, 162960. https://doi.org/10.1155/2012/162960.

Prado-Jean, A., Couratier, P., Druet-Cabanac, M., Nubukpo, P., Bernard-Bourzeix, L., Thomas, P., et al. (2010). Specific psychological and behavioral symptoms of depression in patients with dementia. *International Journal of Geriatric Psychiatry, 25*(10), 1065–1072. https://doi.org/10.1002/gps.2468.

Pretorius, C., Walker, S., & Heyns, P. M. (2009). Sense of coherence amongst male caregivers in dementia. *Dementia, 8*(1), 79–94. https://doi.org/10.1177/1471301208099046.

Prince, M., Wimo, A., Guerchet, M., Ali, G. C., Wu, Y.-T., & Prina, M. (2015). *World Alzheimer report 2015. The global impact of dementia: An analysis of prevalence, incidence, cost and trends*. Alzheimer's Disease International.

Quinn, C., Clare, L., Pearce, A., & van Dijkhuizen, M. (2008). The experience of providing care in the early stages of dementia: An interpretative phenomenological analysis. *Aging & Mental Health, 12*(6), 769–778. https://doi.org/10.1080/13607860802380623.

Rahe, J., Liesk, J., Rosen, J. B., Petrelli, A., Kaesberg, S., Onur, O. A., et al. (2015). Sex differences in cognitive training effects of patients with amnestic mild cognitive impairment. *Neuropsychology, Development, and Cognition. Section B, Aging, Neuropsychology and Cognition, 22*(5), 620–638. https://doi.org/10.1080/13825585.2015.1028883.

Robinson, C. A., Reid, R. C., & Cooke, H. A. (2010). A home away from home: The meaning of home according to families of residents with dementia. *Dementia, 9*(4), 490–508. https://doi.org/10.1177/1471301210381679.

Romero-Moreno, R., Losada, A., Marquez, M., Laidlaw, K., Fernandez-Fernandez, V., Nogales-Gozales, C., et al. (2014). Leisure, gender and kinship in dementia caregiving: Psychological vulnerability of caregiving daughters with feelings of guilt. *Journals of Gerontology Series B: Psychological Sciences and Social Sciences, 69*, 502–513. https://doi.org/10.1093/geronb/gbt027.

Rose-Rego, S. K., Strauss, M. E., & Smyth, K. A. (1998). Differences in the perceived well-being of wives and husbands caring for persons with Alzheimer's disease. *The Gerontologist, 38*(2), 224–230. https://doi.org/10.1093/geront/38.2.224.

Roth, D. L., Fredman, L., & Haley, W. E. (2015). Informal caregiving and its impact on health: A reappraisal from population-based studies. *The Gerontologist, 55*(2), 309–319. https://doi.org/10.1093/geront/gnu177.

Russel, R. (2001). In sickness and in health: A qualitative study of elderly men who care for their wives with dementia. *Journal of Aging Studies*, *15*(4), 351–367. https://doi.org/10.1016/S0890-4065(01)00028-7.

Sánchez, A., Millán-Calenti, J. C., Lorenzo-López, L., & Maseda, A. (2013). Multisensory stimulation for people with dementia: A review of the literature. *American Journal of Alzheimer's Disease & Other Dementias*, *28*(1), 7–14. https://doi.org/10.1177/1533317512466693.

Scerri, A., & Scerri, C. (2013). Nursing students' knowledge and attitudes towards dementia—A questionnaire survey. *Nurse Education Today*, *33*(9), 962–968. https://doi.org/10.1016/j.nedt.2012.11.001.

Scerri, A., & Scerri, C. (2019). Outcomes in knowledge, attitudes and confidence of nursing staff working in nursing and residential care homes following a dementia training programme. *Aging & Mental Health*, *23*(8), 919–928. https://doi.org/10.1080/13607863.2017.1399342.

Scerri, A., Innes, A., & Scerri, C. (2017). Dementia training programmes for staff working in general hospital settings—A systematic review of the literature. *Aging & Mental Health*, *21*(8), 783–796. https://doi.org/10.1080/13607863.2016.1231170.

Scerri, A., Innes, A., & Scerri, C. (2020). Person-centered dementia care in acute hospital wards—The influence of staff knowledge and attitudes. *Geriatric Nursing*, *41*(3), 215–221. https://doi.org/10.1016/j.gerinurse.2019.09.001.

Scerri, A., Sammut, R., & Scerri, C. (2021). Formal caregivers' perceptions and experiences of using pet robots for persons living with dementia in long-term care: A meta-ethnography. *Journal of Advanced Nursing*, *77*, 83–97. https://doi.org/10.1111/jan.14581.

Schultz, R., & Martire, L. M. (2004). Family caregiving of persons with dementia: Prevalence, health effects, and support strategies. *American Journal of Geriatric Psychiatry*, *12*, 240–249. https://doi.org/10.1097/00019442-200405000-00002.

Shin, J. H. (2015). Doll therapy: An intervention for nursing home residents with dementia. *Journal of Psychosocial Nursing and Mental Health Services*, *53*(1), 13–18. https://doi.org/10.3928/02793695-20141218-03.

Smyth, W., Fielding, E., Beattie, E., Gardner, A., Moyle, W., Franklin, S., et al. (2013). A survey-based study of knowledge of Alzheimer's disease among health care staff. *BMC Geriatrics*, *13*, 2. https://doi.org/10.1186/1471-2318-13-2.

Spector, A., Thorgrimsen, L., Woods, B. O. B., Royan, L., Davies, S., Butterworth, M., et al. (2003). Efficacy of an evidence-based cognitive stimulation therapy programme for people with dementia: Randomised controlled trial. *British Journal of Psychiatry*, *183*(3), 248–254. https://doi.org/10.1192/bjp.183.3.248.

Spector, A., Thorgrimsen, L., Woods, B., & Orrell, M. (2006). *Making a difference: An evidence-based group programme to offer cognitive stimulation therapy (CST) to people with dementia*. Hawker Publications.

Spector, A., Orrell, M., & Goyder, J. (2013). A systematic review of staff training interventions to reduce the behavioural and psychological symptoms of dementia. *Ageing Research Reviews*, *12*(1), 354–364. https://doi.org/10.1016/j.arr.2012.06.005.

Spector, A., Revolta, C., & Orrell, M. (2016). The impact of staff training on staff outcomes in dementia care: A systematic review. *International Journal of Geriatric Psychiatry*, *31*(11), 1172–1187. https://doi.org/10.1002/gps.4488.

Stokes, L., Combes, H., & Stokes, G. (2015). The dementia diagnosis: A literature review of information, understanding, and attributions. *Psychogeriatrics*, *15*(3), 218–225. https://doi.org/10.1111/psyg.12095.

Stoner, C. R., Lakshminarayanan, M., Durgante, H., & Spector, A. (2019). Psychosocial interventions for dementia in low- and middle-income countries (LMICs): A systematic review of effectiveness and implementation readiness. *Aging & Mental Health*, 1–12. Advance online publication https://doi.org/10.1080/13607863.2019.1695742.

Surr, C. A., & Gates, C. (2017). What works in delivering dementia education or training to hospital staff? A critical synthesis of the evidence. *International Journal of Nursing Studies*, 75, 172–188. https://doi.org/10.1016/j.ijnurstu.2017.08.002.

Surr, C. A., Gates, C., Irving, D., Oyebode, J., Smith, S. J., Parveen, S., et al. (2017). Effective dementia education and training for the health and social care workforce: A systematic review of the literature. *Review of Educational Research*, 87(5), 966–1002. https://doi.org/10.3102/0034654317723305.

Swinkels, J., Tilburg, T. V., Verbakel, E., & Broese van Groenou, M. (2019). Explaining the gender gap in the caregiving burden of partner caregivers. *Journals of Gerontology, Series B: Psychological Sciences and Social Sciences*, 74(2), 309–317. https://doi.org/10.1093/geronb/gbx036.

Tamres, L. K., Janicki, D., & Helgeson, V. S. (2002). Sex differences in coping behavior: A meta-analytic review and an examination of relative coping. *Personality and Social Psychology Review*, 6(1), 2–30. https://doi.org/10.1207/S15327957PSPR0601_1.

Tatangelo, G., McCabe, M., Macleod, A., & Konis, A. (2018). I just can't please them all and stay sane: Adult child caregivers' experiences of family dynamics in care-giving for a parent with dementia in Australia. *Health & Social Care in the Community*, 26(3), e370–e377. https://doi.org/10.1111/hsc.12534.

Teel, C. S., & Carson, P. (2003). Family experiences in the journey through dementia diagnosis and care. *Journal of Family Nursing*, 9(1), 38–58.

Tornatore, J. B., & Grant, L. A. (2002). Burden among family caregivers of persons with Alzheimer's disease in nursing homes. *The Gerontologist*, 42(4), 497–506. https://doi.org/10.1093/geront/42.4.497.

Ulstein, I. D., Sandvik, L., Wyller, T. B., & Engedal, K. (2007). A one-year randomized controlled psychosocial intervention study among family carers of dementia patients—Effects on patients and carers. *Dementia and Geriatric Cognitive Disorders*, 24(6), 469–475. https://doi.org/10.1159/000110740.

Utsumi, K., Fukatsu, R., Yamada, R., Takamaru, Y., Hara, Y., & Yasumura, S. (2020). Characteristics of initial symptoms and symptoms at diagnosis in probable dementia with Lewy body disease: Incidence of symptoms and gender differences. *Psychogeriatrics*, 20(5), 737–745. https://doi.org/10.1111/psyg.12586.

van der Steen, J. T., Smaling, H. J., van der Wouden, J. C., Bruinsma, M. S., Scholten, R. J., & Vink, A. C. (2018). Music-based therapeutic interventions for people with dementia. *Cochrane Database of Systematic Reviews*, 7(7). https://doi.org/10.1002/14651858.CD003477.pub4, CD003477.

Van Mierlo, L. D., Van der Roest, H. G., Meiland, F. J. M., & Dröes, R. M. (2010). Personalized dementia care: Proven effectiveness of psychosocial interventions in subgroups. *Ageing Research Reviews*, 9(2), 163–183. https://doi.org/10.1016/j.arr.2009.09.002.

Van Mierlo, L. D., Meiland, F. J., Van der Roest, H. G., & Dröes, R. M. (2012). Personalised caregiver support: Effectiveness of psychosocial interventions in subgroups of caregivers of people with dementia. *International Journal of Geriatric Psychiatry*, 27(1), 1–14. https://doi.org/10.1002/gps.2694.

van Uffelen, J. G., Paw, M. J. C. A., Hopman-Rock, M., & van Mechelen, W. (2007). The effect of walking and vitamin B supplementation on quality of life in community-dwelling adults with mild cognitive impairment: A randomized, controlled trial. *Quality of Life Research*, 16(7), 1137–1146. https://doi.org/10.1007/s11136-007-9219-z.

Vikstrom, S., Josephsson, S., Stigsdotter-Neely, A., & Nygard, L. (2008). Engagement in activities: Experiences of persons with dementia and their caregiving spouses. *Dementia*, *7*(2), 251–270. https://doi.org/10.1177/1471301208091164.

Wimo, A., Gauthier, S., & Prince, M. (2018). *Global estimates of informal care*. Alzheimer's Disease International. https://www.alz.co.uk/adi/pdf/global-estimates-of-informal-care.pdf.

Wipfli, B. M., Rethorst, C. D., & Landers, D. M. (2008). The anxiolytic effects of exercise: A meta-analysis of randomized trials and dose-response analysis. *Journal of Sport & Exercise Psychology*, *30*(4), 392–410. https://doi.org/10.1123/jsep.30.4.392.

Woods, B., Thorgrimsen, L., Spector, A., Royan, L., & Orrell, M. (2006). Improved quality of life and cognitive stimulation therapy in dementia. *Aging & Mental Health*, *10*(3), 219–226. https://doi.org/10.1080/13607860500431652.

Woods, B., O'Philbin, L., Farrell, E. M., Spector, A. E., & Orrell, M. (2018). Reminiscence therapy for dementia. *Cochrane Database of Systematic Reviews*, *3*(3). https://doi.org/10.1002/14651858.CD001120.pub3, CD001120.

World Health Organization. (2017). *Global action on public health response to dementia 2017–2025*. https://www.who.int/mental_health/neurology/dementia/action_plan_2017_2025/en/.

World Health Organization. (2019). *Delivered by women, led by men: A gender and equity analysis of the global health and social workforce*. https://apps.who.int/iris/bitstream/handle/10665/311322/9789241515467-eng.pdf.

Xing, Y., Wei, C., Chu, C., Zhou, A., Li, F., Wu, L., et al. (2012). Stage-specific gender differences in cognitive and neuropsychiatric manifestations of vascular dementia. *American Journal of Alzheimer's Disease & Other Dementias*, *27*(6), 433–438. https://doi.org/10.1177/1533317512454712.

Yilmaz, C. K., & Aşiret, G. D. (2020). The effect of doll therapy on agitation and cognitive state in institutionalized patients with moderate-to-severe dementia: A randomized controlled study. *Journal of Geriatric Psychiatry and Neurology*, 891988720933353. Advance online publication https://doi.org/10.1177/0891988720933353.

Zwijsen, S. A., Kabboord, A., Eefsting, J. A., Hertogh, C. M., Pot, A. M., Gerritsen, D. L., et al. (2014). Nurses in distress? An explorative study into the relation between distress and individual neuropsychiatric symptoms of people with dementia in nursing homes. *International Journal of Geriatric Psychiatry*, *29*(4), 384–391. https://doi.org/10.1002/gps.4014.

CHAPTER 14

Sex and gender differences in caregiving patterns and caregivers' needs

Klara Lorenz-Dant[a] and Mary Mittelman[b],
[a]*Care Policy and Evaluation Centre, The London School of Economics and Political Science, London, United Kingdom*
[b]*Department of Psychiatry, NYU Grossman School of Medicine, New York, NY, United States*

What are the patterns of care?

Despite societal changes including increases in male longevity, which have led to an increase in the number of older men available to provide care to their wives (OECD, 2019, p. 66; Public Health England, 2017), as well as the emancipation movements that have enabled a greater proportion of women to engage in the labor force and have, therefore, reduced the number of female fulltime homemakers, unpaid care remains largely a female responsibility (Ferrant, Pesando, & Nowacka, 2014; Scott & Clery, 2013). It is thus perhaps not surprising that the majority of unpaid care for people with Alzheimer's disease and other dementias around the world is provided by wives, daughters, and daughters-in-law, the largest proportion of whom are aged 50 years and older (Alzheimer's Association, 2019, p. 31; Bartlett et al., 2018, p. 15; Custodio et al., 2017; Erol, Brooker, & Peel, 2015; Kim, Kim, & An, 2016; Prince and The 10/66 Dementia Research Group, 2004; Toribio-Diaz et al., 2013).

Alzheimer's Disease International (ADI) recently published estimates of the proportion of unpaid dementia care provided by women around the world. The report estimates that in North America, 71% of unpaid care is provided by women (Wimo, Gauthier, & Prince, 2018, p. 6). Bott, Sheckter, and Milstein (2017, p. 757) also commented that "the best long-term care insurance in [the US] is a conscientious daughter." ADI further reports that the proportion of female unpaid caregivers in Latin America ranges from 74% in Southern Latin America to 91% in Tropical Latin America (Wimo et al., 2018, p. 6). Other examples from Latin America and the Caribbean, including studies conducted in Argentina, Brazil, Chile, Colombia, Guatemala, Mexico, Panama, Peru, Uruguay, Venezuela, and Cuba, also report this high proportion of female caregivers (from 70% to more than 80%) in dementia-specific studies (Custodio et al., 2017; Prince and The 10/66 Dementia Research Group, 2004, p. 173; Slachevsky et al., 2013). This pattern remains consistent among estimates for Africa and the Middle East. ADI estimates that 71% of unpaid care in

North Africa and the Middle East for people with dementia is provided by women. This proportion increases to 81% in Sub-Saharan Africa (Wimo et al., 2018, p. 6). More variation in the provision of dementia care by gender can be found in Asia. While it is estimated that just over half of unpaid care (55%) is provided by female caregivers in East Asia, this percentage increases to more than 70% in Central (71%) and South Asia (77%) and to over 80% in the high-income Asia Pacific region (81%) and Southeast Asia (86%). A high proportion of female caregivers can also be found in Australasia (72%), while the male/female division of unpaid dementia caregivers appears more even in Oceania (55% female) (Wimo et al., 2018, p. 6). As across Asia, considerable variability can also be found among European countries. While women provide the majority of unpaid dementia care, the percentage is higher in Central (74%) and Eastern Europe (82%) than in Western Europe (66%) (Wimo et al., 2018, p. 6). These findings are supported by dementia-specific studies from Spain and Italy, which report that about 70% of unpaid caregivers are women (Lavarone et al., 2014; Toribio-Diaz et al., 2013).

Despite the fact that women continue to carry the main responsibility of unpaid care, studies that have focused on female caregivers of people living with dementia consistently conclude that female caregivers remain largely "invisible" in society and that the literature on dementia care does not generally pay attention to gender differences (Bartlett et al., 2018, p. 15; Erol et al., 2015, p. 7; Savitch, Abbott, & Parker, 2015, p. 12).

Women continue to be expected to care whether they want to or not

Even though many male and female caregivers express the explicit wish to support their relatives with dementia, more women than men experience being pushed into fulfilling the socially ascribed female caring and nurturing role. In most cultures, the socialization of women as "natural" caregivers begins in infancy when girls are encouraged to play with dolls to develop nurturing and caring behaviors, while boys are encouraged to develop fighting and protecting behaviors (Savitch et al., 2015, p. 23). Despite educational emancipation in many countries, the cultural expectation of women continues to embrace traditional caring values in fulfilling their roles as nurturing wives and mothers (Toepfer, Foster, & Wilz, 2014, p. 242) (the cultural and familial aspect of caregiving is discussed in Chapter 13). While some women, usually those with higher-socioeconomic status and educational attainment, may be able to reduce their care involvement if they wish to do so, women with low socioeconomic status and less educational attainment frequently become the "natural" family caregivers (Toribio-Diaz et al., 2013, p. 99). A study from Cyprus reported that women did not necessarily choose to care, but experienced societal expectation to conform to their nurturing and caring "female nature" (Papastavrou et al., 2007, pp. 452–453). Moreover, many women experience guilt when they decide not to provide care (Friedemann & Buckwalter, 2014, p. 315; Toepfer et al., 2014, p. 242).

Among immigrant groups in Western countries, traditional values are especially salient. A study of Turkish, Moroccan, and Surinam Creole female caregivers living in the Netherlands found that the provision of family care increased the respect for women within the community, and caregivers emphasized feeling satisfaction from providing care that was based on their religious values (van Wezel et al., 2016, p. 77). An American study conducted in Florida including a large number of Latin and Caribbean caregivers found that male caregivers felt less burden and depression than women, who believed caregiving to be a female duty (Friedemann & Buckwalter, 2014, p. 322).

The concept of the family as a reciprocal unit where children pay back for sacrifices parents made earlier in their life through care has also been identified among Sri Lankan caregivers (Watt et al., 2014, p. 845). Similarly, reports from Nigeria emphasized that children are viewed as a form of social protection, placing duty and moral obligation on adult children, primarily on female offspring (Uwakwe, 2006; World Health Organization and Alzheimer's Disease International, 2012). Filial piety was also expressed by caregivers from other countries, including South Africa, the United States, Brazil, the Netherlands and the United Kingdom (Greenwood & Smith, 2019, p. 15).

However, other research (Greenwood & Smith, 2019; Quinn, Clare, & Woods, 2010) noted that the notion of the concept of filial piety was less likely to be explicitly expressed among caregivers from Western cultures, but rather that motivation to care, regardless of culture, is based on long-standing family relationships and the desire to reciprocate for care received in the past. A study from Spain, for instance, reports that most unpaid caregivers offer care out of moral duty and gratitude to the care recipient, to maintain the relative's dignity, and for personal satisfaction. However, 25.4% of caregivers responded that they provided care because someone had to and 15.5% explained that they provided care due to insufficient funds for residential care (Toribio-Diaz et al., 2013, pp. 97–98). Similarly, Da Roit (2007) links reduced involvement by Italian middle-class daughters with more opportunities and willingness to organize paid care rather than increased commitment by male caregivers. The aforementioned study of female immigrant caregivers in the Netherlands echoed this notion, showing that while older women emphasized that care should be provided by the family, some younger caregivers understood caring as taking responsibility to ensure "that good care is provided" (van Wezel et al., 2016, p. 76).

Pressure to care was also experienced by lesbian caregivers, even in cases where the caregivers' sexuality had caused previous tensions in family relationships. Lesbian caregivers further perceived greater pressure to care than their heterosexual or married siblings as it was felt that their personal relationships and responsibilities were comparatively less important (Price, 2011, p. 1293).

Men become an increasingly important caregiver group

As pointed out earlier, increasing male longevity creates a situation in which a growing number of husbands are available to support their wives with care needs, leading to a growing proportion of older male caregivers (White, 2013). In fact, in the United Kingdom, there are more male than female caregivers among the oldest old, most of whom are husbands supporting their wives (Dahlberg, Denmack, & Bambra, 2007; ONS, 2013; Vlachantoni, 2010). Data from the British Household Panel survey showed that in the age group 65 and older, men provided more hours of care on average than women (Carmichael & Ercolani, 2014, p. 403).

We have identified studies from the United States, Canada, Portugal, the United Kingdom, and South Africa that focused on husbands providing dementia care. Husbands in all studies were reported to express their commitment to caring for their wives. Many reported a deeply rooted motivation based on marital commitment as well as feelings of gratitude and reciprocity for the care and support they received from their wives throughout often long-standing marriages (Atta-Konadu, Keller, & Daly, 2011, p. 311; Boyle, 2013a, p. 236; Pretorius, Walker, & Heyns, 2009, pp. 89–90; Ribeiro & Paul, 2008, p. 170). Some of these husband caregivers also expressed religious reasons as motivating factors (Pretorius et al., 2009, pp. 89–90). For some, the gaining of new skills, receiving recognition and gratitude from their wives, families, and extended networks, as well as finding personal meaning in these activities became a source of purpose and pride in their lives (Boylestein & Hayes, 2012; Ribeiro & Paul, 2008, pp. 174, 176).

Studies investigating the role of sons in the provision of dementia care have found distinct patterns. Sons usually only take on the role of the main caregiver if there is no one else to take on the responsibility or if they are single (Campbell, 2010; Frehlih, 2019, pp. 1140–1141; Friedemann & Buckwalter, 2014). It was reported that sons provided the fewest direct care tasks in comparison to spouses or daughters (Friedemann & Buckwalter, 2014, p. 322). A Canadian study found that a close relationship to their parent as well as socioeconomic aspects, such as financial need or unemployment influenced sons' decisions to become caregivers (Campbell, 2010, p. 80). This study found considerable differences in the involvement of never married and married sons. Never married sons were more likely to live with their parent, to provide personal care in the home, even when the parent became incontinent and required more demanding personal care tasks, and to report that their care responsibility took on a central role in their lives (Campbell, 2010, pp. 79–80).

In many studies, men were more likely to take on a "managerial" approach, often indicating that their professional experience provided them with relevant skills. For example, in two Canadian studies, married sons reported their care responsibilities as one of the "dimensions in their lives." Male caregivers also received practical and emotional support from their female relatives (Campbell, 2010, p. 81; Grigorovich et al., 2016, p. 4). Some sons reported difficulties with the provision of personal care, particularly for their mothers (Campbell, 2010, p. 78). Similar to husbands, sons are given considerable recognition for their involvement in parental care "in ways that women who engage in the same caregiving activities are not" (Campbell, 2010, p. 81).

Sex and gender differences in the care provided

The amount and type of care provided to people living with Alzheimer's disease and other dementias is largely determined by the care needs of the person, which are likely to change over the course of the disease (Friedemann & Buckwalter, 2014, p. 329; Pinquart & Sörensen, 2006).

Emerging evidence reports gender-related differences in the time spent caring and the tasks performed.

Time

In addition to the fact that a larger proportion of women globally provide unpaid dementia care, women have been found to spend more time providing care than men (Alzheimer's Association, 2019; Ferrant et al., 2014; Pinquart & Sörensen, 2006, p. 38). Research further suggests that men frame care work differently. It has been argued that men generally characterize household tasks as "care work," while women may not classify these tasks, many of which they have provided throughout their lives, as "care work." Thus, men may count more tasks as care work than women do (Savitch et al., 2015, p. 24).

Tasks

The type of care tasks male and female caregivers take on has also been investigated.

In an analysis of the intake data for a large longitudinal study conducted in New York City, Mittelman (2003, p. 275) found that many spouse caregivers had taken over the tasks previously carried out by their husbands and wives. Other literature added that there may be some differences in the type of tasks women and men volunteer to provide as well as in self-expectation (Pinquart & Sörensen, 2006, p. 38).

These studies focus on differences in care patterns between husbands and wives. First, studies note that many older women view the provision of personal care tasks as an extension of responsibilities they carried out while raising children. For older husbands in traditional marriages, the provision of personal care, particularly to a woman, may be a new experience requiring them to learn new skills (Calasanti & Bowen, 2006). One study argues that the increase in workload for men, therefore, seems comparatively greater (Savitch et al., 2015, p. 24). Husbands described having to learn new skills that involved not just household tasks, such as cooking, washing, cleaning, and shopping, but also taking responsibility for their wives' personal care (Pretorius et al., 2009).

Studies focusing on husbands explored how they, in particular, responded when they found it difficult to take on their wives' former roles. Some placed their partner with dementia in residential care, other couples changed their joint living situation or found alternative resources, such as meals from formal providers, or support from other (female) family members (Atta-Konadu et al., 2011, pp. 308, 313; Hong & Coogle, 2016). The fluidity with which gender-specific roles can shift between men and women may depend on cultural context and age of caregiver. Furthermore, in families with high socioeconomic status, as found in one American study, husbands can afford to delegate tasks to paid caregivers (Calasanti & King, 2007, p. 520).

Boyle (2013b) qualitatively studied gender differences in husbands and wives caring for their spouses with dementia in England. The author noted that in "husband-dominated" partnerships, wives living with dementia in almost a third of the cases investigated continued maintaining the household, whether they wished to or not, and received reminders of their duties by their husbands who "managed" the tasks. Furthermore, both husbands and wives overstated the men's involvement in household tasks. While Boyle interpreted women's gratitude to their caregiver as a potential sign of vulnerability in the relationship, other researchers argued that this might be due to women having a better understanding of the nature of domestic work and as a result showing greater appreciation of its value (Calasanti & Bowen, 2006, p. 262). Boyle's study further found that husbands only took on household responsibilities when their wives were no longer able to maintain them (Boyle, 2013b, 2014). Similarly, other research found that husbands felt that they preserved their male identity by being "in charge" of the care situation (Ribeiro, Paúl, & Nogueira, 2007). Women, on the other hand, took "facilitative" approaches, engaging their husbands in everyday decision making, such as what to eat as well as actively involving them in activities (Boyle, 2013a, pp. 232–233). However, when making important decisions (e.g., residential respite care, attendance of day care), both wives and husbands excluded their spouses with dementia (Boyle, 2013a, p. 239).

The aforementioned study among migrant communities in the Netherlands also identified a gendered conceptualization of care tasks. Particularly among Turkish and Moroccan families, men were less often involved in the provision of care. However, family care is preferred to paid care and when provided by men, tends to be only in the same "family line." As in other cultures, men were more often involved in managerial aspects of care (van Wezel et al., 2016, p. 77).

What are the implications of providing dementia care?
Positive outcomes

Positive aspects of caregiving have only been explicitly evaluated in recent studies, despite the fact that, anecdotally, many caregivers have expressed the wish to provide care and have reported feelings of satisfaction, pride, feeling close to the person with dementia, "doing the right thing," and the wish to reciprocate in long-established relationships (Erol et al., 2015). These feelings appear to be particularly common among immigrant caregivers with traditional values; for example, female caregivers of Turkish, Moroccan, and Surinamese Creole origin in the Netherlands emphasized that they experienced satisfaction and fulfillment from their role. The concept of fulfillment was greatest among those who emphasized religious and culture aspects (van Wezel et al., 2016, p. 70, 78). The importance of religiosity in helping caregivers to find meaning in their role was also found among caregivers in the United Kingdom and female caregivers in Sri Lanka (Quinn, Clare, & Woods, 2012; Watt et al., 2014). Other studies have reported that daughters reporting satisfaction from their caring role emphasized attachment and placed great value on the concept of family (Day, Anderson, & Davis, 2014, p. 802; Newman et al., 2019, p. 10).

Another group that often described positive outcomes from their caregiver role, as pointed out above, were husbands, who described increased self-worth from learning new skills, receiving recognition and gratitude from their wives, and social honor from family and friends (Lloyd, Patterson, & Muers, 2014, pp. 1554–1555; Ribeiro & Paul, 2008; Sampson & Clark, 2016). The older men in the Portuguese study who reported positive outcomes reflected on long-standing marriages and close relationships prior to their wives' illness, described problem-focused coping strategies, and the ability to "draw broader meanings from their situation" (Ribeiro & Paul, 2008, p. 169). One study found that men with more traditional values regarding "emotional closeness … success, power, and competition" reported greater gain from their new roles in providing care (Baker, Robertson, & Connelly, 2010, p. 324). The authors hypothesized that men with less traditional views may have already had domestic and childcare responsibilities, so that providing care for an ill relative did not involve as much of a role change (Baker et al., 2010, p. 325).

A Canadian study investigating the experience of sons caring for a parent with dementia found that some of the never-married sons, in particular, extracted great value, purpose, and worth from their care responsibility (Campbell, 2010, p. 77; Frehlih, 2019). However, all sons reported positive outcomes, such as the development of closer family relationships, personal growth, satisfaction, "greater 'patience,' 'understanding' or 'tolerance'" as well as increased resilience and resourcefulness from their care responsibilities (Campbell, 2010, p. 78; Grigorovich et al., 2016, p. 5).

A review of qualitative research found that personal growth was reported by all family caregivers but wives. Male caregivers were more likely to report gaining in humility when asked about personal growth. Wives, on the other hand, were more likely to identify spiritual growth than other caregivers. Both husbands and wives identified intimacy and relationship gains as positive outcomes from their care commitment (Lloyd et al., 2014, pp. 1550–1551).

Negative outcomes of caregiving

While many women and men experience positive outcomes from providing care, there is a large body of evidence that the provision of dementia care also bears the risk of negative outcomes. Caregivers report that the provision of care "was unexpectedly tiring, time-consuming, emotionally trying and frustrating at times" (Newman et al., 2019, p. 9). The most well-researched outcomes include caregiver burden as well as mental and physical health implications.

Caregiver burden

There is a great deal of literature investigating the burden of unpaid caregivers of people with dementia. The main message is that women, particularly wives, experience substantial burden.

Research across countries reports that women experienced the most burden when caring for a relative with dementia (Akpinar, Küçükgüçlü, & Yener, 2011; Bartlett et al., 2018; Chappell, Dujela, & Smith, 2015, p. 637; Friedemann & Buckwalter, 2014; Gibbons et al., 2014; Lavarone et al., 2014; Pillemer, Davis, & Tremont, 2018; Pinquart & Sörensen, 2006; Pöysti et al., 2012; Prince et al., 2012). For example, the female caregivers in immigrant communities in the Netherlands described caring as a major effort. They found both the mental and physical deterioration of their relative and the impact their care responsibility had on their personal life burdensome. Some explained that family expectations limited their choice in how to provide care and "the freedom to share the burden of care with professionals" (van Wezel et al., 2016, p. 78).

Greater burden has also been associated with the intensity of care provided, the age of the caregiver, and self-esteem. Canadian research found that caregivers providing more hours of care were more likely to be younger and to have lower self-esteem (Chappell et al., 2015, p. 634). This matches findings from an American study reporting that caregiver burden was associated with "anger-resentment" toward the care recipient, feelings of "personal time restriction" and reduction in social life. "Emotional lability" of the person with dementia appeared to have a greater effect on caregivers than cognitive impairment (Croog et al., 2006, p. 87). Difficulties with the behavior of the person with dementia, severity, care need, and time spent caring were also found to be associated with caregiver strain in a study in low- and middle-income countries. This study also reported an association between caregiver burden and cutting back on work to provide care in several of the sites (Prince et al., 2012, p. 674, 676). Another study, in which 60% of the sample cared for a person with dementia, reported that in addition to age, ethnicity, spirituality, and care recipient behavior, caregivers with health problems experienced care as more burdensome (Friedemann & Buckwalter, 2014, p. 328).

Mental health

As with burden, in many countries female caregivers of people living with dementia are found to be at greater risk of experiencing psychological distress, depression, and anxiety (Andreakou et al., 2016; Bartlett et al., 2018; Borden & Berlin, 1990; Borsje et al., 2016; Gibbons et al., 2014; Papastavrou et al., 2007, 2009; Pillemer et al., 2018; Pinquart & Sörensen, 2006; Valimaki et al., 2009). An American study that investigated a largely white, college-educated sample found that, for women with a partner with Alzheimer's disease, those who reported being satisfied with intimacy reported fewer symptoms of stress and depression; while for both genders, those caring for a partner with mild dementia reported fewer depressive symptoms than those caring for a person with more severe dementia (Davies et al., 2012, pp. 89, 94).

Two studies identified caregiving daughters as being at greatest risk of developing depression (Romero-Moreno et al., 2014, p. 509; Watson, Tatangelo, & McCabe, 2019). A Spanish study identified daughters as reporting high levels of guilt and found that those with little engagement in leisure activities were at particular risk of depression (Romero-Moreno et al., 2014). As above, the authors suggest that cultural expectations that women provide care may increase the pressure on daughters, who often will also have other competing family and work demands. A Finnish study, on the other hand, did not find any gender difference for caregiver "depression, satisfaction with life, or loneliness" (Pöysti et al., 2012, p. 1), perhaps because gender role expectations are less clearly delineated in Finland.

Physical health

Family caregivers of people with dementia have been found to experience worse physical health than noncaregivers (Dassel & Carr, 2016, p. 444; World Health Organization and Alzheimer's Disease International, 2012, p. 74). An American study on spouse caregivers reported that frailty continued to be greater among caregivers supporting a spouse with dementia at the end of life compared to caregivers of spouses without dementia, both before and after the provision of care had stopped (Dassel & Carr, 2016, p. 449).

Another American study comparing physical health and physiological risks found that wives providing care rated their physical health worse than wives who were not caregivers, while husband caregivers reported better physical health than their counterparts not providing care. However, indicators of physiological risk showed the opposite: husband caregivers exhibited significantly greater physiological risks than noncaregiver husbands, while for wives, no difference was found. The authors suggest that this might be because women may find it easier to disclose health and psychological problems, particularly when experiencing sustained stress (Zhang, Vitaliano, & Lin, 2006, pp. 173–178).

A study on female Latina and non-Latina caregivers of people with dementia in the US found considerable differences between ethnic groups, with Latinas less likely than non-Latinas to report their health as very good or excellent (Rabinowitz & Gallagher-Thompson, 2007, p. 11). A Spanish study identified lower health related quality of life among female caregivers than in the general female population (Argimon et al., 2004, p. 456).

Why do we observe different outcomes for male and female caregivers?

The literature offers a number of interlinked explanations of why women may experience greater care burden as well as greater impact on their physical and mental health. Pinquart and Sörensen suggest that gender differences among caregivers are small, but larger than in the general population, and that these differences could be attributed to women's greater experience of care-related stressors and fewer social resources; notably, greater "readiness to disclose negative feelings and health problems" could explain the greater negative impact reported by women (Pinquart & Sörensen, 2006, p. 39). Similarly, other research suggests that men and women may report emotion in accordance with gender stereotypical expectations but also allude to issues around biases due to sampling of people in contact with services that may influence reporting (Baker & Robertson, 2008). Here, we focus on four aspects that are likely to impact men and women differently: possible differences in coping mechanisms, complex care situations, societal demands, and existing support structures.

Gender differences in coping mechanisms

One argument focuses on gender differences in coping mechanisms, which suggest that women feel greater empathy for their care recipients and are more prone to use emotional coping mechanisms as well as avoidance and escape strategies (Calasanti & King, 2007, p. 526). Other research corroborates the finding that women were more likely to use emotion-focused coping, which led to greater stress and burden (Lavarone et al., 2014, p. 1411).

Men, on the other hand, are understood to be generally more likely to employ problem-solving and task-oriented approaches, including strategies such as "focusing on tasks, blocking emotions, minimizing disruption, and self-medicating" (Calasanti & King, 2007, p. 521; Geiger et al., 2015, pp. 243–244; Hong & Coogle, 2016; Pretorius et al., 2009). These skills, it has been suggested, have been acquired in their professional careers (Lavarone et al., 2014; Papastavrou et al., 2007; Savitch et al., 2015, p. 17). Calasanti and King (2007) argue that women experience greater guilt when using task-oriented approaches. However, an earlier study of spouse caregivers (Borden & Berlin, 1990, p. 607) reported contradictory findings, showing that men and women both used problem-focused approaches "with equal frequency," but that in addition, women were likely to use emotion focused coping, specifically tension reduction and support seeking. In a study among Portuguese husbands, the men reporting problem-based coping rated their health higher than those who used other mechanisms (Ribeiro & Paul, 2008, p. 177). Similarly, an American study among male caregivers found negative associations between emotion-focused and avoidance-focused coping and caregiver burden, but did not find an association between caregiver burden and task-focused coping (Geiger et al., 2015, p. 244). Emotion-focused and avoidance-focused coping mechanisms are not solely gender-based but may be triggered by factors underlying the experience and life circumstances of the caregiver (Geiger et al., 2015, p. 244). There is further evidence that avoidance-based techniques may be a temporary mechanism until caregivers have adjusted to their care responsibility. Newman et al. (2019, pp. 11–12) found that while all participants in their study used physical distancing to "reduce feelings of discomfort and loss" initially, they all eventually found other ways of coping.

Complexity of care situations

A second explanation for gender differences in caring outcomes suggests that female caregivers are exposed to more complex care situations and problem behaviors. Papastavrou et al. (2007, p. 452) showed that the experience of burden was most strongly associated with aggressive behavior by the care recipient. This may be a particular issue for wives in traditional marriages, where husbands with dementia, who had previously been the heads of households, may become aggressive in response to their changing situation. Pinquart and Sörensen's review also found that female caregivers report more behavioral problems from their partner with dementia than their male counterparts (Pinquart & Sörensen, 2006, p. 38). A Canadian study of spouse caregivers reported that caregiving wives reported greater role strain and greater frequency of verbal and nonverbal aggression from care recipients than did caregiving husbands (Gibbons et al., 2014, p. 11). Greater workload for female caregivers due to challenging behavior was also found in an American sample, where the majority of caregivers cared for a person with dementia (Friedemann & Buckwalter, 2014, p. 329).

Societal demands and caregiving

Many studies report that women experience greater social demands and expectations to care and spend more time caring than men (Zhang et al., 2006, p. 178). A Swedish study reports that women ascribe different caregiving roles to themselves throughout their life as daughters, wives, and mothers (Eriksson, Sandberg, & Hellstrom, 2013, p. 162). Other research supports this idea, arguing that men are less expected to provide care and therefore receive greater endorsement and recognition for the task than women, which somewhat protects men against caregiver burden (Lavarone et al., 2014, p. 1411). Furthermore, Calasanti and King (2007, p. 520) found that only wives experienced negative reactions when they used respite care options. The authors further suggest that positive recognition of their efforts may protect men from frustration and that "men's relative lack of stress resulted not from a refusal on their part to perform difficult work but rather from their relative freedom from responsibility for particular expectations or from their wives' feelings" (Calasanti & King, 2007, p. 521).

A qualitative study from the United States noted subtle differences that may be linked to societal expectations. They found that husbands focused on the importance of their wives being fed, rather than worrying about whether they received "enough home cooked meals" (Calasanti & Bowen, 2006, p. 261). Sons' ability to set clear boundaries regarding their time commitment as well as their care tasks was attributed to their perception of the cultural expectation that they are primarily care managers, which enabled them to avoid more time-intensive activities, to practice self-care, and to maintain a social life (Grigorovich et al., 2016, p. 6). In contrast, a study of adult daughters reported that they generally had to navigate between complex care situations and other competing demands, such as their own families, employment, and voluntary commitments. This left them physically exhausted and feeling that they were missing out on things, resulting in what the authors called "compassion fatigue" (Day et al., 2014, p. 801). The argument that traditional cultural expectations of women may increase the pressure on daughters, who often will have other competing family and work demands, was put forward by Romero-Moreno et al. (2014), who also found that daughters were most vulnerable to depression.

Nevertheless, research from a number of countries including Cyprus and Turkey, suggests that men may under-report burden and negative feelings due to the social pressures that force them to uphold narrow concepts of masculinity (Akpinar et al., 2011; Friedemann & Buckwalter, 2014; Papastavrou et al., 2009, p. 42). This argument has also been raised elsewhere (Baker et al., 2010, p. 325). For instance, a study investigating white, middle-class husbands in South Africa found that while participants reported burden on an assessment tool, they did not describe their care experience as burdensome during qualitative interviews (Pretorius et al., 2009, p. 90).

Furthermore, other research suggests that men may experience depression in ways that are not reflected by current diagnostic criteria (Martin, Neighbors, & Griffith, 2013), which may partially explain why male caregivers are reported to experience less depression than female caregivers.

Support structures for unpaid caregivers

The third issue focuses on the differences between male and female caregivers in the availability and use of support. It has been observed that in situations where caregivers are unable to take breaks, they experience greater burden (Chappell et al., 2015, p. 626). Many men and women providing dementia care do not receive any support, while others get emotional and practical help from family members or through voluntary or for-profit organizations.

The results of research on gender differences in support received are mixed. One review suggests that men, in general, are more likely to accept or pay for support and both an American and a Cypriot study found that husbands had more family or paid support than wives as the number of daily care tasks increased (Calasanti & Bowen, 2006, p. 258; Papastavrou et al., 2007; Savitch et al., 2015, p. 24). A study from the Midwestern United States also reported that husbands received more assistance than wives. This study further identified a difference in role perspective. While men viewed themselves as their wife's "helper," women were more likely to identify their caregiver role "as taking over their lives" (Boylestein & Hayes, 2012, p. 607). In the Mittelman study, in which all (predominantly white) participants were spouses or partners of the person with dementia and lived in the New York metropolitan area, a significantly larger number of the male spouse caregivers received help from their adult children (44.4%) than the female spouse caregivers (23.8%). Furthermore, a significantly larger number of female spouse caregivers reported receiving help from no one at all (43.4%) compared to male spouse caregivers (26.5%) (Mittelman, 2003, p. 276). On the other hand, this study identified no gender difference in the amount of paid help husbands and wives received. A study of Canadian spouse caregivers of people with dementia found that while there was no gender difference in the frequency of community service use between spouse caregivers, husbands received more hours of support (Gibbons et al., 2014, pp. 11–12).

Uptake of support may depend not only on the kin relationship between caregiver and care recipient, but also on ethnic background. For example, in an American study of caregivers who were mostly of Hispanic and Caribbean backgrounds, daughters received more support than sons, and adult children received more support than spouses. In this study, unlike the Mittelman report, less support was given to husbands than to wives (Friedemann & Buckwalter, 2014, pp. 323, 329). Among sons providing care, married sons usually received female support while never-married sons usually did not report any family support. Sons generally also rely heavily on support from the formal health sector (Campbell, 2010; Grigorovich et al., 2016).

The influence of culture with regard to the uptake of support has frequently been cited. For example, the aforementioned study by Friedemann and Buckwalter found that the older Hispanic population who had family members nearby received the most family support of the caregivers in the sample (Friedemann & Buckwalter, 2014, pp. 323, 329). Similarly, in many Asian cultures, care remains a family responsibility (World Health Organization and Alzheimer's Disease International, 2012, p. 79).

Some studies tried to disentangle underlying reasons behind these different patterns. A German study reported that many female caregivers had given up leisure activities outside their own home, and that a barrier to taking up support was endorsing what the authors characterized as motherly self-sacrifice (Toepfer et al., 2014, p. 242). Another study argued that handing over care may be more difficult for female caregivers, at least for daughters; feelings of guilt about handing over the care responsibility was associated with higher ratings of depressive symptoms among daughters (Romero-Moreno et al., 2014, p. 510). Male caregivers, on the other hand, were found not only to take breaks when support was available but were found to engage in activities that were meaningful to them in other ways (Grigorovich et al., 2016; Pretorius et al., 2009, p. 89). Furthermore, research from the United Kingdom reported gender differences in caregivers' satisfaction with the care provided by paid caregivers. It found that male caregivers were more likely to agree that the standard of care provided by paid caregivers was excellent, while females were more likely to agree that paid caregivers were not sensitive to their needs (Peel & Harding, 2014, pp. 649–650).

Identified key support needs

The impact the provision of dementia care has on women and men shows clearly that family caregivers require supportive interventions and resources that are culturally, relationally, and gender appropriate (Mittelman, 2003). The WHO global action plan on dementia has identified several important aspects that should be put in place to support family caregivers. This includes the availability of support services, such as information, training, or respite opportunities that address caregiver specific needs and the training of professionals to enable the recognition of caregivers as "essential partners in the planning and provision of care in all settings" in line with the preferences of the person with dementia. The WHO plan on dementia further reiterates the need to "develop and strengthen" the financial support for caregivers through "social and disability benefits" and "policies and legislation against discrimination" (World Health Organization, 2017b, pp. 26–27).

Need for information

Access to information and education is important for all family caregivers of people with dementia. Peer support groups were identified as particularly useful sources of information, especially for knowledge of existing local support structures and advice on how to access them (Grigorovich et al., 2016, p. 5; Potgieter & Heyns, 2006). Potgieter and Heyns (2006, p. 559) suggest that the opportunity for an additional family member to also attend some support group meetings could help them understand the complexity of care and support for people with dementia and understand the need to help the main family caregiver in providing support to create a stronger and well-informed family support network. The results of studies of the NYU Caregiver Intervention make it clear that family involvement and support is key to caregiver wellbeing (Mittelman et al., 2004a; Roth et al., 2005).

Support to address mental health issues

Peer support groups and other psychosocial interventions have been identified as positively contributing to family caregivers' mental health. However, it has been recognized that there is insufficient support for interventions for family caregivers of people with dementia (Potgieter & Heyns, 2006), and the provision of services designed to support people with dementia and their informal caregivers are not expected to increase at the same rate as the increase in those needing these services (Van Mierlo et al., 2012). Some authors have focused on the perception of caregiver support groups as inherently female due to their "emotionally expressive climate" (Erol et al., 2015, p. 37; Pretorius et al., 2009, p. 86). American research, on the other hand, did not find a difference in the use of support groups between men and women (Erol et al., 2015; Sun et al., 2008, p. 943), and the experience of one of the authors (MM) is that in practice, male caregivers are often reluctant to join support groups, but attend them regularly and are willing to share their feelings with others in the group, especially if it is composed entirely of men.

One report suggested that networks to exchange experiences and feelings may be particularly important for women, while men may focus more on identifying information and advice to resolve particular issues (Calasanti & King, 2007, p. 524). It would be important to think about how support networks can better respond to gender-specific needs (Pretorius et al., 2009, p. 92; Rabinowitz & Gallagher-Thompson, 2007, p. 11).

While younger caregivers might have liked to connect with others in similar situations, they were particularly interested in "time-flexible, low-commitment, and drop-in" support structures (Newman et al., 2019, p. 12) as they are more often torn between competing demands than older caregivers, who may have retired and whose children are grown.

Time for themselves—Improved access to caregiver allowance and respite care

A key aspect discussed earlier is that many family caregivers lack the opportunity of pockets of time for themselves. Maintaining and rebuilding old as well as developing new social networks, maintaining, resuming or starting leisure activities, and therefore staying in control of their own lives is important to most family caregivers (Grigorovich et al., 2016). Given the information from studies of gendered expectations discussed throughout this chapter, it is likely that women would particularly benefit from additional support to enable time for themselves, and a change in expectations that makes them willing to take such time, as they have historically been more likely to subordinate their own needs to those of the person with care needs (Frehlih, 2019, p. 1146; Friedemann & Buckwalter, 2014; Pillemer et al., 2018, p. 1165).

Recognition by relevant professionals

The value of the care provided by family members, and particularly women, should be recognized and acknowledged (Akpinar et al., 2011, p. 253). Health and social service professionals can play an important role in enabling family caregivers to access support by providing information, care consultation, and pointing them toward or connecting them with relevant resources (Rubinelli and Diviani focus on communication with patients and caregivers in Chapter 15). It is important that healthcare professionals become more aware of potentially underlying gendered, family, and cultural expectations and values. Healthcare professionals and policy makers need to challenge "their own assumptions that the caregiving responsibility of 'families' is identical to that of 'women'" (Eriksson et al., 2013, p. 164). Friedemann and Buckwalter (2014, pp. 329–330) suggest that that all family caregivers should regularly be assessed for burden and/or depression. Other research also suggests that caregivers, and particularly wives, should be evaluated for potential support need (Chappell et al., 2015, p. 637). Acknowledging family caregivers, actively involving them in decision making processes, and breaking down barriers toward service receipt may go a long way in supporting family caregivers of people with dementia (Potgieter & Heyns, 2006, p. 559).

Barriers to support

Many family caregivers acknowledge that there may be a point at which they require additional support; however, research has found that family caregivers are likely to postpone seeking help from support structures to a point in the future (Eriksson et al., 2013, p. 163). A German study identified the female family caregivers' feeling that they are essential to the person living with dementia as a barrier to agreeing to receive external help (Toepfer et al., 2014, p. 241). Cultural perceptions may also play a role. In Asian cultures, such as China, Korea, and Malaysia, the family is expected to support family members with care needs. The fear of "losing face" and being perceived as not providing appropriate support for the person with dementia may reduce the acceptance of paid support among such caregivers (World Health Organization and Alzheimer's Disease International, 2012, p. 79).

Gendered expectations present another important barrier to accessing support for caregivers. The perceived social expectation for women to identify with the caregiver role can make seeking help and support difficult. Women who identify with their caregiver role may be reluctant to admit the need for support, as it may feel like failure not to carry out this task (Eriksson et al., 2013, p. 163). For some men, the sense that they will be expected to express their emotions may pose a barrier to their seeking help from resources such as support groups (Pretorius et al., 2009, p. 86).

Other key barriers to seeking help and support that have been identified include lack of information and awareness of existing formal support structures, fragmented and scattered support structures that are difficult to access, terminology that prevents family caregivers from identifying themselves as eligible for support, stigma around dementia and negative attitudes toward diagnosis and treatment, stigma associated with asking for help, lack of training on dementia in the health workforce, as well as absence of support structures (Newman et al., 2019, p. 12; World Health Organization and Alzheimer's Disease International, 2012, p. 79).

Designing and delivering effective interventions is not that straightforward

While it is evident that caregivers benefit from support, it is also important to understand which interventions are effective in improving caregivers' wellbeing. One metaanalysis focused on interventions that reduce the burden of family caregivers. It found that only multicomponent interventions were effective in reducing caregiver burden. Interventions that combined emotional support with education on coping strategies that focus on reframing cognitive appraisals were identified as more effective (Williams et al., 2019). Another metaanalysis also concluded that psychosocial interventions generally had a small to moderate effect on caregiver burden, depression, and general health (Teahan et al., 2020).

Does caregiver gender matter with regard to intervention effectiveness?

A small number of studies have focused on whether interventions benefit subgroups differently. One review investigated how frequently caregiver gender and race were explicitly investigated (rather than just controlled for in analyses) among studies focusing on dementia caregiver support interventions that were funded by the National Institute of Health (NIH) in the United States. It was found that 67% of the 46 included studies "did not report results by gender." Among the 15 studies that did investigate the effect of the interventions by gender, just over half (8) reported statistically significant differences between male and female caregivers (Gilmore-Bykovskyi et al., 2018, p. 149).

Studies of the NYU Caregiver Intervention (NYUCI) did explore intervention effectiveness by gender. The original study was specifically for spouse caregivers and demonstrated that the intervention was effective in reducing symptoms of stress and depression in spouse caregivers (Mittelman et al., 2004a, 2004b), and was *equally effective* for men and women (Mittelman et al., 2004b, p. 854). Notably by improving caregiver well-being, the NYUCI enabled spouse caregivers, regardless of gender, to keep their partners with dementia at home for substantially and significantly longer than those who received usual care (median time difference was a year and a half) (Mittelman et al., 2006). Another example of a study that did explore gender differences evaluated the effects of an environmental skill-building program on caregiver wellbeing. The comparison of intervention and control group by gender found that women gained more from the intervention than men. Women who received the intervention reported "less need for help from others, reduced strain from dementia-related behaviours, and improved affect and well-being," while men reported less objective burden (Gitlin et al., 2003).

A literature review of studies that investigated the "personal characteristics of caregivers of people with dementia for whom psychosocial interventions were effective" found that female gender of caregiver was frequently associated with positive intervention outcomes (Van Mierlo et al., 2012, p. 1). The authors point out that the investigation of differences among subgroups can help to customize interventions to the needs of the individual. However, they caution that such studies require large samples, which are expensive and often not feasible (Van Mierlo et al., 2012).

Is this likely to change in future?

The United Nations estimates that in 2019 there were 703 million people aged 65 and over. By 2050, the number of people 65 years and older is projected to increase to 1.5 billion (United Nations, 2019, p. 1). As the number of older people increases, the number of people living with dementia is also projected to increase from about 50 million in 2015 to 152 million in 2050 (World Health Organization, 2017a). The number of older adults, and therefore the number of people with dementia, is expected to rise most quickly in low- and middle-income countries in Northern Africa and Western Asia, Central and Southern Asia, Latin America and the Caribbean, and Eastern and South Eastern Asia, where services for people with dementia and their caregivers are scarce and the main care responsibility continues to lie with family members, who are unpaid, and most of whom are women (Erol et al., 2015; Prince et al., 2015; United Nations, 2019, p. 1).

In order to enable people with dementia to live as well as possible, and to protect their family members from negative health and economic outcomes, it is important that health and long-term care systems around the world recognize the importance of these unpaid caregivers and provide the structural and financial support for effective interventions that address their many needs. (In Chapter 16, Weidner et al. discuss dementia policy and gender in relation to patients and caregivers.) Supportive living environments should also be designed to enable people with dementia to live well if their family members cannot or choose not to provide care.

Even though women around the world have been making progress in achieving greater gender equality, the disproportionate share of women who are providing unpaid care has been identified as a key barrier (United Nations, 2020). The effects of the COVID-19 pandemic on caregivers (see Box 1) has illustrated the precariousness of female advances on equality, as many employed women experienced the double burden of paid and unpaid labor (Power, 2020).

This chapter showed how women continue to be expected to provide unpaid care. While many may gain benefits from caring for an aging relative, there is an

Box 1 The impact of COVID-19 on family caregivers of people with Alzheimer's disease and other dementias

International organizations and researchers have highlighted the negative impact the COVID-19 pandemic has had on decades of progress toward gender equality. Restrictive policies to reduce the spread of the virus have led to the suspension of community services and increased the disproportionate burden of unpaid care, which weighs heavier on women (Mercado, Naciri, & Mishra, 2020; Power, 2020; United Nations, 2020; Wenham et al., 2020). Here, we provide a brief overview of evidence of the impact of the COVID-19 pandemic on family caregivers of people with dementia. While all studies have included substantial proportions of female caregivers (in one study by Giebel, Hanna, et al., 2020, almost all caregivers are women), and an Argentinian study noted that more women than men took on additional care responsibilities for people with dementia, to our knowledge, no analysis so far has been conducted specifically from a gender perspective (Cohen et al., 2020).

Increased demand has negative implications for caregivers

For many caregivers, the COVID-19 pandemic has meant an increase in care responsibility (World Health Organization, 2020). An Alzheimer's Society survey among 1000 caregivers in England found that 73% of caregivers have experienced an increase in care responsibility since COVID-19 restrictions started. This has increased the time family caregivers have spent supporting their relative with dementia by 9.8 hours per week, on average. Before the restrictions started in England on March 23, 2020, about 40% of caregivers reported spending 100 hours or more per week providing care. Since then this has increased to 50% of caregivers. Almost half of caregivers surveyed (45%) reported that they could not provide the level of care the person with dementia required (Alzheimer's Society, 2020, p. 35). Caregivers in India also reported changes to their routines and responsibilities and some were concerned about how they would be able to keep their relative at home and occupied without the distraction and support of social visits (Vaitheswaran et al., 2020).

The Alzheimer's Society survey also found that almost all (95%) caregivers reported a "negative impact on mental and physical health," 69% reported feeling "constantly exhausted," 64% felt anxious, 50% reported having developed sleeping problems, 49% felt depressed, 14% stated "that they had not had time to see a [general practitioner (GP)] about a health problem," and 13% reported having incurred an "injury from caring" (Alzheimer's Society, 2020, p. 30). The study in India echoed negative effects on caregivers' health and difficulty in accessing healthcare. In addition, the latter study highlighted potential economic implications for caregivers; many caregivers had to work from home due to restrictive measures, but reported finding it difficult to combine their work and care responsibilities (Vaitheswaran et al., 2020).

Perhaps not surprisingly, there is evidence of increased caregiver burden and stress since the beginning of the COVID-19 pandemic. A qualitative study among family caregivers of people with dementia in England reported that caregivers experienced stress and fear about taking on care "responsibilities that they did not feel qualified to be doing" as well as an increased care workload and strain (Giebel, Hanna, et al., 2020). Many caregivers in Canada also reported experiencing stress and burnout in managing day to day activities without their usual support network and availability of services (Roach et al., 2020). Similarly, a study of 53 family caregivers of people with dementia in rural Virginia, United States, found that almost half of the caregivers interviewed (47%) "reported high role overload." The odds of experiencing role overload was found to be greater among caregivers who expressed greater concern about COVID-19 and those who did not receive enough support from family and friends (Savla et al., 2020).

Caregivers who endorsed positive aspects of caregiving, such as spending more time with the person with dementia, receiving help from other family members, and the person with dementia being at greater ease if the caregiver spent more time at home, had reduced odds of role overload (Savla et al., 2020). In a survey of 80 family caregivers in Argentina, the reasons for stress and

Box 1 The impact of COVID-19 on family caregivers of people with Alzheimer's disease and other dementias—cont'd

concern depended at least in part on the severity of dementia; caregivers of people with more advanced dementia experienced more stress and burden due to COVID-19, while caregivers of people with mild dementia were concerned about infecting their relative (Cohen et al., 2020). Qualitative research in India and Canada also identified concerns and feelings of anxiety about the risk of infection for both people with dementia and their caregivers (Roach et al., 2020; Vaitheswaran et al., 2020). In India, caregivers described concerns around their relative's adherence to hygiene measures and physical distancing rules, but also worried about what would happen if they themselves became ill and unable to look after their relative or if the person with dementia were to be hospitalized (Vaitheswaran et al., 2020).

Family support
Concern about infection and policies meant to prevent disease spread meant that family and peer support networks that usually supported caregivers often became unavailable. In the Argentinian study, 60% of families reported that they have discontinued visiting their relative with dementia (Cohen et al., 2020). Caregivers in England, India, and Canada emphasized the negative impact the loss of informal support had on their practical and emotional load (Giebel, Hanna, et al., 2020; Roach et al., 2020; Vaitheswaran et al., 2020). The American study found that while 68% caregivers continued to receive some family support through help with shopping or social interaction over the phone or virtually, almost one third of caregivers (32%) felt that they did not receive enough support from their families (Savla et al., 2020). In Canada, those caregivers with continued family support emphasized its importance (Roach et al., 2020).

Recognition of people with dementia as a vulnerable group
Another issue identified in England, the United States, and India was the lack of recognition that people with dementia and their caregivers are members of a vulnerable group, which has policy implications. For example, in India one respondent reported not receiving travel permission to move the person with dementia to a rural home where they could have benefited from safe outside spaces (Vaitheswaran et al., 2020). Caregivers in England reported difficulty in accessing shops, and concerns around risks of infection when the person with dementia had to be taken shopping; even though online shopping was meant to be available for older and vulnerable people, caregivers reported that these services often were inaccessible due to technical difficulties and poor access to webpages (Giebel, Hanna, et al., 2020).

Home care
For people with dementia who had been receiving home care, concerns around risk of infection had to be balanced with caregivers' ability to provide care. Some caregivers in England would have liked to stop paid services out of concern about the many different care workers entering their relative's home and the lack of available personal protective equipment (PPE) for them, but either needed the support from paid caregivers or were concerned about their ability to re-access services at a later point. Some caregivers felt the quality of care had dropped as paid caregivers had less time or provided fewer services due to staff shortages. Other family caregivers undertook drastic changes to care arrangements, such as moving in with the care recipient and switching to remote work arrangements (Giebel, Hanna, et al., 2020). In the Argentinian study, most caregivers kept paid home care (only 28.6% suspended paid caregivers), particularly caregivers of people with more advanced dementia who were very concerned that paid care might become unavailable. However, many Argentinian families decided to stop community-based interventions, such as cognitive or physical therapies (Cohen et al., 2020).

Community services
Reduced availability of community health and long-term care services were reported to affect the health and wellbeing of people with dementia and their caregivers. Most caregivers in the British

Box 1 The impact of COVID-19 on family caregivers of people with Alzheimer's disease and other dementias—cont'd

Alzheimer's Society survey (90% of 975 respondents) reported that the person with dementia experienced interruption to health and long-term care services, most frequently to "GPs, dentists, memory clinics and chiropodists." Furthermore, 83% of respondents reported that the health of the person they cared for had declined since the beginning of the pandemic, among whom 84% thought that this was at least in part due to changes in the care the person with dementia had received (Alzheimer's Society, 2020, p. 34). Another survey of caregivers in England found that reduced support services affected mental wellbeing of caregivers and increased anxiety among people with dementia (Giebel, Lord, et al., 2020). Qualitative studies in England, Canada, and India echoed that some caregivers felt that the person they care for deteriorated faster without the usual stimulation and physical activity available (Giebel, Cannon, et al., 2020; Roach et al., 2020; Vaitheswaran et al., 2020). Most caregivers in India reported behavioral problems of their relative that they found difficult (Vaitheswaran et al., 2020).

Remote service

Caregivers in England and Canada reported use of remote services and generally welcomed them, although they emphasized that they could not replace practical, in-person support (Giebel, Hanna, et al., 2020; Roach et al., 2020). Caregivers in England pointed out that remote services targeted at the person with dementia often required the caregiver to be present instead of providing them with a break, and some people with dementia were unable to participate in virtual services due to their cognitive impairment or because they were unable to access them (Giebel, Hanna, et al., 2020). While caregivers in Canada also reported barriers around accessibility, as well as some barriers due to limited use of body language and nonverbal communication with telephone and videoconferencing, as well as the inability to speak frankly to the health provider if the person with dementia was present, they also noted some advantages: caregivers felt less rushed, liked having a choice between telephone and video calls, and mentioned that they could speak more candidly with the doctor if the person with dementia was not part of the call. Caregivers emphasized the importance of offering assistance to people who are inexperienced in using online technology for communication (Roach et al., 2020).

The future

Caregivers in England and Canada expressed concern about the long-term impact on the availability of care services. They worried about whether the services they had formerly accessed would become available again in the future, how this might affect their employment, and whether the person they care for would still be able to use these services (Giebel, Cannon, et al., 2020; Roach et al., 2020). In addition to a need for expansion of community services post-COVID-19, the Indian study identified caregivers' key short and long-term needs as access to "consultations with a specialist" and "medicines for dementia," guidance and support on engaging people with dementia at home, practical assistance at home, recognition of dementia in social care policies, and ongoing access to remote consultation and telephone support (Vaitheswaran et al., 2020).

abundance of evidence related to the negative effects on caregivers' health and wellbeing in general, and particularly among female caregivers. Societal expectations that unpaid care is inherently female also pose a key barrier to gender equality. The findings presented highlight the need for gender-specific support and interventions as well as for raising awareness of the challenges and needs of unpaid caregivers.

Chapter highlights

- Women, especially daughters, continue to carry the majority of caring responsibility, however, an increasing proportion of older men are caring for their spouses or partners with dementia.
- While many caregivers report positive aspects related to their caregiver role, there is a lot of evidence that the provision of unpaid care is associated with negative health (physical and mental) as well as financial implications, especially if the caregiver is not sufficiently supported by family and formal services, as is more often the case for female caregivers than for males.
- Caregivers should have access to evidence-based supportive interventions to enable them to provide good quality care to people with dementia and to reduce the risk of negative outcomes. These interventions should be tailored to consider gender differences as well as the different abilities and often complex needs of caregivers.

References

Akpinar, B., Küçükgüçlü, Ö., & Yener, G. (2011). Effects of gender on burden among caregivers of Alzheimer's patients. *Journal of Nursing Scholarship*, *43*(3), 248–254.

Alzheimer's Association. (2019). 2019 Alzheimer's disease facts and figures. *Alzheimers Dement*, *15*(3), 321–387.

Alzheimer's Society. (2020). *Worst hit: Dementia during coronavirus*. London. Available from https://www.alzheimers.org.uk/sites/default/files/2020-09/Worst-hit-Dementia-during-coronavirus-report.pdf.

Andreakou, M. I., et al. (2016). Assessment of health-related quality of life for caregivers of Alzheimer's disease patients. *International Journal of Alzheimer's Disease*, 107–114. https://doi.org/10.1155/2016/9213968.

Argimon, J. M., et al. (2004). Health-related quality of life in carers of patients with dementia. *Family Practice*, *21*(4), 454–457. https://doi.org/10.1093/fampra/cmh418.

Atta-Konadu, E., Keller, H. H., & Daly, K. (2011). The food-related role shift experiences of spousal male care partners and their wives with dementia. *Journal of Aging Studies*, *25*(3), 305–315.

Baker, K. L., & Robertson, N. (2008). Coping with caring for someone with dementia: Reviewing the literature about men. *Aging & Mental Health*, *12*(4), 413–422.

Baker, K. L., Robertson, N., & Connelly, D. (2010). Men caring for wives or partners with dementia: Masculinity, straing and gain. *Aging & Mental Health*, *14*(3), 319–327.

Bartlett, R., et al. (2018). Gender, citizenship and dementia care: A scoping review of studies to inform policy and future research. *Health and Social Care in the Community*, *26*(1), 14–26.

Borden, W., & Berlin, S. (1990). Gender, coping, and psychological well-being in spouses of older adults with chronic dementia. *American Journal of Orthopsychiatry*, *60*(4), 603–610.

Borsje, P., et al. (2016). Psychological distress in informal caregivers of patients with dementia in primary care: Course and determinants. *Family Practice*, *33*(4), 374–381. https://doi.org/10.1093/fampra/cmw009.

Bott, N. T., Sheckter, C. C., & Milstein, A. S. (2017). Dementia care, women's health and gender equity—The value of well-time caregiver support. *JAMA Neurology*, *74*(7), 757–758.

Boyle, G. (2013a). Facilitating decision-making by people with dementia: Is spousal support gendered? *Journal of Social Welfare and Family Law*, *35*(2), 227–243.

Boyle, G. (2013b). Still a woman's job: The division of housework in couples living with dementia. *Families, Relationships and Societies*, *2*(1), 5–21.

Boyle, G. (2014). "Can't cook, won't cook": Men's involvement in cooking when their wives develop dementia. *Journal of Gender Studies*, *23*(4), 336–350.

Boylestein, C., & Hayes, J. (2012). Reconstructing marital closeness while caring for a spouse with Alzheimer's. *Journal of Family Issues*, *33*(5), 584–612.

Calasanti, T., & Bowen, M. E. (2006). Spousal caregiving and crossing gender boundaries: Maintaining gendered identities. *Journal of Aging Studies*, *20*(3), 253–263.

Calasanti, T., & King, N. (2007). Taking "women's work" "like a man": Husbands' experiences of care work. *The Gerontologist*, *47*(4), 516–527.

Campbell, L. D. (2010). Sons who care: Examining the experience and meaning of filial caregiving for married and never-married sons. *Canadian Journal on Aging*, *29*(1), 73–84. https://doi.org/10.1017/S071498080999033X.

Carmichael, F., & Ercolani, M. G. (2014). Overlooked and undervalued: The caring contribution of older people. *International Journal of Social Economics*, *41*(5), 397–419. https://doi.org/10.1108/IJSE-02-2012-0046.

Chappell, N. L., Dujela, C., & Smith, A. (2015). Caregiver well-being: Intersection of relationship and gender. *Research on Aging*, *37*(6), 623–645. https://doi.org/10.1177/0164027514549258.

Cohen, G., et al. (2020). Living with dementia: Increased level of caregiver stress in times of COVID-19. *International Psychogeriatrics*, 1–5. https://doi.org/10.1017/S1041610220001593. Buenos Aires, Argentina: Cambridge University Press.

Croog, S. H., et al. (2006). Spouse caregivers of Alzheimer patients: Problem responses to caregiver burden. *Aging & Mental Health*, *10*(2), 87–100.

Custodio, N., et al. (2017). Dementia in Latin America: Epidemiological evidence and implications for public policy. *Frontiers in Neuroscience*, *9*, 221.

Da Roit, B. (2007). Changing intergenerational solidarities within families in a mediterranean welfare state—Eldery care in Italy. *Current Sociology*, *55*(2), 251–269. https://doi.org/10.1177/0011392107073306.

Dahlberg, L., Denmack, S., & Bambra, C. (2007). Age and gender of informal carers: A population-based study in the UK. *Health and Social Care in the Community*, *5*, 439–445.

Dassel, K. B., & Carr, D. C. (2016). Does dementia caregiving accelerate frailty? Findings from the health and retirement study. *Gerontologist*, *56*(3), 444–450. https://doi.org/10.1093/geront/gnu078.

Davies, H. D., et al. (2012). Gender differences in sexual behaviors of AD patients and their relationship to spousal caregiver well-being. *Aging & Mental Health*, *16*(1), 89–101.

Day, J. R., Anderson, R. A., & Davis, L. L. (2014). Compassion fatigue in adult daughter caregivers of a parent with dementia. *Issues in Mental Health Nursing*, *35*(10), 796–804. https://doi.org/10.3109/01612840.2014.917133.

Eriksson, H., Sandberg, J., & Hellstrom, I. (2013). Experience of long-term home care as an informal caregiver to a spouse: Gendered meanings in everyday life for female carers. *International Journal of Older People Nursing*, *8*(2), 159–165.

Erol, R., Brooker, D., & Peel, E. (2015). *Women and dementia—A global research review*. London. Available from https://www.alz.co.uk/sites/default/files/pdfs/Women-and-Dementia.pdf.

Ferrant, G., Pesando, L. M., & Nowacka, K. (2014). *Unpaid care work: The missing link in the analysis of gender gaps in labour outcomes*. Paris. Available from https://www.oecd.org/dev/development-gender/Unpaid:care_work.pdf.

Frehlih, M. (2019). Challenges for men, providing informal care for people with dementia. *Teorija in Praksa*, *56*(4), 1136–1151.

Friedemann, M.-L., & Buckwalter, K. C. (2014). Family caregiver role and burden related to gender and family relationship. *Journal of Family Nursing*, *20*(3), 313–336. https://doi.org/10.1177/1074840714532715.

Geiger, J. R., et al. (2015). Burden among male Alzheimer's caregivers: Effects of distinct coping strategies. *American Journal of Alzheimer's Disease & Other Dementias*, *30*(3), 238–246. https://doi.org/10.1177/1533317514552666. Louisiana State University School of Social Work, Baton Rouge, LA, USA: Sage Publications Inc.

Gibbons, C., et al. (2014). The psychological and health consequences of caring for a spouse with dementia: A critical comparison of husbands and wives. *Journal of Women & Aging*, *26*(3), 3–21. https://doi.org/10.1080/08952841.2014.854571.

Giebel, C., Cannon, J., Hanna, K., Butchard, S., Eley, R., Gaughan, A., … Gabbay, M. (2020). Impact of COVID-19 related social support service closures on people with dementia and unpaid carers: A qualitative study. *Ageing & Mental Health*. https://doi.org/10.1080/13607863.2020.1822292.

Giebel, C., Hanna, K., et al. (2020). Decision-making for receiving paid home care for dementia in the time of COVID-19: A qualitative study. *BMC Geriatrics*, *20*(1), 333. https://doi.org/10.1186/s12877-020-01719-0. BioMed Central.

Giebel, C., Lord, K., et al. (2020). A UK survey of COVID-19 related social support closures and their effects on older people, people with dementia, and carers. *International Journal of Geriatric Psychiatry*, 1–10. https://doi.org/10.1002/gps.5434.

Gilmore-Bykovskyi, A., et al. (2018). Underreporting of gender and race/ethnicity differences in NIH-funded dementia caregiver support interventions. *American Journal of Alzheimer's Disease & Other Dementias*, *33*(3), 145–152.

Gitlin, L. N., et al. (2003). Effects of the home environmental skill-building program on the caregiver-care recipient dyad: 6-month outcomes from the Philadelphia REACH Initiative. *The Gerontologist*, *43*(4), 532–546.

Greenwood, N., & Smith, R. (2019). Motivations for being informal carers of people living with dementia: A systematic review of qualitative literature. *BMC Geriatrics*, *19*(169). https://doi.org/10.1186/s12877-019-1185-0.

Grigorovich, A., et al. (2016). Roles and coping strategies of sons caring for a parent with dementia. *American Journal of Occupational Therapy*, *70*(1), 1–9. https://doi.org/10.5014/ajot.2016.017715.

Hong, S., & Coogle, C. (2016). Spousal caregiving for partners with dementia: A deductive literature review testing Calasanti's gendered view of care work. *Journal of Applied Gerontology*, *35*(7), 759–787.

Kim, J. S., Kim, E. H., & An, M. (2016). Experience of dementia-related anxiety in middle-aged female caregivers for family members with dementia: A phenomenological study. *Asian Nursing Research*, *10*, 128–135.

Lavarone, A., et al. (2014). Caregiver burden and coping strategies in caregivers of patients with Alzheimer's disease. *Neuropsychiatric Disease and Treatment*, *10*, 1407–1413.

Lloyd, J., Patterson, T., & Muers, J. (2014). The positive aspects of caregiving in dementia: A critical review of the qualitative literature. *Dementia*, 1–28. https://doi.org/10.1177/1471301214564792.

Martin, L. A., Neighbors, H. W., & Griffith, D. M. (2013). The experience of symptoms of depression in men vs women—Analysis of the national comorbidity survey replication. *JAMA Psychiatry*, *70*(10), 1100–1106.

Mercado, L., Naciri, M., & Mishra, Y. (2020). *Women's unpaid and underpaid work in the times of COVID-19*. UN Women Asia and the Pacific. Available from https://asiapacific.unwomen.org/en/news-and-events/stories/2020/06/womens-unpaid-and-underpaid-work-in-the-times-of-covid-19#_ftn2. Accessed 5 August 2020.

Mittelman, M. S. (2003). Community caregiving. *Alzheimer's Care Quarterly*, *4*(4), 273–285.

Mittelman, M. S., et al. (2004a). Effects of a caregiver intervention on negative caregiver appraisals of behavior problems in patients with Alzheimer's disease: Results of a randomized trial. *Journals of Gerontology. Series B, Psychological Sciences and Social Sciences*, *59*(1), 27–34. 14722336.

Mittelman, M. S., et al. (2004b). Sustained benefit of supportive intervention for depressive symptoms in Alzheimer's caregivers. *American Journal of Psychiatry*, *161*(5), 850–856. 15121650.

Mittelman, M. S., et al. (2006). Improving caregiver well-being delays nursing home placement of patients with Alzheimer disease. *Neurology*, *67*(9), 1592–1599. 17101889.

Newman, K., et al. (2019). Carers need care too: Recalling the experience of being a young female carer for a relative living with dementia. *Perspectives: The Journal of the Gerontological Nursing Association*, *40*(3), 6–16.

OECD. (2019). *Health at a glance 2019: OECD indicators*. Paris: OECD Publishing Paris. Available from https://www.oecd-ilibrary.org/docserver/4dd50c09-en.pdf?expires=1593435656&id=id&accname=guest&checksum=3FA2A66CDF95D31283F4354B10294651.

ONS. (2013). *The gender gap in unpaid care provision: Is there an impact on health and economic position*. London. Available from https://www.ons.gov.uk/peoplepopulationandcommunity/healthandsocialcare/healthandwellbeing/articles/fullstorythegendergapinunpaidcareprovisionisthereanimpactonhealthandeconomicposition/2013-05-16.

Papastavrou, E., et al. (2007). Caring for a relative with dementia: Family caregiver burden. *Journal of Advanced Nursing*, *58*(5), 446–456.

Papastavrou, E., et al. (2009). Gender issues in caring for demented relatives. *Health Science Journal*, *31*(1), 41–53.

Peel, E., & Harding, R. (2014). "It's a huge maze, the system, it's a terrible maze": Dementia carers' constructions of navigating health and social care services. *Dementia*, *13*(5), 642–661.

Pillemer, S., Davis, J., & Tremont, G. (2018). Gender effects on components of burden and depression among dementia caregivers. *Aging & Mental Health*, *22*(9), 1162–1167.

Pinquart, M., & Sörensen, S. (2006). Gender differences in caregiver stressors, social resources, and health: An updated meta-analysis. *Journal of Gerontology: Psychological Sciences*, *61B*(1), 33–45. https://doi.org/10.1093/geronb/61.1.p33.

Potgieter, J., & Heyns, P. (2006). Caring for a spouse with Alzheimer's disease: Stressors and strengths. *South Africa Journal of Psychology*, *36*(3), 547–563.

Power, K. (2020). The COVID-19 pandemic has increased the care burden of women and families. *Sustainability: Science, Practice and Policy*, *16*(1), 67–73. https://doi.org/10.1080/15487733.2020.1776561.

Pöysti, M. M., et al. (2012). Gender differences in dementia spousal caregiving. *International Journal of Alzheimer's Disease*, 1–5. https://doi.org/10.1155/2012/162960.

Pretorius, C., Walker, S., & Heyns, P. M. (2009). Sense of coherence amongst male caregivers in dementia: A south African perspective. *Dementia: The International Journal of Social Research and Practice*, *8*(1), 79–94.

Price, E. (2011). Caring for mum and dad: Lesbian women negotiating family and navigating care. *International Journal of Geriatric Psychiatry*, *41*(7), 1288–1303.

Prince, M., & The 10/66 Dementia Research Group. (2004). Care arrangements for people with dementia in developing countries. *International Journal of Geriatric Psychiatry*, *19*(2), 170–177.

Prince, M., et al. (2012). Strain and its correlates among carers of people with dementia in low-income and middle-income countries. A 10/66 Dementia Research Group population-based survey. *International Journal of Geriatric Psychiatry*, *27*(7), 670–682.

Prince, M., et al. (2015). *World Alzheimer report 2015: The global impact of dementia—An analysis of prevalence, incidence, cost and trends*. London. Available from https://www.alz.co.uk/research/WorldAlzheimerReport2015.pdf.

Public Health England. (2017). Chapter 1: Life expectancy and health life expectancy. In *Health profile for England*. Available from https://www.gov.uk/government/publications/health-profile-for-england/chapter-1-life-expectancy-and-healthy-life-expectancy.

Quinn, C., Clare, L., & Woods, R. T. (2010). The impact of motivations and meanings on the wellbeing of caregivers of people with dementia: A systematic review. *International Psychogeriatrics*, *22*(1), 43–55.

Quinn, C., Clare, L., & Woods, R. T. (2012). What predicts whether caregivers of people with dementia find meaning in their role? *International Journal of Geriatric Psychiatry*, *27*(11), 1195–1202.

Rabinowitz, Y. G., & Gallagher-Thompson, D. (2007). Health and health behaviors among female caregivers of elderly relatives with dementia: The role of ethnicity and kinship status. *Clinical Gerontologist*, *31*(2), 1–15.

Ribeiro, O., & Paul, C. (2008). Older male carers and the positive aspects of care. *Ageing and Society*, *28*, 165–183. https://doi.org/10.1017/S0144686X07006460.

Ribeiro, O., Paúl, C., & Nogueira, C. (2007). Real men, real husbands: Caregiving and masculinities in later life. *Journal of Aging Studies*, *21*, 302–313. https://doi.org/10.1016/j.jaging.2007.05.005.

Roach, P., et al. (2020). Understanding the impact of the COVID-19 pandemic on well-being and virtual care for people living with dementia and care partners living in the community. *Preprint*. https://doi.org/10.1101/2020.06.04.20122192.

Romero-Moreno, R., et al. (2014). Leisure, gender, and kinship in dementia caregiving: Psychological vulnerability of caregiving daughters with feelings of guilt. *Journals of Gerontology. Series B, Psychological Sciences & Social Sciences*, *69*(4), 502–513.

Roth, D. R., et al. (2005). Changes in social support as mediators of the impact of a psychosocial intervention for spouse caregivers of persons with Alzheimer's disease. *Psychology and Aging*, *20*(4), 634–644. 16420138.

Sampson, M. S., & Clark, A. (2016). "Deferred of chickened out?" Decision making among male carers of people with dementia. *Dementia*, *15*(6), 1605–1621. https://doi.org/10.1177/1471301214566663.

Savitch, N., Abbott, E., & Parker, G. M. (2015). *Dementia: Through the eyes of women*. Available from http://eprints.whiterose.ac.uk/91782/1/dementia_eyes_of_women_full.pdf.

Savla, J., et al. (2020). Dementia caregiving during the "stay-at-home" phase of COVID-19 pandemic. *Journals of Gerontology. Series B, Psychological Sciences and Social Sciences*. https://doi.org/10.1093/geronb/gbaa129.

Scott, J., & Clery, E. (2013). Gender roles: An incomplete revolution? In *British social attitudes: The 30th report*. London: NatCen Social Research. Available from www.bsa-30.natcen.ac.uk.

Slachevsky, A., et al. (2013). The CUIDEME study: Determinants of burden in Chilean primary caregivers of patients with dementia. *Journal of Alzheimer's Disease*, *35*(2), 297–306. https://doi.org/10.3233/JAD-122086.

Sun, F., et al. (2008). The influences of gender and religiousness of Alzheimer disease caregivers' use of informal support and formal services. *Journal of Aging and Health*, *20*(8), 937–953.

Teahan, A., et al. (2020). Psychosocial interventions for family carers of people with dementia: A systematic review and meta-analysis. *Journal of Aging and Health*, *32*(9), 1198–1213.

Toepfer, N. F., Foster, J. L. H., & Wilz, G. (2014). "The good mother and her clinging child": Patterns of anchoring in social representations of dementia caregiving. *Journal of Community and Applied Social Psychology*, *24*, 234–248. https://doi.org/10.1002/casp.2164.

Toribio-Diaz, M. E., et al. (2013). Characteristics of informal caregivers of patients with dementia in Alicante province. *Neurología*, *28*(2), 95–102.

United Nations. (2019). *World population ageing 2019: Highlights*. New York. Available from https://www.un.org/en/development/desa/population/publications/pdf/ageing/WorldPopulationAgeing2019-Highlights.pdf.

United Nations. (2020). *Policy brief: The impact of COVID-19 on women*. New York. Available from https://www.unwomen.org/-/media/headquarters/attachments/sections/library/publications/2020/policy-brief-the-impact-of-covid-19-on-women-en.pdf?la=en&vs=1406.

Uwakwe, R. (2006). Satisfaction with dementia care-giving in Nigeria—A pilot investigation. *International Journal of Geriatric Psychiatry*, *21*, 296–297. https://doi.org/10.1002/gps.1500.

Vaitheswaran, S., et al. (2020). Experiences and needs of caregivers of persons with dementia in India during the COVID-19 pandemic—A qualitative study. *American Journal of Geriatric Psychiatry*, 1–10. https://doi.org/10.1016/j.jagp.2020.06.026.

Valimaki, T. H., et al. (2009). Caregiver depression is associated with a low sense of coherence and health-related quality of life. *Aging & Mental Health*, *13*(6), 799–807.

Van Mierlo, L. D., et al. (2012). Personalised caregiver support: Effectiveness of psychosocial interventions in subgroups of caregivers of people with dementia. *International Journal of Geriatric Psychiatry*, *27*, 1–14. https://doi.org/10.1002/gps.2694.

van Wezel, N., et al. (2016). Family care for immigrants with dementia: The perspectives of female family carers living in the Netherlands. *Dementia*, *15*(1), 69–84.

Vlachantoni, A. (2010). The demographic characteristics and economic activity patterns of carers over 50: Evidence from the English Longitudinal Study of Ageing. *Population Trends*, *141*, 51–73. https://doi.org/10.1057/pt.2010.21.

Watson, B., Tatangelo, G., & McCabe, M. (2019). Depression and anxiety among partner and offspring carers of people with dementia: A systematic review. *The Gerontologist*, *59*(5), e597–e610.

Watt, M. H., et al. (2014). Care-giving expectations and challenges among elders and their adult children in Southern Sri Lanka. *Ageing & Society*, *34*(5), 838–858.

Wenham, C., et al. (2020). COVID-19: The gendered impacts of the outbreak. *Lancet*, *395*(10227), 846–848. https://doi.org/10.1016/S0140-6736(20)30526-2.

White, C. (2013). *2011 census analysis: Unpaid care in England and Wales, 2011 and comparison with 2001*. London. Available from https://webarchive.nationalarchives.gov.uk/20160109213406/http://www.ons.gov.uk/ons/dcp171766_300039.pdf.

Williams, F., et al. (2019). Interventions for reducing levels of burden amongst informal carers of persons with dementia in the community. A systematic review and meta-analysis of randomised controlled trials. *Aging & Mental Health*, *23*(12), 1629–1642. https://doi.org/10.1080/13607863.2018.1515886.

Wimo, A., Gauthier, S., & Prince, M. (2018). *Global estimates of informal care*. London. Available from https://www.alz.co.uk/adi/pdf/global-estimates-of-informal-care.pdf.

World Health Organization. (2017a). *Dementia: A public health priority, infographic*. Available from https://www.who.int/mental_health/neurology/dementia/infographic_dementia/en/. (Accessed 17 October 2020).

World Health Organization. (2017b). *Global action plan on the public health response to dementia: 2017–2025*. Geneva. Available from https://apps.who.int/iris/bitstream/handle/10665/259615/9789241513487-eng.pdf;jsessionid=1CBB8582F88852D36E87588F25F4D873?sequence=1.

World Health Organization. (2020). *Preventing and managing COVID-19 across long-term care services: Policy brief*. Geneva. Available from https://www.who.int/publications/i/item/WHO-2019-nCoV-Policy_Brief-Long-term_Care-2020.1.

World Health Organization and Alzheimer's Disease International. (2012). *Dementia: A public health priority*. Geneva. Available from https://www.who.int/mental_health/publications/dementia_report_2012/en/.

Zhang, J., Vitaliano, P. P., & Lin, H.-H. (2006). Relations of caregiving stress and health depend on the health indicators used and gender. *International Journal of Behavioral Medicine, 13*(2), 173–181.

CHAPTER 15

Gender barriers to communication in Alzheimer's disease

Sara Rubinelli[a,b] and Nicola Diviani[a,b]
[a]*Department of Health Sciences and Medicine, University of Lucerne, Lucerne, Switzerland*
[b]*Person-Centered Health Care and Health Communication Group, Swiss Paraplegic Research, Nottwil, Switzerland*

Introduction

In the triad comprising health professionals, patients, and family caregivers, communication is fundamental to the outcome of the therapeutic relationship (Stewart, 1995; Street, Makoul, Arora, et al., 2009). Indeed, processes of communication are central to healthcare practice and significantly improve accuracy and efficiency of care, recall of information, compliance with therapeutic regimes, and satisfaction for patients, family caregivers, and health professionals. Good communication promotes open dialog between health professionals, patients, and family caregivers (Ong, de Haes, Hoos, et al., 1995; Silverman, 1987). It helps with the accuracy of diagnoses and with identification of the best treatments. For all of these reasons, communication has a significant impact on health outcomes (Silverman, Kurtz, & Draper, 2016).

The study of interpersonal communication in healthcare has advanced greatly in recent decades. There is an extensive body of literature on how to improve this particular area of communication by reflecting on its formats and challenges, barriers, and facilitators, as well as considering the points of view of all relevant stakeholders (Hinz, 2000; Silverman et al., 2016). Thus, several theories, models, guidelines, and recommendations have led to the development of training and education programs that reinforce the communication skills of health professionals and support patients and family caregivers in interacting with health professionals and among themselves (Lloyd, Bor, & Noble, 2018; Silverman, Kurtz, & Draper, 2013).

This chapter addresses interpersonal health communication (IHC) in the complex setting of Alzheimer's disease (AD), and specifically, it focuses on communication that can address gender bias and related barriers that disadvantage patients with AD as well as their caregivers. The objective of this chapter is to present communication strategies that assist health professionals in avoiding gender bias in their interactions and offer strategies for empowering female patients with AD and their family caregivers in their interaction with health professionals. The specific topic of this chapter has not been adequately researched as yet; there is little or no discussion of gendered communication in AD in the literature. Thus, our main approach is to identify useful concepts and strategies within the literature on IHC and AD that can inform recommendations for sound communication as proposed here. Since, as we have just highlighted, this is a field in need of further research, an important part of our text will be devoted to the identification of a research agenda to inform and promote future academic work and professional training. This agenda will include a section on how to study the nature and influence of gender in communication in AD settings.

Communication: Grounding concepts

To address gender-inclusive communication in AD, it is useful to start with a general section that outlines the main aspects involved in interpersonal communication as a human process of interaction. This description is followed by a presentation of what the relevant literature recognizes as the main steps that lead to its effectiveness.

The term "communication" comes from the Latin verb *communico*, meaning "share" or "unite." Communication is, thus, the process of understanding and sharing meaning (Pearson & Nelson, 2000). It is a dynamic activity that, as Jakobson notably described (Waugh, 1980), can be broken down into a series of six constitutive components, namely: the *addresser* (the source) sends a *message* to the *addressee* (the receiver). The message requires a *context*, that is, the surrounding frame that assists in the interpretation of the message. It also requires a *code* that is common to the addresser and the addressee, and a contact, a physical *channel* enabling both to engage in communication.

Thus, to give an example in the field, the doctor and the patient with AD play either the addresser or the addressee in different parts of the consultation. The context is the consultation itself, with its specific features (e.g., the anamnesis); they use the same language, which is the code, and communicate by interpersonal and face-to-face interaction (verbal and nonverbal).

Effective communication involves all six of these different components, and problems can occur in relation to any of them. Thus, for instance, a clear, exhaustive, and understandable message from the doctor to the patient tends toward effectiveness, whereas a message that is unclear and misses important information contributes to unsatisfactory communication.

de Negri, Brown, Hernández, et al. (1997) explained the main factors that contribute to effective IHC. Four are worth reporting below:

(1) Disclosure of sufficient information about the symptoms experienced by the patient in order to build an accurate diagnosis. This is a requirement related to the quality of the patient's message; yet, it presupposes clear communication skills from the doctor (as the addresser of questions and information to the patient), for instance, asking the right questions, using the right tone of voice, appropriate language, and making the patient feel comfortable and "heard."

(2) The identification by the doctor of a treatment that is medically appropriate and agreed upon with the patient. This is the outcome of a decision-making dialog where both the doctor and the patient cooperate in reaching agreement over a therapeutic course of action.

(3) Clear understanding by the patient of his/her health conditions and related treatment. This is an outcome that largely depends on the functioning of all six of Jakobson's main components of communication, especially at the level of the doctor's efforts to guide the patient in gaining new knowledge about their health condition and the treatment, and in understanding the main reasons for proposed treatments.

(4) The establishment of a positive relationship between the doctor and the patient. To this goal, communication—in Jakobson's components form—is also fundamental, as it is the inner process behind the beginning, growth, and development of relationships generally.

Overall, communication has to flourish in a way that can encourage dialog within an atmosphere of care and bridge the different knowledge and experiences that doctors and patients have, respectively. Any distorting influence on this process can make it unsuccessful. As we will see below, gender-biased communication is one of these possible influencers in AD, as well as in all other clinical contexts.

Ethical implications of effective communication

Good interpersonal communication in healthcare—that is, interaction where constructive dialog leads to inclusion of patients and family members—has inherent ethical implications. It reflects ideal processes of care that are nowadays known as "patient-centeredness" and "shared decision-making."

In patient-centered care, patients (often with their families) and health professionals are partners. They collaborate on defining the treatment pathways by disclosing preferences and values. Patients work together with their health professionals, who provide them with the necessary information to make informed decisions about their care. Patient-centered care emphasizes models of treatment where patients are recognized as an individual and, thus, emotional and other support is provided in addition to treatment of their physical symptoms (Epstein & Street, 2011; Oates, Weston, & Jordan, 2000; Taylor, 2009).

This engagement of patients is based on effective ways to involve them in the decision-making process. This process posits as a gold standard that health professionals and patients engage in regulated interaction, where accurate and unbiased medical evidence about options, risks, benefits, and the burdens of each alternative, including no intervention, are discussed with an attitude of mutuality (Barry & Edgman-Levitan, 2012; Elwyn, Frosch, Thomson, et al., 2012). Shared decision-making requires communication skills on the part of both the health professionals and the patients, and must have as its main focus patient goals, preferences, and concerns.

IHC, where the virtues and models of patient-centeredness and shared decision-making are implemented, is ethical in its fostering of four basic principles of biomedical ethics (Beauchamp & Childress, 2001), namely:

(1) *Respect for autonomy*: Patients have to supported in making informed choices that respect their capacities and autonomy (Reid, 2009).
(2) *Beneficence*: Acting for the benefit of patients is the prerogative. This involves a clear balancing between the benefits of treatments against risks and costs and in light of patients' views and wishes (Kinsinger, 2010).
(3) *Nonmaleficence*: Although treatments may involve some form of harm, this harm should not be greater than the expected benefit. Risks and possible harm caused by treatments or interventions must be carefully discussed with patients and their families (Gillon, 1985).
(4) *Patients' right to know*: Engaging patients is linked to information and education provisions, so that shared decisions are made with informed insight (Giesen, 1993).

Overall, the practice of shared decision-making within the framework of patient-centeredness aligns health professionals' recommendations with patients' informed preferences as the center of care.

The background on communication and its standards and ethics, as introduced so far, is important for understanding the topic of gender in communication, which we will now approach, first from a broad perspective, and then with a specific focus on AD. Gender can, indeed, be an obstacle to IHC. As such, it might negatively impact the effectiveness of communication, thereby impeding communication and preventing the fulfillment of ethical standards.

Gender issues in IHC in general and implications for AD

Men are from Mars, Women are from Venus is the title of a famous book by John Gray, who explains common problems in relationships by tracing them back to psychological and behavioral differences between the two sexes (Gray, 2009). For instance, he describes how men and women have different ways of dealing with stressful situations. This book is an example of how gender stereotypes, beliefs, and expectations that people have about the characteristics of women and men span across different cultures in history. Thus, for instance, men are expected to be more assertive while women are expected to be more caring and emotional.

There are main lines of research that provide evidence for the roles that gender might play in doctor-patient relationships, which, at different levels, also involve communication issues. For instance, there is evidence that females might receive diagnoses later compared to men. This suggests that communication leading to a diagnosis might proceed differently with a woman than with a man. For example, in the context of rectal cancer, a study showed that females were more likely to be diagnosed at more advanced stages of the disease (Sarasqueta, Zunzunegui,

Navascues, et al., 2020). In the context of autism, another study demonstrated that women receive a diagnosis of an autism spectrum condition in middle to late adulthood, which is on average later than for men (Leedham, Thompson, Smith, et al., 2020). The Brain Tumour Charity published a report in 2016 showing that, in the context of brain tumors, women, in addition to low-income patients, were more likely to see 10 or more months pass between their first visit to a doctor and a diagnosis (Cision, 2016).

Several factors might be linked to a medically unmotivated delayed diagnosis. A major factor to emphasize here is that the evidence shows that women's reports of pain are more likely to be ignored or receive less attention from health professionals than those of men (Clerc Liaudat, Vaucher, De Francesco, et al., 2018; Hoffmann & Tarzian, 2001). This can translate into the fact that women's complaints about pain might not receive adequate consideration. For IHC, this is a major issue; it may indicate barriers either at the level of women presenting and discussing their symptoms or at the level of consideration by the health professionals, meaning that, for some reason, they do not pay enough attention to what matters to their patients (Hamberg, 2008; National Pain Report, 2020). Related to this, some other studies have argued that women's complaints about symptoms such as pain are often perceived by doctors as an expression of emotional concern rather than physiological pain (Hoffmann & Tarzian, 2001; Samulowitz, Gremyr, Eriksson, et al., 2018; Woodward, Taft, Gordon, et al., 2009).

Findings in line with the above issues were also discussed comprehensively in a systematic review by Sandhu, Adams, Singleton, et al. (2009).

Clearly, the above findings related to possible gender bias can also be observed in the field of brain and mental health and specifically in the context of AD and dementia. Indeed, as Goldfarb et al. reported, it is very important to provide a diagnosis as early as possible (Goldfarb, Sheard, Shaughnessy, et al., 2019). This favors the involvement of patients in early decision-making when the disease is at an early stage, when patients and their families can be better prepared for a process of change in their lives. In addition, women with AD are reported to lose their communication skills quicker than men (Laws, Irvine, & Gale, 2018) and a faster cognitive decline is observed after diagnosis (Ferretti, Iulita, Cavedo, et al., 2018). Thus, delays in diagnosis can inhibit communication exchanges that can establish the building of a partnership between the patient and health professionals. This partnership is an asset to interpersonal communication and, especially in dealing with life-long conditions, is a main source of guidance and support in a context where emotional and psychological challenges can also lead to major distress, depression, and other forms of grief.

Last but not least, there is evidence that in AD, women and men have neuropsychological differences that are of primary relevance for communication (Ryan, Umfleet, Kreiner, et al., 2018). This point is addressed in more detail in Chapter 6 on neuropsychological differences. Specifically, women are subject to more cognitive impairment in immediate and delayed prose memory, and in verbal and semantic fluency. When the disease progresses, major barriers can challenge the communication exchange that is at the basis of a person-centered approach that fully identifies and takes into consideration the beliefs, needs, and preferences of the patient.

Gender differences are also reported among caregivers of people living with dementia (see Chapter 14). Gallicchio et al. reported that women caregivers might experience a higher burden and are more likely to experience symptoms of depression (Gallicchio, Siddiqi, Langenberg, et al., 2002). These findings reinforce the need to communicate with female caregivers as early as possible to identify sources of distress and specific needs.

General strategies for communication with dementia and Alzheimer's patients

As outlined in the previous section, AD can have, among other things, an important impact on the communicative abilities of the affected patients, augmenting existing challenges in communication. These include both the ability to express oneself (including the expression of emotions and feelings) and the ability to understand and process the information received. To ensure that communicative exchanges with AD patients are as successful and effective as possible, it is thus important, for both healthcare professionals and informal caregivers, to tailor the style of communication to the abilities of the patients (Downs & Collins, 2015). Most importantly, as AD is a progressive disease, it is crucial that communication is continuously adapted to changing circumstances. In the following section, we will outline some possible communication strategies that are generally included in established guidelines (see, e.g., Alzheimer's Association, 2020; Alzheimer's Society, 2020) and can be implemented when communicating with AD patients and their caregivers. The overall goal of these strategies is to make communication easier by responding to two specific needs. First, to facilitate the expression of the thoughts, needs and feelings of AD patients so these can be taken into account in treatment-related decisions. Second, these strategies can maximize the accessibility of information for AD patients, thus enabling healthcare professionals and informal caregivers to convey important information.

Communication with AD patients should be focused on conveying dignity and respect (Batsch & Mittelman, 2012). This means not talking down to the person as if he or she were a child nor speaking as if he or she was not there. In general, it is important to speak clearly (e.g., using short and simple sentences, breaking down conversations into smaller segments, or talking about one topic at a time) and calmly (e.g., at a slightly slower pace, allowing plenty of time between sentences, or without raising one's voice) (Judd, 2017). Several studies have shown that humor can be beneficial to communication with AD patients, as it can help lighten the mood, bringing patients and caregivers closer together and relieving pressure (see, e.g., Moos, 2011). Here it is important that one laughs *with* the patient (e.g., about misunderstandings and mistakes) and not *at* him or her.

In addition to these general rules, communication also has to take into account the specific challenges experienced by AD patients, which vary depending on the stage of the disease. The phase of mild AD, which is the initial stage of the disease, is usually characterized by a relatively high level of communication ability (Caramelli, Mansur, & Nitrini, 1998). Individuals in this stage are generally still able to participate in meaningful conversations, although they may tend to repeat facts, feel overwhelmed by excessive stimulation (e.g., when provided a lot of information at once), or struggle to find the right words during conversations. In this phase, as the disease affects each individual in a different way, it is of utmost importance not to make assumptions about a person's ability to communicate because of an AD diagnosis. Concretely, this means continuing to engage in conversations as usual, making sure not to exclude the patients from the conversations, and speaking directly to the person rather than to his or her caregiver or companion. At the same time, however, it is important to consider the possibility of difficulties with expression and understanding, and therefore take the time to listen to the person express his or her thoughts, feelings, and needs, and, when asking questions, to give the person time to respond, without interrupting. During this phase, it is a good idea to directly ask the person what he or she is still comfortable doing and what he or she may need help with (Downs & Collins, 2015). It is also the ideal time to discuss future steps and the individual's wishes with various tools available to facilitate this conversation (see Box 1 for a discussion on the role of advance care planning in this context).

Box 1 The role of advance care planning as a communication tool in AD

There is a moment in the disease trajectory of every individual affected by AD when direct communication with the patient is not possible anymore, or at least it becomes very difficult for the patient to engage in meaningful conversations. This limitation in communication has important implications for patients who are not able to take part in decision-making anymore, but also for their caregivers, who have to take decisions on behalf of their loved ones, sometimes not being fully aware of their preferences.

Advance care planning (ACP) can be a very important and relevant tool in this context. ACP refers to the process of enabling individuals to make plans about their future healthcare and usually involves the designation of a substituted decision maker as well as the completion of an advance care directive, a document specifying the actions that should be taken if the person is no longer able to make decisions for him- or herself. Although evidence on the impact of ACP in the field of dementia is still in its infancy, current findings are promising in terms of several outcomes, ranging from quality of death to healthcare costs (Dening, Jones, & Sampson, 2011; Martinsson, Lundström, & Sundelöf, 2020). Moreover, ACP holds the potential to be a valuable tool to enable communication of the patient's needs and wishes, even when they cannot express themselves anymore. In addition, the use of ACP can contribute to relieving the burden from caregivers, thus facilitating communication about end-of-life issues.

ACP cannot be improvised. As has been suggested, it is the general practitioner's or other health professional's task to seize the right moment for initiating an ACP process, to inform patients and caregivers about ACP and its uses, to test the patient's decision-making capacity, and finally, involve appropriately trained healthcare professionals in the actual ACP consultation process (Bally, Krones, & Jox, 2020). Patient's gender should also be considered in the process, as evidence shows that men and women might have different expectations and attitudes toward ACP (Perkins, Hazuda, & Cortez, 2004).

The phase of moderate AD, often referred to as the middle stage of the disease, is arguably the most challenging phase for communication, as it is usually characterized by a significant decline in some of the patient's abilities, including the ability to communicate (Frank, 1994). In this phase, it is particularly important to avoid all distracting factors from the conversation. In this context, it could, for instance, be helpful to engage in one-to-one conversations in quiet spaces whenever possible. This is also the phase where it is of particular importance to make sure that what is being communicated is as easy as possible to process. This includes, among other things, asking one question at a time, asking yes or no questions instead of open questions (e.g., "Would you like to go to the mall?" rather than "What would you like to do?"), and offering clear, step-by-step instructions for tasks. In this context, it is also important to take advantage of external aids. For instance, giving visual cues and demonstrating tasks can encourage participation. Similarly, writing important things as notes can be helpful when spoken words seem confusing. One last aspect to consider in this phase is the patient's need for reassurance. Here, a useful strategy is to maintain eye contact, which can show that you care about what the patient is saying. It is also important to avoid criticism, corrections, and arguing, if not strictly necessary, as these could interrupt the exchange.

In the phase of severe AD, patients rely more and more often on nonverbal communication, such as facial expressions or vocal sounds (Bayles, Tomoeda, Cruz, et al., 2000). In this phase, where verbal communication is strongly impaired, it is particularly important to find alternative ways to communicate, for instance, by encouraging nonverbal communication (Schiaratura, 2008). This includes asking the patient to point or gesture to illustrate what he or she is saying, or using touch, visuals, sounds, smells, and tastes as a form of communication with the person. It is also important to consider the feeling behind words or sounds, as often the emotions being expressed are more important than what is being said. A person with AD is generally able to read body language. Sudden movements or a tense facial expression may upset or cause distress, and can make communication more difficult. It is thus important to make sure that body language and facial expressions match what is being said. Finally, in this challenging phase of the disease, physical contact can be an important tool for communicating interest and providing reassurance (Parenteau, 2000). Holding a person's hand, putting an arm around them, or even just being there can help reassure a patient in this later stage of AD.

Communicating with caregivers of AD patients

In the more advanced phases of AD, a large part of the communication from healthcare professionals, especially communication involving gathering and providing information, will be directed to the caregivers of the patient. In this case, even if the caregiver does not have any impairment at the level of communication, it is important that dedicated communication strategies are put into place to ensure the effectiveness of the exchange of information. Often caregivers find themselves in a challenging situation when discussing the health of their loved ones. Especially when discussing bad news or issues related to end-of-life, caregivers are likely to experience stress (Allen, Curran, Duggan, et al., 2017). Furthermore, caregivers are often requested to deal with a great amount of new information about medical issues without having a medical background. All these aspects might significantly impact a caregiver's ability to understand and process the advice he or she is given. As shown by research in other fields, this might negatively impact the caregiver's ability to take concrete actions and could result in medication errors, hospital admissions, lack of preventive care, increased use of emergency rooms, and poorer health outcomes overall (Kim, 2021).

For this reason, the same degree of attention dedicated to communication with patients with AD should also be applied to communication with their caregivers. Here, it is advisable to adopt a universal precautions approach. This is a concept that originated in medicine in the context of preventing the transmission of infections. The idea is to always assume that infection could be present and therefore take the necessary precautions (e.g., wearing gloves) at all times. The concept was subsequently adopted by researchers and clinicians working in the field of health literacy (Brown, Ludwig, Buck, et al., 2004). In this context, experts recommend assuming that everyone may have difficulty understanding medical information and instructions from their healthcare provider. Concretely, this means taking steps that are based on the assumption that all patients and their caregivers may have difficulty comprehending health information and accessing health services.

In the specific context of communication with caregivers of AD patients, adopting a universal precautions approach would entail simplifying communication with and confirming comprehension for all caregivers, so that the risk of miscommunication is minimized. There are four main strategies that are now recognized as being effective for reaching this aim by leading institutions in the field: using plain language, using visual aids, recommending and using technology, and using effective teaching methods.

Plain language is defined as written or verbal communication that an audience can understand the first time they read or hear it and aims to ensure that users can find what they need, understand what they find, and use what they find to meet their needs (Stableford & Mettger, 2007). Central elements of plain language include organizing information so the most important points are mentioned first, breaking complex information into smaller and more understandable chunks, using simple language (ideally at a sixth-grade reading level), defining technical or medical terms, and avoiding use of the passive voice.

The use of *visual aids*, such as simple illustrations, images, informational graphics, and videos, has consistently been shown to significantly improve patients' and caregivers' understanding of health information, especially when they are used as a complement to written or verbal communication (Pratt & Searles, 2017). This is especially important since health information that is provided in a stressful or unfamiliar situation is less likely to be retained.

Technology can also be an effective tool for improving communication between healthcare professionals and caregivers (Weiner, 2012). According to recent data, the majority of people use the internet and have a smartphone. This is also increasingly true for people in late adulthood, who are more likely to find themselves in a situation where they care for an AD patient (Anderson & Perrin, 2017). The various technological tools available, such as patient portals, telemedicine solutions, and mobile applications, can greatly help healthcare providers connect more effectively with their patients. Concretely, patient portals can, for instance, give access to critical health information, such as test results and treatment instructions; telemedicine can be used to assess and treat underserved patient populations, such as those with limited mobility or living in rural areas; mobile apps can offer caregivers multiple options for learning about or managing health issues; smartphone apps can collect real-time, personal health-related data to be shared with physicians, provide general health information, and assist with preventive lifestyle strategies.

Overall, it is also important that healthcare professionals apply *effective teaching methods* to improve communication and help caregivers better understand health information. This includes, for instance, asking open-ended questions to assess understanding of written materials, including prescription labels, using the "teach back" communication method (Dinh, Bonner, Clark, et al., 2016) to determine if the person has understood the instructions and can repeat the information in their own words, or applying the "show back" technique when teaching how to use a device or perform a task, to demonstrate correct use (Kountz, 2009). In general, it is essential that healthcare professionals speak slowly when providing instructions and place an emphasis on being respectful and clear without being patronizing.

It must be acknowledged that male and female caregivers are observed to differ in communication styles and coping strategies (Rose-Rego, Strauss, & Smyth, 1998; Russell, 2007; Swinkels, van Tilburg, Verbakel, et al., 2019). Gender-specific needs are therefore to be taken into account when communicating with caregivers. For instance, gender differences in needs and preferences related to technologies among caregivers (see, e.g., Xiong, Ye, Mihailidis, et al., 2020) should be considered when planning technology-based communication interventions (Box 2).

A research agenda in AD, gender, and communication

As outlined in the previous sections, both gender and communication are central topics in AD. Besides being related to differences in the manifestation and progression of AD, gender also has important implications for the success of communication with both patients and their caregivers. We know from research on doctor-patient communication in the context of other health conditions that women and men tend to have different communication styles and preferences when it comes to medical consultations, as well as in regular interactions (Street, 2002). These differences, if not acknowledged and adequately addressed, can have important and long-lasting implications for diagnosis and for the overall success of the communication between patients, their caregivers, and healthcare professionals.

> **Box 2 Information and communication technology and artificial intelligence for supporting people living with AD and other dementias**
>
> In recent years, increasing attention has been devoted to the use of information and communication technology (ICT) and artificial intelligence (AI) to address all sorts of issues related to health and self-management. The field of AD/dementia is no exception to this trend. ICT and AI are indeed seen as promising tools to increase the quality of life of people living with AD/dementia and that of their caregivers (Guzman-Parra, Barnestein-Fonseca, Guerrero-Pertiñez, et al., 2020; Husebo, Heintz et al., 2020). For patients, for instance, digital technology such as touchscreen tablets has been shown to provide a means of delivering concise personalized prompts that combine audio, text, and pictures, helping patients to overcome common difficulties in completing multistep, everyday tasks (Evans, Boyd, Harris, et al., 2020). Technology has also been shown to have the potential to promote the capacity of people with AD and other forms of dementia and support them in coping with cognitive deficits and managing everyday life as independently as possible (Øksnebjerg, Janbek, Woods, et al., 2020).
>
> Although it is widely recognized that ICT and AI are the future, their role to support people with AD and dementia to date has received only limited scholarly attention, and research in the field is generally not characterized by randomized controlled trials, thus leaving their potential largely unexplored (Øksnebjerg et al., 2020). Furthermore, there are several barriers to the use of ICTs, such as inadequate knowledge, negative attitudes, or lack of enthusiasm for new technologies. This is especially true among the elderly, who potentially could be the main beneficiaries of such innovations (Guzman-Parra et al., 2020).
>
> Finally, it is recognized that a sex and gender bias exists in ICT and AI in healthcare: the design of the majority of algorithms neglect the sex and gender dimension and its contribution to health and disease differences among individuals (Cirillo, Catuara-Solarz, Morey, et al., 2020; Parikh, Teeple, & Navathe, 2019). Recent studies show that consideration of sex and gender leads to more effective technological and AI solutions, such as the development and use of digital biomarkers for sensitive and early diagnosis of multiple cognitive domain impairment (MCI) leading to dementia (Buegler et al., 2020). As consideration of sex and gender is imperative for research in AD and other forms of dementia, further research, together with addressing sex and gender bias, is essential to deliver effective and sustainable tools and products that address individual needs and while taking individual differences into account.

Despite its importance, however, the interplay between gender and communication has not yet received much scholarly attention. In the following section, we will therefore outline a research agenda to further our understanding of the issue.

A first line of research should be dedicated to strengthening the evidence base regarding differences between men and women on how AD impacts their ability to engage in communicative exchanges. Based on the limited evidence available and the understanding that AD has different risk factors and pathways for men and women, we can, for instance, expect gender-related differences in the rate or onset of decline of communication abilities. Indeed, various studies have reported a faster brain atrophy and cognitive decline in women, marked gender differences in progression of mild cognitive impairment, as well as, in contrast to what happens among non-cognitively impaired people, lower scores on verbal memory tasks among women diagnosed with AD/dementia (Ferretti et al., 2018; Lin, Choudhury, Rathakrishnan, et al., 2015). To investigate this further, dedicated observational longitudinal studies with a specific focus on communication are necessary.

A second line of research should focus on the exploration of gender differences in the experience of communication. This would include an in-depth investigation of expectations, perceptions, actual conversations, and outcomes (e.g., satisfaction with the exchange) of interpersonal encounters; this should include AD patients, their caregivers, and healthcare professionals. Although standardized quantitative measures can be used to provide important insights, qualitative methods, such as in-depth interviews and observational methods, are particularly well suited to this context and have the potential to provide a rich understanding of patients' subjective lived experiences and of possible barriers and biases related to gender that deserve particular attention.

Last but not least, systematically building on findings from the first two lines of research, research is needed to develop and test tailored interventions to support patients, caregivers, and healthcare professionals in making sure that gender differences are taken into account in communication exchanges and to maximize their effectiveness. For patients, this would include, for instance, the development of gender-specific (technological) tools to support them in the elaboration and delivery of information. For caregivers and healthcare professionals, this could translate into dedicated training that focuses on non-gender-biased communication. Such tools and trainings should be developed in strict collaboration with all relevant stakeholders, and their effectiveness should be evaluated in dedicated RCTs.

Ten lessons learned about health communication avoiding gender biases in AD

As previously highlighted, more research is needed to identify gender-related challenges in the provider-patient relationship in relation to AD. However, we can summarize the content above in the format of "ten lessons learned" about optimal communication in the field. These lessons can form the basis for providers' self-reflection on how to improve their communication with patients with AD and their families.

(1) *Communication toward the fulfillment of standards*. Person-centered communication and shared decision-making are implemented in the medical consultation through optimal communication. There is no person-centered care that does not address patients' points of view, beliefs, and expectations; the aim is to always reach consensus through careful, shared decision-making.

(2) *Ethical standards*. Optimal communication is fundamental to the fulfillment of ethical standards. In particular, autonomy requires functional provider-patient communication, as patients can only make appropriate decisions when they are well-informed about the relevant issues.

(3) *Biases in AD health communication*. Provider-patient with AD communication can be affected by biases, especially during diagnosis and in relation to the way women and men talk about their symptoms and are perceived in relation to this.

(4) *Tailoring communication.* Since AD is progressive, communication needs to be constantly adapted to the linguistic and cognitive skills of the patients living with AD. Since women and men might differ in the different phases of the disease development, specific adaptations need to be made accordingly.

(5) *Phases of the disease.* Communication in AD also has to take into consideration the challenges experienced by patients depending on the stage of the disease. Overall, three main phases are recognized that differ in terms of the abilities that patients can use in their communication efforts: mild, moderate, and severe. This adaptation has to be marked by a process of simplification of communication, especially in terms of information about the status of the health condition and the steps, healthcare plans, and actions to be made. Again, communication has to consider possible different courses of the health condition, not only from patient to patient, but also among genders (with marked differences between how men and women might act and react).

(6) *Nonverbal communication.* Nonverbal communication is considered a main asset when cognitive impairments challenge verbal communication. Special gestures are important to communicate a feeling of care and are essential to capture, for instance, psychological and emotional components of patients' behavior in the consultation. Verbal communication is inherently linked to gender characteristics that have now to be carefully addressed in promoting a functional relationship with patients.

(7) *Stress in provider-family communication.* Gender differences might also occur in how families deal with managing a difficult health condition. Thus, special attention is needed on communication, including about negative information, that is done in a way that minimizes or avoids stress while being attentive to what support and resources male and female caregivers need to assist their loved ones.

(8) *Formats and channels of communication.* Using visual aids and technology-enhanced communication channels is an enrichment of face-to-face communication with patients and families with AD.

(9) *Healthcare practice and research* (a). Health professionals and researchers are invited to contribute with their work to provide further evidence on how AD impacts the ability to engage in communicative exchange and sex and gender differences observed in this regard.

(10) *Healthcare practice and research* (b). Another area where evidence on possible gender biases in communication in the context of AD is in the experience that patients, both male and female, have of interactions with their health professionals. Here, in-depth exploration is needed to capture knowledge, beliefs, and emotions (e.g., fear and anger) of patients and evaluate whether some reactions can be generalized in terms of gender differences for how people deal with this health condition.

Conclusion

Mara Botonis, an Alzheimer's advocate, once said, "If you learn to listen to cues as to how I feel instead of what I say, you will be able to understand me much better." In this chapter, we have highlighted how communication, both verbal and nonverbal, is the main process through which health professionals engage with patients living with AD and their families. As a degenerative health condition that impacts a person's cognitive and linguistic capacities, communication in the healthcare relationship needs continual adaptation, variation, and simplification. In AD, there is also evidence for possible gender differences between female and male patients. These differences occur not only at a physiological level, but can translate into behaviors that have to be carefully identified and considered to avoid gender biases in communication that ultimately impact the quality of care. This is a challenge in provider-patient/family communication, where important lessons can be derived from the extensive literature on healthcare communication. We conclude with an invitation for those active in research to advance knowledge in the field and develop guidelines and recommendations that focus on care of patients, taking into account and addressing their specific characteristics including gender and their autonomy, as well as how to best facilitate families' roles and actions in the process of care.

Chapter highlights

- Gender plays a central role in the diagnosis and the progression of AD, but also impacts interpersonal communication between doctors, patients, and their caregivers.
- Optimal communication is recognized as a main tool for diagnosis and treatment of AD, but current interventions to support patients and caregivers in their communication activities only marginally address gender differences.
- Further in-depth research is needed to investigate how gender impacts communication in the specific context of AD and to identify effective ways to support patients and caregivers through tailored interventions.

References

Allen, A. P., Curran, E. A., Duggan, Á., et al. (2017). A systematic review of the psychobiological burden of informal caregiving for patients with dementia: Focus on cognitive and biological markers of chronic stress. *Neuroscience & Biobehavioral Reviews, 73*, 123–164.

Alzheimer's Association. (2020). *Communication and Alzheimer's*. Alzheimer's disease and dementia https://alz.org/help-support/caregiving/daily-care/communications (Accessed 23 November 2020).

Alzheimer's Society. (2020). *Tips: communicating with someone with dementia*. Alzheimer's Society. https://www.alzheimers.org.uk/about-dementia/symptoms-and-diagnosis/symptoms/tips-for-communicating-dementia. (Accessed 23 November 2020).

Anderson, M., & Perrin, A. (2017). *Technology use among seniors*. Washington, DC: Pew Research Center for Internet & Technology.

Bally, K. W., Krones, T., & Jox, R. J. (2020). Advance care planning for people with dementia: The role of general practitioners. *Gerontology, 66*, 40–46.

Barry, M. J., & Edgman-Levitan, S. (2012). Shared decision making—The pinnacle of patient-centered care. *New England Journal of Medicine, 366*, 780–781.

Batsch, N. L., & Mittelman, M. S. (2012). *World Alzheimer Report 2012: Overcoming the stigma of dementia* (p. 5). Alzheimer's Disease International (ADI).

Bayles, K. A., Tomoeda, C. K., Cruz, R. F., et al. (2000). Communication abilities of individuals with late-stage Alzheimer disease. *Alzheimer Disease & Associated Disorders, 14*, 176–181.

Beauchamp, T. L., & Childress, J. F. (2001). *Principles of biomedical ethics*. USA: Oxford University Press.

Brown, D. R., Ludwig, R., Buck, G. A., et al. (2004). Health literacy: Universal precautions needed. *Journal of Allied Health, 33*, 150–155.

Buegler, M., Harms, R. L., Balasa, M., Meier, I. B., Exarchos, T., Rai, L., … Rampini, M. (2020). Digital biomarker-based individualized prognosis for people at risk of dementia. *Alzheimer's & Dementia: Diagnosis, Assessment & Disease Monitoring, 12*(1), e12073.

Caramelli, P., Mansur, L. L., & Nitrini, R. (1998). Chapter 32—Language and communication disorders in dementia of the Alzheimer type. In B. Stemmer, & H. A. Whitaker (Eds.), *Handbook of neurolinguistics* (pp. 463–473). San Diego: Academic Press.

Cirillo, D., Catuara-Solarz, S., Morey, C., et al. (2020). Sex and gender differences and biases in artificial intelligence for biomedicine and healthcare. *NPJ Digital Medicine, 3*, 1–11.

Cision. (2016). *Women wait longer for brain tumour diagnosis, report finds*. News Powered by Cision. https://news.cision.com/the-brain-tumour-charity/r/women-wait-longer-for-brain-tumour-diagnosis--report-finds,c9894921. (Accessed 23 November 2020).

Clerc Liaudat, C., Vaucher, P., De Francesco, T., et al. (2018). Sex/gender bias in the management of chest pain in ambulatory care. *Women's Health (London, England), 14*, 1745506518805641.

de Negri, B., Brown, D. L., Hernández, O., et al. (1997). *Improving interpersonal communication between health care providers and clients*. Bethesda US (pp. 3–59).

Dening, K. H., Jones, L., & Sampson, E. L. (2011). Advance care planning for people with dementia: A review. *International Psychogeriatrics, 23*, 1535–1551.

Dinh, T. T. H., Bonner, A., Clark, R., et al. (2016). The effectiveness of the teach-back method on adherence and self-management in health education for people with chronic disease: A systematic review. *JBI Evidence Synthesis, 14*, 210–247.

Downs, M., & Collins, L. (2015). Person-centred communication in dementia care. *Nursing Standard, 30*, 37.

Elwyn, G., Frosch, D., Thomson, R., et al. (2012). Shared decision making: A model for clinical practice. *Journal of General Internal Medicine, 27*, 1361–1367.

Epstein, R. M., & Street, R. L. (2011). The values and value of patient-centered care. *Annals of Family Medicine, 9*, 100–103.

Evans, N., Boyd, H., Harris, N., et al. (2020). The experience of using prompting technology from the perspective of people with dementia and their primary carers. *Aging & Mental Health*, 1–9.

Ferretti, M. T., Iulita, M. F., Cavedo, E., et al. (2018). Sex differences in Alzheimer disease—The gateway to precision medicine. *Nature Reviews Neurology, 14*, 457–469.

Frank, E. M. (1994). Effect of Alzheimer's disease on communication function. *Journal of the South Carolina Medical Association (1975), 90*, 417–423.

Gallicchio, L., Siddiqi, N., Langenberg, P., et al. (2002). Gender differences in burden and depression among informal caregivers of demented elders in the community. *International Journal of Geriatric Psychiatry, 17*, 154–163.

Giesen, D. (1993). The patient's right to know—A comparative law perspective. *Medicine and Law, 12*, 553–565.

Gillon, R. (1985). 'Primum non nocere' and the principle of non-maleficence. *British Medical Journal (Clinical Research Ed.), 291*, 130.

Goldfarb, D., Sheard, S., Shaughnessy, L., et al. (2019). Disclosure of Alzheimer's disease and dementia: Patient- and care partner-centric decision-making and communication. *Journal of Clinical Psychiatry, 80*. https://doi.org/10.4088/JCP.MS18002BR1C. Epub ahead of print 19.

Gray, J. (2009). *Men are from Mars, women are from Venus: Practical guide for improving communication.* Zondervan.

Guzman-Parra, J., Barnestein-Fonseca, P., Guerrero-Pertiñez, G., et al. (2020). Attitudes and use of information and communication technologies in older adults with mild cognitive impairment or early stages of dementia and their caregivers: Cross-sectional study. *Journal of Medical Internet Research, 22*, e17253.

Hamberg, K. (2008). Gender bias in medicine. *Women's Health, 4*, 237–243.

Hinz, C. A. (2000). *Communicating with your patients: Skills for building rapport.* Chicago, IL: American Medical Association.

Hoffmann, D. E., & Tarzian, A. J. (2001). The girl who cried pain: A bias against women in the treatment of pain. *Journal of Law, Medicine & Ethics, 28*, 13–27.

Husebo, B. S., Heintz, H. L., Berge, L. I., Owoyemi, P., Rahman, A. T., & Vahia, I. V. (2020). Sensing technology to monitor behavioral and psychological symptoms and to assess treatment response in people with dementia. A systematic review. *Frontiers in Pharmacology, 10*, 1699. https://doi.org/10.3389/fphar.2019.01699.

Judd, M. (2017). Communication strategies for patients with dementia. *Nursing, 47*, 58–61.

Kim, S. (2021). Caregivers' information overload and their personal health literacy. *Western Journal of Nursing Research, 43*(5), 0193945920959086.

Kinsinger, F. S. (2010). Beneficence and the professional's moral imperative. *Journal of Chiropractic Humanities, 16*, 44–46.

Kountz, D. S. (2009). Strategies for improving low health literacy. *Postgraduate Medicine, 121*, 171–177.

Laws, K. R., Irvine, K., & Gale, T. M. (2018). Sex differences in Alzheimer's disease. *Current Opinion in Psychiatry, 31*, 133–139.

Leedham, A., Thompson, A. R., Smith, R., et al. (2020). 'I was exhausted trying to figure it out': The experiences of females receiving an autism diagnosis in middle to late adulthood. *Autism, 24*, 135–146.

Lin, K. A., Choudhury, K. R., Rathakrishnan, B. G., et al. (2015). Marked gender differences in progression of mild cognitive impairment over 8 years. *Alzheimer's & Dementia, 1*, 103–110.

Lloyd, M., Bor, R., & Noble, L. M. (2018). *Clinical communication skills for medicine.* Elsevier Health Sciences.

Martinsson, L., Lundström, S., & Sundelöf, J. (2020). Better quality of end-of-life care for persons with advanced dementia in nursing homes compared to hospitals: A Swedish national register study. *BMC Palliative Care, 19*, 1–9.

Moos, I. (2011). Humour, irony and sarcasm in severe Alzheimer's dementia—A corrective to retrogenesis? *Ageing and Society, 31*, 328–346.

National Pain Report. (2020). *Women in pain report significant gender bias*. National Pain Report. http://nationalpainreport.com/women-in-pain-report-significant-gender-bias-8824696.html. (Accessed 23 November 2020).

Oates, J., Weston, W. W., & Jordan, J. (2000). The impact of patient-centered care on outcomes. *Family Practice, 49*, 796–804.

Øksnebjerg, L., Janbek, J., Woods, B., et al. (2020). Assistive technology designed to support self-management of people with dementia: User involvement, dissemination, and adoption. A scoping review. *International Psychogeriatrics, 32*, 937–953.

Ong, L. M., de Haes, J. C., Hoos, A. M., et al. (1995). Doctor-patient communication: A review of the literature. *Social Science & Medicine, 40*, 903–918.

Parenteau, P. (2000). Communication with Alzheimer patients: A matter of time, caring and contact. *Canadian Alzheimer Disease Review, 5*.

Parikh, R. B., Teeple, S., & Navathe, A. S. (2019). Addressing bias in artificial intelligence in health care. *JAMA, 322*(24), 2377–2378.

Pearson, J. C., & Nelson, P. E. (2000). *An introduction to human communication: Understanding and sharing*. McGraw-Hill.

Perkins, H. S., Hazuda, H. P., & Cortez, J. D. (2004). Advance care planning: Does patient gender make a difference? *American Journal of the Medical Sciences, 327*, 25–32.

Pratt, M., & Searles, G. E. (2017). Using visual AIDS to enhance physician-patient discussions and increase health literacy. *Journal of Cutaneous Medicine and Surgery, 21*, 497–501.

Reid, K. I. (2009). Respect for patients' autonomy. *Journal of the American Dental Association, 140*, 470–474.

Rose-Rego, S. K., Strauss, M. E., & Smyth, K. A. (1998). Differences in the perceived well-being of wives and husbands caring for persons with Alzheimer's disease. *Gerontologist, 38*, 224–230.

Russell, R. (2007). The work of elderly men caregivers: From public careers to an unseen world. *Men and Masculinities, 9*, 298–314.

Ryan, J. J., Umfleet, L. G., Kreiner, D. S., et al. (2018). Neuropsychological differences between men and women with Alzheimer's disease. *International Journal of Neuroscience, 128*, 342–348.

Samulowitz, A., Gremyr, I., Eriksson, E., et al. (2018). "Brave men" and "emotional women": A theory-guided literature review on gender bias in health care and gendered norms towards patients with chronic pain. *Pain Research & Management, 2018*, 6358624.

Sandhu, H., Adams, A., Singleton, L., et al. (2009). The impact of gender dyads on doctor–patient communication: A systematic review. *Patient Education and Counseling, 76*, 348–355.

Sarasqueta, C., Zunzunegui, M. V., Navascues, J. M. E., et al. (2020). Gender differences in stage at diagnosis and preoperative radiotherapy in patients with rectal cancer. *BMC Cancer, 20*, 1–11.

Schiaratura, L. T. (2008). Non-verbal communication in Alzheimer's disease. *Psychologie & Neuropsychiatrie du Vieillissement, 6*, 183–188.

Silverman, D. (1987). *Communication and medical practice: Social relations in the clinic*. London: Sage.

Silverman, J., Kurtz, S., & Draper, J. (2013). *Skills for communicating with patients* (3rd ed.). CRC Press. https://www.crcpress.com/Skills-for-Communicating-with-Patients-3rd-Edition/Silverman-Kurtz-Draper/p/book/9781846193651. (Accessed 1 May 2018).

Silverman, J., Kurtz, S., & Draper, J. (2016). *Skills for communicating with patients*. CRC Press.

Stableford, S., & Mettger, W. (2007). Plain language: A strategic response to the health literacy challenge. *Journal of Public Health Policy, 28*, 71–93.

Stewart, M. A. (1995). Effective physician-patient communication and health outcomes: A review. *CMAJ: Canadian Medical Association Journal*, *152*, 1423.

Street, R. L., Jr. (2002). Gender differences in health care provider–patient communication: Are they due to style, stereotypes, or accommodation? *Patient Education and Counseling*, *48*, 201–206.

Street, R. L., Jr., Makoul, G., Arora, N. K., et al. (2009). How does communication heal? Pathways linking clinician–patient communication to health outcomes. *Patient Education and Counseling*, *74*, 295–301.

Swinkels, J., van Tilburg, T., Verbakel, E., et al. (2019). Explaining the gender gap in the caregiving burden of partner caregivers. *Journals of Gerontology. Series B, Psychological Sciences and Social Sciences*, *74*, 309–317.

Taylor, K. (2009). Paternalism, participation and partnership—The evolution of patient centeredness in the consultation. *Patient Education and Counseling*, *74*, 150–155.

Waugh, L. R. (1980). The poetic function in the theory of Roman Jakobson. *Poetics Today*, *2*, 57–82.

Weiner, J. P. (2012). Doctor-patient communication in the e-health era. *Israel Journal Health Policy Research*, *1*, 1–7.

Woodward, H. E., Taft, C. T., Gordon, R. A., et al. (2009). Clinician bias in the diagnosis of posttraumatic stress disorder and borderline personality disorder. *Psychological Trauma Theory Research Practice and Policy*, *1*, 282.

Xiong, C., Ye, B., Mihailidis, A., et al. (2020). Sex and gender differences in technology needs and preferences among informal caregivers of persons with dementia. *BMC Geriatrics*, *20*, 1–12.

CHAPTER

Women and dementia policy: Redressing imbalance through gender transformative policies

16

Wendy Weidner, Paola Barbarino, and Chris Lynch
Alzheimer's Disease International, London, United Kingdom

Dementia is one of the greatest health challenges of our time (Prince et al., 2013). Every 3 seconds someone in the world develops dementia. There are already 50 million people living with it globally and this number is set to treble by 2050, when almost 70% of these individuals will be living in low- and middle-income countries (LMICs) (Alzheimer's Disease International, 2019). Dementia is the 5th leading cause of death globally (World Health Organization, 2018a), yet receives only a fraction of the research focus devoted to other major illnesses, such as cancer or coronary heart disease (Luengo-Fernandez, Leal, & Gray, 2015; Patterson, 2018). It permeates society, with significant costs to health systems, long-term care, and economies as a whole (Prince, Comas-Herrera, Knapp, Guerchet, & Karagiannidou, 2016). It affects entire families, deeply impacting the lives of loved ones, who find their roles shifting from spouse or offspring to that of carer. Yet the most profound impact of dementia is on an individual's personhood: one's memories, abilities, independence, and importantly, relationships.

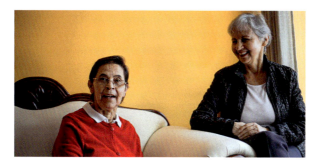

The global figures can be difficult to comprehend and the personal impact overwhelming; but when we drill down into the detail, we find an important truth: that the scales of impact are heavily tipped against women. Dementia disproportionally affects women on a global scale. More women than men develop dementia and a higher

> **Box 1 A word about language and intent.**
> Throughout this chapter, we use the term "sex" to refer to biological differences or characteristics that determine whether an individual is a man or a woman. The term "gender" is used to refer to the societal constructs or meaning we impose on individuals based on those biological differences, i.e., how women are treated because they are perceived to be female (Bamford, 2011b; Criado Perez, 2019a).

percentage of carers for people living with dementia are female (Erol, Brooker, & Peel, 2015a). The impact of stigma and risk factors place an additional burden on women, and women are largely absent from decision-making and policy development that may benefit them (Bamford, 2011a).

This chapter will explore why this imbalance exists and delve into how, through dementia policy, governments can take transformative steps to readjust the sex and gender balance toward equilibrium (Box 1).

Acknowledging the imbalance: Where we are now

It is important to note that although this chapter focuses on the impact of dementia on women and policy implications through a sex and gender lens, it is not meant to imply that the experience of men living with dementia is of less consequence. Each person, regardless of their sex, experiences dementia in a deeply personal way and this is of value. However, exploring the layered and complex impact of dementia on women will help us contextualize the need for gendered approaches for new and better policy structures that can improve quality of life for both sexes.

First, we need to explore some of the key areas that contribute to the complicated relationship of sex, gender, and dementia. Many of these contributing factors are dealt with in more detail in other chapters of this book, but briefly, here are four important truths to remember.

One: More women have dementia

Our global population is aging rapidly, and it is projected to more than double by 2050, reaching over 1.5 billion people over the age of 65. Women tend to live longer than men and, although this gender gap is slowly closing, it is still forecast that by 2050, 54% of people over 65 will be female, increasing slightly to 59% for those over the age of 80 (United Nations, Department of Economic and Social Affairs, Population Division, 2019). As age is the biggest risk factor for dementia, it would follow that more women would be affected. Indeed, in 2016 it was estimated that women made up 62% of all dementia cases globally, while men comprised 38% (Nichols et al., 2019).

While living longer does increase women's risk of developing dementia, it is not the only contributing factor. Statistical models accounting for gender-dependent mortality rates show a 2:1 ratio at any age. In other words, regardless of age, there are twice as many women with Alzheimer's as there are men with the disease (Mosconi, 2020a). Research has revealed that biological differences in male and female brains may influence how disease-related changes occur in the brain (Snyder et al., 2016). Emerging evidence also indicates that when women do develop dementia, their decline is more rapid, both in terms of cognition and in quality of life measures (Carey, 2015; Ferretti, Iulita, Cavedo, et al., 2018). And finally, it seems hormones may play a role. Estrogen is known to have a protective effect on the brain, and the reduced levels as a result of menopause may, in fact, lead to the deficits in brain metabolism found in Alzheimer's disease (Carter, Resnick, Mallampalli, & Kalbarczyk, 2012). (The influence of hormones on dementia is addressed in detail in Chapters 2 and 9.)

Two: More women are carers

Women provide the bulk of both formal and informal care for people living with dementia. In fact, between 60% and 70% of all unpaid dementia carers are women (Alzheimer's Impact Movement, Alzheimer's Association, 2020; Alzheimer's Research UK, 2015a; Erol, Brooker, & Peel, 2015b). In 2015, it was estimated that women, most of whom live in LMICs, contribute to 71% of the annual global hours of informal care—that's 58 billion hours (Wimo et al., 2018). This takes its toll, with 62% of women sharing that they found their caring role to be emotionally stressful, experiencing isolation that can be linked to depression, itself a key risk factor for dementia (Alzheimer's Research UK, 2015b; European Institute of Women's Health, 2019). To make matters worse, women's unpaid caring roles often mean they are left without pensions or access to social protection schemes that could provide a much-needed security net in old age.

In addition, working women who are also carers report negative impacts on their career, with 20% having to reduce working hours to part-time and nearly 19% having to quit work entirely because their caregiving roles become too demanding (Alzheimer's Impact Movement, Alzheimer's Association, 2020; Alzheimer's Research UK, 2015c). Women also make up the majority of the professional or formal care workforce, often with pay that is 10% lower than that of men in a similar role (Erol, Brooker, & Peel, 2015c). (The topic of female caregivers is addressed in further detail in Chapter 14.)

Three: Women with dementia experience added stigma

Stigma around dementia is a huge global challenge. Lack of understanding and knowledge impacts our attitudes, which, in turn, impact our behavior toward people living with dementia. The 2019 World Alzheimer Report indicated that 2 out of 3 people still believe that dementia is a normal part of aging. More surprisingly, 62% of healthcare professionals also believe this to be the case (Alzheimer's Disease International, 2019). The lack of understanding that dementia is a neurological condition can create huge barriers to seeking diagnosis and support. It also clears the way for stigmatized views of individuals who exhibit symptoms and reinforces feelings of fear and shame associated with changed capacity and behavior. Moreover, in some cultures, lack of knowledge and stigma leads to false beliefs about dementia as well as abusive behavior toward those living with the condition (Mkhonto & Hanssen, 2018).

It is widely accepted that women with dementia face "triple jeopardy;" experiencing increased stigma and discrimination due to their age, sex, and neurological condition. Negative attitudes and mistaken beliefs that they are somehow responsible for their symptoms and behavior can impede women from coming forward to seek support or a diagnosis (Bamford, 2011c; Graham et al., 2003). The stigma tied to the diagnosis and the resulting discrimination can bring feelings of isolation, hopelessness, and powerlessness (Erol, Brooker, & Peel, 2015d).

Four: Early education for girls is key for risk reduction

There are opportunities for women to reduce the risk of developing dementia along the whole life course, but strong evidence places emphasis firmly at the beginning, with education. Evidence shows that childhood education and lifelong higher educational attainment actually reduce the risk of dementia. New research suggests that cognitive ability increases with early education, eventually reaching a plateau in late adolescence when the brain has the greatest plasticity (Livingston et al., 2020). However, fewer girls attend primary and secondary school than boys, especially in LMICs, where parents with limited funds are more likely to invest in the education of their sons rather than their daughters. Even today, women still make up two-thirds of the 774 million illiterate adults in the world (Mosconi, 2020b). Beyond the positive impact that education has for brain resilience, access to it is a strong determinant for an individual's life chances and opportunities (Bamford, 2011d). (The role of education as a protective factor is also discussed in Chapter 12.)

It's pretty clear that when it comes to dementia, the scales of fairness do not favor women. They experience more dementia, provide more care for people with dementia, endure more stigma as a result, and some lose access to early education that can reduce risk of dementia in the future. How can we tackle this imbalance? What kind of comprehensive policy framework can address the complex and problematic reality we have just described and how do we go about building it? Before we outline some solutions, it is important to pull back and look at the big picture to understand how we got here in the first place.

Understanding the imbalance: How did we get here

The imbalances experienced by women around dementia do not happen in a vacuum. Inequities exist across many sectors and across global boundaries. To get some perspective, we need to think about the issue of sex and gender in the context of societal norms—what is accepted and what is expected. The truth is, we live in a world that implicitly has a male bias. This is not necessarily ill-intentioned. It is a phenomenon that has developed through historical trends and is perpetuated via socialization, gender stereotypes, and cultural norms (Criado Perez, 2019b).

For example, the masculine default exists in areas as basic as our use of language. In gender-inflected languages, such as French, German, or Spanish, the generic masculine is used to describe a mixed group of people. In other words, you could have a group of 100 female teachers, referred to as "las profesoras," and add one male teacher, and the whole gender reference switches to "los profesores," the male default (Criado Perez, 2019c). Seemingly, small examples that are hardly noticeable until tabulated are all around us. Men have more roles in movies and spend twice as much time as women on screen (Criado Perez, 2019d). In the news media, the amount we hear from women has stagnated recently. In both 2010 and again in 2015, The Global Media Monitoring Project found that "women make up only 24% of persons heard, read about, or seen in newspaper, television and radio news" (World Association for Christian Communication, 2015). One study in the US found that named men outnumbered named women in high-school history textbooks by a ratio of about 18 to 100 (Criado Perez, 2019e). In her book, "Invisible Women: Exposing data bias in a world designed for men," Caroline Criado Perez states it clearly, "what is male becomes universal and what is female becomes niche" (Criado Perez, 2019f).

In this context, it becomes clear that women have an uphill battle ahead. In order to count, they have to be heard. But in order to be heard, they have to prove their issues exist—which requires data—and this is the clincher: if women aren't part of data sets, they become invisible.

Data bias—Women are invisible

Data are important. They provide evidence that legitimizes an issue, proving it exists and is worth investigating. They can help us understand the scale and complexity of a problem and how this impacts on populations. They provide an evidence base that underpins the policies governments develop to address a range of issues, provide solutions, and monitor progress.

It's equally important that data are unbiased, so that we can be sure they are representative of a population. A data gap occurs when part of a population is not included in data collection, giving only part of the picture, rather than the whole. This is particularly true with the gender data gap, which was already recognized almost a half century ago in 1975 at the World Conference of the International Women's Year, when it was acknowledged that there was incomplete data on gender and a lack of solid indicators to measure the situation of women. This helped spur on the launch the first UN Decade for Women (United Nations, 1976).

In 2014, Data2x, a technical and advocacy platform whose goal is to improve gender data collection and use it to guide policy, put out a report mapping gender data gaps in developing countries across five domains of women's empowerment, one of which was health. Although it was found that, in general, health data had good clarity, comparability, and country-coverage, when looking at women's excess disease burdens, such as dementia, there was a noticeable data gap in terms of coverage and complexity (Buvinic, Furst-Nichols, & Koolwal, 2014a). Data2x updated their report in 2020, this time focusing on the Sustainable Development Goals (SDG). Once again, data on aging populations was found to be a pressing gender gap, with women above 49 years old not adequately covered in the SDG monitoring framework. This is of particular concern because of their vulnerability to conditions that occur most often in old age, such as dementia (Data2x, 2020a).

This information gap has a significant knock-on effect. If we are not collecting data on women over 49, i.e., women beyond child-bearing age, then we don't know the condition of their health or disease burden—particularly with regard to dementia—and won't recognize the need to develop policies and devote resources to support them and monitor their health and wellbeing. If older women are not counted, they become invisible.

Research—Patchy progress

Clinical research is central to understanding how the human body works so that we can use this knowledge to improve health outcomes. However, historically, medical interventions and research tend to have been tested and modeled based on their effects on men. This stems from the idea of "bikini medicine," which posits that the only thing that sets women apart from men are their reproductive organs, i.e., what fits below the triangular bikini (Mosconi, 2020c).

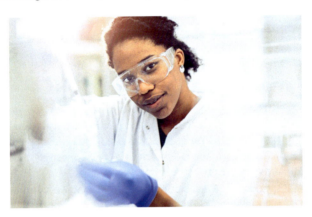

Still, we know men and women are not biologically identical. Their bodies differ in many ways, such as different hormones and genetic factors, that impact on how they respond to medical interventions, such as how they metabolize drugs. One dangerous example is the sleep drug known as Ambien. As late as 2012, women and men had the same recommended dosage, until women began reporting episodes of sleepwalking and even sleep-driving, some resulting in car accidents. A reexamination by the Federal Drug Administration (FDA) ended up cutting the dosage for women by half—meaning that for the previous 20 years, women had been dangerously overmedicated. To make matters worse, it has recently been found that high cumulative dosages of Ambien increase risk of dementia (Mosconi, 2020d).

Unfortunately, in the field of dementia research there has been an equal tendency to ignore sex differences for many years, with women playing a marginal role in clinical studies. More profoundly, women of color were mostly ignored (American Association of Retired Persons, 2020). The result is a data gap that leaves women at a disadvantage and researchers playing catch-up in trying to understand how women respond differently to drugs or treatment options. The situation is even worse for women living with dementia in LMICs, where there has been a historical lack of research and clinical trials. A quick search shows that, at writing, there are currently 851 global clinical trials that are active or recruiting new participants, including females. Only 9% of these are taking place in LMICs (https://clinicaltrials.gov/ct2/results/map?recrs=ad&cond=Dementia&gndr=Female&map=, n.d.).

However, there has been a shift. Tangible progress began in the United States in the 1990s, when the National Institute of Health (NIH) established the Office of Research on Women's Health (ORWH) and the Revitalization Act was passed, requiring women and minorities to be included in any clinical research funded by the NIH (Mager & Liu, 2016). As recently as 2016, the 21st Century Cures Act was passed, endorsing the inclusion of women in clinical research considering sex as a biological variable in research using humans and nonhuman vertebrate animals (National Institute of Health, 2019a). The NIH has also laid out clear objectives in their most recent 5-year strategic plan for women's health research that include the promise of rigorous research, data methods that consider sex and gender influences, increased training, and evaluation (National Institute of Health, 2019b).

Although policy frameworks and legislature endorse inclusion, there is still a lot of catching up to do. More needs to be done to encourage and facilitate inclusion of women of color and ethnic minorities in clinical trials and to ensure global participation, especially in LMICs. We still do not have all the answers about how and why dementia affects men and women differently, but the only way we will learn anything new is by ensuring the inclusion of women in trials and the disaggregation of data to uncover new answers.

Policy and gender—Giving women a voice

On the whole, women are generally forgotten or excluded from decision-making and policy formulation (Bamford, 2011a). Although progress has been made in countries such as Latvia, Spain, and Thailand, globally there still exist significant gaps in opportunities for women to reach parity with men within the political arena that would enable them to influence or make policy (World Economic Forum, 2020).

Over the past 14 years, the World Economic Forum (WEF) has published the Global Gender Gap Report that tracks the progress on relative gaps between women and men in health, education, economy, and politics. In the 2020 report, the WEF tracked progress across 153 countries. In the domain of political empowerment, women were found to be severely under-represented. Women hold only 25% of the 35,127 parliamentary seats across all 153 countries and only 21% of the ministers are women. In some of the countries, there are no women representatives (World Economic Forum, 2020).

Even when women do decide to run for political office, they are often faced with extreme online abuse. Female politicians in Asia and Latin America have indicated that violence against them has made them less likely to seek reelection and more likely to leave office. Equally, more than 75% of British women on a female leadership program noted that online sexist abuse was a key point of consideration when deciding whether or not to pursue political office (Criado Perez, 2019g). Indeed, in their 2020 report on gender data gaps, Data2x added a new data measure focusing on violence against women politicians, as it has become widely acknowledged as both a serious problem and a barrier to women's participation in politics (Data2x, 2020b).

In the global health sector, male authority, particularly from high-income countries, is deeply entrenched in leadership and decision-making roles. In the most recent Global Health 50/50 report, which reviewed 200 global organizations active in health and health policy, it was found that "more than 70% of leaders… are men, more than 80% are nationals of high-income countries and more than 90% were educated in high income countries" (Global Health 50/50, 2020a). This power imbalance aligns with World Health Organization (WHO) data from 2019, which found that women make up 70% of the global health workforce, but hold only 25% of the leadership positions (World Health Organization, 2019a). At executive and board level, where key decisions are made in terms of strategy, women make up only 30% of CEOs and 32% of board chairs. Of these leaders, only 5% come from LMICs (Global Health 50/50, 2020b). And finally, in terms of national governments, only 31% of Ministries of Health are headed up by women (World Health Organization, 2019b). These numbers are stark reminders that despite the fact that women make up the vast majority of the health workforce, they have very little decision making power within the sector itself or in the health organizations that support the sector or develop key policies around it. This creates an environment in which women have less influence than men, where they are disempowered and unable to reach their full potential as leaders.

It's clear that the issue of sex, gender, and dementia is complex. We have seen that dementia disproportionately impacts women, with more women experiencing it or providing care for those who do. We have learned that older women with dementia suffer triple jeopardy due to their age, sex, and health condition and that in some countries, many young girls miss out on opportunities for early education, which has been proven to reduce risk and increase brain resilience. All of this happening in a society where male bias is the default, gender data gaps make women invisible, and women's integration into dementia research has been variable. To top it all off, women hold fewer leadership positions, particularly in health, positions that would enable them to influence policies and enable change.

Unfortunately, there is no silver bullet solution to this very complicated issue. What is required is a multifaceted approach that cuts across sectors and geographical boundaries, one that threads gender through policies and strategies in a proactive and transformative way, ensuring tangible actions and long-term change. This demands a pincer-like movement—one that simultaneously converges from the top, through policy transformation, and the bottom, through grassroots advocacy and action. Let us be clear: this isn't about words, it's about commitment that is transformed into action. This next section will explore some of the ways to readjust the gender imbalance through policy, leadership, and action.

Addressing the imbalance: How do we change and move forward?

Policy transformation does not mean one has to go back to the drawing board and start over. Yet this does not make the challenge any easier. Weaving redefined priorities around gender into existing policies will require political will and commitment to dedicate resources, build capacity, and monitor progress. It will also require broad-based collaboration across governments, civil society, and service providers.

In keeping with our analogy of taking a "pincer-like" approach to change, it's important to start at the top to understand the context provided by existing international frameworks around health policy and explore how they lay the groundwork for focusing on the global health agenda on dementia.

International frameworks

As far back as 1995, when the Beijing Declaration and the Platform for Action declared that "women's rights are human rights" (United Nations, 1996), hopes were held high for a seismic shift in the way policies would be developed in future. The Declaration laid out a new framework for global policy focusing on the rights of women; introducing the concept of "gender mainstreaming" that encouraged governments to include a gender perspective into all policies and programs (United Nations, n.d.-a).

Over the subsequent 25 years, the concept of gender equality has become widely accepted—expected even. The United Nations Educational, Scientific, and Cultural Organization (UNESCO) describes gender mainstreaming as "process rather than a goal" (United Nations Educational, Scientific and Cultural Organization, 2003), implying that it is an ongoing and organic progression that improves with learning. There are some who argue that although the idea of gender mainstreaming is ubiquitous, the term has become technocratic and "lost its bite"—that there still exists a gap between policy rhetoric and real change in the day-to-day lives of women (Pinto, 2019).

In terms of international health policy frameworks, language has changed significantly, with policies espousing "gender-sensitive" or "gender-specific" frameworks or approaches. While this is valuable, it is important to note that older women, and particularly women living with dementia, are still on the periphery.

Sustainable development goals

Adopted by all UN member states in 2015, the Sustainable Development Goals (SDGs) are an ambitious framework of 17 goals to end poverty, improve health and education, reduce inequality, and spur economic growth, with a promise to "leave no one behind." Although the SDGs are not legally binding, all member states are expected to develop national frameworks to meet the goals.

Issues of gender are threaded through each of the 17 SDGs; however, SDG 5 focuses specifically on gender equality. It is broken down into further targets aiming to end discrimination, eliminate violence and harmful practices against women and girls, recognize the value of unpaid care, protect reproductive rights, undertake reforms to give women equal rights to economic resources, empower women via technology, and adopt and strengthen policies to promote gender equality (United Nations, n.d.-b). SDG 3 focuses on health and there is reference to reducing premature mortality from noncommunicable diseases (NCDs) and to promoting mental health and wellbeing. However, dementia is not included as one of the five NCDs listed as indicators, nor under mental health, whose indicator focuses on suicide prevention. Recently, in 2018, mental health and neurological disorders were added to the NCD 5×5 agenda—however, this has still not been made explicit within SDG 3.

Thus, although the SDG gender targets implicitly include older women, their specific complex challenges detailed earlier in this chapter are not included and, under health, dementia is not specifically mentioned either. The worry is that older women, or indeed, women living with dementia, may get lost in the bigger picture or fall through the cracks.

Nevertheless, United Nations (UN) Women is on the case. Their 2018 report, "Turning Promises into Action: Gender Equality in the 2030 Agenda for Sustainable Development," monitors progress toward gender specific targets within the 17 SDGs. The report recognizes the vulnerability of older women, especially those with dementia, who may be subject to discrimination and violence. It especially focuses on the role of women as unpaid carers, particularly those caring for people with dementia, and the need to scale up long-term care support for aging populations. The report calls for improved gender data and analysis, prioritizing gender-responsive resources and policies, and strengthening accountability through gender-responsive processes and institutions (U.N. Women, 2018). This close monitoring is key, as we know that what gets measured gets noticed. Furthermore, what is noticed is more likely to be actioned.

The Convention on the Elimination of All Forms of Discrimination against Women (CEDAW)

The Convention on the Elimination of All Forms of Discrimination against Women (CEDAW) defines discrimination against women and girls and mandates that signatories incorporate gender equality into their domestic legislation. To date, 189 countries have ratified or acceded to the convention and are legally bound to put its provisions into practice and to regularly report on their progress. Over the years, in countries that have ratified the treaty, it has helped to promote gender equality and oppose discrimination in areas such as violence, lack of legal protection, and access to credit, to name a few (UN Human Rights Office of the High Commissioner, n.d.-a).

Adherence to CEDAW is overseen by the Committee on the Elimination of Discrimination against Women (Committee), a group of 23 experts on women's rights from across the globe who meet on a yearly basis to review progress of each member state, to receive communications from groups or individuals reporting violations of the treaty, and to initiate inquiries into serious or systemic violations of women's rights (UN Human Rights Office of the High Commissioner, n.d.-b). The committee also releases general recommendations on the treaty and, although these are not legally binding, they are highly authoritative interpretations of the convention (Corfield, 2017a).

In 1999, the committee published "General recommendation No. 24: Article 12 of the Convention (women and health)" and for the first time, zeroed in on the specific needs of older women, specifically regarding dementia and also in their role as carers. Paragraph 24 reads, "The Committee is concerned about the conditions of health-care services for older women, not only because women often live longer than men and are more likely than men to suffer from disabling and degenerative chronic diseases, such as osteoporosis and dementia, but because they often have the responsibility for their aging spouses. Therefore, States parties should take appropriate measures to ensure the access of older women to health services that address the handicaps and disabilities associated with aging" (United Nations, 1999).

The important point about CEDAW and the committee that oversees it, is that the relationship with the states that have signed the treaty is a two way street. The committee can hold states accountable for any violations, but equally, individuals, or the organizations that represent them (such as nongovernmental organizations (NGOs)), can bring issues or questions to the committee and the committee is required to take action and follow-up. This can be an important advocacy tool for members of the community and NGOs to have the right to request, through the committee, that CEDAW consider recommending that national governments report back and prove change or progress on specific issues, such as requesting that member states include statistical data on the impact of dementia and develop policies that address gender concerns (Bamford, 2011e).

Global Equity Hub

The WHO established the Global Equity Hub (GEH) in 2017. A key focus of the GEH is to achieve the deliverables of the Working for Health five-year action plan and to "accelerate large-scale gender-transformative progress to address gender inequities and biases in the health and social care workforce in order to achieve the SDGs" (World Health Organization, 2019c). The GEH is co-chaired by WHO and Women in Global Health and members include a range of key stakeholders from the global health sector, including intergovernmental and multilateral agencies, civil society, researchers, foundations, and the private sector.

The GEH's work focuses on four priority areas: examining occupational segregation, decent work (ensuring workplaces are free from discrimination and harassment), the gender pay gap, and leadership and governance. They do this by mapping out evidence on good practice, evaluating key data, developing policy briefs and tools, disseminating evidence and guidance through advocacy and social/political dialogue, and facilitating policy implementation through workshops and engagement with key stakeholders (World Health Organization, 2019d).

A key output of the GEH has been the 2019 report, "Delivered by Women, Led by Men: A Gender and Equity Analysis of the Global Health and Social Workforce," which explores gender biases, discrimination, and systemic inequities in the global health workforce. The report provides important evidence and makes recommendations for gender-transformative policy action that will be driven by the Working For Health program, the WHO, the Organization for Economic Cooperation and Development (OECD), and the International Labour Organization (ILO), with support from the GEH.

Although not dementia-focused, the GEH does promote gender-transformative policies that foster female leadership, reduce professional inequalities and pay gaps, and encourage better working conditions for women in the health sector.

G20 Okayama declaration of health ministers 2019

In October 2019, ministers of health from all G20 member countries gathered with representatives of international health organizations to discuss key global issues pertaining to the global health economy. Upon completion of their summit, the health ministers issued a joint declaration, which, although it is not legally binding, is seen as a political statement with a punch.

The 2019 G20 Okayama Declaration of Health Ministers addressed the issues of universal health coverage (UHC), the response to population aging, and the management of health risk and health security. The declaration also recognized the needs of older people with disabilities and their right to healthy aging, in line with the UN Convention on the Rights of Persons with Disabilities. The ministers of health also recognized the important role women play in the health sector workforces, stating they "reaffirm the need to empower women for leadership and management roles in the health workforce" (Okayama Declaration of the G20 Health Ministers, 2019).

For the first time, the G20 declaration focused-in on dementia, adding six dementia-specific articles that highlighted the importance and impact of dementia on the global health economy. For example, paragraph 28 recognizes the global scale of the problem as well as the cost, being equivalent to 1.1% of global gross domestic product (GDP). Paragraph 29 recognizes the endorsement of the Global Action Plan on the Public Health Response to Dementia 2017–2025 (see following section) and goes on to declare, "we commit to developing and implementing multi-sectoral national action plans, adopting integrated approaches on dementia in line with the Global Action Plan to improve the quality of care and the quality of life of people with dementia, their families and caregivers" (Okayama Declaration of the G20 Health Ministers, 2019).

This was an important moment for dementia advocates worldwide. It was a clear recognition of the global cost of the condition, both in economic terms and also for people living with the dementia. Although, once again there was no mention of gender, it was also a rallying call to all governments, committing ministries of health to respond to the Global Action Plan and develop national policies.

Global action plan on the public response to dementia 2017–2025

In May 2017, the 194 member states of the WHO unanimously adopted the Global Action Plan on the Public Health Response to Dementia 2017–2025 (global action plan). The vision of the global action plan is dementia prevention and ensuring people with dementia and their carers live well and receive the care and support they need to fulfill their potential with dignity, respect, autonomy, and equality (World Health Organization, 2017a).

The plan lays out seven action areas that provide a framework for each member state to develop a comprehensive response to dementia in their country. In addition, the plan is grounded in seven crosscutting principles, one of which is equity, declaring that member states should make, "all efforts to implement public health responses to dementia must support gender equity and take a gender-sensitive perspective" (World Health Organization, 2017a). Indeed, the global action plan makes several references to ensuring "gender sensitive approaches, responses, or interventions" throughout the document, particularly in five of the seven action areas looking at dementia awareness, risk reduction, diagnosis and treatment, support for carers, and research (World Health Organization, 2017b).

Yet, is gender sensitivity enough? The WHO have developed a gender responsive assessment scale that lists criteria for assessing the gender responsiveness of a policy, starting at gender-unequal and progressing toward gender-transformative policies that are proactively gender-inclusive and promote equality (Fig. 1).

The Global Action Plan includes gender as an important crosscutting issue and also includes references to gender-sensitive approaches and interventions in several action plans, however it lacks specific recommendations, statements, or actions to actively promote gender. The Global Action Plan is supplemented with a step-by-step guide, "Towards a dementia plan: a WHO guide," to help member states develop their own national dementia plan. The WHO guide does include more gender-specific actions for developing a national plan; with recommendations to research gender inequities in policies, to include gender experts in stakeholder consultations, and to ensure policy activities are gender equitable (World Health Organization, 2018b). When compared to the gender responsiveness assessment scale, the Global Action Plan with the accompanying WHO guide combined could be considered to be gender-specific.

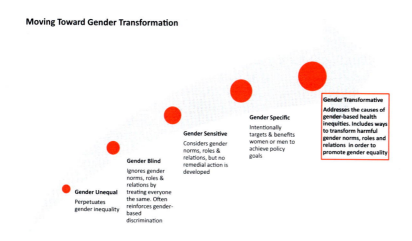

FIG. 1

Gender transformation women and dementia policy.

However, considering that a growing body of evidence has established the disproportionate impact of dementia on women, wouldn't it be innovative to have a global action plan that tunes-in to the needs of the majority of individuals affected by the condition and try to be gender-*transformative*? The following section considers adaptations that could be made to the existing global dementia plan to shift it along the assessment scale toward a more gender-transformative focus.

Toward a gender-transformative global action plan

Imagine that we could encourage a "re-look" at the global action plan, through a gender-transformative lens. Without taking anything away from the existing recommendations or support proposed for vulnerable groups therein—just refocusing to ensure a more proactively gender-equitable and progressive guide to inform policy development. The following is just a start in reimagining the slight changes that could be made to the seven action areas of the global action plan to make it more gender-transformative (see Table 1).

Dementia as a public health priority. In recognizing that dementia is a growing health crisis affecting entire communities, especially in LMICs, it is equally important to consider the disproportionate impact of dementia on women living in these communities. National dementia plans require a coordinated response across multiple government ministries, as the impact of the condition is felt across all sectors. A gender-transformative response should include an examination of gender-based inequities across all sectors of the public economy, above and beyond the health economy. This would require a coordinated response to dementia aligning with the strategic goals of the SDGs. An effective method would be to conduct an in-depth situational analysis to help policy makers understand and recognize gender-specific service gaps, strengths, weaknesses, and opportunities in order to develop priorities that incorporate progressive strategies and solution-focused and measurable actions. An essential component would be to include female leaders across the spectrum of policy, health, long-term care, and the wider economy as stakeholders in policy development. Coupled with this should be the strong advocacy efforts of civil society and NGOs, to amplify the need for change and to put pressure on governments, holding them to account for adding a gender-specific agenda to national dementia plans. Most important would be to include the voices of women living with dementia and those who are providing unpaid family care.

Dementia awareness and friendliness. Effective dementia awareness campaigns take a human rights approach; raising awareness and busting myths and misconceptions about the impact of dementia. This is a perfect environment for fostering a gender-transformative approach, ensuring that awareness campaigns and anti-stigma information include a sex and gender perspective and positive messaging. Educative approaches that reduce the "triple jeopardy" of stigma against women are paramount, using appropriate language and focusing on the voices and experience of women as well

Table 1 National Dementia Plans through a gender transformative lens.

Dementia as a public health priority
- National dementia policies should be interwoven with strategies that acknowledge sex and gender differences in dementia and proactively address gender-specific issues in each action area, with tangible and measurable actions
- Include female leaders in policy development
- Include the voice of women with dementia and increase advocacy

Dementia awareness and friendliness
- Include a sex and gender perspective in dementia awareness and inclusivity campaigns
- Promote educative campaigns to reduce "triple jeopardy" of stigma experienced by women—age, sex, dementia
- Use appropriate language and include female voices

Dementia risk reduction
- Promote early and continuous education for girls
- Encourage female participation in research to understand impacts of sex-based differences in risk, such as hormones or informal caring roles
- Foster women's brain health

Dementia diagnosis, treatment, care and support
- Encourage timely diagnosis—women often seek a diagnosis at later stages than men
- Support must take into account women who live alone with dementia

Support for dementia carers
- Work across sectors to legislate for and facilitate employment/labour rights and support for female carers
- Remove discrimination and ensure fair access to social insurance/protection schemes for women who have provided unpaid care
- Improve dementia training and close the gender pay-gap for professional care workforce

Information system for dementia
- Collect disaggregated data by sex, age, and race/ethnicity in all research; including diagnosis, care, incidence/prevalence, mortality etc.
- Data should have three hallmarks: *quality* (reliable), *coverage* (cross country) and *comparable* (meets international standards)
- Gender data should include cross-cutting issues to provide a holistic picture and enable rounded analysis

Dementia research and innovation
- Facilitate inclusion of women in clinical trials to better understand sex difference, effects, and sex-genotype interactions more frequent in women
- Encourage and promote research focusing on sex-based differences in dementia—focusing on the role of hormones, menopause, and stress

as men. Campaigns can inform, but also model how to best integrate a dementia-inclusive approach in all areas of society, from health to design to public transport, to name a few.

 Dementia risk reduction. Evidence shows that access to early education is an important factor in building brain plasticity and resilience. As a crosscutting feature of the dementia plan, coordinated efforts must be made to ensure young girls have access to early and continuous education. We know that men and women are not biologically identical and may therefore have different risk factors. Risk reduction research needs to encourage female participation in research in order to better understand sex-based differences in risk. Equally, dementia plans should encourage further research into the mental health issues such as stress, anxiety, and depression experienced by women who are unpaid carers, to better understand the risk this poses to their brain health.

 Dementia diagnosis, treatment, care, and support. A timely diagnosis is important as it can open the door to post diagnostic support, but research suggests that early signs of dementia are often overlooked in women. A good place to start would be better training of primary care doctors, as a recent OECD report revealed that physicians average just 12 hours of dementia training during medical school (Organization for Economic Co-operation and Development, 2018); barely enough, particularly if training needs to include how sex and gender may impact the diagnostic process. Diagnosis needs to be followed by joined-up and coordinated post diagnostic support that is not only person-centered, but also gender-specific. Healthcare professionals also need to be trained, supported, and properly resourced to provide gender-transformative interventions that are person-centered and holistic and to empower women with dementia to make informed decisions about their care, especially if they live alone. Dementia is a life-limiting condition and access to good palliative and end of life care that uses a comprehensive, interdisciplinary, and gender-specific approach is essential to ensure dignity and to meet the needs and wishes of the individual as well as to support caregivers (van der Steen et al., 2014).

 Support for dementia carers. Recognizing the key role that women play in providing unpaid care is essential. Access to psychosocial support for carers is necessary, particularly for women who have to juggle complex care responsibilities for both their own families and their elderly parents. Equally, gender-specific support should be provided to men, to encourage and enable them to engage in care, in much the same way that paternity leave has been encouraged in many countries. Coordination across sectors needs to ensure women—and men—working full-time have employment/labor rights to protect their jobs if they need to take temporary leave due to their caring role. Equally important would be to ensure that social protection programs acknowledge the role of women as care providers and that they are given fair access to these schemes. Professional carers of people living with dementia, the majority of whom are women, should have access to appropriate training in dementia care and a key priority should be to close the gender pay gap.

Information systems for dementia. In order to support countries in measuring progress on dementia actions outlined in the global action plan, the WHO developed the Global Dementia Observatory, however, this is not routinely disaggregated. At the very least, data collected should be robust enough to be disaggregated by sex, age, and race/ethnicity in all research; including diagnosis, care, incidence/prevalence, mortality, etc. Data should have three hallmarks: quality (reliable), coverage (cross country), and comparability (meets international standards). Gender data should include crosscutting issues to provide a holistic picture to fully understand the determinants of women's health conditions, such as dementia, and enable rounded analysis (Buvinic, Furst-Nichols, & Koolwal, 2014b).

 Dementia research and innovation. Investment in dementia research is key, particularly in the effort to find a disease-modifying treatment. Taking advantage of recent advancements and inclusion of sex variables in clinical studies, governments need to promote the exploration of sex and gender differences at all levels of research, from basic science to biomedical dementia research and psychosocial and behavioral research. Equally important, governments need to commit resources to research and empower more female scientists to take a lead in dementia research.

In addition to reimagining the global action plan on dementia to make it more gender-transformative, another change to rebalance equality would be to encourage more female leadership in the field of dementia.

Encouraging and empowering female leadership

In her 2018 TED talk on gender balancing in the 21st century, Avivah Wittenberg-Cox, CEO of gender consultancy 20-first, discusses how moving from male dominance to gender balance takes effort; in particular, it takes "will and skill… government policy drives culture and countries can't balance without strong leadership, laws and policies… smart countries redesign policies to create balance" (TED Talks, n.d.).

Women leaders at national and local levels often drive change in health economies. Increasingly, evidence is showing that female parliamentarians are particularly adept at coalition-building and agenda-setting, and are often able to shift legislative focus to prioritize health (Foundation for Innovative New Diagnostics, Women in Global Health, 2020).

In her forward to the WHO report, "Delivered by women, led by men: A gender and equity analysis of the global health and social workforce." Dr. Roopa Dhatt, co-chair of the Gender Equity Hub, discusses a "triple gender dividend" payback that can occur when investing the global health and social workforce with an aim to reduce gender inequities. Global demographics are changing and with that comes increased demand for healthcare. By 2030, we will need approximately 40 million new health and social care jobs, almost half of those in LMICs, in order achieve universal healthcare and the SDGs. Investing in gender-transformative change across the health sector not only benefits women, but creates opportunities for men in areas of the health workforce where they have been traditionally under-represented, such as nursing. The payback can take the form of:

- **Health dividends**: Investing resources into equitable training will enable the development of a skilled workforce, of both men and women, who can competently provide healthcare across the demands of UHC and SDGs by 2030.
- **Gender equality dividends**: Investment in women and in the education of girls for employment will increase equality as women gain income, education, and autonomy (which will have a positive knock-on effect on families and other aspects of development).
- **Development dividends**: Investing in an equitable health workforce can add value and increase productivity through diversification. More new jobs will be created, fueling economic growth (World Health Organization, 2019e).

The bottom line being that investing in gender equality helps improve health and health economies, and the lives of all people and society in general.

The same report goes on to discuss the crucial role that women leaders have in encouraging a positive culture that trickles down into better quality of care. "Addressing gender gaps in leadership leads to a more empowered workforce, improved motivation, reduced attrition, improved quality of care, and better understanding of health systems, which feeds into designing more suitable solutions" (World Health Organization, 2019f). Studies have proved that more women demonstrate transformational leadership qualities, mentoring their subordinates and empowering them to reach their full potential (Eagly & Carli, 2007). Female leadership has the power to expand health agendas, have positive knock-on effects on economies and development, and to transform workforce teams (Box 2).

An absolute precursor to having women in leadership will be assuring young girls have access to early and continued education. Not only has research shown that education has a preventive effect in building brain resilience and reducing risk of developing dementia in later life, it also provides girls and young women with the tools they need to become the leaders of the future.

So, it is clear from the top down, there are a number of international frameworks that include gender-sensitive language and, in some cases, prioritize gender-specific programs. Specifically around dementia, although the Global Action Plan does address gender issues, there are opportunities to go further. By reimagining the Global Action Plan through a gender-transformative lens, there is an opportunity to model best practice for national governments who look to this document for guidance; making the plan a truly gender-transformative document and encouraging the development of equally transformative national plans in member states. We also see that female leadership, when enabled to thrive, can positively alter health economies, benefitting the population as a whole.

Harking back to the pincer analogy, let's explore the sort of transformation that can happen from the "bottom-up."

Box 2 Covid-19 case study.

The year 2020 will be inextricably linked to the Covid-19 pandemic that sent shock waves across the globe; damaging economies, stretching health and long-term care systems to the brink, and leaving behind devastated families.

At the time of writing, the pandemic is still ongoing, with global cases still on the rise. Data and evidence are still emerging, but early evidence shows that elderly people, particularly those living with dementia in long-term care facilities, have been the hardest hit by the pandemic. A recent report indicated that up to 75% of Covid-19 deaths globally in long-term care facilities were individuals with dementia as an underlying health condition (Suárez-González et al., 2020). In Canada alone, 85% of all Covid-19 deaths have been in long-term care, where two thirds of people have dementia (Alzheimer's Disease International, 2020a).

The speed and complex nature of the pandemic has made it difficult to gather data and this is further complicated by inconsistencies across countries in how data are collected. Not surprisingly, disaggregated data—particularly pertaining to women with dementia—is very hard to find. However, in the UK, early evidence showed that, during the pandemic, more female care home residents died of dementia than Covid-19, with 34% of all deaths of female care home residents attributed to dementia compared to 27% attributed to Covid-19 (Alzheimer's Society, 2020).

Emerging data indicates that females are less likely to have and to die from Covid-19, although some evidence indicates that women and older adults may be more susceptible to long Covid (Sudre et al., 2020). On the UN Women's website, as of June 2020, global estimates indicate that marginally more men have had Covid-19, with 54% of men as opposed to 46% women, except for those with 80+ years of age, where women's cases outnumber men's. Of the 53 countries that were able to provide disaggregated data on Covid-19 cases and mortality, only four countries, or 7%, indicated that more females had died of Covid-19 than men (UN Women, 2020a).

Yet, the pandemic has had a significant impact on women. As cited previously in this chapter, women comprise roughly 70% of the healthcare workforce and are therefore at the frontline of many Covid-19 responses, although they still make up only a minority of senior or leadership positions (Care International, 2020). At a global level, women constitute an estimated two-thirds of the health workforce worldwide and make up the majority of nurses and midwives in the 104 countries for which data are available (Boniol et al., 2019). In addition, women are disproportionately affected by pandemic lockdown or confinement measures and resulting school or nursery closures, where the expectation traditionally falls on women to step in and provide at-home care or schooling (Organization for Economic Co-operation and Development, 2020). It is clear that women are contributing significantly to the care response around Covid-19, whether it be within the healthcare sector or through their role as mothers or primary caregivers. And yet, a recent survey by CARE International found that the majority of national-level committees established to respond to Covid-19 do not have equal female–male representation. Interestingly, the same study found that countries with more women in leadership positions are more likely to deliver Covid-19 responses that consider the effects of the crisis on women and girls (Care International, 2020).

As governments begin to cross-compare the impact of their pandemic responses, one theme has emerged. Although the global pandemic experienced in 2020 is far from over, thus far it has become clear that the countries with the most successful Covid-19 responses have one thing in common: they are led by women. Women are heads of state or of government in only 21 countries globally, however, their leadership response to the pandemic has been praised (UN Women, 2020b). Consistently, female leaders have combined quick and decisive action with empathy. Leaders from Germany, Taiwan, New Zealand, Iceland, Finland, Norway, and Demark, to name a few, combined a firm approach, clear communication, and compassion to convince the public to adhere to strict lockdown measures for the public good. In Germany, Angela Merkel based her public communications on science and initiated testing quickly. In Taiwan, Tsai Ing-wen introduced 124 measures to impede the spread of the virus, which has been hailed as "among the world's best"

(Continued)

Box 2 Covid-19 case study—cont'd

pandemic responses. Prime Minister Katrin Jakobsdottir from Iceland introduced free Covid-19 testing, while Norway's Prime Minister, Erna Solberg, used television to speak directly to children and ease their fears (Wittenberg-Cox, 2020). At the time of writing, there are currently only 21 countries around the world that are led by women, that's roughly 10%, and most of these have had relative success in dealing with the pandemic. A recent study reveals this may be due to key characteristics that are common with female leaders: seeing the big picture, being empathetic, and using good communication (Fillion, 2020).

It is clear that the crisis is not over yet and we need to continue to protect and support vulnerable communities as we endure the ongoing pandemic. However, as we move into the future, it would make sense for the other 90% of countries led by men to take a leaf out of the female leadership book: combining strength and empathy for success.

Advocacy from the bottom-up: The role of civil society

When thinking about promoting change from the bottom up, the role of civil society is key. Civil society organizations, such as Alzheimer's associations or NGOs, play an essential role in advocating for people living with dementia and their families and in holding governments to account. Civil society organizations raise awareness of dementia and challenge the stigma faced by people living with dementia, promoting dementia-inclusiveness.

Since 1984, Alzheimer's Disease International (ADI) has been known as the "global voice on dementia," advocating globally for dementia to be a public health priority, challenging stigma, and urging increased research into cure and care for people living with dementia. ADI is a membership organization of 102 Alzheimer's associations worldwide and recently confirmed via correspondence that 59% of these are led by women. The organization has published important data on incidence, prevalence, cost of care, and, in 2015, women and dementia. ADI's advocacy was instrumental in ensuring the adoption of the Global Action Plan, and their role continues in advocating for the development of national dementia plans on a global basis. As of writing, there are only 33 national dementia plans globally (Alzheimer's Disease International, 2020b). In 2017, it was estimated that only 12 of the 29 national dementia plans had gender-sensitive responses (Corfield, 2017b). It is worth noting that many of 33 national dementia plans or strategies were developed before the WHO Global Action Plan was launched. It would be transformative to see gender become a more identifiable part of national plans through their updating, revision, and fine-tuning. Moreover, it is encouraging to see newly adopted plans, such as Canada and Spain's national plans, with gender-specific language and goals (Ministerio de Sanidad, Consumo y Bienestar, 2019; Public Health Agency of Canada, 2019).

ADI's 2015 Women and Dementia report was a systematic review of existing research and focused on the disproportionate impact of dementia on women, in terms of prevalence, but also in terms of their role as family care givers and the impact of this on their own health. It explored how women manage their condition and access support and also the role of women in professional care. The report identified key data gaps, particularly in LMICs. Most importantly, the report was an essential baseline for Alzheimer's associations globally, and for NGOs and other dementia advocates, to use as evidence in their national advocacy, but also as a benchmark from which to measure change (Erol, Brooker, & Peel, 2015e).

Every September, ADI leads and promotes World Alzheimer's Month (WAM) and supports its 100+ members to run campaigns to raise awareness and challenge stigma globally. In 2020, the WAM campaign theme was "Let's talk about dementia," encouraging Alzheimer's associations globally to start a conversation with people they support—or with governments—about why dementia needs to be a priority. Campaigns such as these are an excellent opportunity to encourage the voices of women living with dementia and others to be part of the conversation, to challenge governments to invest in programs that support female carers, to question the gender gap in research and data, and to make a call to action for a national dementia plan that is gender transformative. ADI provides campaign tools and master classes for members to equip them with the means to tackle complex issues in order to run successful campaigns (Alzheimer's Disease International, 2020c). The result is a powerful groundswell—a chorus of people living with dementia and their families/supporters demanding change that is hard to ignore.

Gender-based data

This chapter has revealed serious gender-based data gaps throughout all levels of society. However, there are methods to use and steps to take to slowly address this gap and begin to reveal a fuller, more cohesive picture. In order to do this, we need a full range of data that creates a more robust picture, such as gender statistics. The UN Statistics Division defines gender statistics as the sum of data that:

- are collected and presented by sex as a primary and overall classification;
- reflect gender issues;
- are based on concepts and definitions that adequately reflect the diversity of women and men and capture all aspects of their lives;
- collection methods take into account stereotypes and social and cultural factors that may induce gender bias in the data (United Nations, 2015).

In other words, we need to do more than to just disaggregate data. We need gender data to meet certain criteria. They need to have wide coverage and a level of granularity to enable further disaggregation and analysis. Data need to be rich enough to cut across domains, allowing for observation of patterns, and other factors. Furthermore, they need to be comparable and meet international standards (Buvinic, Furst-Nichols, & Koolwal, 2014c).

We need to make sure that the gender statistics we gather are representative of the complex lived reality of women, particularly those who are living with or caring for someone with dementia. Good gender-based data will not change everything, but they are the solid bedrock that underpins the whole transformation process.

Conclusion

The scales may be unbalanced, but there are steps that can be taken toward achieving equilibrium. It will require a coordinated response across sectors as well as a simultaneous top-down and bottom-up approach. Truly transformative change is multifaceted and interrelated. It is a process that is progressive and cyclical, with one change feeding into and reinforcing the next (see Fig. 2). The field of dementia care has an opportunity to lead such change and to demonstrate how gender inclusiveness can reshape our understanding of dementia and potential treatments as well as how we can develop policies to ensure joined up care and support for people living with dementia and their carers. Key recommendations are to:

- **Close the gender data gap.** We must commit to collecting gender-based data as the foundation for evidence based interventions and decision-making from basic science to care to policy development. We need to do more than just disaggregate data, we need to start using gender statistics with data that meet robust criteria. They need to have wide coverage and a level of granularity to enable further disaggregation and analysis. Data need to be rich enough to cut across domains, allowing for observation of patterns. They need to be comparable and meet international standards. Gender statistics need to be representative of the complex lived reality of women, particularly those who are living with or caring for someone with dementia.
- **Increase gender-based research and clinical trials.** We also need to build upon the advancements made recently to include sex as a biological variable in

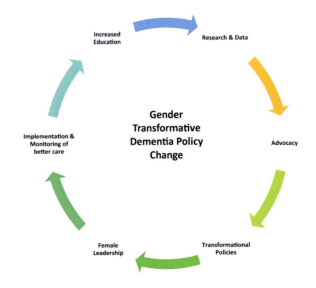

FIG. 2

Gender transformative change women and dementia.

clinical trials and research. More needs to be done to encourage and facilitate inclusion of women of color and ethnic minorities in clinical trials and to ensure global participation, especially in LMICs. Equally, we need to promote training and career development to foster a diverse and equitable scientific workforce and encourage the development of precision medicine.

- **Expand Advocacy.** We need to increase advocacy efforts, particularly through civil society, by targeting UN and other multilateral agencies that exist to protect women's rights and ask for women and dementia to be included in their strategic planning and implementation. We need to target countries that have women-specific governance bodies to increase their awareness of gender imbalances in dementia and their significance in society. In countries that do not have these bodies, civil society should target influential female figures to increase their own awareness and enlist their support to amplify the message around gender transformation.

- **Encourage development of gender-transformational dementia policies.** We need to address the causes of gender inequalities within the dementia sphere, using the Global Action Plan as a framework to enable change. National governments should be committed to strategic and tangible gender-transformative responses and interventions within each of the seven action areas of the Global Plan. These need to be resourced to ensure implementation and measurable to enable evaluation of impact.

- **Promote inclusion of women leaders.** We have seen that female leaders at national and local levels can help drive change in health economies. Women leaders play a crucial role in encouraging a positive culture that trickles down into a better quality of care, and investing in enabling more women and girls to access education for employment will increase equality as women gain income, education, and autonomy (which will have a positive knock-on effect on families and other aspects of development). We need to close the gender gap in political empowerment and ensure women are enabled to seek political office without risk, that health organizations across the sector strive for gender equitable leadership at executive and board level, and that women's voices, talents, and intelligence are recognized and valued in research, advocacy, and policy development. Equally, we need to ensure we are equitable and gender-balanced in listening to the voice of people living with dementia and their carers. Investing in gender equality helps improve health and health economies, and the lives of all people. When given the opportunity, female leadership has the power to expand health agendas, have positive knock-on effects on economies and development, and to transform workforce teams.

- **Foster education of young girls.** Absolutely key to having women in leadership will be ensuring young girls have access to early and continued education. Not only has research shown that education has a preventive effect in building brain resilience and reducing risk of developing dementia in later life, it also provides girls and young women with the tools they need to become the leaders of the future.

Ruth Bader Ginsburg, Associate Justice of the US Supreme Court said, "real change, enduring change, happens one step at a time." We all have a role to play in redressing the imbalanced impact of dementia on women. Whether we are researchers, scientists, health or social care workers, NGO members, policy makers, or someone living with dementia—male or female—all we need to do is take the first step.

Chapter highlights

- Dementia disproportionally affects women on a global scale; they experience more dementia, provide more care for people with dementia, stigma and risk factors place an additional burden on women, and they are largely absent from decision-making and policy development that may benefit them.
- Inequities exist across sectors and global boundaries, impacted by societal norms, gender-biased data, patchy inclusion in research, and exclusion from key leadership roles.
- Changing existing international policy frameworks to include gender priorities requires a multifaceted approach and broad-based collaboration across governments, civil society, and service providers that cuts across sectors and geographical boundaries, requiring political will and commitment to dedicate resources, build capacity, and monitor progress.
- By reimagining the Global Action Plan on Dementia through a gender-transformative lens, there is an opportunity to model best practice for national governments; making the plan a truly gender-transformative document and encouraging the development of equally transformative national plans in member states.
- Top-down approaches in policy reform, political and leadership empowerment, gender-based research, and education are essential, combined with bottom-up approaches through advocacy in civil society, encouraging the voices of people with dementia—especially women—to raise awareness, share their experience and hold governments to account.
- The field of dementia care has an opportunity to lead transformative policy change and to demonstrate how gender inclusiveness can reshape our understanding of dementia and potential treatments as well as how we can develop policies to ensure joined up care and support for people living with dementia and their carers.

References

Alzheimer's Disease International. (2019). *World Alzheimer report 2019: Attitudes to dementia* (p. 13). London: Alzheimer's Disease International.

Alzheimer's Disease International. (2020a). *News release: COVID-19 deaths disproportionately affecting people with dementia, targeted response urgently needed.* https://www.alz.co.uk/media/010920. accessed 01.09.20.

References

Alzheimer's Disease International. (2020b). *From plan to impact III: maintaining dementia as a priority in unprecedented times*. London: Alzheimer's Disease International.

Alzheimer's Disease International. (2020c). *World Alzheimer's Month*. https://www.worldalzmonth.org/. accessed 25.08.20.

Alzheimer's Impact Movement, Alzheimer's Association. (2020). *Women and dementia fact sheet* (pp. 43–44). https://www.aarp.org/content/dam/aarp/health/brain_health/2020/05/gcbh-womens-report-english.doi.10.26419-2Fpia.00102.001.pdf. accessed 31.08.20.

Alzheimer's Research UK. (2015a). *Women and dementia: A marginalised majority* (p. 8). Cambridge: Alzheimer's Research UK.

Alzheimer's Research UK. (2015b). *Women and dementia: A marginalised majority* (pp. 8–9). Cambridge: Alzheimer's Research UK.

Alzheimer's Research UK. (2015c). *Women and dementia: A marginalised majority* (p. 10). Cambridge: Alzheimer's Research UK.

Alzheimer's Society. (2020). https://www.alzheimers.org.uk/news/2020-07-03/ons-figures-show-50-cent-all-covid-19-deaths-care-homes-also-had-dementia. accessed 15.08.20.

American Association of Retired Persons. (2020). *It's time to act: The challenges of Alzheimer's and dementia for women* (p. 18). https://www.aarp.org/content/dam/aarp/health/brain_health/2020/05/gcbh-womens-report-english.doi.10.26419-2Fpia.00102.001.pdf. accessed 20.08.20.

Bamford, S. M. (2011a). *Women and dementia—Not forgotten* (p. 9). London: The International Longevity Centre, UK.

Bamford, S. M. (2011b). *Women and dementia—Not forgotten* (p. 11). London: The International Longevity Centre, UK.

Bamford, S. M. (2011c). *Women and dementia—Not forgotten* (p. 27). London: The International Longevity Centre, UK.

Bamford, S. M. (2011d). *Women and dementia—Not forgotten* (p. 38). London: The International Longevity Centre, UK.

Bamford, S. M. (2011e). *Women and dementia—Not forgotten* (p. 6). London: The International Longevity Centre, UK.

Boniol, M., McIsaac, M., Xu, L., Wuliji, T., Diallo, K., et al. (2019). *Gender equity in the health workforce: analysis of 104 countries*. World Health Organization. https://apps.who.int/iris/handle/10665/311314. License: CC BY-NC-SA 3.0 IGO. accessed 21.12.20.

Buvinic, M., Furst-Nichols, R., & Koolwal, G. (2014a). *Mapping gender data gaps* (pp. 1–16). https://data2x.org/wp-content/uploads/2019/05/Data2X_MappingGenderDataGaps_FullReport.pdf. accessed 18.08.20.

Buvinic, M., Furst-Nichols, R., & Koolwal, G. (2014b). *Mapping gender data gaps* (pp. 11–12). https://data2x.org/wp-content/uploads/2019/05/Data2X_MappingGenderDataGaps_FullReport.pdf. accessed 18.08.20.

Buvinic, M., Furst-Nichols, R., & Koolwal, G. (2014c). *Mapping gender data gaps* (p. 8). https://data2x.org/wp-content/uploads/2019/05/Data2X_MappingGenderDataGaps_FullReport.pdf. accessed 18.08.20.

Care International. (2020). *WHERE ARE THE WOMEN? The conspicuous absence of women in COVID-19 response teams and plans, and why we need them*. https://www.care-international.org/files/files/CARE_COVID-19-womens-leadership-report_June-2020.pdf. accessed 21.12.20.

Carey, B. (2015). *Dementia develops faster in women than in men, study suggests*. https://www.nytimes.com/2015/07/22/health/women-decline-toward-dementia-faster-than-men-study-suggests.html. accessed 14.08.20.

Carter, C. L., Resnick, E. M., Mallampalli, M., & Kalbarczyk, A. (2012). Sex and gender differences in Alzheimer's disease: Recommendations for future research. *Journal of Women's Health, 21*(10), 1018–1023. https://doi.org/10.1089/jwh.2012.3789. accessed 31.08.20.

Corfield, S. (2017a). *Women and dementia: A global challenge* (pp. 21–22). London: GADAA.

Corfield, S. (2017b). *Women and dementia: A global challenge* (p. 16). London: GADAA.

Criado Perez, C. (2019a). *Invisible women: Exposing data bias in a world designed for men* (p. xiii). London: Chatto & Windus.

Criado Perez, C. (2019b). *Invisible women: Exposing data bias in a world designed for men* (p. xii). London: Chatto & Windus.

Criado Perez, C. (2019c). *Invisible women: Exposing data bias in a world designed for men* (pp. 6–7). London: Chatto & Windus.

Criado Perez, C. (2019d). *Invisible women: Exposing data bias in a world designed for men* (p. 10). London: Chatto & Windus.

Criado Perez, C. (2019e). *Invisible women: Exposing data bias in a world designed for men* (p. 12). London: Chatto & Windus.

Criado Perez, C. (2019f). *Invisible women: Exposing data bias in a world designed for men* (p. 11). London: Chatto & Windus.

Criado Perez, C. (2019g). *Invisible women: Exposing data bias in a world designed for men* (pp. 280–281). London: Chatto & Windus.

Data2x. (2020a). *Mapping gender data gaps: An SDG era update, mapping gender data gaps in health* (pp. 1–8). https://data2x.org/wp-content/uploads/2020/03/MappingGenderDataGaps_Health.pdf. accessed 18.08.20.

Data2x. (2020b). *Mapping gender data gaps: An SDG era update, mapping gender data gaps in public participation* (pp. 1–6). https://data2x.org/wp-content/uploads/2020/03/MappingGenderDataGaps_Public.pdf. accessed 20.08.20.

Eagly, A., & Carli, L. L. (2007). *Women and the labyrinth of leadership*. Harvard Business Review. https://hbr.org/2007/09/women-and-the-labyrinth-of-leadership. accessed 25.08.20.

Erol, R., Brooker, D., & Peel, E. (2015a). *Women and dementia: A global research review* (p. 3). London: Alzheimer's Disease International.

Erol, R., Brooker, D., & Peel, E. (2015b). *Women and dementia: A global research review* (p. 13). London: Alzheimer's Disease International.

Erol, R., Brooker, D., & Peel, E. (2015c). *Women and dementia: A global research review* (p. 9). London: Alzheimer's Disease International.

Erol, R., Brooker, D., & Peel, E. (2015d). *Women and dementia: A global research review* (p. 22). London: Alzheimer's Disease International.

Erol, R., Brooker, D., & Peel, E. (2015e). *Women and dementia: A global research review* (pp. 1–50). London: Alzheimer's Disease International.

European Institute of Women's Health. (2019). *Women and dementia in Europe position paper: Addressing the disproportionate burden of dementia on women*. https://eurohealth.ie/wp-content/uploads/2019/01/Women-and-dementia-in-Europe-report-2017.pdf. accessed 02.08.20.

Ferretti, M., Iulita, M. F., Cavedo, E., et al. (2018). Sex differences in Alzheimer disease—The gateway to precision medicine. *Nature Reviews. Neurology, 14*, 457–469. https://doi.org/10.1038/s41582-018-0032-9. https://www.nature.com/articles/s41582-018-0032-9. accessed 10.12.20.

Fillion, S. (2020 June). *The science behind women leaders in fighting covid-19*. Forbes. https://www.forbes.com/sites/stephaniefillion/2020/08/05/the-science-behind-women-leaders-success-in-fighting-covid-19/#695f5c0c749b. accessed 01.09.20.

Foundation for Innovative New Diagnostics, Women in Global Health. (2020 July). *Testing, women's empowerment and universal health coverage. discussion paper*. https://www.finddx.org/wp-content/uploads/2020/07/Discussion-Paper-FIND-WGH-Final.pdf. accessed 25.08.20.

Global Health 50/50. (2020a). *The global health 50/50 report 2020: Power, privilege and priorities* (p. 10). https://globalhealth5050.org/wp-content/uploads/2020/03/Power-Privilege-and-Priorities-2020-Global-Health-5050-Report.pdf. accessed 31.08.20.

Global Health 50/50. (2020b). *The global health 50/50 report 2020: Power, privilege and priorities* (pp. 25–64). https://globalhealth5050.org/wp-content/uploads/2020/03/Power-Privilege-and-Priorities-2020-Global-Health-5050-Report.pdf. accessed 31.08.20.

Graham, N., Lindesay, J., Katona, C., Bertolote, J. M., Camus, V., Copeland, J. R. M., et al. (2003). Reducing Stigma and discrimination against older people with mental disorders; a technical consensus statement. *International Journal of Geriatric Psychiatry, 18*(8), 670–678.

https://clinicaltrials.gov/ct2/results/map?recrs=ad&cond=Dementia&gndr=Female&map=. accessed 21.08.20.

Livingston, G., et al. (2020). Dementia prevention, intervention, and care: 2020 report of the Lancet Commission. *The Lancet, 396*(10248), 413–446. ISSN:0140-6736.

Luengo-Fernandez, R., Leal, J., & Gray, A. (2015). UK research spend in 2008 and 2012: Comparing stroke, cancer, coronary heart disease and dementia. *BMJ Open, 5*. https://doi.org/10.1136/bmjopen-2014-006648, e006648. last accessed 18/12/20.

Mager, N. A., & Liu, K. A. (2016). Women's involvement in clinical trials: Historical perspective and future implications. *Pharmacy in Practice, 14*(1). https://www.pharmacypractice.org/journal/index.php/pp/article/view/708. accessed 21.08.20.

Ministerio de Sanidad, Consumo y Bienestar. (2019). *Social Plan Integral de Alzheimer y otras Demencias (2019-2023)*. https://www.mscbs.gob.es/profesionales/saludPublica/docs/Plan_Integral_Alhzeimer_Octubre_2019.pdf. accessed 31.08.20.

Mkhonto, F., & Hanssen, I. (2018). When people with dementia are perceived as witches. Consequences for patients and nurse education in South Africa. *Journal of Clinical Nursing, 27*, e169–e176. https://onlinelibrary.wiley.com/doi/full/10.1111/jocn.13909. accessed 18.12.20.

Mosconi, L. (2020a). *The XX Brian: The groundbreaking science empowering women to maximise cognitive health and prevent Alzheimer's disease* (p. 21). New York: Avery, an imprint of Penguin Random House.

Mosconi, L. (2020b). *The XX Brian: The groundbreaking science empowering women to maximise cognitive health and prevent Alzheimer's disease* (p. xv). New York: Avery, an imprint of Penguin Random House.

Mosconi, L. (2020c). *The XX Brian: The groundbreaking science empowering women to maximise cognitive health and prevent Alzheimer's disease* (pp. xvi–xvii). New York: Avery, an imprint of Penguin Random House.

Mosconi, L. (2020d). *The XX Brian: The groundbreaking science empowering women to maximise cognitive health and prevent Alzheimer's disease* (p. xxiii). New York: Avery, an imprint of Penguin Random House.

National Institute of Health. (2019a). *Advancing science for the health of women: The trans-NIH strategic plan for women's health research 2019-2023* (pp. 1–8). Washington, DC: NIH.

National Institute of Health. (2019b). *Advancing science for the health of women: the trans-NIH strategic plan for women's health research 2019-2023* (pp. 1–8). Washington, DC: NIH.

Nichols, E., et al. (2019). Global, regional, and national burden of Alzheimer's disease and other dementias, 1990-2016: A systematic analysis for the Global Burden of Disease Study 2016. *Lancet Neurology, 18*(5), 459–480.

(2019). *Okayama Declaration of the G20 Health Ministers*. https://www.mhlw.go.jp/seisakunitsuite/bunya/hokabunya/kokusai/g20/health/img/G20Okayama_HM_EN.pdf. accessed 24.08.20.

Organization for Economic Co-operation and Development. (2018). *Care needed: Improving the lives of people with dementia*. OECD Health Policy Studies.

Organization for Economic Co-operation and Development. (2020). *Women at the core of the fight against COVID-19 crisis* (p. 3). OECD. https://www.oecd.org/coronavirus/policy-responses/women-at-the-core-of-the-fight-against-covid-19-crisis-553a8269/. accessed 21.12.20.

Patterson, C. (2018). *World Alzheimer report 2018—The state of the art of dementia research: New frontiers* (p. 10). London: Alzheimer's Disease International.

Pinto, G. (2019). *Gender mainstreaming: Moving from rhetoric to reality*. https://www.bond.org.uk/news/2019/03/gender-mainstreaming-moving-from-rhetoric-to-reality. accessed 23/8/20.

Prince, M. J., Comas-Herrera, A., Knapp, M., Guerchet, M. M., & Karagiannidou, M. (2016). *World Alzheimer Report 2016: Improving healthcare for people living with dementia—Coverage, quality and costs now and in the future*. London: Alzheimer's Disease International.

Prince, M., Guerchet, M., Prina, M., & Alzheimer's Disease International. (2013). *Policy brief for heads of government: The global impact of dementia 2013-2050* (pp. 1–7). London: Alzheimer's Disease International.

Public Health Agency of Canada. (2019). *Dementia strategy for Canada: Together we aspire*. https://www.canada.ca/en/public-health/services/publications/diseases-conditions/dementia-strategy.html. accessed 31.8.20.

Snyder, H. M., Asthana, S., Bain, L., Brinton, R., Craft, S., Dubal, D. B., et al. (2016). Sex biology contributions to vulnerability to Alzheimer's disease: A think tank convened by the Women's Alzheimer's Research Initiative. *Alzheimer's & Dementia : The Journal of the Alzheimer's Association, 12*(11), 1186–1196. https://alz-journals.onlinelibrary.wiley.com/doi/abs/10.1016/j.jalz.2016.08.004. accessed 14.08.20.

Suárez-González, A., Livingston, G., Low, L. F., Cahill, S., Hennelly, N., Dawson, W. D., et al. (2020). *Impact and mortality of COVID-19 on people living with dementia: cross-country report*. https://ltccovid.org/wp-content/uploads/2020/08/International-report-on-the-impact-of-COVID-19-on-people-living-with-dementia-19-August-2020.pdf. accessed 31.08.20.

Sudre, C., Murray, B., Varsavsky, T., Graham, M., Penfold, R., et al. (2020). *Attributes and predictors of Long-COVID: Analysis of COVID cases and their symptoms collected by the Covid Symptoms Study App*. https://doi.org/10.1101/2020.10.19.20214494. accessed 21.12.20.

TED Talks. *Avivah Wittenberg-Cox*. https://www.ted.com/talks/avivah_wittenberg_cox_gender_balancing_how_countries_companies_and_couples_are_defying_history?utm_source=tedcomshare&utm_medium=email&utm_campaign=tedspread. accessed 25.08.20.

UN Human Rights Office of the High Commissioner. *CEDAW in your daily life*. https://www.ohchr.org/EN/HRBodies/CEDAW/Pages/DailyLife.aspx. accessed 23.08.20.

UN Human Rights Office of the High Commissioner. *Committee on the elimination of discrimination against women*. https://www.ohchr.org/EN/HRBodies/CEDAW/Pages/Introduction.aspx. accessed 24.08.20.

UN Women. (2020a). *COVID-19: Emerging gender data and why it matters*. https://data.unwomen.org/resources/covid-19-emerging-gender-data-and-why-it-matters. accessed 15.08.20.

UN Women. (2020b). *Policy Brief No. 18 Covid-19 and women's leadership: from an effective response to building back better* (p. 3). https://www.unwomen.org/en/digital-library/publications/2020/06/policy-brief-covid-19-and-womens-leadership. accessed 21.12.20.

United Nations. (1976). *Report of the world conference of the international women's year, Mexico City, 19 June-2 July 1975* (p. 32). New York: United Nations. https://digitallibrary.un.org/record/586225?ln=en. accessed 18.08.20.

United Nations. (1996). *Report of the fourth world conference on women, Beijing 4-15 September 1995* (p. 3). https://www.un.org/womenwatch/daw/beijing/pdf/Beijing%20full%20report%20E.pdf. accessed 31.08.20.

United Nations. (1999). *Report of the committee on the elimination of discrimination against women twentieth session (19 January-5 February 1999), twenty-first session (7-25 June 1999), general assembly, official records, fifty-fourth session, supplement no. 38 (A/54/38/Rev.1)* (p. 6). https://www.un.org/womenwatch/daw/cedaw/reports/21report.pdf. accessed 31.08.20.

United Nations. (2015). *Gender statistics manual: Integrating a gender perspective into statistics. What are gender statistics*. https://unstats.un.org/unsd/genderstatmanual/What-are-gender-stats.ashx. accessed 18.08.20.

United Nations. *Beijing declaration and platform for action*. https://www.un.org/womenwatch/daw/beijing/pdf/BDPfA%20E.pdf. accessed 23.08.20.

United Nations. *Sustainable development goals, goal 5: Gender equality*. https://www.un.org/sustainabledevelopment/gender-equality/. accessed 23.08.20.

United Nations, Department of Economic and Social Affairs, Population Division. (2019). *World population ageing 2019: Highlights. (ST/ESA/SER.A/430)* (pp. 9–11). https://www.un.on/development/desa/population/publications/pdf/ageing/WorldPopulationAgeing2019-Highlights.pdf. accessed 31.08.20.

United Nations Educational, Scientific and Cultural Organization. (2003). *UNESCO's gender mainstreaming implementation framework* (pp. 1–3). http://www.unesco.org/new/fileadmin/MULTIMEDIA/HQ/BSP/GENDER/PDF/1.%20Baseline%20Definitions%20of%20key%20gender-related%20concepts.pdf. accessed 23/08/20.

van der Steen, J. T., Radbruch, L., Hertogh, C. M., de Boer, M. E., Hughes, J. C., et al. (2014). European Association for Palliative Care (EAPC). White paper defining optimal palliative care in older people with dementia: A Delphi study and recommendations from the European Association for Palliative Care. *Palliative Medicine, 28*(3), 197–209. https://doi.org/10.1177/0269216313493685. Epub 2013 Jul 4 23828874. accessed 17,12,20.

Wimo, A., Gauthier, S., Prince, M. J., & Alzheimer's Disease International. (2018). *Global estimates of informal care* (p. 15). London: Alzheimer's Disease International.

Wittenberg-Cox, A. (2020 April). *What do countries with the best coronovirus responses have in common?*. Forbes: Women Leaders. https://www.forbes.com/sites/avivahwittenbergcox/2020/04/13/what-do-countries-with-the-best-coronavirus-reponses-have-in-common-women-leaders/#e76eb993dec4. accessed 01.09.20.

Women, U. N. (2018). *Turning promises into action: Gender equality in the 2030 agenda for sustainable development*. https://www.unwomen.org/-/media/headquarters/attachments/sections/library/publications/2018/sdg-report-gender-equality-in-the-2030-agenda-for-sustainable-development-2018-en.pdf?la=en&vs=4332. accessed 23.08.20.

World Association for Christian Communication. (2015). *The global media monitoring project*. http://cdn.agilitycms.com/who-makes-the-news/Imported/reports_2015/highlights/highlights_en.pdf. accessed 31.08.20.

World Economic Forum. (2020). *The global gender gap report 2020* (p. 5). http://www3.weforum.org/docs/WEF_GGGR_2020.pdf. accessed 20/8/20.

World Health Organization. (2017a). *Global action plan on the public health response to dementia 2017–2025* (p. 4). Geneva: World Health Organization. Licence: CC BY-NC-SA 3.0 IGO.

World Health Organization. (2017b). *Global action plan on the public health response to dementia 2017–2025* (pp. 1–32). Geneva: World Health Organization. Licence: CC BY-NC-SA 3.0 IGO.

World Health Organization. (2018a). *Global health estimates 2016: Deaths by cause, age, sex, by country and by region, 2000-2016*. Geneva: World Health Organization. https://www.who.int/healthinfo/global_burden_disease/estimates/en/. accessed 13.08.20.

World Health Organization. (2018b). *Towards a dementia plan: A WHO guide* (pp. 1–65). Geneva: World Health Organization. Licence: CCBY-NC-SA 3.0 IGO.

World Health Organization. (2019a). *Delivered by women, led by men: A gender and equity analysis of the global health and social workforce* (p. 36). Geneva: World Health Organization. Human Resources for Health Observer Series No. 24; Licence: CC BY-NC-SA 3.0 IGO.

World Health Organization. (2019b). *Delivered by women, led by men: A gender and equity analysis of the global health and social workforce* (p. 37). Geneva: World Health Organization. Human Resources for Health Observer Series No. 24; Licence: CC BY-NC-SA 3.0 IGO.

World Health Organization. (2019c). *Delivered by women, led by men: A gender and equity analysis of the global health and social workforce* (p. 9). Geneva: World Health Organization. Human Resources for Health Observer Series No. 24; Licence: CC BY-NC-SA 3.0 IGO.

World Health Organization. (2019d). *Delivered by women, led by men: A gender and equity analysis of the global health and social workforce* (p. 9). Geneva: World Health Organization. Human Resources for Health Observer Series No. 24; Licence: CC BY-NC-SA 3.0 IGO.

World Health Organization. (2019e). *Delivered by women, led by men: A gender and equity analysis of the global health and social workforce* (p. vi). Geneva: World Health Organization. Human Resources for Health Observer Series No. 24; Licence: CC BY-NC-SA 3.0 IGO.

World Health Organization. (2019f). *Delivered by women, led by men: A gender and equity analysis of the global health and social workforce* (p. 39). Geneva: World Health Organization. Human Resources for Health Observer Series No. 24; Licence: CC BY-NC-SA 3.0 IGO.

Index

Note: Page numbers followed by *f* indicate figures, *t* indicate tables, and *b* indicate boxes.

A

Activated response microglia (ARMs), 93
ADT. *See* Androgen deprivation therapy (ADT)
Adult-born dentate neurons, 27–28
Advance care planning (ACP), as communication tool, 427*b*
Advocacy, 443, 449, 458–459
Aerobic exercise, 278
Affective disorders, 190, 196–197
Age-dependent behavioral sex differences, 6–7
Age-related brain volume loss, 128
Aging, 44–45, 163–164
   estrogens and, 39–41, 43–44
   microglia, 89–91
   neurogenesis, 28–30
   physiological sleep changes during, 209–210
   sleep disorders, 209–210
Albumin, 115
Alcohol consumption, 277
   dementia, 188
   during midlife, 187–188
Alcohol dependency, 187–188
Alzheimer's Association International Conference, 274–275
Alzheimer's Disease Assessment Scale-Cognitive Subscale (ADAS-Cog), 369
Alzheimer's Disease Cooperative Study Activity of Daily Living Scale (ADSC-ADL), 195
Alzheimer's Disease International (ADI), 393–394, 401, 408, 458
aMCI. *See* Amnestic mild cognitive impairment (aMCI)
Amnesia, anterograde, 165
Amnestic mild cognitive impairment (aMCI), 37, 130, 148–149
Amyloid-beta, 110–111, 197–198, 211–212, 313–314
Amyloid-beta plaques, 80–82, 108, 113
Amyloid pathogenesis, TREM2 role in, 82
Amyloid positron emission tomography, 148–149
   in dementia, 148–149
   in healthy subjects, 148
Amyloid precursor protein (APP), 35, 80
Androgen, 86–87, 234, 236
Androgen deficiency of aging male (ADAM), 246
Androgen deprivation therapy (ADT), 235, 247–248
Androgen receptor (AR), 32, 49–51, 236
Andropause, 246, 275
Animal-assisted therapy, 373
Animal models, Alzheimer's disease (AD), 3–6, 15–17*t*
   ApoE transgenic mouse models, 10–11
   APP transgenic mouse model, 8–10
   multiple FAD mutation mouse models, 4–5
   mutant APP mouse models, 4
   nontransgenic animals, 12
   other AD mutant models, 5–6
   PSEN1 transgenic mouse models, 8–10
   sex differences in, 6–12
   tau mouse models, 11–12
   tau pathology mouse models, 5
Anterograde amnesia, 165
Antidepressants, in dementia, 197–198
APOE. *See* Apolipoprotein E (APOE)
ApoE transgenic mouse models, 10–11
Apolipoprotein E (APOE), 5–6, 33–34, 250
   AD-related biofluid biomarker, 114
   allele, 34–35, 270–272
   deficiency, 38–39
   expression, 38–39
   microglia, 84, 91–92
Apolipoprotein E4 (ApoE4), 10
APPswe/PSEN1dE9 mouse model, 8–9
APP transgenic mouse model, 8–10
Arcuate fasciculus, 169–170
Aripiprazole, in behavioral and psychological symptoms of dementia (BPSD), 200
Aromatherapy, 373
Artificial intelligence (AI), 431*b*

B

Bed nucleus of stria terminalis (BNST), 90
Behavioral and psychological symptoms of dementia (BPSD), 199–201
   aripiprazole, 200
   benzodiazepines in elderly, 200–201
   caregiver factors, 375
   cholinesterase inhibitors, 200
   environmental factors, 375
   gender differences in, 375
   memantine, 200
   patient factors, 375
   risperidone, 200
   treatment of, 200
Beijing Declaration, 447

Index

Benzodiazepines
  in behavioral and psychological symptoms of dementia (BPSD), 200–201
  for insomnia, 217
Blood-based biomarkers, 116
Blood-brain barrier (BBB), 115
Body mass index (BMI), 195–197, 277, 337–338
BOLD contrast imaging, 132
Bone marrow-derived microglia, 81
BPSD. *See* Behavioral and psychological symptoms of dementia (BPSD)
Braak stages, 199–200
Brain
  metabolism, 137, 145–148
  perfusion, 136, 138, 140
  sex differences in, 109–110
  structure, 126–128, 131, 152–153
BrainAGE index, 46–47
Brain-derived neurotrophic factor (BDNF), 12–13, 45–46, 92–93
Bromodeoxyuridine (BrdU), 31–32, 41–43

C

California Verbal Learning Test (CVLT), 165–166, 170–171
Cardiometabolic risk factors, 275–277
Care
  dementia
    negative outcomes, 399–401
    positive outcomes, 398–399
  patterns of, 393–398
  sex and gender differences in, 396–398
  societal demands and, 403–404
Caregivers, 394–396
  burden, 399–400
  communication, 428–430
  COVID-19 pandemic on, 409, 410*b*
  dementia
    adult child, 364–367
    gender differences in psychosocial interventions, 376–380
    spouses, 362–364
  effective interventions, 408–409
  mental health, 400
  outcomes for male and female, 401–405
  physical health, 401
  supportive interventions, 405–407
  unpaid, support structures for, 404–405
CEDAW. *See* Convention on Elimination of All Forms of Discrimination against Women (CEDAW)
CEE. *See* Conjugated equine estrogen (CEE)
Central autonomic network (CAN), 133–134

CERAD. *See* Consortium to Establish Registry for Alzheimer's disease (CERAD)
Cerebrospinal fluid (CSF) biomarkers
  AD-related biofluid biomarker
    apolipoprotein E gene (APOE) genotype, 114
    genetic factors, 114–115
    sex-related factors, 113–116
  core AD-related biomarkers, 110
    amyloid-beta, 110–111
    neurofilament light chain (NfL), 112
    neurogranin, 112
    phosphorylated tau (P-tau), 111–112
    total tau (T-tau), 111–112
  inflammatory markers, 113
  overview, 111*t*, 112–113
Charlson Comorbidity Index (CCI), 195
Circadian dysfunction, 212
Circadian rhythm, 207–209
Citalopram, for depression, 192
Civil society organizations, 458–459
Clinical trials
  biomarkers role, 319–320
  defined, 309
  differences in AD biomarkers between men and women, 313–315
  efficacy of drugs in men and women, 315–316
  inclusion and exclusion criteria, 317–318
  involving human subjects, 311–312
  preclinical stages, 310–311
  prevalence and pathophysiology of disease in men and women, 312
  safety and pharmacokinetics of drugs in men and women, 316–317
  socioeconomic implications, 318–319
  stages, 310, 310*t*
  women participation, 317–319
Clonazepam, for REM sleep behavior disorder (RBD), 213–214, 222–223, 225
Cognition
  hormones and, 234–237
    dehydroepiandrosterone (DHEA), 236–237
    estrogen, 235
    progesterone, 235–236
    testosterone, 236–237
  hormone therapy (HT) and, 241–242
  menopause and, 237–239
    natural, 237–238
    surgical, 239
Cognitive aging, 282–283
Cognitive behavioral therapy for insomnia (CBTi), 217, 281–282
Cognitive biomarkers, 175
Cognitive decline, 174, 217

diet roles in, 280
17β-estradiol, 46
hormones on risk factors for, 248–252
   depression, 252
   diabetes and impaired glucose tolerance, 251
   metabolic syndrome and inflammation, 251–252
   sleep, 252
   vascular risk and disease, 248–251
synaptic loss, 83
trazodone, 217
Cognitive rehabilitation therapy, 369–370
Cognitive reserve, 166–167, 174–175, 337
Cognitive resilience, 166–168, 335
Cognitive stimulation therapy, 369
Communication, 421
   advance care planning (ACP), 427b
   caregivers, 428–430
   components, 422
   with dementia, 426–428
   effective, ethical implications, 423–424
   gender biases, 432–433
   gender issues in IHC, 424–426
   interpersonal, 421
   nonverbal, 428, 433
   physical contact, 428
   plain language, 429
   technology, 430
   verbal, 428, 433
   visual aids, 429
Conjugated equine estrogen (CEE), 44–45, 241, 243–245, 254
Consortium to Establish Registry for Alzheimer's disease (CERAD), 165, 167
Continuous positive airway pressure (CPAP), 210–211, 220–221
Convention on Elimination of All Forms of Discrimination against Women (CEDAW), 448–449
Coping mechanisms, 401–402
Covid-19 pandemic, 409, 410b, 457b
CVLT. See California Verbal Learning Test (CVLT)

D

Dance/movement therapy, 371
Danish Osteoporosis Prevention Study (DOPS), 249–250
Data2x, 443
Decision-making, 172–173, 213–214, 423
Default mode network (DMN), 133–134
Dehydroepiandrosterone (DHEA), 234, 236–237
Dementia, 79, 439
   activity-based psychosocial interventions
      dance/movement therapy, 371
      exercise, 370–371
      life story work, 372
      music therapy, 371
      visual art-based therapy, 371–372
   alcohol consumption, 277
   alcohol dependency, 187–188
   antidepressants in, 197–198
   associated with early childhood outcomes, 335
   awareness and friendliness, 452–454
   behavioral and psychological symptoms, 199–201
      benzodiazepines in elderly, 200–201
      gender differences in, 375
      treatment of, 200
   care and support, 454
   caregivers, 214–215
      adult child, 364–367
      spouses, 362–364
   communication with, 426–428
   diagnosis, 454
   family dynamics, 361–368
   information systems for, 455
   late life vs. earlier life depression and developmental risk of, 193–195
   modifiable risk factors for
      depression, 190–197
      psychiatric disorders, 187–190
   nonpharmacological therapies for
      animal-assisted therapy, 373
      aromatherapy, 373
      doll therapy, 374
      light therapy, 372–373
      multisensory stimulation therapy, 373–374
   physical inactivity, 278
   polypharmacy, 198–199
   psychosocial interventions, 368–374, 376
      cognitive rehabilitation therapy, 369–370
      cognitive stimulation therapy, 369
      for formal caregivers, 378–380
      for informal caregivers, 376–378
      reminiscence therapy, 370
      validation therapy, 370
   research and innovation, 455
   residential long-term care, 367–368
   risk factors for, 271f, 333, 334f
   risk reduction, 454
   smoking, 277
   support for carers, 454
   treatment, 454
   vascular, 194
Dentate gyrus (DG), 24–26

Depression, 252, 286–288, 345–351
  citalopram for, 192
  defined, 286–287
  diagnostic challenge in elderly, 195–197
  diagnostic criteria, 190, 191*t*
  differentiating neuropsychological patterns in, 195–196, 196*t*
  International Classification of Diseases (ICD-10), 190, 191*t*
  late life *vs.* earlier life, 193–195
  misdiagnosis and underrecognition, 350*b*
  overlapping symptoms in, 195, 195*t*
  risk of developing dementia, 190–197
  social signal transduction theory of, 193
  socioeconomic inequality, 347–350
Detrimental polypharmacy, 197–199
DHEA. *See* Dehydroepiandrosterone (DHEA)
Diabetes, 276
  gender differences, 342–343
  and impaired glucose tolerance, 251
  socioeconomic inequality, 342–343, 344*f*
Diaschisis, 172
Digital biomarkers, 320–321
Dihydrotestosterone (DHT), 49–50, 236
Disease-associated microglia (DAM), 81–82, 94
Doll therapy, 374
Dopamine transporter single photon emission computed tomography (DAT SPECT), 140–141
  in dementia, 142
  in healthy subjects, 141–142
Dorsal attention network (DAN), 133–134
Drug development process, 310, 310*t*
Dyslipidemia, 276

E

Educational attainment, socioeconomic inequality in, 335–336, 336–337*f*
Electrocardiography (ECG), 208
Electroencephalography (EEG), 9, 208
Electromyography (EMG), 208, 222
Electrooculogram (EOG), 208
ENC-DAT, 141–142
Episodic memory, 165
Epworth Sleepiness Scale (ESS), 210–211, 213
17β-Estradiol, 39–43, 45–46
Estrogens, 44–45, 190–193, 234–235, 272, 440–441
  and aging, 39–41, 43–44
  in Alzheimer's disease, 45–46
  and neurogenesis, 41–43
Executive function, 171–175, 176*t*
Exercise, 278–279, 370–371

F

Female leadership, 455–456
^{18}F-Fluoro-DOPA PET imaging, 142
Finnish Geriatric Intervention Study to Prevent Cognitive Impairment and Disability (FINGER), 288–289
^{18}F-fluorodeoxyglucose positron emission tomography (FDG-PET), 145
  in dementia, 146–148
  in healthy subjects, 145–146
Focal vascular aphasias, 170
Follicle-stimulating hormone (FSH), 234
Food and Drug Administration (FDA), 311
Frontoparietal network (FPN), 133–134
Frontotemporal lobar degeneration (FTLD), 5
Functional magnetic resonance imaging (fMRI), 131
  in dementia, 135
  in healthy subjects, 132–135

G

GEH. *See* Global equity hub (GEH)
Gender, 164, 440*b*
  mainstreaming, 447
  sensitivity, 451
  transformation, 460, 460*f*
Gender-based data, 459
Gender-transformative global action plan, 452–455, 453*t*
Gestation, 46–49
Global Action Plan on Public Health Response to Dementia, 450–452, 456, 458
Global equity hub (GEH), 449–450
  development dividends, 456
  gender equality dividends, 456
  health dividends, 456
Global Gender Gap Report, 445
Glucose homeostasis, sex differences in, 7
G20 Okayama Declaration of Health Ministers 2019, 450
Gonadotropin-releasing hormone (GnRH), 234

H

Haloperidol, 213–214
Health professionals, 421–423, 425, 433
Healthy Aging Through Internet Counseling in the Elderly (HATICE) study, 289
Heart and Estrogen/Progestin Replacement Study (HERS), 242
Hemispheric asymmetry reduction in older adults (HAROLD) model, 174
Hippocampal neurogenesis, 26–28
  aging, 28–30, 39–41, 44–45
  estrogens in, 39–41, 43–44

testosterone, 51–52
  Alzheimer's disease, 33–34, 37–38
    animal models, 35–37
    in estrogens, 45–46
    models, 38–39
    parity and, 48–49
    sex differences in, 34–35
    testosterone, 51–52
    transgenic mouse models, 35
  cognition, 44–45
  in dentate gyrus, 24–26
  estrogens, 39–45
    in aging, 39–41, 43–44
    in Alzheimer's disease, 45–46
  parity, 46–48
  sex differences, 30–33
    in Alzheimer's disease, 34–35
    animal models, 35–37
  testosterone, 49–51
Hormone replacement therapy (HRT), 273–274
Hormones, 272–275
  and cognition, 234–237
    dehydroepiandrosterone (DHEA), 236–237
    estrogen, 235
    in men, 246–248
    neuropathological timelines, 238f
    progesterone, 235–236
    testosterone, 236–237
  risk factors for cognitive decline, 248–252
    depression, 252
    diabetes and impaired glucose tolerance, 251
    metabolic syndrome and inflammation, 251–252
    sleep, 252
    vascular risk and disease, 248–251
Hormone therapy (HT), 39–40, 43–45, 52, 235, 239–240
  and cognition, 241–242
  interventional use, 240–242
  preparations, 254
  risk of breast cancer, 245–246, 246f
  side-effect profile, 245–246
  timing hypothesis, 243–245
  in younger women, 242–246
HRT. See Hormone replacement therapy (HRT)
HT. See Hormone therapy (HT)
Humanized APOEe3 (hAPOEe3), 35–36
Hypertension, 276
  gender differences in, 341
  socioeconomic inequality, 340–342, 341–342f
Hypothalamic-pituitary-adrenal axis (HPAA), 283–284
Hypothalamus-pituitary-gonadal (HPG) axis, 234

I

Immediate early genes (IEGs), 27–28
Immune function, sex differences in, 7
Immune system, sex differences in, 85–87
Inflammation, metabolic syndrome and, 251–252
Inflammatory markers, 113
Information and communication technology (ICT), 431b
Insomnia
  benzodiazepines for, 217
  cognitive behavioral therapy, 217
  defined, 215–216
  Montreal Cognitive Assessment (MoCA), 216
  Pittsburgh Sleep Quality Index (PSQI), 216
  risk factor for cognitive impairment, 215–217
  trazodone for, 217
  treatment in elderly, 217
  zolpidem for, 217
Interferon response microglia (IRMs), 93
International Classification of Diseases (ICD-10), 188, 190, 191t
International classification of sleep disorders (ICSD), 209
International frameworks, 447–450
International Menopause Society (IMS), 244–245
Interpersonal health communication (IHC), 421–422, 424–426
Irradiation methods, 27

J

JNPL3 strain, 11–12

K

Ki67 marker, 31–32
Kronos Early Estrogen Prevention Study (KEEPS), 243

L

Lancet Commission on Dementia Prevention, Intervention, and Care (2020), 281–282, 290–291
Language, 168–171, 176t
  connectivity, 169–170
  handedness, 169–170
  laterality, 169–170
  plain, 429
  semantic disruption, 170–171
  semantic dysfunction, 170
Late-onset hypogonadism (LOH), 246
Lewy body dementia (DLB), 375
Lexical-semantic network, 169
Life story work, psychosocial interventions, 372
Lifestyle Interventions and Independence for Elders (LIFE) physical activity trial, 289
Lifestyle interventions, multidomain, 288–290

Light therapy, 213, 372–373
Lipoprotein, 250
Loneliness, 285–286
Low- and middle-income countries (LMICs), 439
Luteinizing hormone (LH), 234

M

MCI. *See* Mild cognitive impairment (MCI)
Medroxyprogesterone acetate (MPA), 235–236, 241–242, 245–246, 254
Melatonin, for REM sleep behavior disorder (RBD), 213–214, 222–223
Memory, 165–168
  decline, 165
  episodic, 165
  verbal
    in Alzheimer's disease (AD), 167
    decline rates, 167–168
    in healthy adults, 165–166
    in mild cognitive impairment (MCI), 165–166
  working, 172–173
Menopausal transition, 40–41, 237, 252–253
Menopause, 40–41, 272–275
  and cognition, 237–239
    natural, 237–238
    surgical, 239
  obstructive sleep apnea syndrome (OSAS) during, 218–220
  reproductive history and timing of, 274–275
Metabolic syndrome, and inflammation, 251–252
Microglia, 80
  aging, 89–91
  detrimental roles, 82–83
    complement, 83
    synapse elimination, 83
  neuroinflammation, 84–85
  protective functions
    TREM2 and Aβ plaques, 80–82
    TREM2 and tau, 82
  sex differences in, 87–89
MicroRNAs (miRNAs), 86
Mild cognitive impairment (MCI)
  Rey Auditory Verbal Learning Test (RAVLT), 166
  verbal memory in, 165–166
Mini Mental State Examination (MMSE) test, 195, 210–211, 369
Montreal Cognitive Assessment (MoCA), 216
MPA. *See* Medroxyprogesterone acetate (MPA)
Multidomain Alzheimer Preventive Trial (MAPT), 288–289
Multidomain lifestyle interventions, 288–290
Multisensory stimulation therapy, 373–374
Music therapy, 371

N

National Institute of Aging and Alzheimer's Association (NIA-AA), 313
National Institute of Health (NIH), 253, 312, 445
Neural reserve, 282–283
Neural resilience, 282–283
Neurodegeneration, 79–80, 82
Neurodegenerative markers, 314–315
Neurofibrillary tangles, 108–110, 113, 115
Neurofilament light chain (NfL), 112, 116
Neurogenesis, hippocampus. *See* Hippocampal neurogenesis
Neurogranin, 112
Neuroimaging biomarkers, 127t
  amyloid positron emission tomography, 148–149
  dopamine transporter single photon emission computed tomography (DAT SPECT), 141–142
  ^{18}F-fluorodeoxyglucose positron emission tomography (FDG-PET), 145–148
  functional magnetic resonance imaging (fMRI), 132–135
  neuroinflammation positron emission tomography, 152
  neurotransmission positron emission tomography, 151–152
  perfusion single photon emission computed tomography (SPECT), 136–140
  structural magnetic resonance imaging, 128–131
  tau positron emission tomography (Tau PET), 150–151
Neuroinflammation, 84–85, 93
Neuro Monitor Index (NMI), 320–321
Neuronal activation, 132
Neuropsychiatric Inventory Questionnaire (NPIQ), 195, 199–200
Neuropsychological assessments, 163–164
Neurotransmission, positron emission tomography, 151–152
Nonpharmacological therapy, for dementia
  animal-assisted therapy, 373
  aromatherapy, 373
  doll therapy, 374
  light therapy, 372–373
  multisensory stimulation therapy, 373–374
Nonrapid eye movement (NREM) sleep, 208, 213
  physiological aging, 209–210
  stages, 209–210
Nontransgenic animals, 12
Nonverbal communication, 428, 433
NREM sleep. *See* Nonrapid eye movement (NREM) sleep
NRLP3 inflammasome, 84
Nutrition, 279–280
NYU Caregiver Intervention (NYUCI), 408–409

O

Obesity
  dementia, 188
  socioeconomic inequality, 337–340, 338f
Obstructive sleep apnea syndrome (OSAS), 218–221
  associated with airway obstruction, 218
  biomarkers in, 220–221
  cognitive impairment, 219–220
  continuous positive airway pressure (CPAP) treatment, 220–221
  in male and female, 218–219
  polysomnography, 219
Office of Research on Women's Health (ORWH), 445
Olfaction, 7–8
Orexin, 211–212
OSAS. See Obstructive sleep apnea syndrome (OSAS)

P

Parity
  and Alzheimer's disease, 48–49
  and neurogenesis, 46–48
Patient-centered care, 423, 432
Perfusion magnetic resonance imaging (PMRI), 134–135
Perfusion single photon emission computed tomography (SPECT), 136
  in dementia, 137–140
  in healthy subjects, 136–137
Personal protective equipment (PPE), 411
Pharmacotherapy, in elderly, 197–199
Phosphorylated tau (P-tau), 111–112
Physical activity, 278–279, 337–340, 339f
Pipamperone, 213–214
Pittsburgh Sleep Quality Index (PSQI), 210–211, 213, 216
Plain language, 429
Policy transformation, 446–447
Polypharmacy, dementia, 198–199
Polysomnography, 208, 219, 222
Poverty, old-age, 346–347
Prevention of Dementia by Intensive Vascular Care (PreDIVA), 288–289
Primary progressive aphasias (PPA), 170
Progesterone, 86–87, 190–193, 235–236
Prospective Epidemiological Risk Factor (PERF) study, 242
Prostaglandin E2 (PGE2), 88–89
PSEN1 transgenic mouse models, 8–10
PSQI. See Pittsburgh Sleep Quality Index (PSQI)
Psychiatric disorders, as modifiable risk factors for dementia, 187–190
Psychosocial interventions, dementia, 368–374
  activity-based
    dance/movement therapy, 371
    exercise, 370–371
    life story work, 372
    music therapy, 371
    visual art-based therapy, 371–372
  cognitive rehabilitation therapy, 369–370
  cognitive stimulation therapy, 369
  gender differences in, 376
    for formal caregivers, 378–380
    for informal caregivers, 376–378
  reminiscence therapy, 370
  validation therapy, 370
Pulse oximetry, 208

Q

Quality of life, 368–369
Quality of Life Scale for Alzheimer's Disease (QoL-AD), 195

R

Randomized controlled trials (RCTs), 288–289, 311–312
Rapid eye movement (REM) sleep, 208, 213
Reminiscence therapy, 370
REM sleep. See Rapid eye movement (REM) sleep
REM sleep behavior disorder (RBD)
  clonazepam for, 213–214, 222–223
  defined, 222
  melatonin for, 213–214, 222–223
  polysomnography, 222
  prevalence, 223
  secondary, 221–222
  sex- and gender-related differences, 223
  sundown syndrome associated with, 224–225
  α-synucleinopathies, 221–223
  zolpidem for, 222–223
Resting state-functional magnetic resonance imaging (RS-fMRI), 133
Revitalization Act, 445
Rey Auditory Verbal Learning Test (RAVLT), 165–166, 170–171
Risperidone
  in behavioral and psychological symptoms of dementia (BPSD), 200
  in dementia, 213–214

S

SDGs. See Sustainable Development Goals (SDGs)
Selective serotonin reuptake inhibitors (SSRIs), 192, 197–198, 221–222
Semantic deficits, 170–171
Semantic encoding, 170–171

Semantic vulnerability, 170–171
Sex, 164, 440b
Sex steroid hormones, 7–8
Sex steroids, 86–87
Shared decision-making, 423
"Show back" technique, 430
Sleep, 207–209
  architecture, 212–213
  chronic disturbance in, 252
  sex- and gender-related differences in, 210–211
Sleep deprivation, 211–212
Sleep disorders, 209–215, 212f
  aging, 209–210
  caregiver's burden, 214–215
  defined, 209
  international classification of, 209
  sex- and gender-related differences in, 210–211
  sleep architecture, 212–213
  treatment, 213–214
Sleep Disturbance Inventory (SDI), 213
Sleep disturbances, 280–282
Sleep-wake cycle, 200, 211–213
Smoking, 188, 277
Snoezelen therapy, 373–374
Social isolation, 188, 285–286, 345–351
Social signal transduction theory of depression, 193
Social support, 345–351
Social threats, 193
Society for Women's Health Research, 210
Socioeconomic inequality
  in awareness, 343–345
  in behavioral risk factors, 337–340
  in clinical depression, 347–350, 349f, 350b
  in clinical risk factors, 340–345
  in cognitive reserve, 337
  diabetes, 342–343, 344f
  in educational attainment, 335–336, 336–337f
  hypertension, 340–342, 341–342f
  living arrangements and marital status, 351
  obesity, 337–340, 338f
  physical activity, 337–340, 339f
  in social isolation and loneliness, 350–351
Stem cells, 25f, 28–29, 31–32
Steroids, sex, 86–87
Streptozotocin (STZ), 12
Stress
  aberrant response, 284
  axes, 283–285
  sex and gender differences in, 284–285
Structural magnetic resonance imaging
  in dementia, 129–131
  in healthy subjects, 128–129
Sundown syndrome, 213–214, 224–225

Surface model-based segmentation, 128
Sustainable Development Goals (SDGs), 443, 447–448
Sympatho-adrenomedullary axis (SAMA), 283
Synaptic loss, 83
α-Synucleinopathies, 221–223
Systolic Blood Pressure Intervention Trial-Memory and Cognition in Decreased Hypertension (SPRINTMIND), 289

T

Tau, 82, 314
Tau mouse models, 5, 11–12
Tau positron emission tomography (Tau PET), 150–151
^{99m}Tc-ECD SPECT, 136–137, 138f
"Teach back" communication method, 430
Telemedicine, 430
Testosterone, 87, 193, 234–237, 275
  in aging, 51–52
  in Alzheimer's disease, 51–52
  and neurogenesis, 49–51
  therapy, 236
Toll-like receptors (TLRs), 84
Total tau (T-tau), 111–112
Transforming growth factor beta (TGF-β) signaling, 84
Transgenic mouse models, 35
Transgenic rat model (TgF344-AD), 36–37
Trazodone, for insomnia, 217
Triggering receptor expressed on myeloid cells-2 (TREM2)
  in amyloid pathogenesis, 82
  and Aβ plaques, 80–82
  signaling, 81
  and tau, 82
Triple transgenic AD mouse model (3xTg-AD)
  age-dependent behavioral, 6–7
  in glucose homeostasis, 7
  hormonal-related factors, 7–8
  in immune function, 7
  lifespan, 8
  olfaction, 7–8

U

United Nations Educational, Scientific, and Cultural Organization (UNESCO), 447
Universal health coverage (UHC), 450
Unmet Needs Model, 368
US National Sleep Foundation, 210

V

Validation therapy, 370
Vascular dementia, 194